Neuroendocrinology

VOLUME 5: CONCEPTS IN NEUROSURGERY

Neuroendocrinology

VOLUME 5: CONCEPTS IN NEUROSURGERY

EDITORS

DANIEL L. BARROW, M.D.

Associate Professor and
Deputy Chief of Neurological Surgery
Emory School of Medicine
Atlanta, Georgia

WARREN R. SELMAN, M.D.

Associate Professor
Department of Neurological Surgery
University Hospitals of Cleveland
Cleveland, Ohio

SERIES EDITORS

Fremont P. Wirth, M.D.
Robert A. Ratcheson, M.D.

SERIES ASSOCIATE EDITORS

Robert L. Grubb, Jr., M.D.
Julian T. Hoff, M.D.
Martin H. Weiss, M.D.

**Sponsored by the
Congress of Neurological Surgeons**

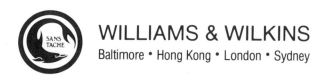

WILLIAMS & WILKINS
Baltimore • Hong Kong • London • Sydney

Accurate indications, adverse reactions, and dosage schedules for drugs are provided in this book, but it is possible that they may change. The reader is urged to review the package information data of the manufacturers of the medications mentioned.

Printed in the United States of America

Library of Congress Cataloging-in-Publication Data

Neuroendocrinology / editors Daniel L. Barrow and Warren R. Selman; sponsored by
   the Congress of Neurological Surgeons.
      p.   cm.—(Concepts in neurosurgery ; v. 5)
   Includes index.
   ISBN 0-683-07665-5
   1. Neuroendocrinology.   2. Neurosurgery.   I. Barrow, Daniel L. and Selman, Warren
   R.   II. Congress of Neurological Surgeons.   III. Series.
   [DNLM: 1. Endocrine Glands—innervation.   2. Endocrine Glands—
physiopathology.   3. Endocrine Glands—secretion.   W1 C0459RK v. 5]
RC649.N48 1992
616.4—dc20
DNLM/DLC
for Library of Congress   92-5836
                                                                                    CIP

                                                                 92 93 94 95 96
                                                        1 2 3 4 5 6 7 8 9 10

Series Foreword

The Congress of Neurological Surgeons was founded in 1951 with the primary purposes of maintaining high standards of neurosurgery and promoting continuing education. Although the emphasis has been on the needs of the resident in training and the younger neurosurgeon, the programs of the Congress have benefited not only neurosurgery but also the neuroscience fields in general.

To help provide for the continuing education needs of its members, the Congress began publication in 1953 of an annual volume entitled *Clinical Neurosurgery,* which presents in detail the invited presentations made at the annual meeting of the organization. This volume has become an important reference source for neurosurgeons. Then in 1977, after several years of planning, the Congress began publication of a monthly journal entitled *Neurosurgery,* which proved to be an outstanding addition to the medical literature.

Now, under the direction of Doctors Fremont P. Wirth and Robert A. Ratcheson, the Congress is embarking on another publication series entitled *Concepts in Neurosurgery.* The goals of this publication, as proposed by Dr. Ratcheson during his term as President of the Congress, are to provide a monograph that will cover a specific area in depth with basic scientific knowledge and theory applied to practical neurosurgical issues. For the resident in training this publication can supplement the educational program or provide knowledge in an area that might not be covered in depth in a training program. For the trained neurosurgeon, each monograph will provide the opportunity to review recent knowledge about a practical subject and supply up-to-date information in an important area of neurosurgery.

The Congress has selected as editors Doctors Wirth and Ratcheson, two individuals who have been members of the Executive Committee for several years and have recently been officers. They have also had considerable experience with educational programs. They will be aided by associate editors, Doctors Robert L. Grubb, Julian T. Hoff, and Martin Weiss, who also have had broad experience with publications and continuing education endeavors.

The Congress is again providing a leadership role in an important area that will benefit all of neurosurgery.

Robert G. Ojemann, M.D.

Foreword

This is the fifth volume in the *Concepts in Neurosurgery* series. It represents the ongoing commitment of the Congress of Neurological Surgeons to continuing education in neurosurgery. The editors, Daniel Barrow and Warren Selman, have organized this volume to address the scientific basis and related clinical application of current neuroendocrinological principles. The section on basic neuroendocrinology deals with hypothalamic control, the molecular biology of hormone synthesis, and hormonal effects on the immune system and brain. A distinguished group of experts elucidate these areas and, in the clinical section, present current concepts of endocrine dysfunction, neuropathology, and therapeutic considerations, among others.

This monograph accomplishes the aims of *Concepts in Neurosurgery*. It will provide neurosurgical practitioners and trainees with current concepts and their scientific foundations. The publication of this volume by the Congress of Neurological Surgeons is anticipated to benefit neurosurgery and enhance the care of our patients.

Fremont P. Wirth, M.D., F.A.C.S.
Robert A. Ratcheson, M.D., F.A.C.S.

Preface

The optimal management of patients who have pituitary dysfunction continues to be both challenging and controversial. The choice of the most effective and appropriate treatment for common disorders, such as adenomas, requires a thorough understanding of not only the clinical manifestations of pituitary tumors, but also the basic mechanisms of their growth and control. A variety of treatment options other than surgery are currently available to deal with patients who suffer from pituitary tumors. Recent advances in the understanding of gene expression in relation to pituitary tumors and hormone production will undoubtedly influence the future management of these lesions. This text first details the scientific foundation of neuroendocrinology and then emphasizes diagnostic neuroendocrinology. Both perspectives provide a foundation from which a subsequent analysis of patient management can be appreciated.

Neuroendocrinology, the fifth volume of the *Concepts in Neurosurgery* series, is intended to bring into focus the tremendous growth in our understanding of the basic scientific and clinical aspects of the endocrine system, particularly as it relates to the function of the nervous system. In the opening chapters of this volume, the contributors concisely detail the control of pituitary secretion by examining the role of the hypothalamus, neuropharmacological regulation, and the molecular biology of hormone synthesis. Part I concludes with a discussion of the effects of hormones on brain function.

Part II provides a detailed analysis of the clinical evaluation of disorders in the regulation of the specific pituitary hormones, including prolactin, growth hormone, thyroid-stimulating hormone, the gonadotrophs, and antidiuretic hormone. Special attention is devoted to the neuro-ophthalmological examination and the optimal use of radiological studies in the evaluation of patients who have neuroendocrine disorders. The neuropathology of endocrinological dysfunction, including disorders of the hypothalamus, the pituitary gland, and the effector glands, is also presented.

This volume concludes with a discussion of therapeutic considerations which is intended to provide a rationale for the use of medical, surgical, or radiation therapy in patients who have pituitary adenomas.

Acknowledgments

We wish to express our gratitude to the authors and to Cara Kaufman, Carole Pippin and Charles Zeller of Williams & Wilkins for their patience, and to Stephanie Del Vecchio and Wendy Barringer for their perseverance.

Daniel Barrow, M.D.
Warren Selman, M.D.

Contributors

SERIES EDITORS

Fremont P. Wirth, M.D.
Neurological Institute of Savannah
Director, Neurosurgical and Neurological
  Intensive Care Unit
St. Joseph's Hospital
Savannah, Georgia

Robert A. Ratcheson, M.D.
Professor and Chief Division of Neurological
  Surgery
Case Western Reserve University
University Hospitals of Cleveland
Cleveland, Ohio

SERIES ASSOCIATE EDITORS

Robert L. Grubb, Jr., M.D.
Professor of Neurological Surgery
Washington University School of Medicine
St. Louis, Missouri

Julian T. Hoff, M.D.
Professor of Surgery
Head, Section of Neurosurgery
University of Michigan Hospital
Ann Arbor, Michigan

Martin H. Weiss, M.D.
Professor and Chairman
Department of Neurosurgery
LAC/USC Medical Center
Los Angeles, California

VOLUME EDITORS

Daniel L. Barrow, M.D.
Associate Professor and Deputy Chief of
  Neurological Surgery
Emory School of Medicine
Atlanta, Georgia

Warren R. Selman, M.D.
Associate Professor
Department of Neurological Surgery
University Hospitals of Cleveland
Cleveland, Ohio

CONTRIBUTORS

Baha M. Arafah, M.D.
Associate Professor, Medicine
Case Western Reserve University
Division of Endocrinology and Hypertension
University Hospitals of Cleveland
Cleveland, Ohio

Daniel L. Barrow, M.D.
Associate Professor and Deputy Chief of
  Neurological Surgery
Emory School of Medicine
Atlanta, Georgia

Peter McL. Black, M.D., Ph.D.
Neurosurgeon-in-Chief
Brigham and Women's Hospital
The Children's Hospital
Boston, Maine

Ronald Burde, M.D.
Professor and Chairman, Department of
  Ophthalmology
Albert Einstein College of Medicine/
  Montefiore Medical Center
Bronx, New York

William F. Chandler, M.D.
Professor of Surgery
Section of Neurosurgery
Taubman Health Care Center
Ann Arbor, Michigan

P. Murali Doraiswamy, M.D.
Department of Psychiatry
Duke University Medical Center
Durham, North Carolina

Shereen Ezzat, M.D.
Assistant Professor of Medicine
Division of Endocrinology & Metabolism
The Wellesley Hospital
Toronto, Ontario, CANADA

Jacob I. Fabrikant, M.D., Ph.D.
Professor of Radiology
Donner Laboratory and Donner Pavilion
University of California at Berkeley
Berkeley, California

James C. Hoffman, M.D.
Professor of Radiology
Chief, Division of Neuroradiology
Emory University School of Medicine
Atlanta, Georgia

Samir Kailani, M.D.
Fellow
Department of Medicine
Division of Endocrinology and Hypertension
University Hospitals of Cleveland
Cleveland, Ohio

K. Ranga Krishnan, M.D.
Associate Professor of Psychiatry
Head, Division of Biological Psychiatry
Duke University Medical Center
Durham, North Carolina

Anne Klibanski, M.D.
Associate Professor, Medicine
Neuroendocrine Unit
Medical and Neurosurgical Services
Massachusetts General Hospital and
   Harvard Medical School
Boston, Maine

Edward R. Laws, Jr., M.D.
Professor of Neurosurgery
University of Virginia
Charlottesville, Virginia

Richard P. Levy, M.D., Ph.D.
Assistant Professor of Radiology
Donner Laboratory and Donner Pavilion
University of California at Berkeley
Berkeley, California

Ian E. McCutcheon, M.D.
Assistant Professor of Neurosurgery
The University of Texas
   M.D. Anderson Cancer Center
Houston, Texas

Dennis C. Matzkin, M.D.
Resident
Department of Ophthalmology
Albert Einstein College of Medicine/
   Montefiore Medical Center
Bronx, New York

Paul B. Nelson, M.D.
Professor, Department of Neurosurgery
Presbyterian-University Hospital
Pittsburgh, Pennsylvania

Charles B. Nemeroff, M.D., Ph.D.
Chief, Division of Biological Psychiatry
Professor of Psychiatry and Pharmacology
Duke University Medical Center
Durham, North Carolina

Edward H. Oldfield, M.D.
Chief, Surgical Neurology Branch
NINDS
Bethesda, Maryland

Robert B. Page, M.D.
Professor of Surgery and Neuroscience Anatomy
Penn State College of Medicine
   University Hospital
Hershey Medical Center
Hershey, Pennsylvania

Mary H. Samuels, M.D.
Assistant Professor, Medicine
Department of Medicine
Division of Endocrinology
University of Texas Health Sciences Center
San Antonio, Texas

Toshiaki Sano, M.D., Ph.D.
Assistant Professor, Department of Pathology
University of Tokushima School of Medicine
Tokushima, JAPAN

Warren R. Selman, M.D.
Associate Professor
Department of Neurological Surgery
Case Western Reserve University
University Hospitals of Cleveland
Cleveland, Ohio

Steven A. Smith, M.D.
Senior Associate Consultant, Endocrinology
May Clinic Jacksonville
Instructor in Medicine, Mayo Medical School
Jacksonville, Florida

Marc Thibonnier, M.D., M.Sc.
Associate Professor of Medicine
  and Pharmacology
Division of Endocrinology and Hypertension
School of Medicine
Case Western Reserve University
Cleveland, Ohio

Shozo Yamada, M.D., Ph.D.
Head Neurosurgeon
Department of Neurosurgery
Toranomon Hospital
Tokyo, JAPAN
Nicholas T. Zervas, M.D.
Chief, Neurosurgical Service
Massachusetts General Hospital
Boston, Massachusetts

Contents

PART 1

Basic Neuroendocrinology

Hypophysiotropic Regulation of Anterior Pituitary Hormones: Cellular and Molecular Mechanisms

SHEREEN EZZAT, M.D.

INTRODUCTION

Classically, the pituitary gland has been viewed as a compartmentalized organ with five discrete cell types. Somatotrophs, lactotrophs, thyrotrophs, gonadotrophs, and corticotrophs were regarded as being under the influence of unique releasing factors from the hypothalamus. Increasing evidence, however, suggests that pituitary cells are capable of producing more than one hormone. For example, growth hormone (GH) and prolactin (Prl), and GH and thyroid-stimulating hormone (TSH) have been reported to be expressed by the same cells in nonadenomatous human pituitary cells (69). Similarly, the characterization of hypothalamic factors has highlighted their effects on multiple anterior pituitary hormone secretion (51). Furthermore, isolation of authentic hypothalamic peptides outside the hypothalamic-pituitary system has led to their classification change from hypothalamic factors to hypophysiotropic hormones. In addition, responsiveness of the pituitary to hypothalamic influences appears to be further modulated by a unique endocrine milieu established by the pituitary's target hormones and growth factors (47).

With this premise, recent progress in the understanding of the cellular and molecular mechanisms of hypothalamic regulation of the anterior pituitary hormones is summarized in this chapter.

PITUITARY GONADOTROPINS

Pituitary gonadotropins are a family of glycoprotein hormones that includes luteinizing hormone (LH) and follicle-stimulating hormone (FSH). Recent evidence suggests that human chorionic gonadotropin (hCG) may also be expressed in the fetal (102) and adult (60) human pituitary and, therefore, may also be a member of this group. Structurally these peptides are composed of non-covalently bound heterodimers. The α-subunit is shared commonly by all members of this family and is synthesized and secreted in excess quantities of the heterodimers (15, 68). The β-subunit, however, confers unique immunological and biological properties to each hormone. Separately, these subunits possess no biological potency.

α-Subunit Gene

Mammalian pituitary gonadotropin α-subunit is the product of a single gene consisting of four exons and three intronic sequences that vary in size from 8 to 16.5 kilobase (kb) (56). Species differences in the size of the first intron interrupt the 5'-untranslated region and contribute to the genomic length variation. Nevertheless, there is at least 70% sequence homology between the mouse, rat, bovine, and human α-subunit coding regions. The mature messenger RNA (mRNA) product is approximately 0.8 kb in size. Human α-mRNA is translated into a 20–22 kilodalton (kd), 116 amino acid peptide which includes a 24 amino acid signal peptide. The α-subunit also undergoes posttranslational glycosylation with the addition of multiple N-linked complex carbohydrate moieties (126). The incorporation of a third carbohydrate chain appears to retard further association of α with β-subunits (103). Transcriptional regulation of the human α-subunit gene is conferred by an 18-base pair palindromic, cyclic adenosine monophosphate or cAMP-consensus sequence situated on the 5'-flanking region (41). Studies are currently underway to address the possible differential regulation of α-subunit gene expression in different pituitary cell types.

β-LH/CG Genes

Human LH and HCG are 82% homologous. Unlike other β-glycoproteins, however, β-HCG is encoded for by at least 7 separate genes. This gene family, one member of which encodes for β-LH, is situated as a cluster on chromosome 19 (16, 133). The β-LH gene is approximately 1.5 kb in length with three exons and two short (352 and 233 kb) introns that encode a 121 amino acid mature protein and a 24 amino acid signal peptide. Despite the high degree of sequence homology ($> 90\%$) upstream from the translational start site, the β-LH and β-HCG genes differ significantly. The β-HCG genes are devoid of consensus (adenosine-tyrosine-rich region located upstream from site of initiation of transcription) boxes and employ different promoters from those for β-LH (64). This implies that unique tissue-specific transcription factors may act on different enhancer sites on these genes with very similar coding regions. Finally, a point mutation in the termination codon of the β-LH gene, along with an insertion of two nucleotides downstream from the termination codon of the ancestral gene, have led to a 24 codon extension which translates into a 24 amino acid carboxyterminal extension not present on other β glycoprotein hormones. Gene transfer experiments have demonstrated that the rat β-LH 5'-flanking region contains an estrogen-responsive element very similar to that on the Prl gene (124).

β-FSH Gene

β-FSH is encoded for by a highly conserved single gene of three exons and two introns. Unique to β-FSH, however, is a well-documented "CAGT" sequence (Cys-Ala-Gly-Tyr) at the exon-2 intron-2 junction in nearly all mammalian species (105). This sequence may be involved in glycoprotein subunit interactions and stability. The β-FSH gene is also unusual in possessing an extremely long (1.5 kb) 3'-untranslated region (55) which may be important for RNA stability. In addition to the 1.7 kb mRNA species of the bovine and rat, the human β-FSH gene is transcribed into three other mRNA transcripts that result from multiple alternative donor splicing sites (63).

Regulation of Gonadotropin Secretion

Gonadotropin-releasing hormone (GnRH) is a decapeptide (Glu-His-Trp-Ser-Tyr-Gly-Leu-Arg-Pro-Gly-amide) that binds to pituitary gonadotroph cell membranes. GnRH neurons are primarily located in the anterior (preoptic) and tuberal (arcuate nucleus) regions of the hypothalamus (18). Projections from these neurons pass through the median eminence to terminate near the hypophyseal-portal capillary system. Other central nervous system projections of GnRH-containing neurons are present in the amygdala, hippocampus, periaqueductal region, and posterior pituitary.

The relative amounts of LH and FSH secreted by the gonadotroph in response to GnRH is a function of the frequency and concentration of administration of the decapeptide. Infrequent (every 3 hrs) or large amplitude pulses of GnRH produce a greater LH and FSH response than frequent (every 1 hr) or small amplitude pulses (67). Rapid pulses also result in a greater LH than FSH response (141). These phenomena are likely caused by the slower clearance of FSH from the circulation (10) coupled with alterations in the number of GnRH receptors (25). Responsiveness of the gonadotroph to GnRH is diminished in humans following brief periods of estrogen, progesterone, or corticosteroid administration (33). The physiological relevance of the GnRH-associated peptide derived from the GnRH precursor molecule remains to be elucidated (100).

After many years of search, the peptides responsible for modulating gonadotropin suppression have been identified (87). Inhibins are glycoprotein hormones composed of two heterodimers sharing a common α-subunit. They are ubiquitously expressed in the gonads, hypothalamus, brain, and pituitary (115). Purified inhibin attenuates GnRH-mediated gonadotropin stimulation possibly by suppressing GnRH-induced receptor upregulation on gonadotrophs (27). Similarly, immunoneutralization with anti-inhibin antibodies increase basal and GnRH-stimulated gonadotropin secretion in the rat (114). Dimers of homologous inhibin β-subunits (B_AB_A or B_BB_B) stimulate FSH secretion and are termed activins (22). In addition, a recently isolated single chain glycosylated peptide, follistatin, suppresses FSH secretion (121). Regulation of gonadotropin secretion is summarized in Figure 1.1.

At the cellular level, GnRH results in maximal release of gonadotropins from rat pituitary cells at 3 hrs with an ED_{50} dose of about 3 nM (28). Although Ca^{2+} is not required for GnRH receptor binding, its absence from the culture medium leads to cell refractoriness to this hypophysiotropic peptide (83). Pharmacological manipulation of cellular calcium stores suggests that Ca^{2+} is mobilized from the extracellular pool by GnRH stimulation. GnRH also stimulates the cytosolic translocation of the Ca^{2+}-binding protein, calmodulin, to the plasma membrane (26). This Ca^{2+}-mediated signalling pattern appears to be potentiated by diacylglycerols. Accordingly, GnRH-activated receptors stimulate membrane inositol phospholipid hydrolysis to produce diacylglycerols, which in turn activates protein kinase C synthesis. Thus, receptor binding affects calmodulin and protein kinase C activation which act synergistically to induce gonadotropin secretion (27) (Fig. 1.2).

Regulation of Gonadotropin Biosynthesis

The effects of GnRH on gonadotropin biosynthesis are less clear. Earlier in vitro studies had indicated that GnRH induces the glycosylation of LH without significantly increasing synthesis of the apoprotein (76). However, actinomycin D-induced protein

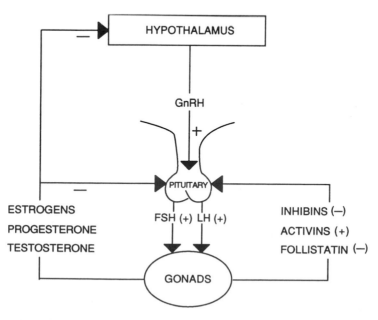

Figure 1.1. Schematic model of hypothalamic-pituitary-gonadal axis. Stimulatory and inhibitory factors are indicated by ($+$) and ($-$) symbols, respectively. (Adapted and modified from Gherib, S.D., Wierman, M.E., Shupnik, M.A., et al. Molecular biology of the pituitary gonadotropins. Endocr. Rev., *11*:177-199, 1990.)

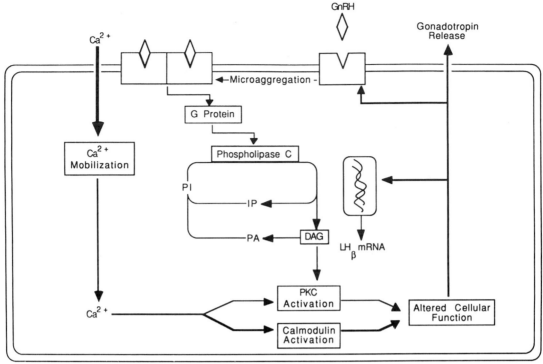

Figure 1.2. GnRH signal transduction pathways that mediate gonadotropin secretion. The GnRH receptor's binding to the gonadotroph facilitates intracellular calcium mobilization, whereas G protein activation induces phospholipase C, which in turn hydrolyzes phospholipid inositol (PI) to produce diacylglycerol (DAG). DAG stimulates protein kinase C (PKC) which, with Ca^{2+}-activated calmodulin, mediates peptide synthesis and secretion. (Reprinted with permission from Conn, P.M. and Crowley, W.F. Gonadotropin-releasing hormone and its analogues. N. Engl. J. Med., *324*.93–103, 1991.)

inhibition attenuates GnRH-mediated LH release. This suggested that intermediate mRNA synthesis was contributory to GnRH-LH induction. GnRH also stimulates amino acid incorporation into α- and β-LH subunits (130). This effect appears to be further enhanced by the presence of estradiol possibly by upregulating GnRH receptor numbers (107). More recently, low concentrations (10^{-10}M) of GnRH have been shown to induce β-LH mRNA accumulation in dispersed rat anterior pituitary cells (3). This effect appears to be also enhanced by protein kinase C.

In the ovariectomized ewe model, surgical interruption of the hypothalamic-pituitary stalk results in significant suppression of α- and β-LH mRNA levels in the pituitary (58). Restoration of subunit mRNA accumulation can be achieved in these animals by GnRH pulsatile administration (59). Frequent (every 8 min) pulses of GnRH increase α but not β-LH or β-FSH mRNA levels, whereas pulses every 120 min increase β-FSH only (57). Intermediate frequency (every 30 min) pulses increase mRNA levels of all subunit species.

THYROTROPIN-STIMULATING HORMONE

TSH Peptide and Gene Structure

TSH belongs to the family of pituitary glycoprotein hormones because it shares the same α-subunit. β-TSH is approximately 18 kd in molecular weight and contains a single N-linked complex carbohydrate group (105). Posttranslational modification of TSH is also under thyrotropin-releasing hormone (TRH) influence to the extent that glycosylation of TSH alters its bioactivity and metabolic clearance (138). Unlike the α-subunit, free TSH β-subunits are not detectable in the circulation.

The entire human β-TSH gene was cloned in 1988 (142). It is composed of three exons (3.9 kb) and two introns (0.45 kb), which differs from the mouse β-TSH gene. Unlike the rat and mouse genes, the human β-TSH gene appears to have a single transcriptional start site (142). A first exon ($+23$ to $+37$) thyroid hormone response element confers responsiveness of the human β-TSH gene to triiodothyronine (T3) regulation (142).

Regulation of β-TSH Secretion

The most significant hypophysiotropic regulators of circulating TSH include TRH, dopamine, and somatostatin (somatotropin release inhibitory factor). TRH is the first hypophysiotropic peptide to have been characterized structurally. This tripeptide (phyroglutamyl-histidyl-proline amide) stimulates the release of TSH and Prl. Besides its role in the hypothalamus, this peptide functions as an ubiquitous neurotransmitter throughout the central nervous system, pancreas, gastrointestinal tract, gonads, and placenta (94).

The TSH response to TRH stimulation is seen over a wide range of concentrations (10^{-11} to 10^{-7} M) and is modulated by circulating thyroid hormone levels. This effect has been ascribed to a concordant change in the number of TRH receptors with changes in thyroid hormone levels (94). The mechanism of TRH stimulation of pituitary hormone secretion has been most extensively studied in radiolabelled GH cells. TRH receptor interaction leads to enhanced hydrolysis of phosphatidylinositol 4,5-biphosphate (IP_2) by phospholipase C that leads to the production of 1,2-diacylglycerol and inositoltriphosphate (IP_3) (92). The latter two compounds serve as second messengers to transduce and amplify the cell-signalling pathway that leads to increased hormone secretion (11). Diacylglycerol enhances Ca^{2+} and phospholipid-dependent protein kinase C action, whereas IP_3 helps mobilize intracellular calcium pools (101). Basal intracellular Ca^{2+} concentration of approximately 120 nM rises to 500 nM within seconds of TRH stimulation. The second phase of sustained Ca^{2+} elevation is considered to be the result of enhanced influx of the cation through voltage-dependent membrane channels (53). The net effect is coupling of hypophysiotropic ligand-receptor binding with an elevation in cytoplasmic free Ca^{2+} which is critical for hormone secretion.

In addition to TRH, the hypothalamic tetradecapeptide somatotropin release-inhibiting factor suppresses the nocturnal TSH rise in euthyroid subjects (137) and attenuates TRH-induced TSH secretion (79). Furthermore, somatostatin neutralization by specific somatostatin antibodies results in increased release of both GH and TSH (134). The role of somatostatin in regulating TSH secretion is further complicated by studies that demonstrate a biphasic response of somatostatin receptor number following clonal pituitary cell exposure to TRH (119). Chronic treatment of these pituitary cells with TRH results in a decrease in somatotropin release-inhibiting factor receptor number without change in receptor affinity (119). The net effect of TRH and somatotropin release-inhibiting factor on TSH regulation is summarized in Figure 1.3.

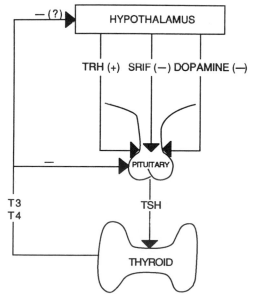

Figure 1.3. Schematic representation of hypothalamic-pituitary-thyroid hormone modulatory interactions. (Adapted and modified from Morley, J.E. Neuroendocrine control of thyrotropin secretion. Endocr. Rev., 2:396–436, 1981.)

Regulation of β-TSH Gene Expression

TRH directly stimulates TSH biosynthesis as evidenced by enhanced radiolabelled amino acid incorporation into rat TSH (140). TRH treatment of dispersed primary rat pituitary cells in culture results in an equal increase in β-TSH and α-subunit mRNA levels (123). Stimulation occurs within 30 min and reaches 2- to 5-fold over control (183). This effect appears to be partly explained by an associated increase in the transcriptional rate of the TSH gene by TRH.

By contrast, dopamine treatment of cultured pituitary cells decreases TSH mRNA levels while suppressing transcription of the β-TSH and α-subunit gene transcription rate by 60%–75% (29, 123). Dopamine also reverses TRH-induction of TSH gene transcription (123). Although cAMP treatment results in little alterations in TSH mRNA transcription, it can ameliorate the effect of dopamine on the TSH gene (123). These findings have been further corroborated by the demonstration of reduction in intracellular cAMP levels with dopamine treatment of pituitary cells. The role of cAMP or protein kinase C-dependent transactivating factors in mediating the effect of hypophysiotropic hormones on the β-TSH gene remains the subject of ongoing studies.

PROOPIOMELANOCORTIN

ACTH Peptide and Gene Structure

Proopiomelanocortin is a polypeptide that is posttranslationally processed in anterior pituitary corticotroph cells into ACTH, β-lipotropin (β-LPH), and β-melanocyte-stimulating hormone (β-MSH) (44). In the intermediate lobe melanotroph, proopiomelanocortin is cleaved into α-MSH, corticotropin-like intermediate lobe peptide, γ-LPH, and acetyl β-endorphin (56). The different biological properties of proopiomelanocortin-derived molecules dictate a complex regulatory system of proopiomelanocortin secretion and gene expression in the pituitary. Sequencing of genomic DNA from several mammalian species indicates that only one functional gene encodes for proopiome

lanocortin (80). This gene is composed of three exons and two large (2–4 kb) intronic sequences (132). Exon 1 is approximately 100 nucleotides in length and is largely comprised in the 5'-untranslated region of proopiomelanocortin mRNA. Exon 2 begins the peptide coding region of the mRNA that includes signal peptide and N-terminal amino acids. Exon 3 encodes all biologically active proopiomelanocortin-derived peptides, including ACTH. Expression of the proopiomelanocortin gene extends beyond the pituitary to include the hypothalamus, brain, adrenal medulla, spleen, and gonads (24, 80). Variations in primary transcript sizes reflect alternative transcriptional (alternative promoters) as well as posttranscriptional (alternative splicing sites) processing (71). Pituitary, hypothalamic, and macrophage mRNAs are approximately 1.1 kb in size. An additional smaller transcript is expressed in equal proportion in the anterior and intermediate lobes of the rat anterior pituitary (80).

Regulation of Proopiomelanocortin-Derived Peptide Secretion

The cellular signalling mechanisms that lead to proopiomelanocortin-derived peptide secretion have been studied best in the AtT20 clonal mouse corticotroph tumor cell line. Corticotropin-releasing hormone (CRH) that binds to membrane receptors activates adenylate cyclase through a coupled stimulatory guanine nucleotide-binding protein (G_s) (104). The associated increase in intracellular cAMP is considered to be instrumental in enhanced peptide secretion through a Ca^{2+}-dependent protein kinase A (75). Inhibition of this kinase results in AtT20 cell refractoriness to CRH (110). Glucocorticoids also rapidly inhibit CRH-stimulated proopiomelanocortin-derived peptide secretion in perfused mouse and rat pituitaries (13). In contradistinction, other hypophysiotropic hormones such as arginine vasopressin do not act on the pituitary corticotroph through the adenylate cyclase pathway (112). Instead, enhanced phosphoinositol turnover leads to the mobilization of intracellular calcium and activation of protein kinase C.

Regulation of Proopiomelanocortin Synthesis and Gene Expression

In the adrenalectomized animal model, pituitary proopiomelanocortin mRNA levels rise in a time-dependent fashion following surgery (96). Additional surgical interruption of the paraventricular nucleus results in a decrease in the levels of proopiomelanocortin mRNA (19). Furthermore, corticosterone replacement of these lesioned adrenalectomized rats has no effect on anterior pituitary proopiomelanocortin mRNA accumulation (34). What has been suggested by these data is that the inhibitory effect of glucocorticoids on proopiomelanocortin regulation is at least partly mediated by the effect of glucocorticoids on the hypothalamus. Chronic IV administration of CRH in intact rats results in 2- to 3-fold induction in proopiomelanocortin mRNA expression in the anterior pituitary (19). Pretreatment of these animals with dexamethasone abolishes this effect.

In vitro, the treatment of primary anterior pituitary or AtT20 cells with glucocorticoids results in a reduction of proopiomelanocortin mRNA accumulation. This effect is detectable after 10 hrs of treatment and is maximal with dexamethasone followed by cortisol and corticosterone after 36 hrs of exposure (43). Nevertheless, the magnitude of inhibition of proopiomelanocortin mRNA by glucocorticoids is only half that demonstrated in vivo, which suggests an additional effect of steroids at the hypothalamic level. CRH directly stimulates proopiomelanocortin mRNA accumulation in dispersed primary anterior and intermediate lobe pituitary cells (77). In AtT20 cells, this effect can be duplicated by 8-bromo-cAMP or phorobol-ester (110). Furthermore, phosphodiesterase inhibition elevates proopiomelanocortin mRNA expression in these cells (110). Although arginine vasopressin potentiates CRH-induced increases in cAMP levels and ACTH secretion (2), this hypophysiotropic peptide decreases proopiomelanocortin primary transcript levels in rat anterior pituitary cells (73). Arginine vasopressin also attenuates the stimulatory effect mediated by CRH on proopiomelanocortin expression (73). In melanotrophs, the dopamine agonist bromocriptine, potently inhibits intermediate lobe proopiomelanocortin mRNA levels (30). This effect can be blocked with pertussis toxin (8). Thus, CRH and dopamine can be viewed as dual hypophysiotropic peptides acting through membrane-coupled G-proteins to differentially regulate melanotroph proopiomelanocortin gene expression.

GROWTH HORMONE

The Growth Hormone Family

The GH family of polypeptide hormones includes pituitary and placental GH as well as chorionic somatomammotropin (CS) (formerly known as placental lactogen). The human GH genes are situated as a cluster of five closely linked genes on the long arm of chromosome 17 (q 22–24) (23). GH-N is normally the only transcriptionally active GH gene in the pituitary (92). Human CS is encoded for by two highly homologous genes: CS-A and CS-B (7). Recently, a distinct peptide of 13 amino acids, placental GH, has been demonstrated to be the product of the variant GH gene (GH-V) (49). The fifth gene, CS-like (CS-L), is considered to be an orphan pseudogene with no known product (23).

Pituitary Growth Hormone Peptide and Gene Structure

The general organization of the GH genes includes a five exon, four intron sequence (23). The initially transcribed pre-mRNA encodes a 217 amino acid prehormone. On cleavage of a 26 amino acid signal peptide, a mature 191 amino acid (22 kd) polypeptide is secreted. Alternative splicing of the second intron leads to a shorter 14 amino acid (20 kd) variant, which represents 10% of the pituitary GH content. Exon 1 contains 60 nucleotides of the 5′-untranslated region and the first three codons of the signal peptide. Exon 2 codes for the remainder of the signal peptide and the first 31 amino acids of the mature hormone. Exons 3 and 4 encode the remaining sequence of the GHs. Exon 5 encodes amino acids 127 to 191 and extends for 100 nucleotides 3′ to the termination signal.

Regulation of GH Secretion

Although the secretory patterns of GH have been extensively studied, the specific metabolic events that trigger neuromodulatory centers remain to be elucidated. Nevertheless, it is currently believed that most GH secretory stimuli involve neural activation of any of the following: ventromedial nucleus, arcuate nucleus, and limbic system. The net effect of these signals is enhanced release of GH-releasing hormone (GHRH) from the median eminence of the hypothalamus (35).

GHRH is an ubiquitously expressed hypophysiotropic hormone that is cleaved from a 107 and a 108 amino acid (13 kd) precursor to equipotent peptides that vary in length from 29 to 44 amino acid residues (50). In fact, GHRH was first isolated from two pancreatic tumors associated with ectopic GHRH production and clinical acromegaly (113, 135). Cloning and sequencing of this human pancreatic GHRH has since confirmed its identity to that from the hypothalamus (90). This single-copy gene, which has been mapped to chromosome 20, undergoes alternative splicing to yield the two forms of GHRH prohormones (89). GHRH immunoreactivity in the circulation likely represents extrahypothalamic GHRH production, GHRH metabolites, and nonspecific immunoreactivity. Nevertheless, sufficiently high levels are present in patients who harbor ectopic-GHRH-producing tumors (117). Furthermore, GHRH is closely homologous to other polypeptides, including vasoactive intestinal peptide and histadyl-isoleucine (PHI-27).

GHRH selectively binds to normal somatotroph membranes (120). Glucocorticoid treatment potentiates the GH response to GHRH in vitro. This is the result of glucocorticoid-mediated GHRH receptor up-regulation in addition to direct stimulation of GH gene transcription (45, 120). Unlike other hypophysiotropic factors, sustained exposure to GHRH leads to only partial loss of response (12). This is supported by the development of somatotroph hyperplasia and acromegaly in patients who have sustained GHRH hypersecretion from ectopically produced GHRH (117). Receptor binding leads to activation of a membrane-coupled stimulatory G-protein (Ga1), which in turn activates the enzyme, adenylate cyclase. The resulting rise in cAMP leads to GH secretion (17). The cotreatment of pituitary cells with cAMP analogues, cholera toxin or forskolin, and GHRH does not lead to further increase in the GH response (17). This information supports the role of cAMP in mediating GHRH-induced GH secretion. Calcium channel blockers, however, can completely inhibit GHRH-induced GH secretion without altering cAMP levels (14). Thus, calcium mobilization distal to cAMP generation appears also to play a role in GHRH-mediated GH secretion. As with other anterior pituitary hormones, phospholipase C, diacylglycerol, and phorbol esters stimulate peptide secretion (97).

Preformed GH appears to be packaged in an immediately releasable pool and another pool that is responsive to sustained stimulation (129). The immediately releasable pool exhibits particular sensitivity to such secretagogues as prostaglandin E_2 (PGE_2), dibutyryl cyclic AMP as well as potassium (17). The association between GHRH and the prostaglandin system was first suggested on the basis of the observation that GHRH-induced GH secretion is coupled with enhanced PGE_2 release from rat pituitaries (48). Furthermore, cyclooxygenase inhibitors attenuate GHRH-induced GH secretion, an effect that can be reversed by PGE_2. The additive effect of GHRH and PGE_2 on GH secretion, however, suggests that these two agents act in distinct manners (17). In addition, the in vitro responsiveness of pituitary somatotrophs is age dependent. The increased responsiveness of somatotrophs from immature rats to GHRH does not appear to be influenced by thyroid hormone (46) but can be further elicited by TRH or dibutyryl cAMP treatment (131).

Conversely, somatotropin release inhibitory factor (somatostatin) exhibits profound inhibitory effects on GH secretion. The interaction between GHRH, somatostatin, and the GH target growth factor IGF-1 on GH secretion is conceptually depicted in *Figure 1.4*. This decapeptide is widely expressed throughout the nervous system as well as the gastrointestinal tract, pancreas, and genitourinary system, among others (109). Somatostatin was originally believed to be synthesized as a prohormone that is cleaved into somatostatin-28 and subsequently to the bioactive peptide somatostatin-14 (118). Subsequent studies, however, have revealed that somatostatin-14 and somatostatin-28 display varying activities in different tissues (109). In addition to its inhibitory effect on GH, somatostatin interferes with the release of TSH and almost all extraneural peptides from somatostatin receptor-expressing tissues (21). In neural tissues, somatostatin is present in appreciable concentrations throughout the hypothalamus, thalamus, cortex, brainstem, and spinal cord (108). The physiological significance of this inhibitory peptide on the hypothalamic-pituitary system is supported by multiple lines of evidence. Mediobasal hypothalamic deafferentation results in increased somatic growth rate, GH secretion, and decreased somatostatin concentrations in the isolated area (109). Hypothalamic somatostatin is under neuroexcitatory influence by acetylcholine, dopamine, and neurotensin. Variable effects have been noted with other neurotransmitters, whereas GABA appears to predominantly inhibit somatostatin release (109).

Somatostatin binds to specific membrane receptors that are closely coupled to inhibitory G-proteins (Fig. 1.5). Receptor binding is associated with inhibition of adenylate cyclase activity and cAMP levels (128). The cellular effects of somatostatin, however, appear to be also associated with impairment of intracellular calcium uptake. Somatostatin can also block calcium inophore-mediated GH secretion as well as the cations efflux from the cell (70). The addition of calcium in culture medium reverses somatostatin's inhibitory effects (78).

Regulation of GH Synthesis

Ablation of GHRH-containing hypothalamic neurons results in decreased pituitary GH content and circulating levels (91). Conversely, GHRH stimulates GH gene transcription (6) in addition to increasing GH mRNA accumulation in dispersed rat pituitary cells (54). These effects can be mimicked with cAMP or forskolin (5), thus highlighting the integrated role of the adenylate cyclase system in GHRH-stimulated GH synthesis. In contradistinction, however, calcium mobilization does not influence GH gene transcription (5). Unlike GHRH, somatostatin has no appreciable effects on GH mRNA accumulation (52).

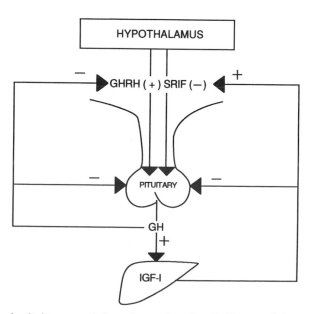

Figure 1.4. Hypothalamic-pituitary-growth factor interactions. Insulin-like growth factor 1 (IGF-1), somatotropin release inhibitory factor (SRIF, somatostatin) growth hormone (GH), and growth hormone-releasing factor (GHRH) are considered to be the primary physiological regulators of this system. (Adapted and modified from Melmed, S. N. Engl. J. Med., *14*:966-967, 1990.)

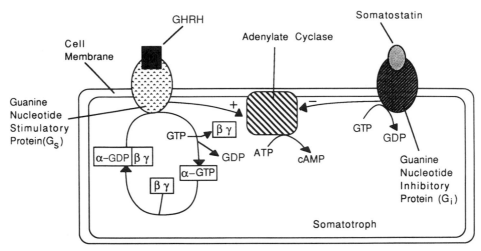

Figure 1.5. Membrane receptor and G proteins in the somatotroph. GHRH and somatostatin binding to their respective surface receptors is associated with activation of stimulatory (G_s) and inhibitory (G_i) signals on adenylate cyclase and therefore cAMP production.

PROLACTIN

Gene Structure and Peptide Heterogeneity

This lactotroph-derived 198 amino acid polypeptide is encoded by a single copy gene on human chromosome 6 (122). Recent evidence suggests that the selective activation of the Prl and GH genes is mediated by Pit-1 (GHF-1) (61). Pit-1 is a 33 kd pituitary transcription factor normally expressed in somatotrophs, lactotrophs, and thyrotrophs (82). This protein shares significant sequence homology with a highly conserved region, referred to as homeodomain, which has been described in other early developmental and position-specific regulatory genes (116). Association of Pit-1 to a distal (-1831 to -1530 bp) (98) and a proximal (-422 to $+33$ bp) (99) enhancer on the Prl gene results in enhanced expression. Furthermore, sequences that flank the distal enhancer appear to contribute to the specificity and regulatory features of this family of transcription factors (116). Identification of Pit-1 is helping explain the molecular basis of the ontogeny of somatotroph and lactotroph development from their progenitor stem cell and mammosomatotroph. Because hypothalamic hormones are known to influence the proportion of GH- and Prl-expressing cells, the interaction between hypophysiotropic factors and pituitary transcription factors such as Pit-1 is currently under investigation.

Prl bears only 16% sequence homology with GH (92). Like GH, however, Prl belongs to a subfamily of molecular variants that differ in immunological and biological potency (74). Following synthesis on the polyribosome in the rough endoplasmic reticulum, the precursor molecule undergoes cleavage. The resultant fragments are packaged into the secretory granules of the golgi apparatus. In the rat, small or monomeric Prl is loosely coupled to cytoplasmic organelles (136). Big or polymeric Prl is stored mainly in secretory granules (136). An additional small molecular-weight variant (21 kd) of rat Prl has been suggested to be the result of alternative site gene splicing (125). Prl also undergoes posttranslational glycosylation whereby a less bioactive molecule is generated (84). It remains to be shown whether morphologically distinct lactotroph subpopulations release unique Prl variant forms.

Dopaminergic Regulation of Prl Secretion

Dopamine is the primary hypophysiotropic factor responsible for maintaining the predominantly inhibitory hypothalamic influence on Prl secretion (9). Dopaminergic pathways originate in the substantia nigra, giving rise to the mesolimbic and nigrostriatal projections. Within the hypothalamus, the tuberoinfundibular pathway appears to be responsible for control of Prl secretion (9). Newly synthesized dopamine in the median eminence is released with a predominance in centrally located vessels in the hypophyseal-portal circulation (112). An inverse relationship between hypothalamic dopamine turnover rates and Prl levels during the rat estrous cycle is now well established (72). Conversely, intracisternally or systemically administered Prl results in stimulated dopamine discharge (4). Despite structural similarity between dopamine and other catecholamines, dopamine binds specifically to its unique set of receptors (9). D1 receptors induce adenylate cyclase activity and are predominantly expressed in the caudate nucleus and parathyroid glands. D3 receptors are presumed presynaptic dopamine autoreceptors. D2 receptors, however, display either a decrease or no effect on cAMP production and are primarily situated in the anterior and intermediate lobes of the pituitary (9). D2 receptors also exhibit dual binding affinities which appear to be modulated by guanine nucleotides (72). Dopamine binding is associated with functional activation of the inhibitory guanine nucleotide regulatory protein and the high-affinity form of the D2 receptor (31). The resultant inhibition of adenylate cyclase activity, cAMP accumulation, and Prl release can be reversed with pertussis toxin treatment (32). Dopamine's inhibitory effect on Prl release, however, persists despite elevated intracellular cAMP levels (37). This suggests that other second messenger systems may, at least, be equally as important as cAMP in mediating dopamine's effects on the lactotroph. Indeed, Prl secretion is stimulated by increased calcium concentrations and is attenuated by the cation's depletion or addition of a calcium channel blocker (81). Dopamine also inhibits calcium-dependent lactotroph action potentials (9). The effect of dopaminergic agents on cytoplasmic calcium concentrations is varied. This is possibly because of functional lactotroph heterogeneity. Inhibition of calcium-calmodulin-sensitive cAMP generation may be an additional mechanism of dopamine action (139).

As in other signal transduction pathways,

cell membrane phosphoinositide metabolism plays an important role in the cellular regulation of Prl secretion. Earlier studies had suggested that dopamine and bromocriptine inhibit basal and TRH-stimulated phosphoinositol turnover (20). This effect, however, does not appear to be caused by the direct inhibition of phospholipase C (65). Instead, chronic D2 receptor activation appears to be associated with attenuation of the rate of phosphorylation of PI to PI-4P (mediated by phosphoryl-transferase) and PI-4P to PIP_2 (65).

Hypothalamic Prl-Stimulatory Factors

The observation that stress stimulates Prl secretion in dopamine-blocked rats is one of several lines of evidence that suggests the existence of a Prl-stimulatory factor(s). In particular, two physiologically relevant hypothalamic peptides have been described, including TRH and vasoactive intestinal peptide. TRH has been implicated in suckling-induced (39) and the rat proestrous-associated Prl surge (40). An inverse relationship between TRH secretion and hypophyseal-portal blood dopamine concentrations has also been described (38). The stimulatory effect of TRH on Prl secretion and gene transcription is mediated by activated protein kinase C and intracellular calcium release (95). Estradiol that binds to its cytoplasmic receptor directly interacts with a distal enhancer element on the 5′-flanking region of the Prl gene (88). In particular, the distal enhancer region (-1713 to -1495) on the rat Prl promoter appears to confer cAMP, TRH, and estrogen responsiveness (36).

Vasoactive intestinal peptide and peptide histidine isoleucine are cleavage products of pro-vasoactive intestinal peptide (62). Fibers for this prohormone originate from the paraventricular hypothalamic nuclei. Vasoactive intestinal peptide is also locally synthesized in lactotrophs, which suggests a possible paracrine role for vasoactive intestinal peptide in the regulation of Prl. In vitro, vasoactive intestinal peptide directly stimulates Prl release from rat pituitary (1) and human prolactinoma cells (127). Unlike TRH, vasoactive intestinal peptide retains the ability of repeated TRH treatment to induce Prl secretion in cells continuously exposed to dopa-

subunit messenger ribonucleic acids and LH secretion. Mol. Endocrinol., *2*:338–343, 1988.

58. Hamernik, D.L., Crowder, M.E., Nilson, J.H., *et al.* Measurement of messenger ribonucleic acid for gonadotropins in ovariectomized ewes after hypothalamic-pituitary disconnection. Endocrinology, *119*:2704–2710, 1986.

59. Hamernik, D.L. and Nett, T.M. Gonadotropin-releasing hormone increases the amount of messenger ribonucleic acid for gonadotropins in ovariectomized ewes after hypothalamic-pituitary disconnection. Endocrinology, *122*:959–966, 1988.

60. Hoermann, R., Spoeth, G., Moncayo, R., *et al.* Evidence of the presence of human chorionic gonadotropin (hCG) and free β-subunit of hCG in the human pituitary. J. Clin. Endocrinol. Metab., *71*:179–186, 1990.

61. Ingraham, H.A., Albert, V.R., Chen, R., *et al.* A family of pou-domain and pit-1 tissue specific transcription factors in pituitary and neuroendocrine development. Annu. Rev. Physiol., *52*:773–791, 1990.

62. Itoh, N., Obeta, K., Yanaihara, N., *et al.* Human preprovasoactive intestinal peptide contains a novel PHI-27-like peptide, PHM-27. Nature, *304*:547–549, 1973.

63. Jameson, J.L., Becker, C.B., Lindell, C.M., *et al.* Human follicle-stimulating hormone β-subunit gene encodes multiple messenger ribonucleic acids. Mol. Endocrinol., *2*:806–815, 1988.

64. Jameson, J.L., Lindell, C.M., and Habener, J.F. Evaluation of different transcriptional start sites in the human luteinizing hormone and chorionic gonadotropin β-subunit genes. DNA, *5*:227–234, 1986.

65. Jarvis, W.D., Judd, A.M., and Macleod, R.M. Attenuation of anterior pituitary phosphoinositide metabolism by the D_2 dopamine receptor. Endocrinology, *123*:2793–2799, 1988.

66. Kaji, H.K., Chihara, K., Abe, H., *et al.* Effect of passive immunization with antisera to vasoactive intestinal polypeptide and peptide histidine isoleucine amide on 5-hydroxy-L-tryptophan-induced prolactin release in rats. Endocrinology, *117*:1914–1919, 1985.

67. Knobil, E. The neuroendocrine control of the menstrual cycle. Recent Prog. Horm. Res., *36*:53–88, 1980.

68. Kourides, I.A., Landon, M.B., Hoffman, B.J., *et al.* Excess production of free α relative to β subunits of the glycoprotein hormone in normal and abnormal human pituitary glands. Clin. Endocrinol., *12*:407–416, 1980.

69. Kovacs, K., Horvath, E., Asa, S.L., *et al.* Pituitary cells producing more than one hormone. Trends Endocrinol. Metab., *1*:104–107, 1989.

70. Kraicer, J. and Spence, J.W. Release of growth hormone from purified somatotrophs: use of high K^+ and the ionophore A23187 to eliminate interrelations among Ca^{++}, adenosine 3',5'-monophosphate, and somatostatin. Endocrinology, *108*:651–657, 1981.

71. Lacaze-Masmonteil, T., de Ketzer, Y., Luton, J.P., *et al.* Characterization of proopiomelanocortin transcripts in human nonpituitary tissues. Proc. Natl. Acad. Sci. USA, *84*:7261–7265, 1987.

72. Lambert, S.W.J. and Macleod, R.M. Regulation of prolactin secretion at the level of the lactotroph. Physiol. Rev., *70*:279–318, 1990.

73. Levin, N., Blum, M., and Roberts, J.L. Modulation of basal and corticotropin-releasing factor-stimulated proopiomelanocortin gene expression by vasopressin in rat anterior pituitary. Endocrinology, *125*:2957–2966, 1989.

74. Lewis, U.J. Variants of growth hormone and prolactin and their posttranslational modifications. Annu. Rev. Physiol., *46*:33–42, 1984.

75. Litvin, Y., Pamantier, R., Fleischer, N., *et al.* Hormonal activation of the cAMP dependent protein kinases in AtT20 cells. J. Biol. Chem., *259*:10296–10302, 1984.

76. Liu, T.C., Jackson, G.L., and Gorski, J. Effects of synthetic gonadotropin-releasing hormone on incorporation of radioactive glucosamine and amino acids into luteinizing hormone and total protein by rat pituitaries in vitro. Endocrinology, *98*:151–163, 1976.

77. Loeffler, J.P., Kley, N., Pittas, C.W., *et al.* Corticotropin-releasing factor and forskolin increase proopiomelanocortin messenger RNA levels in rat anterior and intermediate cells in vitro. Neurosci. Lett., *62*:383–387, 1985.

78. Login, I.S., Judd, A.M., and Macleod, R.M. Association of $^{45}Ca^{2+}$-mobilization with stimulation of growth hormone (GH) release by GH-releasing factor in dispersed normal male rat pituitary cells. Endocrinology, *118*:239–243, 1986.

79. Lucke, C., Hoffken, B., and Von Zur Muhlen, A. The effect of somatostatin on TSH levels in patients with primary hypothyroidism. J. Clin. Endocrinol. Metab., *41*:1082–1084, 1975.

80. Lumblad, J.R. and Roberts, J.L. Regulation of proopiomelanocortin gene expression in pituitary. Endocr. Rev., *9*:135–158, 1988.

81. Macleod, R.M. and Fontham, E.H. Influence of ionic environment on the in vitro synthesis and release of pituitary hormones. Endocrinology, *86*:863–869, 1970.

82. Mangalan, H.J., Albert, V.R., Ingraham, H.A., *et al.* A pituitary POU domain protein, Pit-1, activates both growth hormone and prolactin promoters transcriptionally. Genes Dev., *3*:946–958, 1989.

83. Marian, J. and Conn, P.M. GnRH stimulation of cultured pituitary cells requires calcium. Mol. Pharmacol., *16*:196–201, 1979.

84. Markoff, E., Sigel, M.B., Lacour, B.K., *et al.* Glycosylation selectively alters the biological activity of prolactin. Endocrinology, *123*:1303–1306, 1988.

85. Martinez de la Escalera, G., Guthrie, G.J., and Weiner, R.I. Transient removal of dopamine potentiates the stimulation of prolactin release by TRH but not VIP: stimulation via Ca^{2+}/protein kinase C pathway. Neuroendocrinology. *47*:38–45, 1988.

86. Martinez de la Escalera, G. and Weiner, R.I. Mechanisms by which the transient removal of dopamine regulation potentiates the prolactin-releas-

ing action of thyrotropin-releasing hormone. Neuroendocrinology, *47:*186–193, 1988.

87. Mason, A.J., Hayflick, J.S., Ling, N., *et al.* Complimentary DNA sequences of ovarian follicular fluid inhibin show precursor structure and homology with transforming growth factor *β.* Nature, *318:*659–663, 1985.

88. Maurer, R.A. Estradiol regulates the transcription of the prolactin gene. J. Biol. Chem., *257:*2133–2136, 1982.

89. Mayo, K.E., Cerelli, G.M., Lebo, R.V., *et al.* Gene encoding human growth hormone-releasing factor precursor. Structure, sequence, and chromosomal assignment. Proc. Natl. Acad. Sci. USA, *82:*63–67, 1985.

90. Mayo, K.E., Vale, W., Rivier, J., *et al.* Expression-cloning and sequence of a cDNA encoding human growth hormone-releasing factor. Nature, *306:*86–88, 1983.

91. Millard, W.J., Martin Jr., J.B., Audet, J., *et al.* Evidence that reduced growth hormone secretion observed in monosodium glutamate-treated rats is the result of a deficiency in growth hormone-releasing factor. Endocrinology, *110:*540–550, 1982.

92. Miller, W.L. and Eberhardt, N.L. Structure and evolution of the growth hormone gene family. Endocr. Rev., *4:*97–130, 1983.

93. Minamitani, N.T., Minamitani, T., Lechan, R.M., *et al.* Paraventricular nucleus mediates prolactin secretory responses to restraint stress, ether stress, and 5-hydroxy-L-tryptophan injection in the rat. Endocrinology, *120:*860–877, 1987.

94. Morley, J.E. Neuroendocrine control of thyrotropin secretion. Endocr. Rev., *2:*396–436, 1981.

95. Murdoch, G.H., Waterman, M., Evans, R.M., *et al.* Molecular mechanisms of phorbol ester, thyrotropin-releasing hormone and growth factor stimulation of prolactin gene transcription. J. Biol. Chem., *260:*11852–11858, 1985.

96. Nakanishi, S., Kita T., Taii, S., Imura, H., *et al.* Glucocorticoid effect on the level of corticotropin messenger RNA activity in rat pituitary. Proc. Natl. Acad. Sci. USA, *74:*3283–3286, 1977.

97. Negro-Vilar, A. and Lapetina, E.G. 1,2-dideacanoyl-glycerol and phorbol 12,13-dibutyrate enhance anterior pituitary hormone secretion in vitro. Endocrinology, *117:*1559–1564, 1985.

98. Nelson, C., Albert V.R., Elshotz, H., *et al.* Activation of cell-specific expression of rat growth hormones and prolactin genes by a common transcriptional factor. Science, *239:*1400–1405, 1988.

99. Nelson, C., Crenshaw, E.B., Franco, R., *et al.* Discrete cis-active genomic sequences dictate the pituitary cell type specific expression in rat prolactin and growth hormone genes. Nature, *322:*557–562, 1986.

100. Nikolics, K., Mason, A.J., Szonyi, E., *et al.* A prolactin-inhibiting factor within the precursor for human gonadotropin-releasing hormone. Nature, *316:*511–517, 1985.

101. Nishizuka, Y. The role of protein kinase C in cell surface signal transduction and tumor production. Nature, *308:*693–698, 1984.

102. Odell, W.D., Griffin, J., Bashey, H.M., *et al.* Secretion of chorionic gonadotropin by cultured human

pituitary cells. J. Clin. Endocrinol. Metab., *71:*1318–1322, 1990.

103. Parsons, T.H. and Pierce, J.G. Free α-like material from bovine pituitaries: restoration of the ability to reassociate with native LH-*β* (abstract). Fed. Proc., *42:*1799, 1983.

104. Perrin, M.H., Haas, Y., Rivier, J.E., *et al.* Corticotropin-releasing factor binding to the anterior pituitary receptor is modulated by divalent cations and guanyl nucleotides. Endocrinology, *118:*1171–1179, 1986.

105. Pierce, J.G. and Parsons, T.F. Glycoprotein hormones: structure and function. Annu. Rev. Biochem., *50:*465–495, 1981.

106. Prysor-Jones, R.A., Sliverlight, J.J., Jenkins, J.S., *et al.* Vasoactive intestinal polypeptide and dopamine in the hypothalamus and pituitary of aging rats with prolactinomas. Acta. Endocrinol., *116:*150–154, 1987.

107. Ramey, J.W., Highsmith, R.F., Wilfinger, W.W., *et al.* The effects of gonadotropin-releasing hormone and estradiol on luteinizing hormone biosynthesis in altered rat anterior pituitary cells. Endocrinology, *120:*1503–1513, 1987.

108. Reichlin, S. Somatostatin. N. Engl. J. Med., *309:*1556–1563, 1983.

109. Reichlin, S. Somatostatin. In: *Brain Peptides,* edited by D.T. Krieger, M. Brownstein, and J.B. Martin, p. 711. New York, Wiley, 1983.

110. Reisine, T., Rougon, G., Barbet, J., *et al.* Corticotropin-releasing factor-induced adreno-corticotropin hormone release and synthesis is blocked by incorporation of the inhibition of cyclic AMP-dependent protein kinase into anterior pituitary tumor cells by liposomes. Proc. Natl. Acad. Sci. USA, *82:*8261–8265, 1985.

111. Raymond, V., Leung, P.C.K., Veilleux, R., *et al.* Vasopressin rapidly stimulates phosphatidic acid-phosphatidylinositol turnover in rat anterior pituitary cells. Febbs. Lett., *182:*196–200, 1985.

112. Reymond, M.J., Speciale, S.G., and Porter, J.C. Dopamine in plasma of lateral and medial hypophysial portal vessels: evidence for regional variations in the release of hypothalamic dopamine into hypophysial portal blood. Endocrinology, *112:*1958–1963, 1983.

113. Rivier, J., Spies, J., Thorner, M., *et al.* Characterization of a growth hormone releasing factor from a human pancreatic islet tumor. Nature, *300:*276–278, 1982.

114. Rivier C., Rivier J., and Vale, W. Inhibin-mediated feedback control of follicle-stimulating hormone secretion in the female rat. Science, *234:*205–208, 1986.

115. Roberts, V., Meunier, H., Vaughan, J., *et al.* Production and regulation of inhibin subunits in pituitary gonadotropes. Endocrinology, *124:*552–554, 1989.

116. Rosenfeld, M.G. POU-domain transcription factors: pou-er-ful developmental regulators. Genes Dev., *5:*897–907, 1991.

117. Sano, T., Asa, S.L., and Kovacs, K. Growth hormone-releasing hormone-producing tumors: clinical, biochemical, and morphological manifestations. Endocr. Rev. *9:*357–373, 1988.

118. Schally, A.V., DuPont, A., Arimura, A., *et al.* Isolation and structure of somatostatin from porcine hypothalami. Biochemistry. *15:*509–514, 1976.

119. Schonbrunn, A., and Tashjian, A.H. Modulation of somatostatin receptors by thyrotropin-releasing hormone in a clonal pituitary cell strain. J. Biol. Chem., *255:*190–198, 1980.

120. Seifert, H., Perrin, M., Rivier, J., *et al.* Growth hormone-releasing factor binding sites in rat anterior pituitary membrane homogenates: modulation by glucocorticoids. Endocrinology, *117:*424–426, 1985.

121. Shimasak, S., Koga, A., Esch, F., *et al.* Primary structure of the human follistatin precursor and its genomic organization. Proc. Natl. Acad. Sci. USA, *85:*4218–4222, 1988.

122. Shull, J.D., and Gorski, J. The hormonal regulation of prolactin gene expression: an examination of mechanism controlling prolactin synthesis and the possible relationship of estrogen to these mechanisms. Vitam. Horm., *43:*197–249, 1986.

123. Shupnik, M.A., Greenspan, S.L., and Ridgway, E.C. Transcriptional regulation of thyrotropin subunit genes by thyrotropin-releasing hormone and dopamine in pituitary cell cultures. J. Biol. Chem., *261:*12675–12679, 1986.

124. Shupnik, M.A., Weinmann, C.M., Notides, A.C., *et al.* An upstream region of the rat luteinizing hormone β gene binds estrogen receptor and confers estrogen responsiveness. J. Biol. Chem., *264:*80–86, 1989.

125. Sinha, Y.N., and Jacobsen, B.P. Structural and immunologic evidence for a small molecular weight (21K) variant of prolactin. Endocrinology, *123:*1364–1370, 1988.

126. Smith, P.L. and Baenziger, J.U. A pituitary N-acetylgalactosamine transferase that specifically recognizes glycoprotein hormones. Science, *242:*930–933, 1988.

127. Spada, A., Nicosia S., Corteslazzi L., *et al.* In vitro studies on prolactin release and adenylate cyclase activity in human prolactin-secreting pituitary adenomas. Different sensitivity of macro- and micro adenomas to dopamine and vasoactive intestinal peptide. J. Clin. Endocrinol. Metab., *56:*1–10, 1983.

128. Spada, A., Vallar, L., and Grammattasio, G. Presence of an adenylate cyclase dually regulated by somatostatin and human pancreatic growth hormone (GH)-releasing factor in GH-secreting cells. Endocrinology, *115:*1203–1209, 1984.

129. Stachura, M.E. and Tyler, J.M. Growth hormone-releasing factor-44 specificity for components of somatotroph and lactotroph immediate release pool substructures. Endocrinology, *120:*1719–1726, 1987.

130. Starzec, Z., Counis, R., and Justisz, M. Gonadotropin-releasing hormone stimulates the synthesis of the polypeptide chains of luteinizing hormone. Endocrinology, *119:*561–565, 1986.

131. Szabo, M. and Cuttler, L. Differential responsiveness of the somatotroph to growth hormone-releasing factor during early neonatal development in the rat. Endocrinology, *118:*69–73, 1986.

132. Takahashi, H., Hakamata, Y., Watanabe, Y., *et al.* Complete nucleotide sequence of the human corticotropin-β-lipotropin precursor gene. Nucleic Acids Res., *11:*6847–6858, 1983.

133. Talmadge, K., Boorstein, W.R., and Fiddes, J.C. The human genome contains seven genes for the β subunit of chorionic gonadotropin but only one gene for the β-subunit of luteinizing hormone. DNA, *2:*281–289, 1983.

134. Tamjasin, P., Kozbur, Y., and Florsheim, W.A. Somatostatin in the physiologic feedback control of thyrotropin secretion. Life Sci., *19:*657–660, 1976.

135. Thorner, M.O., Perryman, R.L., Cronin, M.J., *et al.* Somatotroph hyperplasia. Successful treatment of acromegaly by removal of a pancreatic islet tumor secreting a growth hormone-releasing factor. J. Clin. Invest., *70:*965–977, 1982.

136. Torres, A.I. and Aoki, A. Release of big and small molecular forms of prolactin: dependence upon dynamic state of the lactotroph. J. Endocrinol., *114:*213–220, 1987.

137. Weeke, J., Hansen, A.P., and Lundbaek, K. Inhibition by somatostatin of basal levels of serum thyrotropin (TSH) in normal men. J. Clin. Endocrinol. Metab., *41:*168–171, 1975.

138. Weintraub, B.D., Stannard, B.S., Magner, J.A., *et al.* Glycosylation and posttranslational processing of thyroid-stimulating hormone: clinical implications. Recent Prog. Horm. Res., *41:*577–606, 1985.

139. Weiss, B., Prozialeck, W., Cimino, M., *et al.* Pharmocological regulation of calmodulin. Ann. NY. Acad. Sci., *356:*319–345, 1980.

140. Wilber, J.F. Stimulation of ^{14}C-glucosamine and ^{14}C-alanine incorporation into thyrotropin by synthetic thyrotropin-releasing hormone. Endocrinology, *89:*873–877, 1971.

141. Wildt, L., Hausler, A., Marshall, G., *et al.* Frequency and amplitude of gonadotropin-releasing hormone stimulation and gonadotropin secretion in the rhesus monkey. Endocrinology, *109:*376–385, 1981.

142. Wondisford, F.E., Raslovick, S., Moates, J.M., *et al.* Isolation and characterization of the human thyrotropin β-subunit gene: differences in gene structure and promoter function from murine species. J. Biol. Chem., *263:*12538–12542, 1988.

CHAPTER 2

Antidiuretic Hormone: Regulation, Disorders, and Clinical Evaluation

MARC THIBONNIER, M.D., M.SC.

INTRODUCTION

The antidiuretic hormone, vasopressin (AVP), is a nonapeptide with a ring structure and a disulfide bond that plays a major role in the homeostasis of body fluid volume and osmolality as well as in the maintenance of arterial blood pressure (10, 31). All these actions are mediated through the activation of specific membrane-bound receptors located at the surface of the target cells (33). On the basis of pharmacological and functional studies, Michell et al. proposed, in 1979 (19) to individualize two types of AVP receptors. This classification, widely referred to as V_1-vascular and V_2-renal AVP receptors, was recently amended when several authors reported that AVP receptors present in the anterior pituitary had a slightly different pharmacological profile in the binding characteristics of AVP analogues (15, 17, 29). They are called $V1_b$ receptors to distinguish them from the classical $V1_a$-vascular receptors. As the cloning of AVP receptors nears, the elucidation of sequences of receptors will undoubtedly facilitate and extend the classification of AVP receptors, following the example of the family of α and β adrenergic receptors.

The main action of AVP occurs in the kidneys, where it increases the transepithelial water permeability of the collecting ducts through binding to the V_2-renal AVP receptors, the activation of adenylate cyclase, protein kinase A-dependent protein phosphorylations, the depolymerization of F-actin, and the mobilization of vesicles called aggrephores that contain water channels (38). Vasoconstriction, the other major action of AVP, is mediated by the activation of the V_1-vascular receptors, the mobilization of intracellular calcium and influx of extracellular calcium, the activation of phospholipases A_2, C, and D, the production of inositol triphosphate and diacylglycerol, and protein kinase C-dependent protein phosphorylations (34). In addition, AVP exerts a wide array of physiological effects, including the stimulation of glycogenolysis and neoglucogenesis, corticotropin release, urea and sodium reabsorption, blood platelet aggregation, coagulation factors release, the firing rate of certain neurons, and cell growth and proliferation (32).

SYNTHESIS AND SECRETION OF AVP

The gene that encodes the AVP peptide and its associated neurophysin has been isolated. This gene is composed of three exons separated by two introns (20, 25) (Fig. 2.1). The first exon contains the nucleotide sequence that encodes the signal peptide, immediately followed by the AVP nonapeptide, then a tripeptide spacer (glycine-lysine-arginine where the endoprotease cleavage of the precursor takes place), and, finally, the first nine amino acids of the N-terminus of neurophysin II. The second exon codes for the highly conserved region of neurophysin, followed by a single arginine, and a C-terminal 39 amino acid glycopeptide. The neurophysin is involved in the sorting-packaging and

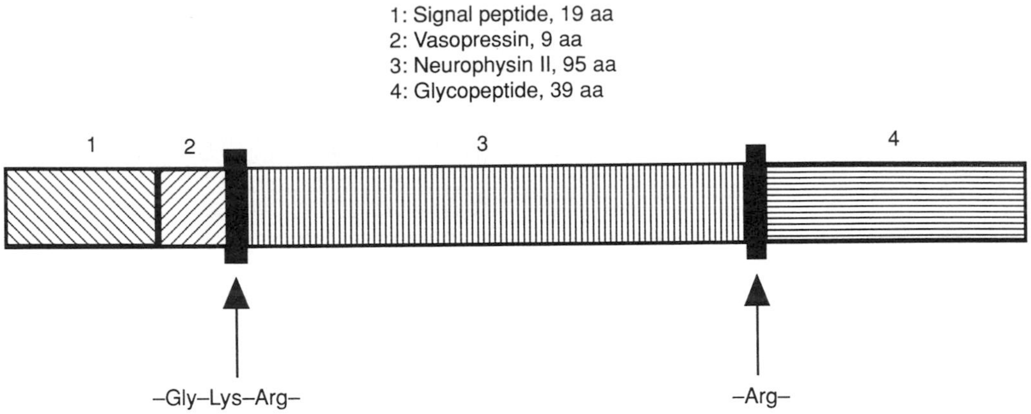

1: Signal peptide, 19 aa
2: Vasopressin, 9 aa
3: Neurophysin II, 95 aa
4: Glycopeptide, 39 aa

Figure 2.1. Structure of the gene coding for vasopressin and its related neurophysin.

transport of AVP, whereas the glycopeptide is thought to be an hypothalamic Prl-releasing factor (21). The expressed AVP mRNA is processed to mature mRNA with no evidence for alternative splicing mechanisms. Therefore, the amino acid sequence of the AVP precursor is directly related to the positions of the structural codons found in the gene. Synthesis occurs in the ribosomes, and the initial posttranslational modifications of the precursor take place in the rough endoplasmic reticulum, i.e., a cotranslational removal of the signal peptide and an N-asparaginyl-high mannose glycosylation of the glycopeptide. The eight disulfide bonds of the precursor are also presumably formed in the rough endoplasmic reticulum. The next posttranslational event occurs in the Golgi apparatus with removal of the high mannose chain and terminal glycosylation of the precursor. The endoproteolytic cleavages that release the individual peptides seem to occur in the neurosecretory vesicles themselves, which contain all the enzymes necessary for the conversion of the AVP precursor into the final peptides. Two endoproteolytic cleavage sites exist in the glycine-lysine-arginine sequence immediately following the AVP sequence, and at the single arginine residue that separates the neurophysin from the glycopeptide. The three peptide moieties of the AVP precursor are transported along the axons of the hypothalamo-neurohypophyseal nerve tract at a rate of 2–3 mm/hr. The complexes are then stored in granules and are eventually secreted by the nerve terminals in the posterior pituitary. The secretion is initiated by action potentials that reach the cell bodies of the nerve tracts. These action potentials trigger the influx of calcium across the membrane. AVP and neurophysin II are released by exocytosis into the blood stream. There are also caudal projections of AVP and oxytocin fibers to the brain stem, the nucleus of the tractus solitarii, the dorsal motor nucleus of the vagus, and throughout the gray matter of the spinal cord.

The development of labeled cDNA probes and the techniques of Northern blot, hybridization, and in situ hybridization have allowed the topographic localization of the AVP gene expression in specific sets of hypothalamic magnocellular neurons (vasopressinergic neurons), which are distinct from those expressing the oxytocin gene (oxytocinergic neurons). The specific AVP mRNA is isolated in supraoptic, paraventricular, and suprachiasmatic nuclei. In situ hybridization experiments have shown that AVP and oxytocin genes are expressed exclusively in vasopressinergic and oxytocinergic neurons, with no coexpression of both peptides in the same neuron. The number of neurons that express these two peptides is rather limited: approximately 5,000 vasopressinergic and 3,500 oxytocinergic neurons. The paraventricular nucleus not only contains magnocellular neurons but also parvocellular neurons that contain several peptidergic neurotransmitters, including AVP and oxytocin. These parvocellular neurons include one class ending in the external zone of the median eminence, on the capillary loops of the portal system, from where secreted peptides may reach the anterior pituitary. In this class of parvicellular neurons, AVP colocalizes with corticotropin-releasing hormone (CRH) and is involved in adrenocorticotrophic hormone (ACTH) release (40). The other class of parvicellular neurons projects toward neuronal targets in the brain stem and the spinal cord.

The AVP-containing neurons of the suprachiasmatic nucleus receive afferent signals from the retina and project to the organum vasculosum of the lamina terminalis, the preoptic area, the dorsomedial hypothalamus, and the paraventricular nuclei of the thalamus and hypothalamus. Other vasopressinergic neurons in the rat brain become apparent after colchicine treatment; they are located in the nucleus of the stria terminalis and in the medial amygdala as well as the locus coeruleus. These multiple locations mediate the role played by AVP in the regulation of ACTH release, body temperature, and hormonal circadian rhythms.

Expression of the AVP gene is also observed in several extrahypothalamic tissues, including the cerebellum, the adrenal glands, and the reproductive organs (13). Furthermore, the AVP mRNA is transported along the axons from the hypothalamus to the posterior pituitary gland. The possibility of direct expression of the AVP gene in the posterior pituitary has also been proposed (18). The length of the poly(A) tail at the 3' end of the AVP mRNA varies with the degree of transcription and the site of expression. For instance, the poly(A) tail is longer when the message is expressed in the hypothalamus than in the peripheral organs (14).

Recent studies using cDNA hybridization techniques have shown that stimuli such as dehydration or salt loading in rats increased the level of hypothalamic AVP mRNA 2- to 20-fold, suggesting that the regulation is occurring at the transcriptional level (9). Interestingly enough, the osmotic stimulation increased the mRNA expression in the supraoptic and paraventricular nuclei, but not in the suprachiasmatic nuclei.

The expression of the AVP gene is controlled by several cis- and trans-acting elements that modulate the activity of the vasopressin gene promoter (20). Several putative cis-acting elements have been identified upstream of the transcription initiation

site of the AVP gene. They include a glucocorticoid response element, a cAMP response element, and four AP-2 binding sites. Gel shift assays suggest the existence of transacting proteins in the hypothalamus that can specifically bind to a DNA fragment that harbors three putative AP-2 binding sites. One or all of these AP-2 binding sites may activate the transcription of the AVP gene through an increase in cAMP because it has been established that cAMP is involved in the control of the AVP gene transcription in relation to osmotic stimulation (9).

Recombinant DNA studies have isolated the genetic defect present in the Brattleboro rat afflicted by the absence of pituitary and serum AVP, which leads to the so-called neurogenic type of diabetes insipidus (27). The mutant AVP gene displays a single nucleotide base deletion in the second exon that encodes the highly conserved region of neurophysin II. This deletion does not prevent transcription and translation. It generates instead a different reading frame that produces a hormone precursor that still contains AVP but is characterized by an altered C-terminus and the loss of five out of 14 cysteine residues (Fig. 2.2). The mutated precursor is no longer transported through the intracellular organelles and is retained in the rough endoplasmic reticulum. This posttranslational block explains the lack of AVP in the neurohypophysis.

REGULATION OF VASOPRESSIN SECRETION

Monoamines, amino acids, and peptides modulate the activity of vasopressinergic magnocellular neurons of the hypothalamic supraoptic nuclei and the paraventricular nuclei. Extensive studies in the rat have led to the following findings (6, 8, 16, 24): Noradrenergic ascending pathways arise from the caudal ventrolateral medulla (i.e., the A1 adrenergic cell group) to project onto the supraoptic nuclei and paraventricular nuclei and activate vasopressinergic neurons in response to hypovolemic or hypotensive stimuli. The excitability of AVP-secreting neurons is enhanced by α agonists and depressed by β agonists. Norepinephrine and α agonists provoke membrane depolarization and bursting activity pattern partly through re-

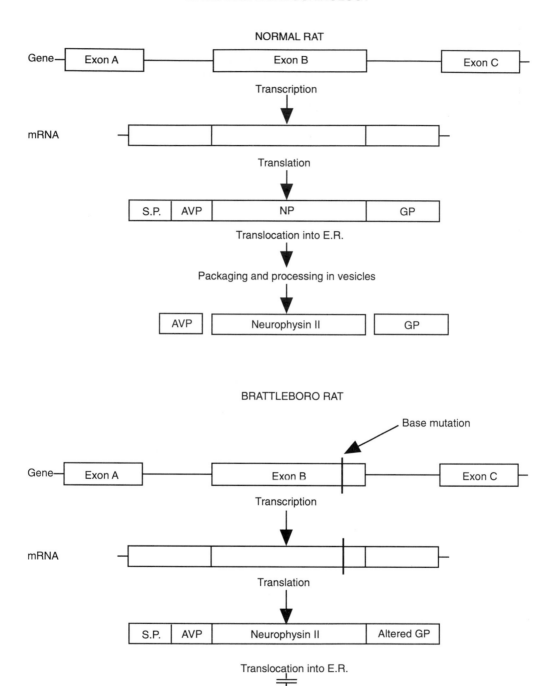

Figure 2.2. Transcription, translation, and processing of the vasopressin precursor in normal and Brattleboro rats. S.P., signal peptide; AVP, vasopressin; NP, neurophysin II, GP, glycopeptide, E.R., endoplasmic reticulum.

duction in a transient outward potassium conductance. Both catecholamine and non-catecholamine peptidergic neurons of the nucleus tractus solitarii excite vasopressinergic neurons in the supraoptic nuclei. Neurons in the subfornical organ and the organum vasculosum of the lamina terminalis stimulate vasopressinergic neurons of the supraoptic nuclei and paraventricular nuclei in response to osmotic stimuli but not hypovolemia. The subfornical organ neurons seem to be sensitive to angiotensin II. Lesions of the AV3V area of the anterior ventral third ventricle reduce the sensitivity of supraoptic nuclei neurons to osmotic stimuli. Neurons in the diagonal band of Broca are responsible for a potent GABA$_a$ receptor-mediated inhibition of the supraoptic nuclei vasopressinergic neurons. The lateral septum and the amygdala are also associated with an inhibitory response of vasopressinergic neurons. Stimulation of the lateral olfactory tract activates AVP-secreting cells, and dopaminergic afferents mediate AVP secretion through D2 receptors. The role of endogenous opioids in AVP regulation is still unclear, but κ agonists inhibit the electrical activity of supraoptic nuclei neurons and reduce AVP secretion. Acute noxious stimuli excite the hypothalamic vasopressinergic neurons, whereas chronic stimuli seem to display an inhibitory effect (23).

Since the classical studies of Verney in 1947 (39), the concept that cerebral osmoreceptors control AVP secretion has been well established, but the precise anatomical location of the osmoreceptors and the nature of the stimulus (alteration of sodium concentration versus change in cell volume) have been widely debated (36). The sodium receptor theory is negated by the fact that an infusion of sucrose (which reduces sodium concentration) can stimulate AVP release. The supraoptic nuclei and paraventricular nuclei are located within the blood-brain and blood-CSF barriers and do not synthesize AVP in response to brain tissue dehydration induced by infusion of glucose or urea. These observations suggest that the magnocellular neurons or other neurons located within the barriers may not be the osmoreceptors. There is evidence that osmoreceptors are located in a circumventricular organ and

shrink in response to hyperosmolar stimuli such as sodium chloride or sucrose, triggering thirst and AVP release (36). As indicated above, the subfornical organ and organum vasculosum of the lamina terminalis neurons are osmosensitive and the AV3V area is also involved in the osmoregulation of AVP secretion. To reconcile the different theories, Thrasher *et al.* (36) proposes that the forebrain circumventricular organ (organum vasculosum of the lamina terminalis and subfornical organ regions) provides the major osmosensitive input to the supraoptic nuclei and paraventricular nuclei vasopressinergic neurons, which by themselves are osmosensitive but only at a higher threshold.

The anatomical and pharmacological factors described above mediate the physiological control of AVP secretion (28). The most important and sensitive controller of AVP secretion under physiological conditions is the effective plasma osmotic pressure (26). Once plasma osmolality reaches a set point or threshold, plasma AVP rises steeply in direct relation to plasma osmolality. An alteration of plasma osmolality as small as 1% is sufficient to provoke a significant release of AVP, modifying urine flow and osmolality. The slope of the relationship between plasma osmolality and plasma AVP varies from one person to another and is modulated by numerous factors including blood volume and blood pressure status, steroid hormones, and other characteristics that directly affect AVP secretion. As mentioned above, not all plasma solutes are equally potent. Although sodium and its anions as well as mannitol and sucrose are potent osmostimuli, increases in plasma glucose or urea do not alter plasma AVP in healthy subjects. These discrepancies are presumably related to the particular location of the osmoreceptors and to the fact that the true signal is an osmotically induced dehydration of the osmoreceptors.

The secretion of AVP is also altered by changes in blood volume and blood pressure. The corresponding afferent pathways arise in pressure-sensitive receptors located in the cardiac atria, the large arteries, and the pulmonary bed. They travel through the vagal and glossopharyngeal nerves and connect in the nucleus tractus solitarii with noradrenergic neurons projecting toward the supra-optic nuclei and paraventricular nuclei. The hemodynamic regulation of AVP secretion is characterized by the following pattern:

- It is mainly an inhibitory input because its elimination leads to an acute rise in AVP and arterial pressure.
- It is not as sensitive as the osmoregulation because decreases in blood pressure or blood volume greater than 10% are required to significantly alter AVP secretion.
- It often leads to a large release of AVP beyond levels required to induce maximum antidiuresis.
- It often mediates the effects of diverse pathological conditions and pharmacological agents (congestive heart failure, liver cirrhosis, nephrosis, positive pressure breathing, diuretics, isoproterenol, norepinephrine, nicotine, nitroprusside, trimethaphan, histamine, bradykinin, morphine).

Other conditions stimulate AVP secretion. Nausea can provoke a rapid and massive AVP release through a pathway that involves the chemoreceptor trigger zone in the area postrema of the medulla. Such an event is blocked by the dopamine antagonists fluphenazine, haloperidol, and promethazine. Emesis mediates at least partly the release of AVP noted with vasovagal reactions, keto-acidosis, acute hypoxia, motion sickness, and various drugs such as cyclophosphamide. A profound hypoglycemia triggers AVP release possibly through an intracellular deficiency of glucose or its metabolites. The renin-angiotensin system stimulates AVP release through a central mechanism that potentiates the osmoregulatory system. Pain, physical exercise, fever, and stress are associated with AVP release through poorly defined mechanisms. Severe hypoxemia markedly enhances AVP secretion, even in the absence of hypotension. Hypercapnia by itself may also trigger AVP release independently of hypoxia or hypotension. Finally, numerous pharmacological agents alter AVP secretion or renal actions as described in the following section.

DISORDERS OF AVP SECRETION AND THEIR CLINICAL EVALUATION

Deficient AVP Secretion

The etiologies of diabetes insipidus (the elimination of large amounts of dilute urine) can be classified in three main categories (Table 2.1).

Neurogenic diabetes insipidus is the most frequent cause of AVP deficiency and relates to various congenital or acquired pathologies listed in Table 2.1. More than 80% of the vasopressin-producing neurons or pathways must be destroyed to produce a permanent diabetes insipidus. After surgery, the vasopressin deficiency may be transient, with return to a normal urine output within a week. In many patients, the AVP deficiency is idiopathic and may occur on a familial basis.

Nephrogenic diabetes insipidus results from a renal insensitivity to the antidiuretic action of AVP. This could be an acquired de-

TABLE 2.1.
Causes of Diabetes Insipidus

1. Neurogenic Diabetes Insipidus (vasopressin deficiency)
   Familial (autosomal dominant)
   Acquired
     Idiopathic
     Trauma
     Surgery (hypophysectomy, removal of suprasellar tumors)
     Tumor (craniopharyngioma, metastasis, lymphoma, cysts)
     Granuloma (sarcoidosis, histiocytosis)
     Infectious (meningitis, encephalitis)
     Vascular (aneurysm, Sheehan's syndrome, vascular occlusion)
     Autoimmune
2. Nephrogenic Diabetes Insipidus (AVP insensitivity)
   Familial (X-linked recessive)
   Acquired
     Chronic renal disease (pyelonephritis, obstructive uropathy, amyloidosis, sickle cell disease, polycystic kidney disease, sarcoidosis)
     Hypokalemia
     Hypercalcemia
     Sjögren's syndrome
     Drugs (lithium, demeclocycline, methoxyflurane, colchicine)
3. Psychogenic Diabetes Insipidus (primary polydipsia)
   Idiopathic (resetting of the osmostat)
   Psychogenic

ficiency from a number of chronic renal diseases that affect the medulla and the collecting duct system (i.e., chronic pyelonephritis), or other conditions that alter the urinary concentrating capacity (i.e., ion disturbances, drug therapy). Congenital nephrogenic diabetes insipidus is a rare disease associated with an insensitivity of the renal tubule adenylate cyclase to AVP. It is transmitted by an X-linked pattern, occurring most commonly in male patients. In this group of diseases, plasma AVP is normal or increased.

Psychogenic diabetes insipidus or potomania leads to a reduced AVP secretion that results from excessive water consumption. This condition may be related to a primary defect in the osmoregulation of thirst or, more often, to psychiatric disorders such as schizophrenia.

The differential diagnosis of diabetes insipidus rests on simple tests.

Plasma and Urine Osmolalities

Measurement of urine osmolality reveals a low value (<200 milliosmoles/kg), which rules out polyuria from osmotic diuresis. In both neurogenic and nephrogenic diabetes insipidus, plasma osmolality is increased, whereas it is diluted in potomania.

Water Deprivation Test

A water deprivation test with careful monitoring of body weight, blood pressure, urine volume, and osmolality shows no rise in urine osmolality and no reduction in urine flow in both neurogenic and nephrogenic types of diabetes insipidus, whereas urine osmolality increases above plasma osmolality level in potomania. The water deprivation test should be terminated if body weight falls by more than 3%.

Hypertonic Saline Infusion

Measurements of urine osmolality before and during a hypertonic saline infusion can differentiate between neurogenic and nephrogenic diabetes insipidus on the one hand (in which urine osmolality is subnormal and remains inappropriately low in reference to plasma osmolality or plasma sodium during the saline infusion), and psychogenic diabe-

tes insipidus on the other hand (in which urine osmolality does increase in response to the saline challenge).

Plasma Vasopressin Radioimmunoassay

Plasma AVP can be measured by a sensitive radioimmunoassay at baseline and during a water deprivation test and hypertonic saline infusion. In neurogenic diabetes insipidus, plasma AVP remains abnormally low. In nephrogenic diabetes insipidus, plasma AVP is normal or high and responds normally to water deprivation or saline infusion. In psychogenic diabetes insipidus, plasma AVP is low to start with but does increase with the osmotic stimuli.

Therapeutic Challenge

A therapeutic trial with 5 units of AVP subcutaneously or 1 μg of 1-(3-mercaptopropanoic acid)8-D-AVP (DDAVP) intravenously, intramuscularly, or subcutaneously shows within 1 hr an increase in urine osmolality in neurogenic diabetes insipidus but no alteration of urine osmolality and flow in nephrogenic diabetes insipidus. If urinary output decreases and urine osmolality increases but polydipsia persists with development of hyponatremia, psychogenic diabetes insipidus is the most likely diagnosis.

Excessive Vasopressin Secretion

An increase in AVP secretion may occur in many clinical settings, either as an appropriate response to an osmotic stimulus or as a response to other stimuli unrelated to the osmotic status of the patient. In the latter category, plasma AVP concentration is inappropriately high for the corresponding plasma osmolality or plasma sodium concentration. Syndromes of osmotically inappropriate AVP secretion are usually divided into three categories based on the patient's intravascular and extracellular fluid volume status (Table 2.2).

1. Hypervolemic hyponatremia is characterized by a reduced effective blood volume but an increased interstitial volume with edema. Congestive heart failure, decompensated liver cirrhosis, glomerulo-

TABLE 2.2.
Causes of Hyponatremia

1. Hypervolemic hyponatremia (edematous states)
   Urinary sodium > 20 mmol/L
     Acute and chronic renal failure

   Urinary sodium < 10 mmol/L
     Cardiac failure
     Liver cirrhosis
     Nephrotic syndrome

2. Hypovolemic hyponatremia
   Urinary sodium > 20 mmol/L
     Diuretic excess
     Mineralocorticoid deficiency
     Salt-losing nephropathy
     Renal tubular acidosis
     Ketonuria
     Osmotic diuresis

   Urinary sodium < 10 mmol/L
     Late diuretic phase
     Vomiting
     Diarrhea
     Cathartic abusers
     Third space burns
     Pancreatitis
     Peritonitis
     Muscle trauma

3. Euvolemic hyponatremia
   Urinary sodium > 20 mmol/L
     Drugs
     Glucocorticoid deficiency
     Hypothyroidism
     Pain, stress
     SIADH

nephritis, and nephrotic syndrome belong in this category.

2. Hypovolemic hyponatremia corresponds to situations in which both blood volume and interstitial volume are reduced. Use or abuse of diuretics is the most frequent cause of hyponatremia with impaired water excretion. Fluid reabsorption is increased in the renal proximal tubule, whereas the maximum urinary dilution capacity is altered in the distal tubule. Adrenal insufficiency also provokes hypovolemia, hyponatremia, and impaired water excretion. Other conditions associated with hypovolemic hyponatremia include vomiting, diarrhea, renal tubular acidosis, medullary cystic disease of the kidney, burns, peritonitis, and pancreatitis.

3. Euvolemic hyponatremia, called the syndrome of inappropriate secretion of antidiuretic hormone or (SIADH), is characterized by normal or slightly increased volumes but no edema. Causes of SIADH are divided into three main categories: neoplastic, nonneoplastic, and pharmacological as listed in Table 2.3. In patients whose SIADH is of neurological origin, the coexistence of schizophrenia or other psychotic disorders may worsen the sever-

ity and incidence of the syndrome if psychogenic polydipsia is present.

The dynamic exploration of AVP secretion during water loading, hypertonic saline infusion, or both have led Zerbe et al. (41) to distinguish at least four types of osmoregulatory abnormalities in patients who have SIADH. Type A, found in about 25% of all patients, is characterized by large, erratic fluctuations in plasma AVP that occur independently of alterations of plasma osmolality. In type B, present in another 25% of patients, plasma AVP remains excessive and constant until plasma osmolality rises into the normal range. Beyond that point, plasma AVP rises in relation to a further increase in plasma osmolality. Type C is the most common pattern, found in 35% of cases. It is characterized by plasma AVP levels closely correlated with plasma osmolality but with an osmotic threshold significantly shifted to the left, suggesting a resetting of the osmostat. In type D, less common than the other three types, AVP secretion falls within the normal dynamic range and its etiology remains unclear (renal supersensitivity to AVP action or secretion of another antidiuretic factor).

The proper evaluation of a patient who has

hyponatremia rests on the following elements:

- complete history and physical examination
- review of the orders and medications on board
- assessment of body weight, fluid volume status, and oral and parenteral intakes
- measurement of plasma electrolytes and osmolality, urine volume, electrolytes, and osmolality
- assessment of cardiac, hepatic, and renal functions
- acid-base status evaluation and plasma uric acid measurement.

With this information at hand, one is able to complete the eight steps described below. Step 1 is to identify hyponatremia. Usually, hyponatremia is revealed by routine measurements of plasma electrolytes, but it may be responsible for various signs and symptoms including lethargy, apathy, disorientation, muscle cramps, agitation, anorexia, nausea, abnormal sensorium, depressed tendon reflexes, Cheyne-Stokes respiration, hypothermia, pathological reflexes, pseudobulbar palsy, seizures, and even coma. These signs and symptoms are often overlooked in the postoperative period, and hyponatremia is revealed by a review of laboratory results. Step 2 eliminates a false hyponatremia. If plasma sodium is measured by flame photometry rather than by ion-selective electrode, a falsely low plasma sodium may be associated with a normal plasma osmolality (hyperlipidemia, hyperproteinemia, use of glycine solution) or an increased plasma osmolality (hyperglycemia and mannitol infusion). Step 3 is performed to exclude hypovolemic and edematous etiologies of hyponatremia as listed in Table 2.2. Step 4 will identify the pharmacological agents listed in Table 2.3 that alter AVP release, actions, or both. At step 5, pituitary, thyroid, and adrenal diseases can be ruled out easily. Step 6 will exclude nonosmotic release of AVP in a context of hypotension, stress, or pain. Step 7 confirms the biological profile of true SIADH as defined by:

- plasma hyponatremia, hypo-osmolality, and hypo-uricemia

TABLE 2.3.
Causes of the Syndrome of Inappropriate Secretion of Antidiuretic Hormone

1. Neoplastic
   Bronchogenic carcinoma
   Lymphoma
   Sarcoma
   Carcinoma of the duodenum, pancreas, prostate, bladder, and ureter
   Mesothelioma
   Thymoma
   Brain tumors
2. Nonneoplastic
   Pulmonary diseases
       Bacterial, viral, parasitological pneumonia
       Aspergillosis
       Tuberculosis, pulmonary abscess
       Asthma, positive pressure breathing, pneumothorax
       Cystic fibrosis
   Central nervous system diseases
       Bacterial or viral meningitis or encephalitis, Guillain-Barré syndrome, Rocky Mountain fever
       Head trauma, subdural or subarachnoid hemorrhage or hematoma, cavernous sinus thrombosis
       Brain abscess
       Acute intermittent porphyria
       Peripheral neuropathy
       Psychosis, delirium tremens
       Cerebral and cerebellar atrophy, hydrocephalus
       Cerebrovascular accidents
       Multiple sclerosis
       Sarcoidosis
   Endocrine disease
       Myxedema
       Idiopathic
3. Pharmacological
   Vasopressin and vasopressin analogues, oxytocin
   Bromocriptine
   Vincristine, cisplatinum, cyclophosphamide
   Chlorpropamide, tolbutamide
   Thiazide diuretics
   Clofibrate
   Carbamazepine
   Nicotine
   Phenothiazines, haloperidol, tricyclic antidepressants
   Monoamine oxidase inhibitors, isoproterenol
   Morphine, barbiturates
   Acetaminophen, indomethacin

- urine hyperosmolality
- urinary sodium excretion >20 mmol/L
- normal pituitary, thyroid, and adrenal functions
- normal renal function.

Radioimmunoassay of plasma AVP, water loading, and saline infusion tests are usually not required to make the diagnosis of SIADH. Finally, step 8 will identify the cause of SIADH as listed in Table 2.3.

Such a systematic approach to the evaluation of patients who have hyponatremia is warranted because hyponatremia (defined as a serum sodium <130 mmol/L) is the most frequent electrolyte abnormality found in a hospital population, with an incidence of 1%, and is associated with a 60-fold increase in mortality rate when compared to normonatremic patients (1). Hyponatremia is even more frequent in the subgroup of postoperative patients, afflicting about 4% of them. However, despite the high incidence of hyponatremia, permanent neurological damage appears to be relatively rare. Nonetheless, it is well established that both hyponatremia and rapid correction of hyponatremia can cause neurological dysfunction and damage. The ideal mode of correction of hyponatremia is the subject of much controversy. In particular, the ideal rate of correction of hyponatremia has been hotly debated (2). Until this debate is concluded, however, a conservative, gradual approach to correction of hyponatremia is warranted.

Cerebral Consequences of Untreated Hyponatremia

In experimental and clinical situations, excess water will cause cerebral edema with a subsequent increase in intracranial pressure. In 1935, Helwig et al. (11) reported the first fatal case of water intoxication in a 50-year old woman who received 9 liters of water following a cholecystectomy. Her brain was uniformly enlarged and swollen with compression of the ventricles and obliteration of the subarachnoid space. Similar findings with brain stem herniation were reported in more recent series (4). However, the dramatic alterations of the brain associated with acute hyponatremia are encountered much less frequently than expected if osmotic equilibrium is achieved solely by water diffusion into the brain. Several adaptive processes are triggered to buffer cerebral swelling. The water increment in brain content in the first 6 hrs after water loading is only 40% of what should be expected, based on typical osmosis (12). Because brain and plasma remain in osmotic equilibrium, the adaptation is occurring promptly after the initiation of acute hyponatremia. There is evidence that the flow of fluid from the interstitial space of the brain into cerebrospinal fluid is increased (12). Water entering the brain as a consequence of hyponatremia increases the interstitial space pressure, with formation of a pressure gradient driving fluid into the CSF. The excess CSF thereafter reenters the systemic circulation. This adaptative mechanism is not observed in newborn puppies in which a compliant skull accommodates more cerebral swelling and less pressure build-up (22). A second defense mechanism becomes operative within hours of the induction of hyponatremia, i.e., the loss of cell solutes, primarily potassium. Sodium and chloride content within brain cells decreases within 30 minutes, whereas brain potassium reduction takes 3 hrs. The loss of brain electrolytes is usually limited to 15% to 20% of total content, suggesting that other osmolytes are involved in the process. As a matter of fact, there is a decrease in total brain amino acid content, reaching up to 70% of the total amount for the amino acid taurine. The contribution of amino acids on a molar basis is greater than that of potassium.

Correction of Hyponatremia

There is no standard process to correct hyponatremia (6). The clinician has to consider the following parameters in his or her therapeutic decision-making:

- the heterogeneity of neurological consequences of hyponatremia
- the presence or absence of symptoms
- the acuteness or chronicity of hyponatremia.

Arieff et al. (3) have identified several factors that are associated with the development of permanent brain damage in patients who have symptomatic hyponatremia (Table 2.4). Hyponatremia that develops quickly requires prompt correction; hyponatremia that develops slowly calls for a slower pace of correction. Rapid correction rates in the range of 2 mmol/L/hr have been found to be safe so long as the total increase in plasma sodium over the first 24 to 48 hrs does not exceed 25 mmol/L (5). This is equivalent to an average 0.5 to 1 mmol/L/hr for 24 to 48 hrs, which

TABLE 2.4.
Factors Predisposing to the Development of Permanent Brain Damage in Patients with Severe Symptomatic Hyponatremia[a]

1. Female sex
2. Episode of hypoxia-anoxia such as respiratory arrest with seizures
3. Alteration of serum sodium of more than 20 to 25 mmol/L within the initial 24 hrs of therapy
4. Associated medical conditions altering the blood-brain barrier, such as hepatic cirrhosis or metastatic cancer
5. Correction of serum sodium to normonatremic or hypernatremic levels
6. Delayed therapy for symptomatic hyponatremia
7. Potassium depletion

[a]Reproduced with permission from Arieff, AI. Hyponatremia, convulsions, respiratory arrest, and permanent brain damage after elective surgery in healthy women. N. Engl. J. Med., *314:*1529–1535, 1986.

has been found to be relatively safe in other studies (30). At no time should the correction rate exceed 2.5 mmol/L/hr. The rate at which serum sodium will increase is not only related to the rate and amount of hypertonic saline given but also to the rate of excretion of free water. In a patient who is excreting free water, the rise in serum sodium can exceed the values calculated from the rate and amount of saline infusion. Needless to say that repeated evaluations of the patient status as well as measurements of plasma and urine osmolalities and urine output are mandatory to avoid these pitfalls.

ACKNOWLEDGMENTS

This work was supported by grants RO1 HL39757 and PO1 HL41618 from the National Institutes of Health.

REFERENCES

1. Anderson, R.J., Chung, H.M., Kluge, R., et. al. Hyponatremia: prospective analysis of its epidemiology and the pathogenic role of vasopressin. Ann. Intern. Med., *102:*164–168, 1985.
2. Arieff, A.I. Consequences of rapid versus slow correction in vasopressin-mediated hyponatremia. In: *Vasopressin: Cellular and Integrative Functions,* edited by A.W. Cowley, J.F. Liard, and D.A. Ausiello, pp. 227–234. New York, Raven Press, 1988.
3. Arieff, A.I. Hyponatremia, convulsions, respiratory arrest, and permanent brain damage after elective surgery in healthy women. N. Engl. J. Med., *314:*1529–1535, 1986.
4. Arieff, A.I., Llach, F., and Massry, S.G. Neurological manifestations and morbidity of hyponatre-
mia: correlation with brain water and electrolytes. Medicine, *55:*121–129, 1976.
5. Ayus, J.C., Krothapalli, R.K., and Arieff, A.I. Treatment of symptomatic hyponatremia and its relation to brain damage. N. Engl. J. Med.,*317:*1190–1195, 1987.
6. Berl, T. Treating hyponatremia: damned if we do and damned if we don't. Kidney Intern, *37:*1006–1018, 1990.
7. Blessing, W.W., and Willoughby, J.O. Excitation of neuronal function in rabbit caudal ventrolateral medulla elevates plasma vasopressin. Neurosci. Lett., *58:*189–194, 1985.
8. Buijs, R.M., Hermes, M.L.H.J., Kalsbeek, A., et al. Vasopressin distribution, origin, and functions in the central nervous system. In: *Vasopressin, Third International Vasopressin Conference,* edited by S. Jard and R. Jamison, pp. 149–158. London, John Libbey and Company, 1991.
9. Carter, D.A., and Murphy, D. Cyclic nucleotide dynamics in the rat hypothalamus during osmotic stimulation: in vivo and in vitro studies. Brain Res., *487:*350–356, 1988.
10. Goldsmith, S.R. Vasopressin as vasopressor. Am. J. Med., *82:*1213–1219, 1987.
11. Helwig F.C., Schutz C.B., and Curry D.E. Water intoxication. Report of a fatal human case, with clinical, pathologic and experimental studies. JAMA, *104:*1569–1575, 1935.
12. Hochwald, G.M., Wald, A., and Malhan, C. The sink action of cerebrospinal fluid volume. Effect on brain water content. Arch. Neurol., *33:*339–344, 1976.
13. Ivell, R. Vasopressin and oxytocin gene expression in the mammalian ovary and testis. In: *Vasopressin, Third International Vasopressin Conference,* edited by S. Jard and R. Jamison, pp. 31–38. London, John Libbey and Company, 1991.
14. Ivell, R., and Richter, D. The gene for the hypothalamic peptide hormone oxytocin is highly expressed in the bovine corpus luteum: biosynthesis, structure and sequence analysis. EMBO J, *3:*2351–2354, 1984.
15. Jard, S., Gaillard, R.C., Guillon, G., et al. Vasopressin antagonists allow demonstration of a novel type of vasopressin receptor in the rat adenohypophysis. Mol. Pharmacol., *30:*171–177, 1986.
16. Jard, S., and Jamison, R. (eds) *Vasopressin, Third International Vasopressin Conference.* London, John Libbey and Company, 1991.
17. Knepel, W., Götz, D., and Fahrenholz, F. Interaction of rat adenohypophyseal vasopressin receptors with vasopressin analogues substituted at positions 7 and 1: dissimilarity from the V_1 vasopressin receptor. Neuroendocrinology, *44:*390–396, 1986.
18. Lehmann, E., Hänze, J., Pauschinger, M., et al. Vasopressin mRNA in the neurolobe of the rat pituitary. Neurosci. Lett., *111:*170–175, 1990.
19. Michell, R.H., Kirk, J.C., and Billah, M.M. Hormonal stimulation of phosphatidylinositol breakdown with particular reference to the hepatic effects of vasopressin. Biochem. Soc. Trans., *7:*861–865, 1979.
20. Mohr, E., and Richter, D. Regulation of vasopres-

sin gene expression. In: *Recent Advances in Basic and Clinical Neuroendocrinology,* edited by F.F. Casanueva and C. Dieguez, pp. 95–106. Amsterdam, Elsevier, 1989.

21. Nagy, G., Mulchahey, J.J., Smyth, D.G., *et al.* The glycopeptide moiety of the vasopressin-neurophysin precursor is neurohypophyseal prolactin releasing factor. Biochem. Biophys. Res. Comm., *151:*524–529, 1988.
22. Nattie, E.E. and Edwards, W.H. Brain and CSF water in newborn puppies during acute hypo- and hypernatremia. J. Appl. Physiol., *51:*1086–1091, 1981.
23. Onaka, T., and Yagi, K. Bimodal effects of noxious stimuli on vasopressin secretion in rats. Neurosci. Res., *6:*143–148, 1988.
24. Renaud, L.P., and Bourque, C.W. Neurophysiology and neuropharmacology of hypothalamic magnocellular neurons secreting vasopressin and oxytocin. Prog. in Neurobiol., *36:*131–169, 1991.
25. Richter, D., Mohr, E., and Schmale, H. Molecular aspects of the vasopressin gene family: evolution, expression, and regulation. In: *Vasopressin, Third International Vasopressin Conference,* edited by S. Jard and R. Jamison, pp. 3–11. London, John Libbey and Company, 1991.
26. Robertson, G.L., and Berl, T. Pathophysiology of water metabolism. In: *The Kidney,* edited by B.M. Brenner and F.C. Rector, pp. 385–432, Philadelphia, Saunders, 1986.
27. Schmale, H., Boroviak, B., Holtgreve-Grez, H., and Richter, D. Impact of altered protein structures on the intracellular traffic of mutated vasopressin precursor from Brattleboro rats. Eur. J. Biochem., *182:*621–627, 1989.
28. Schrier, R.W., Berl, T., and Anderson, R.J. Osmotic and non-osmotic control of vasopressin release. Am. J. Physiol., *236:*321–337, 1979.
29. Schwartz, J., Derdowska, Il, Sobocinska, M., *et al.* A potent new synthetic analog of vasopressin with relative agonist specificity for the pituitary. Endocrinology, *129:*1107–1109, 1991.
30. Sterns, R.H. Severe symptomatic hyponatremia: treatment and outcome. Ann. Intern. Med., *107:*656–664, 1987.
31. Thibonnier, M. La vasopressine l'hormone antidiurétique. La Presse Médicale, *16:*481–485, 1987.
32. Thibonnier, M. Signal transduction of V_1-vascular vasopressin receptors. Regulatory Peptides, *38:*1–11, 1992.
33. Thibonnier, M. Vasopressin agonists and antagonists. Hormone Research, *34:*124–128, 1990.
34. Thibonnier, M., Bayer, A.L., Simonson, M.S., and Kester, M. Multiple signaling pathways of V_1-vascular AVP receptors of A_7r_5 cells. Endocrinology, *129:*2845–2856, 1991.
35. Thrasher, T.N. Role of forebrain circumventricular organs in body fluid balance. Acta Physiol. Scand., *136*(Suppl 583):141–150, 1989.
36. Thrasher, T.N., Brown, C.J., Keil, L.C., and Ramsay, D.J. Thirst and vasopressin release in the dog: an osmoreceptor or sodium receptor mechanism? Am. J. Physiol., *238:*R333–R339, 1980.
37. Thrasher, T.N., and Ramsay, D.J. Anatomy of osmoreception. In: *Vasopressin, Third International Vasopressin Conference,* edited by S. Jard and R. Jamison, pp. 267–278, London, John Libbey and Company, 1991.
38. Verkman, A.S., Zhang, R., Wang, Y.X., *et al.* The vasopressin-sensitive water channel in toad bladder: functional localization in endosomes and mRNA expression in Xenopus oocytes. In: *Vasopressin, Third International Vasopressin Conference,* edited by S. Jard and R. Jamison, pp. 85–93. London, John Libbey and Company, 1991.
39. Verney, E.B. The antidiuretic hormone and the factors which determine its release. Proc. R. Soc. London Ser. B, *135:*25–106, 1947.
40. Wolfson, B., Manning, R.W., Davis, L.G., *et al.* Colocalization of corticotropin releasing factor and vasopressin mRNAs in neurons after adrenalectomy. Nature, *315:*59–61, 1985.
41. Zerbe, R.L., Stropes, L., and Robertson, G.L. Vasopressin function in the syndrome of inappropriate antidiuresis. Ann. Rev. Med., *31:*315–327, 1980.

CHAPTER 3

Neuropharmacology of Anterior Pituitary Control

ROBERT B. PAGE, M.D.

INTRODUCTION

Hormone-secreting neurons that arise in the hypothalamus and terminate in the neurohypophysis can be viewed as the lower motor neurons of the neuroendocrine system. The epithelial cells in the anterior pituitary gland are its motor units. Each functionally distinct clone manufactures and releases a unique hormone profile. Thyrotropes secrete thyroid-stimulating hormone (TSH), gonadotropes secrete follicle-stimulating hormone (FSH), luteinizing hormone (LH), or both, corticomelanotropes secrete either adrenocorticotrophic hormone (ACTH) and β-lipotropin or melanocyte-stimulating hormone (MSH) and β-endorphin, somatotropes secrete growth hormone (GH), and lactotropes secrete prolactin (Prl). Direct innervation of mammalian anterior pituitary epithelial cells has not been found. Peptide hormones released from axon terminals into the portal system are carried from the neurohypophysis to the adenohypophysial cells to regulate their function (147, 148).

Large (magnocellular) neurons in the supraoptic nuclei, paraventricular nuclei, and accessory nuclei project through the supraopticohypophysial tract to the caudal pole of the neurohypophysis, the neural lobe, where they terminate in the perivascular space of fenestrated capillaries. Some magnocellular neurons in each hypothalamic nucleus synthesize arginine vasopressin (AVP) and neurophysin II, whereas others secrete oxytocin and neurophysin I. Dynorphin and/or angiotensin II are often colocalized with AVP. Immunohistochemistry has demonstrated colocalization of met-enkephalin, proenkephalin, cholecystokinin (CCK), and corticotropin-releasing hormone (CRH) in oxytocin-synthesizing neurons. Whereas most of the neural lobe's venous drainage is to the systemic circulation, some blood drains, by capillary and short portal routes, to the adjacent pars distalis; the hormones it contains in the neural lobe may regulate the function of the epithelial cells in a small region of the pars distalis next to the neural lobe (68, 146, 148).

Small (parvicellular) neurons arise in the medial basal hypothalamus (MBH) and in the preopticoseptal region and project to the rostral pole of the neurohypophysis, the median eminence, where they terminate in the perivascular space of the fenestrated capillaries of its primary plexus. TSH secretion is stimulated by the release of TRH from parvicellular axon terminals. ACTH secretion is stimulated by CRH (with supplemental stimulation by AVP (176)) released from terminals of another population of small neurosecretory cells. GH secretion is regulated by a stimulating hormone (growth hormone-releasing hormone [GHRH]) and an inhibiting hormone (somatostatin), each of which is secreted from a separate neuronal population. Somatostatin inhibits the release of TSH from thyrotropes (127) as well as the release of GH from somatotropes. LH and FSH are both stimulated by the secretion of gonadotropin-releasing hormone (GnRH). Prl secretion is inhibited by dopamine release, and in some circumstances stimulated by TRH (148). The MBH and preoptic area constitute a hypophysiotropic area that regulates anterior pituitary function (217). The peptide hormones released by its "lower motor neurons" (210) into the primary capillary plexus are carried by capillary routes into the pars tuberalis above the diaphragm sella and by restricted portal routes to the pars distalis within the sella turcica (146).

This discussion of the neuropharmacology of anterior pituitary control will focus on the "suprasegmental" regulation of parvicellular neurosecretory systems. Three issues will be addressed: the disposition of relevant nuclear groups within the hypothalamus, the input into neurosecretory cell groups from sources both within and outside the hypothalamus, our present understanding of the neurotransmitter(s) and neuromodulator(s) released by each extrasegmental system at synapses with these hypophysiotropic neurons. The purpose of this chapter is to review the progress made in these areas within the last 10 years and to relate findings, where appropriate, to clinical situations that neurosurgeons face. Most of the work presented is derived from experimental studies performed in the rat; any difference from the human state will be cited when known.

PARCELLATION OF THE PREOPTIC AREA AND HYPOTHALAMUS

Longitudinal Preoptic and Hypothalamic Zones

When the hypothalamus is parcellated into a grid of longitudinally oriented zones, several functional relationships become evident. Szentagothai et al. (217) called attention to the unique morphological characteristics of the periventricular zone that extends from the preoptic area to the mamillary bodies and surrounds the third ventricle. Subsequent studies have confirmed their hypothesis that small neurosecretory cells that terminate in the median eminence and regulate anterior pituitary function originate within this periventricular zone (148). Discrete clusters of parvicellular neurons whose axons project to the median eminence are found in the anterior periventricular hypothalamic nucleus, the paraventricular nu-

cleus, and the arcuate nucleus. In addition, two regions that regulate biological rhythms (the suprachiasmatic nucleus, which regulates circadian rhythm, and the anteroventral periventricular preoptic nucleus, which regulates the pulse of GnRH secretion during the estrus cycle) and two circumventricular organs (the organum vasculosum of the lamina terminalis and the subfornical organ) lie in the periventricular zone (Table 3.1).

A medial zone contains well-defined nuclei that receive ascending input from the brain stem and descending input from the limbic system. Its nuclei project into the periventricular zone and back to the limbic telencephalon, to the brain stem, and to the spinal cord. It is thus situated to coordinate endocrine, autonomic, and behavioral responses to internal and external stimuli. The lateral zone is the extension of the reticular formation into the hypothalamus (210). It contains the medial forebrain bundle, which interconnects the mesencephalic reticular formation with the septum and other limbic regions. It has rich connections with the nuclei of the periventricular zone.

Coronal Preoptic and Hypothalamic Areas

The preoptic area extends through all three zones. It lies anterior to a line drawn from the posterior border of the optic chiasm to the posterior border of the anterior commissure and posterior to the level of the lamina terminalis. The periventricular preoptic nucleus contains two regions (the subfornical organ and the organum vasculosum of the lamina terminalis) that lack a blood-brain barrier and are believed to provide windows though which the brain can sense the contents and physical properties of blood (251). In the preoptic area, neurosecretory cells that project to the median eminence are not restricted to a cluster of cells within a single nucleus in the periventricular zone. The medial zone includes a complex group of nuclei including the medial preoptic nucleus, which contains a sexually dimorphic region (Table 3.1). The medial preoptic area projects into the periventricular zone.

The hypothalamic anterior and tuberal areas also extend through all three longitu-

TABLE 3.1.
Hypothalamic Cell Groups[a]

	Preoptic Area	Anterior Hypothalamic	Tuberal Region	Mammillary Region
Periventricular zone	**Periventricular preoptic nucleus**	**Anterior periventricular nucleus**	Posterior periventricular nucleus	Posterior periventricular nucleus
	Median preoptic nucleus	Suprachiasmatic nucleus	Arcuate nucleus	
	Anteroventral preoptic nucleus	Paraventricular nucleus		
	Organum vasculosum of the lamina terminalis			
Medial zone	Medial preoptic area	Anterior hypothalamic area	Tuberal area	Premammillary nucleus
	Medial preoptic nucleus		Ventromedial nucleus	Tuberomammillary nucleus
	Anterodorsal Preoptic nucleus		Dorsomedial nucleus	Mammillary complex
	Strial area			
	Parastrial area			
	Posterior dorsal Preoptic nucleus			
Lateral zone	Lateral preoptic nucleus	Lateral hypothalamic area	Lateral hypothalamic area	
	Magnocellular preoptic nucleus	Supraoptic nucleus		Lateral hypothalamic area

[a]Modified from Swanson, L. W. The hypothalamus. In: Handbook of Chemical Neuroanatomy, vol 5, pp. 1–124, edited by Bjorkland, A., Hokfelc, T., Swanson, L. W. Amsterdam-New York-London, Elsevier, 1987. Nuclei containing neurosecretory cells are indicated by bold type. The medial preoptic area includes those nuclei in bold italics.

dinal zones. They contain aggregations of neurosecretory cells that are for the most part confined within nuclear groups in the periventricular zone. These neuronal clusters are found in the anterior periventricular nucleus and paraventricular nucleus in the anterior hypothalamic area and in the arcuate nucleus in the tuberal area. The medial zone contains the dorsal medial nucleus and ventromedial nucleus, which in turn project heavily into the periventricular zone.

Fiber Pathways in the Hypothalamus

A periventricular pathway courses from the preoptic area to the mamillary region. It unites the nuclear groups in the periventricular zone. Rostrally it receives input from the posterior periventricular area and the medial zone and caudally from the dorsal longitudinal fasciculus. The median forebrain bundle passes through all levels of the preoptic-hypothalamic region in the lateral zone. Major descending inputs arise in the amygdala, the olfactory tubercle, and the medial zone. Major ascending inputs arise in the ventral tegmental and parabrachial regions of the brain stem. The fornix carries fibers from the subiculum to the region of the ventromedial and arcuate nuclei. The stria terminalis carries fibers from the amygdala to the region of the ventromedial nuclei (148, 210).

NEUROSECRETORY CELL GROUPS IN THE PERIVENTRICULAR ZONE

Nuclei in the Periventricular Zone

The arcuate nucleus lies on either side of the third ventricle in the tuberal area just above the median eminence (Fig. 3.1). The projections to the median eminence are aminergic, cholinergic, γ-aminobutyric acid (GABAergic), and peptidergic, and their path is the tuberoinfundibular tract.

Dopaminergic cells lie in the periventricular (dorsomedial) region of the arcuate nucleus, where they constitute the A_{12} ami-

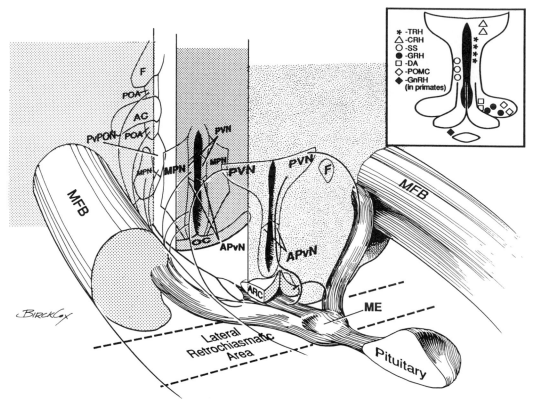

Figure 3.1. Schematic view of the preoptic area and the medio-basal hypothalamus in the rat. POA = preoptic area, PvPON = preoptic periventricular nucleus, MPN = medial preoptic nucleus, PVN = paraventricular nucleus, APvN = anterior periventricular nucleus, ARC = arcuate nucleus, F = fornix, AC = anterior commissure, OC = optic chiasm, MFB = medial forebrain bundle, ME = median eminence. Periventricular and lateral retrochiasmatic components of the "tuberoinfundibular tract" are illustrated. Inset: Coronal section of the medial basal hypothalamus. In rats, GnRH neurons lie scattered in the septal-preoptic region. In primates, most of the GnRH cells lie in the hypothalamus, with the majority lying along the ventral hypothalamic tract and between the arcuate nucleus and the median eminence. In rats and primates, the other hypophysiotropic neurosecretory neurons lie in discrete hypothalamic nuclear groups: star = TRH cells, triangle = CRH cells, open circle = somatostatin cells, black circle = GRH cells, open diamond = POMC cells, black diamond = GnRH cells in the primate. (Modified from Palkovits M. Neuropeptides in the median eminence: their sources and destinations. Peptides., *3*:299–303, 1982.)

nergic cell group of Ungerstedt (241) (Fig. 3.1 inset). They are identified by the presence of immunoreactive tyrosine hydroxylase (ir-TH) and the absence of immunoreactive-dopamine β-hydroxylase (ir-DBH) and immunoreactive phenylethanolamine-N-methyl-transferase (ir-PNMT). Other neurotransmitters identified within neuronal cell bodies in the arcuate nucleus are acetylcholine (ACh) and GABA. GABAergic neurons are identified by the presence of immunoreactive-GABA or glutamic acid dehydrogenase (ir-GAD) (226, 224). GABA cell bodies and terminals have been identified in the ar-

cuate nucleus, and GABA-containing terminals have also been identified in the neurohemal contact zone of the median eminence (226). Destruction of the arcuate nucleus by neonatal administration of monosodium glutamate markedly reduces GABA immunostaining in the median eminence, suggesting a significant input from that source (224). Some cells costore dopamine and GABA (39). Cholinergic neurons are best identified by the immunohistochemical demonstration of choline acetyltransferase (117). ACh is colocalized with dopamine in some cells in the arcuate nucleus (234).

Cholinergic neurons are present in the arcuate nucleus and also project to the median eminence via the tuberoinfundibular tract (218).

Peptidergic cells mostly lie in the ventrolateral region of the arcuate nucleus (Fig. 3.1 inset). Some of these cells synthesize GnRH (143) and others synthesize proopiomelanocortin or its posttranslational products which include ACTH and endorphins (154). Whereas neurons that are immunoreactive proopiomelanocortin or immunoreactive neuropeptide Y (ir-NPY)-positive are restricted to the arcuate nucleus, ir-GnRH-positive neurons are found in the adjacent ventromedial nuclei as well as in the arcuate nucleus (129). Neuropeptide Y (NPY) can be visualized in arcuate nucleus cell bodies by immunohistochemistry following colchicine treatment (28). Immunoreactive-substance P was found in cells in the arcuate nucleus following lesion placement in the median eminence or colchicine treatment (152). Neurotensin is colocalized with some ir-DBH neurons and with some ir-GnRH-positive cells (66). All these cell types, whether they contain dopamine, GABA, neurotensin, NPY, substance P, GnRH, or proopiomelanocortin project to the median eminence in the tuberoinfundibular tract (Fig. 3.1).

The roles of dopamine as a Prl inhibiting factor and that of GHRH as a GH-releasing factor have been well established (12, 129). The role of the other neuropeptides and neurotransmitters in the arcuate nucleus has not; but evidence is accumulating that they can act at three distinct sites by three distinct mechanisms. First, they can act as hormones and be carried by the portal system to the anterior pituitary gland, after being released from terminals in the median eminence, to regulate anterior pituitary cell function directly. Second, they can act in a paracrine fashion after being released from terminals in the median eminence and alter the release of neurohormones from neighboring terminals (65). Third, they can act in a transmitter fashion after release from synaptic terminals in the arcuate nucleus, paraventricular nucleus, periventricular nucleus, or preoptic area to modify the activity of tuberoinfundibular neurons. Examples of each of these mechanisms will be subsequently cited.

Consideration of the GABAergic tuberoinfundibular system serves as a model to demonstrate the potential sites of action of neurotransmitters or neurohormones in the tuberoinfundibular tract.

Ultrastructural studies have identified ir-GABA terminals that make synapses with dopaminergic somata and dendrites in the arcuate nucleus (102, 245). GABA neurons can depress the function of tuberoinfundibular dopaminergic neurons by synaptic activity in the arcuate nucleus, inhibit the release of neurohormones or neurotransmitters from neighboring terminals by paracrine action in the median eminence, and inhibit the release of hormones from the epithelial cells by endocrine action in the pituitary gland (119).

The hypothalamic anterior periventricular nucleus lies along the surface of the third ventricle, between the preoptic periventricular nucleus and the posterior periventricular nucleus (Figs. 3.1 & 3.2). Peptidergic and aminergic cells from the anterior periventricular nucleus project to the median eminence via periventricular paths. The periventricular projection from the anterior periventricular nucleus to the median eminence joins the projection from the arcuate nucleus and is included in the term "tuberoinfundibular tract".

Most of the somatostatin neurons that project to the median eminence are found in the preoptic ventricular nucleus and anterior periventricular nucleus (86). In addition, ir-enkephalin, ir-neurotensin, ir-CRH, ir-GABA and ir-TH cells lie in the anterior periventricular nucleus (210). The dopaminergic cells form the A_{14} cell group and do not project to the median eminence. Ultrastructural examination has demonstrated that ir-GABA axons synapse with ir-TH somata and dendrites in the periventricular nucleus (245). It is not certain that local GABAergic neurons are the source of the ir-GABA terminals found to synapse with ir-TH neurons in the paraventricular nucleus (226). At this time, little more is known about the connections of neurons within this nucleus.

The hypothalamic paraventricular nucleus contains both parvicellular and magnocellular neurosecretory cells that project to the neurohypophysis by periventricular and lateral retrochiasmatic routes (Fig. 3.1). The

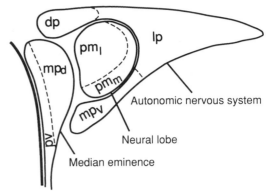

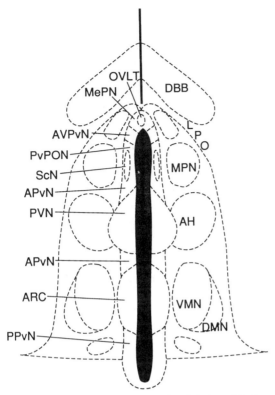

Figure 3.2. Schematic horizontal (axial) view of the hypothalamus. The distribution of the nuclei in the periventricular and medial zones of the preoptic area-medial basilar hypothalamus complex. OVLT = organum vasculosum of the lamina terminalis, DBB = diagonal band of Broca, MePN = median preoptic nucleus, AVPvN = anteroventral preoptic periventricular nucleus, PvPON = preoptic periventricular nucleus, ScN = suprachiasmatic nucleus, APvN = anterior periventricular nucleus, PVN = paraventricular nucleus, ARC = arcuate nucleus, MPN = medial preoptic nucleus, VMN = ventromedial nucleus, DMN = dorsomedial nucleus. (From Swanson L.W. The hypothalamus. In: Handbook of chemical neuroanatomy, vol 5:1–124. Eds. Bjorklunn, A., Hokfelt, T., Swanson, L.W. 1987

Figure 3.3. Coronal section of the paraventricular nucleus in the rat with identification of subdivisions. pm_l = posterior magnocellular (lateral) subdivision, pm_m = posterior magnocellular (medial) subdivision. dp = dorsal parvicellular, lp = lateral parvicellular, mp_d = medial parvicellular (dorsal), mp = medial parvicellular (ventral) subdivisions, and pv = periventricular (parvicellular) subdivision. (From Swanson L.W. and Sawchenko P.E. Hypothalamic integration: organization of the paraventricular and supraoptic nuclei. Ann. Rev. Neurosci., 6:269–324, 1983.)

neurons within the nucleus are parcellated into discrete groups according to (a) neuronal size, (b) protein hormone(s) synthesized, and (c) pattern of afferent input and efferent projections (214, 215). Magnocellular neurons project through the lateral retrochiasmatic area to join the supraopticohypophysial tract and pass onto the caudal end of the neurohypophysis (the neural lobe). The largest magnocellular group lies in the center of the posterior part of the paraventricular nucleus (Fig. 3.3).

Neurosecretory cells that project to the median eminence lie in the periventricular and medial parvicellular subdivisions of the paraventricular nucleus (142, 174, 214) and project to the medial third of the median eminence by periventricular and lateral retrochiasmatic routes (149). These projections, along with those from the anteroventral preoptic periventricular nucleus and the arcuate nucleus, complete the composition of the "tuberoinfundibular tract."

CRH-containing cell bodies lie in the medial parvicellular dorsal subdivision of the paraventricular nucleus. Their axons terminate in the median eminence (142, 174). Adrenalectomy stimulates synthesis and release of CRH (163), whereas corticosterone administration decreases mRNA levels in CRH cells (216). Ether stress elevates plasma ACTH levels in the rat, presumably by activating CRH cells. Lesions to the paraventricular nucleus abolish this response (16). CRH-containing neurons respond to hemorrhage with an increased release of CRH into portal blood (164). AVP has been colocalized with CRH in neurosecretory cells (166, 177, 254). The coexpression of AVP with CRH is increased after adrenalectomy (93, 185). Some CRH cells also costore angiotensin II. The coexpression of angiotensin II in CRH cells is also increased after adrenalectomy. This observation has functional significance because AVP potentiates the stimulatory effect of CRH on corticotropes several-fold (47) and because angiotensin II can directly release ACTH from corticotropes (203, 204). CRH cells have also been found to colocalize with enkephalin, dynorphin, neurotensin, GABA, and CCK (125, 165, 210).

TRH cells lie in the periventricular and adjacent regions of the medial subdivision of the paraventricular nucleus and may respond to circulating levels of thyroid hormone (262). Their secretion stimulates both thyrotropes and lactotropes. Neurosecretory cells that contain vasoactive intestinal peptide also lie in the medial and periventricular subdivisions of the paraventricular nucleus. Vasoactive intestinal peptide is a member of the glucagon/secretin superfamily of brain-gut peptides. It is costored with peptide histidyl isoleucine. Both these products are synthesized together on the same precursor (48). These cells also project to the median eminence, where they terminate amid capillaries in the external plexus (49). Vasoactive intestinal peptide is released into the portal system and acts upon the lactotrope as a Prl-releasing factor (127) mediating the proestrus Prl surge in the rat (137), the Prl response to suckling (50), and the Prl response to stress (51).

Cells in the periventricular zone of the paraventricular nucleus project to the median eminence via a periventricular route, whereas those in the medial parvicellular subdivision pass with magnocellular axons through the lateral retrochiasmatic zone (Fig. 3.1). Both pathways are considered to be components of the tuberoinfundibular tract.

The septal-preoptic area is the site of GnRH cells that project to the median eminence in mammals, with the exception of primates. However, GnRH-containing neurons are not restricted to the periventricular zone or to a single nuclear group (54, 196, 252). In the rat, GnRH cells that project to the median eminence are fairly concentrated in the periventricular preoptic nucleus; but they are also found in the medial preoptic area, the lateral preoptic area, and even in the medial septum and the diagonal band of Broca (2). Retrograde transport studies after application of wheat germ agglutinin to the median eminence demonstrate that only about 60% of ir-GnRH cells in the rat project to the median eminence (53). Neurons containing GnRH are not present in the arcuate nucleus of rodents or other animals that have an estrus cycle. The situation is different in primates, where GnRH-containing neurons have been found along the course of the preoptic-infundibular tract. A cluster of GnRH-containing neurons lies just beneath the arcuate nucleus and above the median eminence in the monkey (55).

In summary, with the exception of GnRH-secreting neurons, hypophysiotropic parvicellular neurosecretory cells lie in well defined sites within specific hypothalamic nuclei and project to the median eminence by the tuberoinfundibular tract. GnRH neurons are more scattered within nuclear groups in the septal-preoptic region, in the anterior hypothalamus, and (in the primate) in the tuberal hypothalamus. They project to the median eminence by the preoptic infundibular tract. Colocalization of amines with peptides and transmitters is common in hypophysiotropic neurons. The costored neurotransmitters and neurohormones act by synaptic, paracrine, and endocrine mechanisms to coordinate the secretory activity of the parent neuron with that of other neurons participating in the neuroendocrine response to changes in the internal milieu or external environment.

Circumventricular Organs within the Periventricular Zone

The circumventricular organs that are of interest in this discussion are the median eminence, the organum vasculosum of the lamina terminalis, and the subfornical organ. Unlike the median eminence, which is a motor organ, the organum vasculosum of the lamina terminalis and the subfornical organ are sensory organs (251). The organum vasculosum of the lamina terminalis lies above the optic chiasm in the lamina terminalis, within the periventricular zone of the preoptic area. It is composed of specialized ependymal cells, fenestrated capillaries, neurons, and axon terminals. The firing rate of neurons in the organum vasculosum of the lamina terminalis was altered when slices of the anterior preoptic area containing the organum vasculosum of the lamina terminalis were perfused with solutions containing differing concentrations of sodium chloride. The majority of cells increased their firing rates with increased NaCl concentrations and decreased them with decreased concentrations of NaCl (247). Although a direct projection from the organum vasculosum of the lamina terminalis to the magnocellular region within the paraventricular nucleus and to the supraoptic nucleus has been identified (197, 215, 237), neurophysiologic evidence suggests that a polysynaptic pathway with a relay in the medial preoptic nucleus is involved (59). In addition to responding to the plasma osmolarity, the organum vasculosum of the lamina terminalis responds to the blood-borne concentration of interleukin-1 β and mediates the ACTH response to elevated levels of this cytokine. The proposed mechanism is locally mediated in the adjacent periventricular preoptic area by prostaglandins and employs projections to the parvicellular neurosecretory regions of the paraventricular nucleus to stimulate CRH release and hence elevate plasma ACTH (60, 61, 62).

The subfornical organ is a circumventricular organ that lies in the median preoptic nucleus in the periventricular zone of the preoptic area. Whereas the organum vasculosum of the lamina terminalis lies in the lamina terminalis just above the optic chiasm, the subfornical organ lies just behind the lamina terminalis beneath the foramen of Monro. It projects by precommissural fibers to the organum vasculosum of the lamina terminalis and the median preoptic nucleus and by postcommissural fibers to the medial septum, the diagonal band of Broca, and the magnocellular nuclei of the hypothalamus (63, 64, 65, 66). Tanaka et al. (67) reviewed the evidence that the subfornical organ responds to the circulating levels of angiotensin II by regulating AVP secretion from magnocellular neurons. Angiotensin II receptors have been demonstrated in the subfornical organ and some of its fiber projections express angiotensin II (8, 68). Immunoreactive angiotensin II cells lie in and around the subfornical organ and project to

nuclear groups in the periventricular zone (69). Immunoreactive angiotensin II cells also project to the supraoptic nucleus (70). This observation raises the possibility that cells that respond to angiotensin II project to neurosecretory hypothalamic nuclei and employ angiotensin II at synapses to stimulate magnocellular neurosecretory cells (70). Although a synaptic relay in the medial septum appears to be present in the pathway through which the subfornical organ regulates magnocellular AVP neurons (67), a direct pathway from the subfornical organ to the paraventricular nucleus appears to be employed by the subfornical organ to regulate the response of CRH neurons in the parvicellular neurosecretory region of the paraventricular nucleus to changes in the circulating angiotensin II levels and, hence, to changes in blood pressure (42, 43).

Communication between Nuclei in the Periventricular Zone

While interconnections between nuclear groups in the periventricular zone are presumably abundant, the proximity of these nuclear groups makes the study of their interconnections by classical retrograde and anterograde tracing techniques difficult. Projections from the suprachiasmatic nucleus to the periventricular nucleus have been identified by tract tracing techniques and are believed to express vasoactive intestinal peptide. Within the periventricular nucleus, their terminal field is limited to the dorsal medial parvicellular subdivision, where CRH cells are abundant. This projection provides a means to entrain the circadian rhythm of ACTH and, hence, cortisol secretion to the light-dark cycle (189). Somatostatin-containing neurons in the periventricular area send projections to the arcuate nucleus to synapse with GRH neurons (110, 255). A direct inhibitory role of somatostatin on GHRH neurons and somatotropes in the pituitary gland seems likely (86). Proopiomelanocortin cells that originate in the arcuate nucleus project to the paraventricular nucleus, where they terminate in the vicinity of both large and small oxytocin containing cells (i.e., in the dorsal and medial parvicellular subdivisions and in the anterior magnocellular subdivision) (191). Tyrosine hydroxylase-containing cells from the arcuate nucleus and the paraventricular nucleus also project into the paraventricular nucleus where they synapse with somata and dendrites in all subdivisions (113). The function of these last two projections is unknown.

NUCLEI IN THE MEDIAL ZONE

The nuclear groups in the medial zone of the preoptic area project into the periventricular zone (197, 209, 237). This region is an important integrative site of input from the brain stem (from which it relays sensory information concerning taste and such visceral sensory information as blood pressure and volume status) and the limbic telencephalon (from which it relays sensory information concerning odor and input from neocortical and limbic regions) (210). The medial preoptic area has been implicated in the control of gonadotropin release. Lesions in the medial preoptic area abolish cyclic gonadotropin release in the rat. Steroid-sensitive neurons are present in the medial preoptic area (44, 157). At least some of these are GABA-ergic (252). Immunoreactive GAD-containing cells synapse with GnRH cells (101) and this relationship (along with the direct effect it has on gonadotropes) may be the basis of estrogen's negative feedback effect. The medial preoptic area also has been involved in the regulation of Prl secretion. Stimulation of the medial preoptic area inhibits the surge of Prl in rats on the afternoon of proestrus, presumably through activation of projections from the medial preoptic area to dopaminergic neurons in the arcuate nucleus (158). The medial preoptic area has been involved in the control of ACTH secretion. Stimulation of the medial preoptic area increases the firing rate of neurons in the periventricular nucleus and the circulating levels of corticosterone (179). The result should not be surprising, in view of the previously discussed pathway from the organum vasculosum of the lamina terminalis to the medial preoptic area to the periventricular nucleus that mediates ACTH secretion from the pituitary gland.

The medial preoptic area is divided into several nuclear groups (see Table 3.1), of which the most important for this discussion are the medial preoptic nucleus and the anteroventral periventricular preoptic nucleus.

The anteroventral periventricular preoptic nucleus lies just lateral to the optic chiasm in the rat and appears to be essential for the cyclic release of gonadotropin in the estrus cycle. The medial preoptic area is parcellated into a medial, a lateral, and a central subdivision. The central subdivision is sexually dimorphic, being much larger in the male rat. Each subdivision in the medial preoptic nucleus and each nuclear group in the medial preoptic area is characterized by a unique field of peptidergic and aminergic terminals and by a unique profile of aminergic and peptidergic neurons (199, 200, 201). The central and medial subnuclei of the medial preoptic nucleus project by the periventricular route and by the medial forebrain bundle to all the nuclei of the periventricular zone. They have dense projections to the parvicellular subdivisions of the periventricular nucleus and to the arcuate nucleus, but scant projections to the suprachiasmatic nucleus.

The medial zone of the tuberal hypothalamic area is occupied by the dorsal median nucleus and ventromedial nucleus. They are at present viewed as sites of integration of input from limbic and brain stem sites, with subsequent relay into the periventricular nucleus. The ventromedial nucleus receives a significant input from the lateral hypothalamic zone (the medial forebrain bundle, fornix, and stria terminalis). The major output from the ventromedial nucleus is to the amygdala (from which it also receives a major input). Reciprocal connections unite the ventromedial nucleus with the dorsal medial nucleus. A major output from the dorsal median nucleus is to the periventricular nucleus. Projections from the dorsal median nucleus to the periventricular nucleus are segregated. Those from the medial portion of the anterior dorsal median nucleus course into the magnocellular region of the periventricular nucleus to sites where oxytocin cells are found (189). Those from the dorsomedial region of the dorsal median nucleus project to the parvicellular region of the periventricular nucleus. Major ascending and descending pathways funnel into the median forebrain bundle and have access to the magnocellular and parvicellular subdivisions of the periventricular nucleus by this route: from the median forebrain bundle to the ventromedial nucleus to the dorsal median nucleus and on to the periventricular nucleus (229).

DIFFUSE INTRINSIC NEURONAL SYSTEMS IN THE HYPOTHALAMUS (Table 3.2)

Some neuronal populations in the periventricular zone do not appear to be confined to classical nuclear groups. Cholinergic neurons are scattered throughout the hypothalamus except for a prominent group in the arcuate nucleus (218). Some cholinergic cells lie dorsal to the supraoptic nucleus and are thought to synapse with dendrites of the AVP cells in the supraoptic nucleus. This arrangement of cholinergic neurons provides the foundation for central cholinergic stimulation of vasopressin secretion from the neural lobe (117, 123). Glutamate-containing neurons are found scattered throughout the hypothalamus. Immunoreactive glutamate axons and terminals form a dense

plexus in the hypothalamus. The presence of ir-glutamate in terminals with large granular vesicles suggests colocalization of glutamate and peptide hormones within the same cell (241). Putative glutaminergic terminals have been demonstrated to make synaptic contact with dendrites and somata in the supraoptic nucleus (124). Demonstration of glutaminergic synapses with other neurosecretory cell types can be expected. GABA-containing cells are similarly distributed in the hypothalamus (247) and their terminals make abundant local synapses (244). GABA terminals synapse on the somata and dendrites of magnocellular neurosecretory cells in the supraoptic nucleus (230, 231, 243), on GnRH cells in the preoptic area (252, 74), on dopaminergic cells in the A_{12} and A_{14} cell groups (in the arcuate nucleus and periventricular nucleus respectively) (102, 225, 231, 245), on somatostatin neurons in the anterior periventricular nucleus (256), and may synapse on CRH neurons in the periventricular nucleus (174).

ASCENDING NEURONAL SYSTEMS

Noradrenergic and Adrenergic Systems

These systems arise outside the hypothalamus in the brain stem (188, 215). They originate in the region of the lateral reticular nucleus (the A_1 and C_1 cell groups in the ventrolateral medulla, the dorsal motor nucleus and the nucleus and tractus solitarius (the A_2 and C_2 cell groups), and the A_6 cell group in the locus ceruleus (27). The C_1 and C_2 cell groups contain epinephrine and are identified by the localization of ir-PNMT within their cell bodies. The A_1 and A_{12} cell groups contain norepinephrine and are identified by the presence of ir-DBH but not ir-PNMT. The epinephrine cell groups lie in a more rostral location than the norepinephrine groups in the nucleus and tractus solitarius and ventrolateral medulla (161). Medullary projections ascend as the ventral noradrenergic bundle of the central tegmental tract (64, 78, 213). Pontine projections ascend in the dorsal noradrenergic bundle. Epinephrine and norepinephrine projections reach all the neurosecretory cell groups in the periventricular zone and extend into the medial zone (151, 201). They also extend into

TABLE 3.2.
Afferents to the MPOA-MBH

	SON	PVN(m)	PVN(p)	PvN	ARC	MPOA
OVLT	+	+				+
SFO	+	+				+
SON	+					
PVNm						
PVNp						
PvN					+	
ARC	+	+	+	+		+
MPOA	+	+	+	+	+	
DMN		+	+			
HIPP	+	+	+			
SEPT	+	+	+			+
AMY			+			+
BNST			+			+
RAPHE	+	+	+		+	+
LC					+	
VLM	+	+				+
DVC			+			+

OVLT = organum vasculosum of the lamina terminalis, SFO = subfornical organ, SON = supraoptic nucleus, PVNm = magnocellular paraventricular nucleus, PVNp = parvicellular paraventricular nucleus, PvN = periventricular nucleus, ARC = arcuate nucleus, MPOA = medial preoptic area including the medial preoptic nucleus, DMN = dorsal medial nucleus, HIPP = hippocampus, AMY = amygdala, BNST = bed nucleus of the stria terminalis, RAPHE = raphe nuclei, LC = locus ceruleus, VLM = ventrolateral medulla, DVC = dorsal vagal complex

the median eminence where they terminate in the internal zone (78).

Innervation of the paraventricular nucleus by these cell groups has been well established. Noradrenergic innervation extends to all the parvicellular subdivisions and to those regions of the magnocellular subdivisions where AVP cells reside. The A$_1$ projection terminates in the magnocellular subdivisions of the paraventricular nucleus and also in the AVP-containing regions of the supraoptic nucleus through collaterals (20, 253). The A$_2$ projection terminates in the medial parvicellular subdivision of the paraventricular nucleus, whereas the A$_6$ projection terminates in the periventricular zone. These regions are the respective sites of CRH and TRH neurosecretory cells (27). Adrenergic projections terminate in the parvicellular but not the magnocellular subdivisions. The dorsal subdivision of the periventricular nucleus that projects to the spinal cord is the most heavily innervated by adrenergic terminals from medullary C$_1$ and C$_2$ cell groups. The terminal field of the C$_1$ and C$_2$ cell groups is the same (26), as opposed to the differing terminal fields of the A$_1$ and A$_2$ projections. Electron microscopic studies have demonstrated synapses between nonadrenergic terminals and dendrites of magnocellular AVP neurons (113, 198) and between ir-DBH and ir-PNMT terminals and parvicellular somata and dendrites in the periventricular nucleus (100). NPY is colocalized with norepinephrine or epinephrine in cell bodies that lie in the caudal medulla but not in those catecholaminergic cells that lie in the locus ceruleus (190).

Norepinephrine injected into the supraoptic nucleus or periventricular nucleus stimulated the release of AVP from the neural lobe (100). Stimulation of the ventrolateral medulla excited phasic firing of AVP cells in the supraoptic nucleus (29), as did stimulation of the nucleus and tractus solitarius. However, the latency in the latter case was considerably greater than in the former, leading to the postulate that information concerning blood pressure and volume status, relayed to the nucleus and tractus solitarius over the IXth and Xth cranial nerves, is relayed to the ventrolateral medulla and then, via noradrenergic neurons, to the magnocellular neurons in the supraoptic nucleus and paraventricular nucleus to stimulate the release of AVP from the neural lobe (31, 32). Although attractive, the hypothesis is not secure because α blockade does not block the excitation of magnocellular AVP cells following A$_1$ stimulation (30).

When injected into the paraventricular nucleus, norepinephrine stimulated corticosterone release (99). Although there has been, in the past, debate over the effect of norepinephrine and epinephrine on the hypothalamic-pituitary-adrenal axis, there now seems to be acceptance of the proposition that these catecholamines are stimulatory when they interact with hypothalamic neurons or corticotropes (161, 184). Numerous studies demonstrate a role for this ascending catecholaminergic pathway in the regulation of the hypothalamic-pituitary-adrenal axis. Caudal deafferentation of the hypothalamus reduced the expression of CRH mRNA (60). Stimulation of the ventral noradrenergic bundle increased the CRH content of portal blood, a response that was blocked by the administration of an α blocker (159). Stimulation of the A$_2$ cell group increased firing rate in about 70% of periventricular nucleus neurons that had projections to the median eminence. However, only about 50% of these cells displayed short latencies and the excitatory effect was not abolished by the administration of an α antagonist (182). Studies of the role of the ascending catecholaminergic systems in the stimulation of AVP and CRH evoke cotransmission with NPY as an explanation for their finding that α adrenergic blockade does not block the response of medullary stimulation (30, 181). Further studies will be necessary to see if NPY is also an active agent at the synapses between these "aminergic" terminals and the somata and dendrites of large and small neurosecretory cells in the periventricular nucleus.

From the above discussion, it can be concluded that the noradrenergic and adrenergic input into the periventricular nucleus that ascends from the brain stem is stimulatory to resident magnocellular AVP- and parvicellular CRH-containing neurosecretory cells. This same ascending input appears to also be stimulatory to the GnRH cells in the medial zone (252).

Serotonergic Systems

Serotonin-containing neurons arise in the midbrain raphe and enter the hypothalamus by the periventricular route and through the median forebrain bundle. They provide a major input into preoptic area (200) and the arcuate nucleus (51) and a lesser one to the paraventricular nucleus (215). Serotonin terminals form a dense plexus in the lateral subdivision of the medial preoptic nucleus of the rat (200). This subdivision is larger in the female than in the male (202). Although serotonergic (5-HT) neurons synapse with GnRH neurons in the preoptic area of the rat (91), their role in the regulation of GnRH neurons is not yet known because both inhibitory and excitatory responses have been reported (196). In the arcuate nucleus, 5-HT terminals synapse with dopaminergic neurons (92). They may play a role in regulation of Prl secretion as the blockade of serotonin synthesis blocks the suckling reflex (252). Serotonin terminals also appose ir-NPY cell bodies and dendrites without synaptic specializations and lie close to ir-proopiomelanocortin cell bodies and dendrites in the arcuate nucleus (52). Serotonin terminals are sparce in the paraventricular nucleus but are present in the parvicellular regions and in the oxytocin regions of the magnocellular subdivisions (215).

Peptidergic Systems

A recent report also demonstrates a peptidergic pathway from the caudal nucleus and tractus solitarius (A_2 region) to the paraventricular nucleus that contains inhibin, somatostatin, and enkephalin (186). The role of this peptidergic projection is not yet known.

DESCENDING NEURONAL SYSTEMS

Limbic Input

Telencephalic input to the hypothalamus is relayed through the temporal lobe. Neocortical input converges in the entorhinal area upon hippocampal structures. Outflow from the hippocampus originates in Ammon's horn and in the subiculum and passes through the fornix. Precommissural fibers (carrying projections from Ammon's horn)

terminate in the septum, from which there is a projection into the medial preoptic nucleus (202) and a massive input into the hypothalamus via the medial forebrain bundle (212). Most postcommissural fibers (carrying projections from the subiculum) pass on to the mammillary body, but some diverge to terminate in the region of the ventromedial nucleus and arcuate nucleus as the corticohypothalamic tract (211). From the amygdala efferent fibers join the stria terminalis and terminate in the bed nucleus of the stria terminalis (261) and in the cell-poor zone around the ventromedial nucleus (58).

Electrophysiologic studies demonstrate projections to the paraventricular nucleus and supraoptic nuclei from the septum and the amygdala (140, 158). Retrograde tracing studies confirm these observations (189, 197). The major limbic input to the supraoptic nuclei and paraventricular nucleus arises in the bed nucleus of the stria terminalis (from the amygdala). The bed nucleus of the stria terminalis sends a projection into the magnocellular regions in the paraventricular nucleus and the supraoptic nuclei and also sends a far denser projection into the parvicellular subdivisions of the paraventricular nucleus. Input from the amygdala can also reach magnocellular neurosecretory cells in the supraoptic nucleus and paraventricular nucleus parvicellular neurosecretory cells in the paraventricular nucleus by projections through the stria terminalis to the ventromedial nucleus and, thence, to the dorsal medial nucleus to the paraventricular nucleus. Tracing studies show terminations of these projections from the dorsal medial nucleus in the cell-poor regions around the supraoptic nucleus and paraventricular nucleus but not within these nuclear groups (189). Synapses between terminals of cells arising in the lateral septum and amygdala, with AVP-containing dendrites lying just outside the boundaries of the paraventricular nucleus have been demonstrated (198).

Stimulation of the dorsal hippocampus or the lateral septum inhibited spontaneous firing of about 40% of the recorded neurons in the paraventricular nucleus that projected to the median eminence. Only about 10% were stimulated (180). Hippocampectomy resulted in an increase in CRH mRNA and an increase in plasma corticosterone (59). Fornix transection resulted in AVP hypersecretion and resistance of CRH to the suppressive effects of high levels of glucocorticoids during stress (183). Thus, because the stria terminalis was divided during fornix transection, the hippocampus and/or amygdala is believed to exert an inhibitory influence upon the CRH cells in the parvicellular subdivisions of the paraventricular nucleus. The neurotransmitters and neuropeptides employed are not known.

THE ROLE OF BIOGENIC AMINES IN THE REGULATION OF NEUROSECRETORY CELLS (Table 3.3)

Norepinephrine

Norepinephrine is believed to stimulate CRH release in vivo (161). Injection of norepinephrine into the third ventricle increased CRH release into portal blood (159). Incubated hypothalamic fragments that were perfused with media containing norepinephrine released CRH in a dose-dependent manner. Whether this stimulatory effect is mediated by α or β receptors (or both) has not as yet been clarified (77, 239). Norepinephrine terminals do synapse on CRH soma and dendrites in the paraventricular nucleus (68, 52). Ascending norepinephrine-containing neurons are presumed to regulate CRH release from neurosecretory terminals in the median eminence via these contacts upon CRH so-

mata and dendrites in the paraventricular nucleus and not by a paracrine action in the median eminence. However, it should be borne in mind that norepinephrine also stimulates corticotropes directly via β receptors (161) and that noradrenergic systems arising in the brain stem project to the median eminence as well as to the hypothalamus and the preoptic area (refer to the section on adrenergic and nonadrenergic systems). Norepinephrine released into the portal circulation from terminals in the median eminence can reach adrenergic receptors on corticotropes that contain β adrenergic receptors (184). Norepinephrine stimulates ACTH release by stimulating CRH-secreting cells in the hypothalamus and corticotropes in the pituitary gland.

Norepinephrine probably stimulates TSH and growth hormone release. Projections from the locus ceruleus (A_6 cell group) terminate in the regions of the anterior paraventricular nucleus and periventricular subdivision of the paraventricular nucleus where TRH neurosecretory cells are found (27). Immunoreactive DBH and ir-PNMT terminals have been found to be closely associated with ir-TRH cells in the paraventricular nucleus (105, 112); and ir-PNMT terminals have been found to synapse with ir-somatostatin neurons in the anterior paraventricular nucleus (109). Abolition of the cold-induced TSH response in the rat by the blockade of norepinephrine synthesis or the blockade of α receptors has been reported

TABLE 3.3.
Afferents to Neurosecretory Neurons

	ACTH	TSH	GH		FSH/LH	Prl
	CRH	TRH	GHRH	Somatostatin	GnRH	Dopamine
Norepinephrine	+ (161)[a]	+ (97)	+ (129)		+ (253)	
Dopamine		+ (103)		+ (104)		
5-HT	+ (95)	+ (22)	+ (24)	− (155)	+ (253)	− (253)
Acetylcholine	+ (95)			− (135)	+ (175)	
Glutamate						
GABA	− (7)	− (79)		− (258)	− (253)	− (253)
Angiotensin II	+ (136)				+ (205)	
Neurotensin				+ (195)		+ (236)
Vasoactive intestinal peptide				+ (171)		
Substance P	− (41)					
NPY	+ (95)			+ (173)	+ (84)	
Opioids	− (262)	− (80)			− ((85))	− ((169))

[a]Numbers in parentheses indicate supporting references.

(140), as has the enhancement of the TSH response to cold by clonidine—an α agonist (72). α Adrenergic (clonidine) stimulation of GH release from the rat's pituitary was blocked by pretreatment with an antibody to GHRH (128).

Norepinephrine is believed to stimulate GnRH release (252). Sawyer et al. (193) demonstrated in 1947 that an adrenergic blocking agent administered following coitus blocked ovulation in the rabbit. Norepinephrine turnover in the medial preoptic nucleus, suprachiasmatic nucleus, arcuate nucleus, and median eminence of the rat increased just before and during the LH surge on the afternoon of proestrus (11). A decrease in the concentration of nuclear estrogen receptors in the preoptic area and hypothalamus of the ovariectomized estrogen-primed guinea pig occurred after α adrenergic blockade. Norepinephrine turnover increased in the preoptic area concurrent with the LH surge induced by estrogen treatment of ovariectomized rats (11). The concentration of nuclear androgen receptors in the preoptic area of the male rat decreased with dopamine-β-hydroxylase inhibition (55). The increased turnover of norepinephrine in the preoptic area, which associated with the LH surge and ovulation, has been taken as strong evidence that norepinephrine regulates GnRH release (11). Intraventricular administration of norepinephrine (and epinephrine)-stimulated LH release in estrogen-progesterone treated ovariectomized rats. However, ir-DBH terminals have not been found to synapse with GnRH cells in the septal-preoptic area complex in the rat (252); and the terminal fields of serotonin projections, not norepinephrine projections, overlap the sites of GnRH cells (73).

The argument that epinephrine is involved in the regulation of GnRH cells in the septal-preoptic region of the rat is reviewed by Kalra (83). He noted that administration of a PNMT antagonist (an inhibitor of the conversion of norepinephrine to epinephrine) on the morning of proestrus blocked ovulation and the LH surge. Work in his laboratory has demonstrated that intraventricular epinephrine (but not norepinephrine) stimulated LH release on the afternoon of proestrus. He proposes that norepinephrine may act on the GnRH cell at preoptic or hypothalamic sites, whereas epinephrine may act at the site of GnRH nerve terminals in the median eminence (82).

Dopamine

The role of dopamine as a neurohormone (Prl-inhibiting factor) is clear (12). Its role as a neurotransmitter or neuromodulator in the preoptic area and hypothalamus, however, is murky. Immunoreactive TH cells in the arcuate nucleus (the A_{12} cell group) and in the preoptic ventricular nucleus (the a_{14} cell group) project into the regions where TRH- and somatostatin-containing cells abide (113) and into the preoptic area (74). Ultrastructural studies demonstrate synapses on somata and dendrites in the parvicellular divisions of the paraventricular nucleus and in the anterior periventricular nucleus (see section on circumventricular organs within the periventricular zone). Dopamine stimulated the release of somatostatin from hypothalamic fragments in a dose-dependent fashion (104) and thus is believed to suppress GH secretion from the pituitary gland. Regulation of other neuroendocrine motor neurons is more problematic. Stimulation of TRH release from hypothalamic fragments (103) but inhibition of TRH release from frog skin preparations (15) have been reported. In the paraventricular nucleus, ir-TH terminals synapse on CRH neurons (111), but the microinjection of dopamine into the paraventricular nucleus of awake rats produced no change in plasma cortisol levels (99). Although ir-TH terminals are closely related to GnRH neurons in the preoptic area, their role in the regulation of GnRH secretion is unclear (196, 252). Dopamine has been reported to both inhibit and stimulate the release of GnRH from incubated hypothalami (168, 227), leading to the suggestion that either two different neuronal populations are involved (each stimulated under the unique conditions of a particular experiment) or that the status of dopamine receptors in the preoptic area-MBH varies with the gonadal steroid milieu of the animal (168).

Serotonin

Serotonin stimulates the release of ACTH from the pituitary by directly stimulating corticotropes and by stimulating the release of CRH from terminals in the median eminence (7, 95). Early evidence for a stimulatory role of 5-HT in the release of ACTH is reviewed by Kreiger (96). Intraperitoneal or subcutaneous administration of serotonin agonists elevated plasma corticosterone levels in a dose-dependent manner (95). Incubation of hypothalamic fragments in the presence of 5-HT or its agonists stimulated the release of CRH. This response was blocked by specific serotonergic antagonists (18, 61, 138). The mechanism of this stimulatory effect is not understood, but it is not likely to be due to transmission across excitatory synapses between 5-HT terminals in the paraventricular nucleus and CRH neurosecretory cells. This proposal will be strengthened by the demonstration of synapses between serotonergic and CRH cells on ultrastructural study (7).

Serotonin stimulates the release of GH. Serotonin terminals synapse on somatostatin neurons (90). Serotonin blocked the secretion of somatostatin induced in fetal hypothalamic cultures following the addition of the cholinergic agonist carbachol (155). A second mechanism by which 5-HT can stimulate GH release is through interaction with the noradrenergic system by stimulation of GHRH neurons. An intact serotonin central system is necessary for noradrenergic stimulation of GHRH release (24). It is not known if both norepinephrine and 5-HT neurons synapse with GHRH neurons, or if the catecholaminergic and indolaminergic neurons are related to the GHRH neuron in series.

The role of serotonin in the regulation of TRH neurons has been a matter of debate, with both stimulatory and inhibitory roles being championed (34, 97, 115). Serotonin stimulated the release of TRH from hypothalamic fragments (22).

Although the density of serotonergic terminals in the medial preoptic nucleus is high (200), and serotonergic terminals are closely related to GnRH cells in the preoptic area (73), the role of serotonin in the regulation of GnRH cells is not clear. The argument for a stimulatory role is reviewed by Weiner et al. (252). The problem of deciding what is the function of a particular substance in the regulation of neurosecretory systems is nicely illustrated by the observation that stimulation of the dorsal and medial raphe nuclei (two sites that project serotonin fibers into the septopreoptic area) had opposite effects upon the LH surge and the timing of ovulation in the female rat. Stimulation of the dorsal raphe nucleus facilitated the LH surge in proestrus. This effect can be explained by a direct excitation of GnRH cells by 5-HT terminals at axodendritic or axosomatic synapses in the preoptic area. Stimulation of the medial raphe nucleus blocked the LH surge in proestrus. This inhibitory effect was abolished by prior intraventricular injection of the GABA antagonist bicuculline. The authors concluded that the inhibitory effect of medial raphe nucleus stimulation was mediated by GABA interneurons in the preoptic area (133).

Serotonin is involved in spontaneous phasic Prl elevations (95) and in the stimulation of Prl release in response to suckling (252). Microinjection of 5-HT in the medial basal hypothalamus increased plasma Prl levels in the rat (258). Lesion of the dorsal raphe nucleus reduced hypothalamic 5-HT concentrations and the plasma level of Prl achieved after suckling (10). Several mechanisms have been proposed. Immunoreactive 5HT terminals synapse with dopaminergic neurons in the rat's arcuate nucleus (92). Serotonin terminals in the arcuate nucleus also synapse with GABA-containing neurons (74, 245). It has been proposed that the serotonin stimulates GABA neurons which, in turn, inhibit tuberoinfundibular dopaminergic neurons and, hence, increase Prl release from lactotropes (2). Serotonin also stimulates vasoactive intestinal peptide release from the hypothalamus in vitro (194). Vasoactive intestinal peptide, in turn, stimulates the release of Prl from lactotropes (95).

ACh

CRH release is stimulated by ACh in vitro and in vivo (95). Release from hypothalamic fragments was dose-dependent and blocked by atropine (207, 219, 238, 62). Release of CRH from dissociated diencephalic cell cultures was also stimulated by ACh. The stimulation was also blocked by atropine (63). ACh injection into the third ventricle elevated the portal concentration of CRH in the rat (162). Thus, there is solid evidence that CRH, like AVP (62, 172), is stimulated by ACh. Although synapses between dendrites and ir-ACh-containing terminals have been demonstrated in the supraoptic nucleus (117, 123), to date, synapses between ir-ACh terminals and small neurosecretory cells in the periventricular nucleus expressing CRH have not been shown to exist.

GnRH released from fragments of the medial basal hypothalamus was stimulated by the addition of ACh to the medium (175). Atropine, given on the morning of proestrus, blocks ovulation in the rat (192). ACh levels in the preoptic area of the rat fluctuate as a function of the estrus cycle. They rise abruptly during the afternoon of proestrus (37). Estrogen-concentrating cells are found in the preoptic area (252). It is currently postulated that rising levels of estrogen on the afternoon of proestrus induce an increase in choline acetyltransferase and, hence, stimulate GnRH release (37). (Refer to discussion of norepinephrine in stimulation of GnRH cells in section on norepinephrine.)

GH secretion increases following the administration of ACh or its agonist through a muscarinic receptor mechanism. Muscarinic antagonists block the response of somatotropes to GHRH. The argument that ACh suppresses somatostatin release is reviewed by Muller (135).

Excitatory Amino Acids

Although glutamate systems will probably turn out to be very important in the regulation of neurosecretory neurons (242), little is known today about how they regulate anterior pituitary function. The argument that terminals utilizing glutamate synapse on magnocellular neurons in the supraoptic nucleus is made convincingly by Meeker et al. (124). Glutamate stimulated the activity of AVP neurons in hypothalamic slices (50). The evidence for a stimulatory role of glutamate on AVP-secreting neurons is reviewed by Renaud and Bourquet (172). Recent studies demonstrated release of somatostatin from cultured fetal diencephalic neurons (221) and increased LH release after intravenous administration of glutamate to monkeys (122).

GABA

The intraventricular administration of GABA reduced the concentration of CRH in the portal blood of rats (162). GABA blocked the stimulation of CRH release from hypothalamic fragments that accompanies the addition of ACh to the medium (61). It does not inhibit release of ACTH from pituitary cells in vitro (7). GABA probably inhibits CRH neurosecretory neurons by the presynaptic inhibition of excitatory extrasegmental neurons.

TSH was lowered by the intraventricular injection of GABA, and the incubation of pituitary fragments with GABA did not alter TSH release into the medium (79). It is tentatively concluded that GABA inhibits TRH release and hence TSH secretion.

GABA inhibits the pulsatile and steroid-induced release of LH in ovariectomized rats (252, 133). The intraventricular administration of GABA also decreased norepinephrine turnover in the preoptic area of the rat (1, 45, 98), a necessary event that accompanies the LH surge (11). The intraventricular administration of GABA antagonists potentiated the plasma LH rise in response to the intraventricular injection of norepinephrine (56). These results are commensurate with the hypothesis that GABA neurons that synapse on GnRH neurons in the preoptic area (101) can inhibit the response of those neurons to norepinephrine (or epinephrine) and/or inhibit the release of norepinephrine or epinephrine from terminals by presynaptic inhibition (56). Some authors have reported a stimulation of GnRH release upon perfusion of hypothalamic fragments with GABA or its agonists (118, 141). It seems probable that this effect is mediated at the level of the arcuate nucleus or the median eminence and is due to the inhibition of endogenous opioid systems that are believed to modulate GnRH release (56). Gonadal steroid receptors are present on GABA cells in the preoptic area (253). It is likely that GABA neurons exert a tonic inhibitory control over GnRH neurons in the septal-preoptic area complex, either directly or by presynaptic inhibition of noradrenergic terminals, that is responsive to gonadal steroid levels (see also discussion in section on opioid peptides).

Prl and GH are stimulated by GABA through similar mechanisms. GABA inhibits the inhibitory tuberoinfundibular, dopaminergic, and somatostatin systems (257, 145, 98). Synapses between GABAergic terminals and dopaminergic (102) and somatostatinergic (81, 256) neurons have been reported. Serotonergic enhancement of GABAergic activity may be a means by which ascending serotonin pathways stimulate Prl release (2). In addition to the effects of GABA on the neurosecretory neurons that project to the median eminence, one must consider the direct inhibitory effect of GABA on lactotropes. The tuberoinfundibular GABA system releases GABA into portal blood, which is carried to the pars distalis. Lactotropes have receptors for GABA and are inhibited by it (135). GABA stimulates Prl release through hypothalamic synapses that have dopaminergic neurons, and directly inhibits Prl release from lactotropes (167).

THE ROLE OF PEPTIDE HORMONES IN THE REGULATION OF NEUROSECRETORY CELLS

Angiotensin II

Angiotensin II is believed to stimulate the release of CRH from neurosecretory cells whose nuclei lie in the medial parvicellular subdivision of the paraventricular nucleus (136). It stimulated the release of immunoreactive CRH from incubated rat hypothalami (208). Its iontophoretic application of angiotensin II in the anterior hypothalamus excited (increased the frequency of firing of) 23/47 neurons that responded to glutamate (233). Intraventricular administration of angiotensin II stimulated the release of ACTH in a dose-dependent fashion and the response was blocked by saralasin (an angiotensin II antagonist) pretreatment (136).

ACTH release is stimulated by increased angiotensin II plasma levels. Although it can directly stimulate the release of ACTH from corticotropes in vitro (203, 204), in vivo studies suggest that the direct stimulation of corticotropes by angiotensin II is not an important mechanism by which it regulates ACTH release (136). Presently, it is believed

that receptors in the subfornical organ respond to increasing plasma levels of angiotensin II by stimulating the activity of angiotensin II neurons in the vicinity of the subfornical organ. First, it acts from the systemic circulation by stimulating receptors in the subfornical organ (210) to activate angiotensin II-containing neurons (42) that, in turn, act upon CRH neurosecretory neurons in the paraventricular nucleus, where angiotensin II receptors have been identified (210, 57). Angiotensin II neurons, activated by systemic angiotensin II, stimulate neurosecretory cells to release CRH which, in turn, causes the release of ACTH from corticotropes. The anatomy of the intrinsic angiotensin II system (reviewed in the section on circumventricular organs within the periventricular zone) is compatible with this construct. Other supporting evidence includes the observation that angiotensin II receptors are present in the subfornical organ and paraventricular nucleus (57, 210), that stimulation of the subfornical organ activated neurons in the paraventricular nucleus that project to the median eminence (42), and that systemic administration of angiotensin II activated cells in the subfornical organ that project to the paraventricular nucleus (42).

Preliminary evidence suggests that angiotensin II stimulates the release of LH from the pituitary by stimulating the release of GnRH (205). Intraventricular administration of angiotensin II increased the plasma LH level in rats, and intraventricular administration of saralasin on the afternoon of proestrus blocked the LH surge. Because the intravenous administration of angiotensin II did not cause an elevation of plasma LH and, because intravenous saralasin did not disrupt the LH response to GnRH, the authors concluded that the effect of angiotensin II was central. The effect of angiotensin II depends upon the steroidal milieu of the brain. Intraventricular infusion of angiotensin II into ovariectomized female rats decreased plasma levels of LH. Following estrogen administration, the same intraventricular infusion increased circulating LH levels. This scenario resembles the response of ovariectomized female rats to the intraventricular administration of norepinephrine. The observation that α adrenergic blockade blocked the effect of intraventricular angiotensin II provides further evidence that angiotensin II stimulates the release of GnRH through the stimulation of norepinephrine release (46).

Neurotensin

Immunoreactive neurotensin cell bodies have been found in the paraventricular and arcuate nuclei in the cat and in the periventricular, paraventricular, and arcuate nuclei in the rat (75). Many of these cells colocalize neurotensin with peptide neurohormones or amine neurotransmitters and project to the median eminence (66). Neurotensin stimulated the release of somatostatin (195) and dopamine (235) from perifused hypothalamic fragments. These fragments included the median eminence. Intraventricular neurotensin inhibited the release of Prl and the effect was abolished by dopamine blockade (95). These observations suggest that neurotensin plays a role in the regulation of GH and Prl release at the level of the terminals of the tuberoinfundibular tract in the median eminence. The result is especially interesting because neurotensin is costored with dopamine in tuberoinfundibular neurons.

Vasoactive Intestinal Peptide

Vasoactive intestinal peptide, a member of the glucagon superfamily that also includes GnRH and peptide histidyl isoleucine, has been found in neurons that lie in the parvicellular regions of the paraventricular nucleus and project to the median eminence (see section on nuclei in the periventricular zone). Vasoactive intestinal peptide stimulated the release of somatostatin from the perifused rat hypothalamus (195) and from rat diencephalic cells dispersed in cell culture (153, 222). It also stimulated somatostatin mRNA synthesis in cultured fetal diencephalic cells (171). Vasoactive intestinal peptide has been reported to stimulate GnRH release from hypothalamic fragments in vitro (144) but to inhibit LH secretion in vivo after intraventricular injection (4, 206). It is premature to reach any conclusions on the mechanism of action of vasoactive intestinal peptide on GnRH release.

Vasoactive intestinal peptide is also found in cells of the suprachiasmatic nucleus, a nuclear group in the anterior periventricular hypothalamus that is concerned with the entrainment of circadian rhythms (3, 170, 182). A strong vasoactive intestinal peptide projection terminates in the paraventricular nucleus and it is conjectured that it may play a role in the circadian rhythm of CRH secretion (210).

Substance P

Substance P is a member of the tachykinin family and is present in the hypothalamus. Neurons that contain substance P have been demonstrated in the arcuate, ventromedial, and a number of other hypothalamic nuclei after colchicine treatment (152). Projections from the adrenergic and noradrenergic cell groups in the brain stem that also contain substance P terminate in the paraventricular nucleus (14). Substance P has been found to inhibit the release of CRH by K^+ from perifused hypothalamic fragments. Intraventricular injection depressed plasma ACTH levels in urethane anesthetized rats (23). Third ventricular injection of an antibody to substance P raised plasma GH levels in awake rats suggesting that GH levels are tonically inhibited by substance P. This interaction is believed to occur at the hypothalamic level (6); however, it is not known whether the effect of substance P is to stimulate somatostatin release or depress GRH release either directly or through the mediation of an interneuron. A similar paradigm was employed to study the effect of substance P on gonadotropin secretion (5). Intraventricular injection of an antibody to substance P depressed both FSH and LH levels in rat plasma. Because substance P did not alter gonadotropin release when incubated with pituitary cells, the authors concluded that the stimulatory effect of substance P on gonadotropin release from the pituitary gland was at the level of the hypothalamus. From experiments trying to determine the effects of substance P on gonadotropin release, the authors concluded that the stimulatory effect of substance P on gonadotropin release from the pituitary gland was at the level of the hypothalamus. As results of experiments trying to determine the effects of substance P on gonadotropin release are contradictory, it is too early to come to a firm conclusion as to its central effect.

NPY

NPY is closely related to pancreatic polypeptide and is widely distributed in the mammalian central and peripheral nervous systems (49). It is classified with the pancreatic peptide family of peptides. Within the diencephalon, cell bodies that contain ir-NPY are found in the arcuate nucleus and project to the median eminence where they terminate in its internal zone (33). High levels of NPY have been recovered from portal blood (120). The NPY cells in the arcuate nucleus also project to the parvicellular subdivision of the paraventricular nucleus. Ablations of the arcuate nucleus markedly reduced, but did not abolish, immunostaining of NPY terminals in the paraventricular nucleus (8). Extrahypothalamic NPY projections from the medulla to the parvicellular subdivisions of paraventricular nucleus are present and originate predominantly from the adrenergic C_1 and C_2 cell groups. These NPY projections, unlike those from the arcuate nucleus, co-store epinephrine (38, 190). Projections from the A_1 cell group (with colocalized norepinephrine) innervate the subfornical organ and the magnocellular subdivisions of the paraventricular nucleus (190). NPY terminals have been demonstrated to make synaptic contact with parvicellular CRH (114) and TRH (236) neurons and with magnocellular AVP cells in the paraventricular nucleus (70). NPY terminals are found throughout the MBH and medial zone and make synaptic contact with GnRH cells in the latter region (28, 33).

Intracisternal NPY elevated the level of plasma ACTH in rats (53), and intraventricular NPY raised plasma ACTH levels in dogs (69). Administration of the same nanomolar doses of NPY by the intravenous route had little effect. Direct injection of NPY into the paraventricular nucleus raised ACTH and corticosterone levels in rats (248). NPY stimulated the release of CRH from hypothalamic fragments in a dose-dependent manner (239). It has not been established whether NPY directly stimulates CRH neurons or whether it stimulates the release of norepi-

nephrine (240) which, in turn, stimulates CRH neurons.

NPY injected into the third ventricle of awake, unrestrained rats lowered plasma GH levels. Incubation of hypothalamic fragments with NPY stimulated release of somatostatin (173).

NPY stimulates the release of GnRH, but its effect depends upon the hormonal status of the animal (121). NPY stimulated release of GnRH from hypothalamic slices harvested from ovariectomized rats treated with estrogen. The GnRH response increased if the rats had been treated with estrogen plus progesterone, and reversed if the ovariectomized rats were not steroid treated (25). Administration of NPY into the MBH of ovariectomized female rabbits (does) reduced the amplitude and frequency of GnRH pulses, whereas the same procedure in intact does increased the amplitude and frequency of GnRH pulses (89). In vitro experiments in rabbits confirmed that NPY superfusion of hypothalamic fragments from normal does stimulate GnRH release, whereas the same procedure performed on hypothalamic fragments from normal does stimulates GnRH release, whereas the same procedure performed on hypothalamic fragments of ovariectomized does has no effect (88).

Opioid Peptides

Three different gene families comprise the opioid peptide group. The endorphins are derived from proopiomelanocortin, the enkephalins from proenkephalin, and the dynorphins from prodynorphin. Cells in the arcuate nucleus that contain β-endorphin are its major source of fibers and terminals throughout the hypothalamus and the preoptic area (249). Enkephalin neurons are present in the arcuate, suprachiasmatic, ventromedial, and dorsomedial hypothalamic nuclei (126). All the sources of enkephalin fibers in the hypothalamus have not been established as yet. Extrahypothalamic sites may also contribute fibers. Dynorphin is present in magnocellular neurons in the supraoptic nucleus, paraventricular nucleus, and accessory hypothalamic nuclei. The distribution of fibers and terminals is widespread (40).

Although the administration of morphine to humans is associated with an elevation in plasma ACTH (95), the incubation of hypothalamic fragments with either endorphin, enkephalin, or dynorphin suppressed the release of CRH (261). Opioid peptides have also been reported to inhibit the spontaneous (80) and K$^+$-stimulated (223) release of TRH from incubated hypothalamic fragments. The story is not a simple one, however, as small intraventricular doses of β-endorphin have been reported to stimulate release of TSH, whereas larger doses were without effect. Enkephalin reduced plasma levels of TSH (169). Opiates and opioid peptides stimulate the release of GH in rats, dogs, and humans through a hypothalamic site. However the effect is probably not due to a direct effect of the opiates or opioids on GHRH or somatostatin neurons. It is an indirect effect on GHRH neurons mediated by interneurons (134).

Proopiomelanocortin neurons synapse on GnRH neurons in the primate (239). Opioid peptides inhibit the release of GnRH in vivo (228, 250) and in vitro (36). Neutralization of the central effects of opioid peptides by intraventricular injection of naloxone increased plasma levels of FSH and LH in lactating rats (228). Neutralization of β-endorphin and met-enkephalin by hypothalamic injection of antibodies to those opioid peptides elevated plasma levels of LH in sheep (250). Neurons that express opioid peptides may act directly on GnRH neurons at sites in the preoptic area, at the level of the arcuate nucleus, or in the median eminence (250). Alternatively, they may inhibit the activity of noradrenergic neurons that excite GnRH neurons (13, 253, 243).

Opioid peptides stimulate the release of Prl by inhibiting the release of dopamine from tuberoinfundibular neurons (35, 95). The effect is probably direct, as proopiomelanocortin neurons have been found to synapse with dopaminergic neurons in the arcuate nucleus of the rat (13, 132).

REPRISE

Neuropharmacologic Control of the CRH Neuron

CRH neurons lie in the medial parvicellular subdivision of the paraventricular nucleus and project to the median eminence. They release CRH in a rhythmic phasic pattern, under basal conditions, and acutely in response to stimulation. Steroid hormone levels modulate the release of CRH. In addition, there is a circadian rhythm to CRH release that is reflected in the patterns of ACTH and glucocorticoid plasma levels (7). Biogenic amines that stimulate the release of CRH from neurosecretory terminals in the median eminence include the catecholamines norepinephrine and epinephrine, the indolamine serotonin, the excitatory amino acids glutamine and aspartamine, and the excitatory neurotransmitter ACh. The evidence that norepinephrine and/or epinephrine act at the level of the CRH soma or its dendrites has been reviewed (section on norepinephrine). Some of the catecholaminergic cells that arise in the medulla and project to the parvicellular subdivision of the paraventricular nucleus are characterized by the presence of steroid receptors (187). This finding suggests that stimulation of the CRH neurons in the paraventricular nucleus from adrenergic cells in the medulla is modified by steroid feedback mechanisms. Although dopamine-containing terminals synapse with GRH cells in the paraventricular nucleus, the role of dopamine in the regulation of these cells has not been established. Serotonin stimulates the release of CRH (section on serotonin), but the site and the mechanism of action remain unknown (7). The source of catecholaminergic and indolaminergic terminals is the brain stem. Glutaminergic systems may well be found to play a major role in the stimulation of CRH (73), but the source of the fibers, the sites of the terminals, and the action of glutamine on CRH neurons have yet to be defined. ACh stimulates CRH release, but once again, the source of the fibers, their mode of termination, and the mechanism of action remain obscure.

Peptides also stimulate CRH release. The evidence that angiotensin II stimulates CRH release is presented in the section on angiotensin II. Angiotensin II-containing neurons lie in the region of the subfornical organ and project into both the parvicellular and magnocellular subdivision of the paraventricular nucleus. Although synapses between angiotensin II terminals and CRH soma or dendrites have not as yet been reported, electro-physiologic evidence suggests that direct in-nervation of CRH neurons by angiotensin II terminals occurs (43). NPY also stimulates CRH release, but it has yet to be determined whether it does so independently or through the mediation of norepinephrine release. The site of NPY activity appears to be in the paraventricular nucleus, and the source of the terminals is either the arcuate nucleus of the hypothalamus or the C_1, C_2, or A_2 catecholaminergic cell groups in the medulla.

Specific neuropeptides and neurotrans-mitters, such as GABA, inhibit the release of CRH. GABA neurons are present through-out the hypothalamus. A particularly dense aggregation is present in the arcuate nucleus. GABA terminals lie just outside the paraven-tricular nucleus and may contact dendrites of CRH cells (174). Although AVP potentiates the action of CRH on corticotropes in the pi-tuitary gland (176), it inhibits the release of CRH from terminals in the median emi-nence (160). Substance P has also been found to inhibit CRH release (see section on sub-stance P) but little is known about the origin of its fibers, its site, or its mode of action. Whereas the systemic administration of opi-ates increases plasma ACTH and glucocor-ticoid levels, centrally acting opioid peptides inhibit the release of CRH (150).

Neuropharmacologic Control of the TRH Neuron

TRH neurons lie in the periventricular subdivision of the paraventricular nucleus and in the anterior periventricular nucleus and project to the median eminence. Their neurosecretion of TRH may be responsive to plasma T_4 levels through interactions in the median eminence (262). Catecholamines (norepinephrine and dopamine) and indo-lamines (5-HT) stimulate TRH release (sec-tions on norepinephrine, dopamine, and serotonin). The proximity of ir-DBH and ir-5-HT terminals and of ir-TH to TRH neu-rons suggests that these mechanisms are physiologic. The dopaminergic system is in-trahypothalamic, whereas the noradrenergic and indolaminergic systems arise in the brain stem. GABA and opioid peptides inhibit the release of TRH.

Neuropharmacologic Control of GHRH and Somatostatin Neurons

GHRH neurons are found in the arcuate and ventromedial nuclei of the rat hypothal-amus. Somatostatin neurons are found in the periventricular preoptic nucleus and in the anterior periventricular nucleus of the hy-pothalamus (see section on nuclei in the peri-ventricular zone). Their interaction regulates the release of GH from somatotropes in the pituitary gland. GHRH stimulates GH re-lease, whereas somatostatin inhibits it. The release of GH is pulsatile (116). Peaks of GH release are accompanied by increased GHRH release and decreased somatostatin release. Troughs are the mirror image (129). Somatostatin neurons synapse with GHRH neurons at the level of the arcuate nucleus (110). Somatostatin can inhibit GH secre-tion from somatotropes directly or by inhi-bition of GHRH neurons (86).

Norepinephrine stimulates the release of GH by stimulating the release of GHRH (see section on norepinephrine). In contrast, do-pamine appears to stimulate the release of somatostatin (see section on dopamine). Stimulation of serotonin receptors in the hy-pothalamus of the awake rat stimulates re-lease of GH (259). The evidence that 5-HT stimulates the release of GHRH and inhibits the release of somatostatin is reviewed by Millard (129). It is well accepted that ACh stimulates the release of GH, but the mech-anisms have to be clarified. Preliminary data suggest inhibition of somatostatin release, but the mechanisms (whether direct or via interneurons) have yet to be worked out (134).

GABA inhibits the release of somatostatin and thus stimulates the release of GH. The site of action is at the cell bodies and den-drites, where synapses between GABA ter-minals and somatostatin soma and dendrites have been recorded.

Vasoactive intestinal peptide, a member of the glucagon superfamily, of which GnRH is also a member, stimulates the release of so-matostatin and thus inhibits the release of GH. The site and mechanism of stimulation (whether direct or through interneurons) re-mains to be elucidated. NPY, a member of the pancreatic polypeptide family, also stim-ulates the release of somatostatin and inhibits the release of GH from somato-tropes.

Neuropharmacologic Control of the GnRH Neuron

GnRH neurons lie in the septal-preoptic region and not in the MBH in rodents. The situation is different in primates, where GnRH neurons lie in well-defined clusters above the optic chiasm, medial to the supra-optic nuclei, and interposed between the ar-cuate nucleus of the hypothalamus and the infundibular lip of the neurohypophysis. They are also scattered along the ventral hypothalamic tract that carries their pro-jections to the median eminence. In the primate, most of the GnRH neurons lie in the MBH, not in the preoptic area (48).

GnRH neurons project to the median em-inence where they release GnRH in a pulsa-tile pattern under basal conditions. The site of the GnRH "pulse generator" is the site of the GnRH neurons—the preoptic area in rats and rabbits and the MBH in primates. The amplitude and frequency of elevations of plasma LH levels was correlated with the phasic hourly (circhoral) pattern of discharge of neurons in the MBH of monkeys (94). The amplitude of these pulses increases following ovariectomy (252). Superimposed upon this phasic pattern of LH release is the surge of LH that accompanies ovulation. Following bilateral destruction of the arcuate nucleus, the normal menstrual cycle can be restored in the monkey by the administration of GnRH at a frequency of one pulse per hour. Knobil (94) interprets this observation to mean that the secretion of GnRH is permis-sive but not causal in the generation of the LH surge in the primate. On the other hand, the rise in GnRH release that occurs on the afternoon of proestrus just prior to ovulation in the rat, and the induction of GnRH release and subsequent ovulation induced by the ad-ministration of cupric acetate suggest that an increase in GnRH release causes the LH surge that results in ovulation in the rat (85).

Norepinephrine and epinephrine are held to stimulate GnRH release in the female rat. The evidence that the stimulatory effect of es-trogens on GnRH release is mediated by the catecholaminergic system ascending from the brain stem has been reviewed in the sec-tion on norepinephrine.

Serotonin terminals synapse with GnRH neurons in the preoptic area of the rat (91). A stimulatory role for serotonin has been pro-posed (see section on serotonin).

ACh stimulates the release of GnRH from hypothalamic fragments. Its role in the estro-gen-induced surge of GnRH on the after-noon of proestrus is reviewed in the section on ACh.

The role of the excitatory amino acids in the control of GnRH release is only begin-ning to come under scrutiny. N-methyl D-as-partic acid (NMDA) stimulates LH release in the monkey. Its administration to ovariec-tomized monkeys elicits increased phasic fir-ing from the pulse generator accompanied by LH pulses. Central NMDA blockade inhibits pulse generator activity (94).

GABA inhibits the pulsatile release of GnRH. Its role in mediating (gonadal) ste-roid effects is reviewed in the section on GABA.

Angiotensin II stimulates the release of GnRH, presumably by acting on norepi-nephrine afferents. The site of this interac-tion is not known.

NPY terminals synapse with GnRH cells in the rat and NPY stimulates the release of GnRH from normal rats but not from ovari-ectomized rats. Treatment of ovariecto-mized rats with E_2 or E_2 + progesterone restores the ability of NPY to stimulate GnRH release.

Opioid peptides inhibit the release of GnRH from the rat in vivo and in vitro (see section on opioid peptides). Opiate admin-istration inhibits the pulsatile release of LH in monkeys and the effect is reversed by the administration of naloxone (71). Proopi-omelanocortin terminals synapse with GnRH neurons in the primate (232). Stress-initiated inhibition of LH release is believed to be modulated by GnRH-stimulated β-en-dorphin release, with subsequent inhibition of GnRH release (17, 156). Sahu et al. (178) present evidence to support the hypothesis that, in the rat, a decrease in opioid tone ini-tiated by a rise in plasma E_2 levels on the af-ternoon of proestrus allows increased NPY and (concurrent or consequent) increased catecholamine release, with resultant GnRH stimulation and consequent ovulation. Further work will be necessary to determine if this postulate is applicable to the initiation of cyclic ovulation in the human female.

Neuropharmacologic Control of Dopamine, TRH, and Vasoactive Intestinal Peptide Neurons

Prl release from lactotropes is regulated by one inhibitory hormone (dopamine) and two stimulatory hormones (TRH and vasoactive intestinal peptide.) Serotonin mediates the increase in Prl release that occurs with suckling by stimulating vasoactive intestinal peptide and TRH release and inhibiting dopamine release. The latter effect is perhaps mediated by a GABA interneuron. Opioid peptides inhibit dopamine release from tuberoinfundibular neurons. Because β-endorphin neurons are stimulated by CRH, opioid inhibition of dopamine release mediates the increased secretion of Prl seen during stress. Neurotensin inhibits Prl release by stimulating dopamine release from tuberoinfundibular neurons.

NEUROSURGICAL CORRELATIONS

Anatomical Considerations

Lesions or surgery of the intrasellar pituitary gland put the motor units of the neuroendocrine system at risk. Tumors or surgery in the neighborhood of the pituitary stalk also endanger these units because of the possibility of damage to the portal system. Surgery and pathology at the floor of the third ventricle endanger the terminals of the lower motor neurons in the median eminence and, hence, endanger all anterior pituitary (motor) functions. Surgery within the third ventricle puts the cell bodies of the neuroendocrine system's motor neurons at risk because they lie in a periventricular location. However, since the removal of a large craniopharyngioma from the sella and the stalk endangers the end organ, damage to its innervation by the removal of the capsule from the walls of the third ventricle may escape detec-

tion. Segmental and motor unit dysfunction accompany lesions to the sella, stalk, and third ventricle.

Extrasegmental defects will only be manifest when the pituitary gland, its blood supply, and its innervation are intact. Pathology or surgery at a distance from the pituitary may cause unexpected extrasegmental deficits in pituitary function. Injury to the lamina terminalis will involve the organum vasculosum of the lamina terminalis and disrupt a sensory function in the neuroendocrine system—the ability to sense plasma osmolality. Damage slightly higher in the region of the subfornical organ will alter the ability of the paraventricular nucleus to sense circulating levels of angiotensin II and, hence, deprive CRH cells of input concerning vascular volume.

The effects of unilateral damage of the ventrolateral medulla on pituitary function have not been evaluated, but some effect upon AVP release from the neural lobe and CRH and GnRH release in response to vascular depletion might be expected.

Temporal lobectomy, for epilepsy, trauma, or tumor can be expected to alter the response of the pituitary to stress and, perhaps, to alter aspects of reproductive function. In the light of recent findings, renewed clinical study of patients following temporal lobectomy will have to focus not on basal ACTH or cortisol levels, but on the ACTH response to stress and the modification of that response by circulating glucocorticoid levels. The presence of normal AM and PM cortisol levels is not sufficient to document freedom from suprasegmental defects in the hypothalamic-pituitary-axis.

Surgery at the entrance to the Isle of Reil, deep within the Sylvian fissure, beneath the anterior perforated space, is routinely performed for a variety of lesions. This is the region of the septum, a major relay from medial temporal lobe structures to the hypothalamus. It is not known if subtle defects in neuroendocrine function can occur following successful surgery in this region.

Endocrine dysfunction is not overt in patients with posterior fossa lesions, although subtle defects have not been sought. The ascending catecholaminergic and peptidergic systems could be at risk in the terminal stages and their dysfunction may become manifest in the Cushing response.

As neurosurgeons, we are used to carrying out sophisticated neurological examinations and tests to separate sensory from motor dysfunction or segmental from suprasegmental pathology. We are not used to performing an analogous task in the neuroendocrine evaluation of patients.

Pharmacological Considerations

Whereas the use of long-acting analogues of hypothalamic inhibiting hormones (i.e., dopamine, somatostatin) has met with varying degrees of success, the modification of normal or neoplastic pituitary secretion by the alteration of extrasegmental input has had little success. The use of serotonin inhibitors in the medical management of Cushing's disease has not stood the test of time.

Of the drugs employed in neurosurgical practice, steroids and opiates are the most likely to alter pituitary function at both pituitary and suprasegmental levels. Glucocorticoids suppress feedback mechanisms at the piutitary level but can also be expected to alter noradrenergic input from the brain stem to CRH cells and input from steroid sensitive cells in the limbic lobe. Systemic opiates can be expected to stimulate Prl release and inhibit GnRH release and to stimulate ACTH (even though in vitro experiments demonstrate that opioids inhibit CRH release) and GH release.

It can be surmised that, although much is known about the neuropharmacology of intrinsic hypothalamic systems and systems ascending from the brain stem, little is known about the neuropharmacology of systems that project to the preoptic area and MBH from the temporal lobe. Progress in the study of these pathways can be expected in the next several years.

REFERENCES

1. Adler B.A., and Crowley W.R. Evidence for gamma-aminobutyric acid modulation of ovarian hormonal effects of luteinizing hormone secretion and hypothalamic catecholamine activity in the female rat. Endocrinology, *118*:91–7, 1986.
2. Afione S., Duvilanski B., Seilicovigh A., Lasaga M., Diaz M.D.C., and Debeljuk L. Effects of serotonin on the Hypothalamic-pituitary gabaergic system. Brain. Res. Bull., *25*:245–249, 1990.
3. Albers H.E., Stopa E.G., Zoeller R.T., Kauere J.S., King J.C., Fink J.S., Mobtaker H., and Wolfe H. Day-Night variation in prepro vasoactive intestinal peptide/peptide histidine isoleucine MRNA within the rat suprachiasmatic nucleus. Mol. Brain Res., *7*:85–89, 1990.
4. Alexander M.J., Clifton D.K., Steinder R.A., Vasoactive intestinal polypeptide effects a central inhibition of pulsatile luteinizing hormone secretion in ovariectomized rats. Endocrinology., *117(5)*:2134–2139, 1985.
5. Arisawa M., Depalatis L., Ho R., Snyder G.D., Yu W.H., Pan G., McCann S.M. Stimulatory role of substance P on gonadotropin release in ovariectomized rats. Neuroendocrinology., *51*:523–529, 1990.
6. Areswaa M., Snyder G.D., Depalatis L., Ho R.H., Xu R.K., Pan G., McCann S.M. Role of substance P in suppressing growth hormone release in the rat. Proc. Natl. Acad. Sci. USA., *86*:7290–7294, 1989.
7. Assenmacher I., Szafarczyk A., Alonso G., Ixart G., Barbanel G. Physiology of neural pathways affecting CRH secretion. Ann. N.Y. Acad. Sci., *512*:149–161, 1987.
8. Bai F.L., Yamano M., Shiotani Y., Emson P.C., Smith A.D., Powell J.F., Tohyama M. An arcuato-paraventricular and dorsomedial hypothalamic neuropeptide Y-containing system which lacks noradrenaline in the rat. Brain Res., *369*:172–175, 1985.
9. Barbabel G., Ixart G., Szafarczyk A., Malaval F., Assenmacher I. Intrahypothalamic infusion of interleukin-1 Beta increases the release of corticotropin-releasing hormone (CRH 41) and adrenocorticotropic hormone (ACTH) in free-moving rats bearing a push-pull cannula in the median eminence. Brain Res., *516*:31–36, 1990.
10. Barofsky A-L., Taylor J., Massari V.J. Dorsal raphe-hypothalamic projections provide the stimulatory serotonergic input to suckling-induced prolactin release. Endocrinology., *113*:1894–1903, 1983.
11. Barracluogh C.A., Wise P.M. The role of catecholamines in the regulation of pituitary luteinizing hormone and follicle-stimulating hormone secretion. Endoc. Rev., *3*:91–119, 1982.
12. Ben-Jonathan N. Dopamine: a prolactin-inhibiting hormone. Endoc. Rev., *6(4)*:564–589, 1985.
13. Bicknell R.J. Endogenous opioid peptides and hypothalamic neuroendocrine neurons. J. Endocrinology., *107*:437–466, 1985.
14. Bettencourt J., Benoit R., Sawchenko P. Distribution and origins of substance p-immunoreactive projections to the paraventricular and supra-optic nuclei: partial overlap with ascending catecholaminergic projections. J. Che. Neuroanat., *4*:63–78, 1991.
15. Bolaffi J., Jackson I. Regulation of thyrotropin-releasing hormone secretion from frog skin. Endocrinology., *110*:842–846, 1982.
16. Bruhn T.O., Plotsky P.M., Vale W.W. Effect of paraventricular lesions of corticotropin-releasing factor (CRF)-like immunoreactivity in the stalk-

median eminence: studies on the adrenocorticotropin response to ether stress and exogenous CRF. Endocrinology., *114:*57–62, 1984.

17. Burns G., Almeida F.X., Passarelli F., Herz A. A two-step mechanism by which corticotropin-releasing hormone releases hypothalamic b-endorphin: the role of vasopressin and G-proteins. Endocrinology., *125(3):*365–1372, 1989.

18. Calogero A.E., Bernardini R., Margioros A.N., Bagdy G., Gallucci W.T., Munson P.J., Tamarkin L., Tomai T.P., Brady L., Gold P.W., Chrousos G.P. Effects of serotonergic agonists and antagonists on corticotropin-releasing hormone secretion by explanted rat hypothalami. Peptides., *10:*189–200, 1989.

19. Castren E., Saaverdra J.M. Angiotensin II receptors in paraventricular nucleus, subfornical organ, and pituitary gland of hypophysectomized, adrenalectomized, and vasopressin-deficient rats. Proc. Natal. Acad. Sci. USA., *86:*725–729, 1989.

20. Caverson M.M., Ciriello J. Electrophysiological identification of neurons in ventrolateral medulla sending collateral axons to paraventricular and supraoptic nuclei in the cat. Brain Res., *305:*375–379, 1984.

21. Ceccatelli S., Tsuruo Y., Hokfelt T., Fahrenkrug J., Dohler K-D. Some blood vessels in the rat median eminence are surrounded by a dense plexus of vasoactive intestinal polypeptide/peptide histidine isoleucine (VIP/PHI) immunoreactive nerves. Neurosci. Lett., *84:*29–34, 1988.

22. Chen Y.F., Ramirez V.D. Serotonin stimulates thyrotropin-releasing hormone release from superfused rat hypothalami. Endocrinology., *108:*2359–2366, 1981.

23. Chowdrey H.S., Jessop D.S., Lightman S.L. Substance P stimulates arginine vasopressin and inhibits adrenocorticotropin release in vivo in the rat. Neuroendocrinology., *52:*90–93, 1990.

24. Conway S., Richardson L., Speciale S., Mohoerek R., Mauceri H., Krulich L. Interaction between norepinephrine and serotonin in the neuroendocrine control of growth hormone release in the rat. Endocrinology., *126:*1022–1030, 1990.

25. Crowely W.R., Kalra S.P. Neuropeptide Y stimulates the release of luteinizing hormone-releasing hormone from medial basal hypothalamus in vitro: modulation by ovarian hormones. Neuroendocrinology., *46:*97–103, 1987.

26. Cunningham E.T., Bohn M.C., Sawchenko P.E. Organization of adrenergic inputs to the paraventricular and supraoptic nuclei of the hypothalamus in the rat. J. Comp. Neurol., *292:*651–657, 1990.

27. Cunningham M.M., Sawchenko P.E. Anatomical specificity of noradrenergic inputs to the paraventricular and supraoptic nuclei of the rat hypothalamus. J. Comp. Neurol., *274:*60–76, 1988.

28. Danger J.M., Tonon M.C., Jenks B.G., Pierre-Saint S., Martel J.C., Fasolo A., Breton B., Quirion R., Pelletier G., Vaudry H. Neuropeptide Y: localization in the central nervous system and neuroendocrine functions. Fundam. Clin. Pharmacol. *4:*307–340, 1990.

29. Day T.A., Renaud L.P. Electrophysiological evidence that noradrenergic afferents selectively facil-itate the activity of supraoptic vasopressin neurons. Brain Res. *303:*233–240, 1984.

30. Day T.A., Renaud L.P., Sibbald J.R. Excitation of supraoptic vasopressin cells by stimulation of the A1 noradrenaline cell group: failure to demonstrate role for established adrenergic or amino acid receptors. Brain Res., *516:*91–98, 1990.

31. Day, T.A., Sibbald J.R. A1 cell group mediates solitary nucleus excitation of supraoptic vasopressin cells. Am. J. Physiol., *257:*R1020–R1026, 1989.

32. Day T.A., Sibbald J.R. Solitary nucleus excitation of supraoptic vasopressin cells via adrenergic afferents. Am. J. Physiol., *254(4PT2):*R711–716, 1988.

33. De Quidt M.E., Enson P.C. Distribution of neuropeptide Y-like immunoreactivity in the rat central nervous system-II. Immunohistochemical Analysis. Neuroscience., *18:*545–614, 1986.

34. DeGreef W.J., Vooght J.L., Visser T.J., Lamberts S.W.J., Van Der Shoot P. Control of prolactin release induced by suckling. Endocrinology., *121:*316–322, 1987.

35. Dobson, P.R.M., Brown B.L. Involvement of the hypothalamus in opiate-stimulated prolactin secretion. Regulatory Peptides. *20:*305–310, 1988.

36. Drouva S.V., Epelbaum J., Tapia-Arancibia L., Laplante E., Kordon C. Opiate receptors modulate LHRH and SRIF release from mediobasal hypothalamic neurons. Neuroendocrinology., *32:*162–167, 1981.

37. Egozi Y., Kloog Y., Sokolovsky M. Acetylcholine rhythm in the preoptic area of the rat hypothalamus is synchronized with the estrous cycle. Brain Res., *383:*310–313, 1986.

38. Everitt B.J., Hokfelt T., Terenius L., Tatemoto K., Mutt V., Goldstein. Differential co-existence of neuropeptide Y (NPY)-like immunoreactivity with catecholamines in the central nervous system of the rat. Neuroscience., *11:*443–462, 1984.

39. Everitt B.J., Hokfelt T., Wu J-Y, Goldstein J. Coexistence of tyrosine hydroxlase-like gamma-aminobutyric acid-like immunoreactivities in neurons of the arcuate nucleus. Neuroendocrinology., *39:*289–191, 1984.

40. Fallon J.H., Leslie F.M. Distribution of dynorphin and enkephalin peptides in the rat brain. J. Comp. Neurol., *249:*293–36, 1986.

41. Faria M., Navarra P., Tsagarakis S., Besser G.M., Grossman A.B. Inhibition of CRH-41 release by substance P, but not Substance K, from the rat hypothalamus in vitro. Brain Res., *538:*76–78, 1991.

42. Ferguson A.V. Systemic angiotensin acts at the subfornical organ to control the activity of paraventricular nucleus neurons with identified projection to the median eminence. Neuroendocrinology., *47:*489–497, 1988.

43. Ferguson A.V., Day T.A., Renaud L.P. Subfornical organ efferents influence the excitability of neurohypophyseal and tuberoinfundibular nucleus neurons in the rat. Neuroendocrinology., *39:*423–428, 1984.

44. Freeman M. The ovarian cycle of the rat. In: *The Physiology of Reproduction,* edited by E. Knobil and E. Neill, Ch. 45, pp. 1893–1928, New York, Raven Press, 1988.

45. Fuchs E., Stock K.W., Vijayan E., Wuttke W. In-

volvement of catecholamines and glutamate in gabaergic mechanism regulatory to luteinizing hormone and prolactin secretion. Neuroendocrinology., *38:*484–489, 1984.

46. Ganong W.F. Angiotensin II in the brain and pituitary: contrasting roles in the regulation of adenhypophyseal secretion. Horm. Res., *31:*24–31, 1989.

47. Gillies G.E., Linton E.A., aowry P.J. Corticotropin releasing activity of the new CRF is potentiated several times by vasopressin. Nature., *299:*355–357, 1982.

48. Goldsmith P.C., Song T. The gonadotropin-releasing hormone containing ventral hypothalamic tract in the fetal rhesus monkey (macaca mulata). J. Comp. Neurol., *257:*130–139, 1987.

49. Gray T., Morley J.E. Neuropeptide Y: anatomical distribution and possible function in mammalian nervous system. Life Sci., *38:*389–401, 1986.

50. Gribkoff V.K., Dudek F.E. Effects of excitatory amino acid antagonists on synaptic responses of supraoptic neurons in slices of rat hypothalamus. J. Neurophysiology., *63:*60–71, 1990.

51. Gruber K., McRae-Degueurce A., Wilkin L.D., Mitchell L.D., Johnson A.K. Forebrain and brainstem afferents to the arcuate nucleus in the brain: potential pathways for the modulation of hypophyseal secretions. Neurosci. Lett., *75:*1–5, 1987.

52. Guy J., Pellitier G. Neuronal interactions between neuropeptide Y (NPY) and catecholaminergic systems in the rat arcuate nucleus as shown by dual immunocytochemistry. Peptides., *9:*567–570, 1988.

53. Haas, D.A., George S.R. Neuropeptide Y administration acutely increases hypothalamus corticotropin-releasing factor immunoreactivity: lack of effect in other rat brain regions. Life Sciences., *41*2725–2731, 1987.

54. Halasz B., Kiss J., Molnar J. Regulation of the gonadotropin-releasing hormone (GnRH) neuronal system: morphological aspects. J. Steroid Biochem., *33:*663–668, 1989.

55. Handa R.J., Resko J.A., Alpha-adrenergic regulation of androgen receptor concentration in the preoptic area of the rat. Brain Res., *482:*312–320, 1989.

56. Hartman R.D., He J.-R., and Barraclough C.A. Gamma-Aminobutyric acid-A and -B receptor antagonists incrasing luteinizing hormone-releasing hormone neuronal responsiveness to intracerebroventricular norepinephrine in ovariectomized estrogen-treated rats. Endocrinology., *172:*1336–1345, 1990.

57. Healy D.P., Maciejewski A.R., Printz M.P. Localization of central angiotensin II receptors with (^{125}I)-SAR[1], ILE[8]-Angiotensin II: periventricular sites of the anterior third ventricle. Neuroendocrinology., *44:*15–21, 1986.

58. Heimer L., Nauta W.J.H. The hypothalamic distribution of the stria terminalis in the rat. Brain Res., *12:*284–297, 1969.

59. Herman J.P., Schafer M.K.H., Young E.A., Thompson R., Douglass J., Akil H., Watson S.J. Evidence for hippocampal regulation of neuroendocrine neurons of the hypothalamo-pituitary-adrenocortical axis. J. Neurosci., *9:*3072–3082, 1989.

60. Herman J.P., Weigand S.J., Watson S.J. Regulation of basal corticotropin-releasing hormone and arginine vasopressin messenger ribonucleic acid expression in the paraventricular nucleus: effects of selective hypothalamic deafferentations. Endocrinology., *127*2408–2417, 1990.

61. Hillhouse E.W., Milton N.G.N. Effect of noradrenal and gamma-aminobutyric acid on the secretion of corticotropin-releasing factor 41 and arginine vasopressin from the rat hypothalamus in vitro. J. Endocrinol., *122:*719–723, 1989.

62. Hillhouse E.W., Milton G.N. Effect of acetylcholine and 5- hydroxytryptamine on the secretion of corticotrophin-releasing factor-41 and arginine vasopressin from the rat hypothalamus in vitro. J. Endocrinol. *122:*713–718, 1989.

63. Hillhouse E., Reichlein S. Acetylcholine stimulates the secretion of corticotropin-releasing factor from primary dissociated cell cultures of the rat telecephalon and diencephalon. Brain Res., *506:*9–13, 1990.

64. Hokfelt T., Elde R., Fuxe K., Johansson O., Ljungdahl A., Goldstein M., Luft R., Efendic S., Nilsson G., Terenius L., Ganten D., Jeffcoate S.L., Rehfeld J., Said S., Perez De LaMora M., Possani L., Rapia R., Teran L., Palacios R. Aminergic and peptidergic pathways in the nervous system with special reference to the hypothalamus. In: *The Hypothalamus.,* Edited by S. Riechlin, R.J. Baldessarini, J.B. Martin, pp. 69–135, New York, Raven press, 1978.

65. Hokfelt T., Fahrenkrug J., Tatemoto K., Mutt V., Werner S., Hutling A-L., Terenius L., Chang K.J. The PHI (PHI-27)/corticotropin-releasing factor/enkephalin immunoreactive hypothalamic neuron: possible morphological basis for integrated control of prolactin, corticotropin, and growth hormone secretion. Proc. Natl. Acad. Sci. USA., *80:*895–898, 1983.

66. Hokfelt T., Meister B., Melander T., Everitt B. Coexistence of classical transmitters and peptides with special reference to the arcuate nucleus. Advances in Biochemical Pharmacology., *93:*21–34, 1987.

67. Honda K., Negoro H., Higuchi T., Tadokoro Y. Activation of neurosecretory cells by osmotic stimulation of anteroventral third ventricle. Am. J. Physiol., *252:*R1039–R1045, 1987.

68. Hyde J.F., and Ben-Jonathan N. Characterization of prolactin-releasing factor in the rat posterior pituitary. Endocrinology., *122:*2533–9, 1988.

69. Inoue T., Inui A., Minoru O., Noriaki S., Manabu O., Hideki M., Nobuhiko M., Munetada O., Shigeaki B. Effect of neuropeptide Y on the hypothalamic-pituitary-adrenal axis in the dog. Life Sci., *44:*1043–1051, 1987.

70. Iwai C., Ochiai H., Nakai Y. Electron-microscopic immunocytochemistry of neuropeptide Y immunoreactive innervation of vasopressin neurons in the paraventricular nucleus of the rat hypothalamus. Acta Anat., *136:*279–284, 1989.

71. Jaffe R.B., Plosker S., Marshall L., Martin M.C. Neuromodulatory regulation of gonadotropin-re-

leasing hormone pulsatile discharge in women. Am. J. Obstet. Gynecol., *163(5,Pt.2):*1727–1731, 1990.

72. Jaffer A., Searson A., Russel V.A., Taljaard J.J.F.T. The effect of selective noradrenergic denervation on thyrotropin secretion in the rat. Neurochemical Res., *14:*13–16, 1990.

73. Jennes L., Beckman W.C., Stumpf W.E., Grzanna R. Anatomical relationships of serotoninergic and noradrenalinergicprojections with the GNRH system in septum and hypothalamus. Exp. Brain. Res., *46:*331–338, 1982.

74. Jennes L., Stumpf W.E., Tappaz M.L. Anatomical relationships of dopaminergic and gabaergic systems with the GNRH-systems in the septo-hypothalamic area. Exp. Brain. Res., *50:*91–99, 1983.

75. Jh H., Rao J.K., Prasad C., Jayaraman A. Distribution pattern of cell bodies and fibers with neurotensin like immunoreactivity in the cat hypothalamus. J. Comp. Neurol., *272:*269–279, 1988.

76. Jhamandas J.H., Lind R.W., Renaud L.P. Angiotensin II may mediate excitatory neurotransmission from the subfornical organ to the hypothalamic supraoptic nucleus: an anatomical and electrophysiological study in the rat. Brain Res., *487:*52–61, 1989.

77. Joanny P., Steinberg J., Zamora A.J., Conte-Devolx B., Millet Y., Oliver C. Corticotropin-releasing factor release from in vitro superfused and incubated rat hypothalamus. Effect of potassium, norepinephrine, and dopamine. Peptides., *50:*81–87, 1989.

78. Jonsson G., Fuxe K., Hokfelt T. On the catecholamine innervation of the hypothalamus, with special reference to the median eminence. Brain Res., *40:*271–281, 1972.

79. Jordan D., Poncet C., Veisseire M., Mornex R. Role of GABA in the control of thyrotropin secretion in the rat. Brain Res., *268:*105–110, 1983.

80. Jordan D., Veisseire M., Borson-Chazot F., Mornex R. In vitro effects of endogenous opiate peptides of thyrotropin function: inhibition of thyrotropin-releasing hormone release and absence of effect on thyrotropin release. Neurosci. Lett., *67:*289–294, 1986.

81. Kakucsa I., Tappaz M.L., Gaal G., Stoeckel M.E., Makara G.B. Gabaergic innervation of somatostatin-containing neurosecretory cells of the anterior periventricular hypothalamic area: a light and electron microscopy double labelling study. Neuroscience., *25:*585–593, 1988.

82. Kalra S.P. Catecholamine involvement in preovulatory LH release: reassessment of the role of epinephrine. Neuroendocrinology., *40:*139–144, 1985.

83. Kalra S.P. Neural circuitry involved in control of LHRH secretion: a model for the preovulatory LH release. In: *Frontiers in Neuroendocrinology.* vol. 9. Editors W.F. Ganong and L. Martini, pp. 31–75, New York, Raven Press, 1986.

84. Kalra S.P., Allen L.G., Sahu A., Kalra P.S., Crowley W.R. Gonadal steroids and neuropeptide Y-opioid-LHRH axis. J. Steroid Biochem., *30(1–6):*185–193, 1988.

85. Kalra P.S., Kalra S.P. Steroidal modulation of the

regulatory neuropeptides: leutinizing hormone releasing hormone, neuropeptide Y and endogenous opioid peptides. J. Steroid Biochem., *25(5B)*733–740, 1986.

86. Katakami H., Downs T.R., Frohman L.A. Inhibitory effect of hypothalamic medial preoptic area somatostatin on growth hormone-releasing factor in the rat. Endocrinology., *123:*1103–1109, 1988.

87. Katsuura G., Arimura A., Koves K., Gottschall P.E. Involvement of organum vasculosum of lamina terminalis and preoptic area in interleukin 1B-induced ACTH release. Am. J. Physiol., *258:*E163–E171, 1990.

88. Khorram O., Pau K.Y.F., Speis H.G. Release of hypothalamic neuropeptide Y and effects of exogenous NPY on the release of hypothalamic and pituitary gonadotropins in intact and ovariectomized does in vitro. Peptides., *9:*411–417, 1988.

89. Khorram O., Pau K.Y.F., Spies H.G. Biomodal effects of neuropeptide on hypothalamic release of gonadotropin-releasing hormone in conscious rabbits. Neuroendocrinology., *45:*290–297, 1987.

90. Kiss J., Csaky A., Halasz B. Demonstration of serotoninergic axon terminals on somatostatin-immunoreactive neurons of the anterior periventricular nucleus of the rat hypothalamus. Brain Res. *442:*23–32, 1988.

91. Kiss J., Halasz B. Demonstration of serotoninergic axons terminating on luteinizing hormone-releasing hormone neurons in the preoptic area of the rat using a combination of immunocytochemistry and high resolution autoradiography. Neuroscience., *14(1):*69–78, 1985.

92. Kiss J. Halasz B. Synaptic connections between serotoninergic axon terminals and tyrosine hydroxylase-immunoreactive neurons in the arcuate nucleus of the rat hypothalamus. A combination of electron microscopic autoradiography and immunocytochemistry. Brain Res., *364:*284–294, 1986.

93. Kiss J.Z., Mezey E., Skirboll L. Corticotropin-releasing factor-immunoreactive neurons of the paraventricular nucleus become vasopressin positive after adrenalectomy. Proc. Natl. Acad. Sci. USA., *81:*1854–1858, 1984.

94. Knobil E. The GnRH Pulse "Generator". Am. J. Obstet. Gyn., *163:*1721–1727, 1990.

95. Koenig J.I. Pituitary gland: neuropeptides, neurotransmitters and growth factors. Toxicol. Pathol., *17:*256–265, 1989.

96. Krieger D.T. Serotonin regulation of ACTH secretion. Ann. N.Y. Acad. Sci., *297:*527–535, 1977.

97. Krulich L. Neurotransmitter control of thyrotropin secretion. Neuroendocrinology., *35:*139–147, 1982.

98. Lamberts R., Vijayan E., Graf M., Mansky T., Wuttke W. Involvement of preoptic-anterior hypothalamic gaba neurons in the regulation of pituitary LH and prolactin release. Exp. Brain Res., *52:*356–362, 1983.

99. Leibowitz S.F., Diaz S., Tempel D. Norepinephrine in the paraventricular neuclus stimulates cortocosterone release. Brain Res., *496:*219–227, 1989.

100. Leibowitz S.F., Eidelman D., Suh J., Diaz S., Saldek C.D. mapping study of noradrenergic stimu-

lation of vasopressin release. Exp. Neurol., *110*:298–305, 1990.

101. Leranth C., Maclusky N.J., Sakamoto H., Shanabrough M., Naftolin F. Glutamic acid decarboxylase-containing axons synapse on LHRH neurons in the rat medial preoptic area. Neuroendocrinology., *40*:536–539, 1985.

102. Leranth C.S., Sakamoto H., Maclusky N.J., Shanabrough M., Naftolin F. application of avidin-ferritin and peroxidase as contrasting electron-dense markers for simultaneous electron microscopic immunocytchemical labelling for glutamic acid decarboxlyase and tyrosine hydroxylase in the rat arcuate nucleus. Histochemistry., *82*:165–168, 1985.

103. Lewis B.M., Dieguez C., Lewis M.D., Scanlon M.F. Dopamine stimulates release of thyrotrophin-releasing hormone from perfused intact rat hypothalamus via hypothalamic D2-receptors. J. Endocrinol., *115*:419–424, 1987.

104. Lewis B.M., Dieguez C., Lewis M., Hall R., Scanlon M.F. Hypothalamic D2 receptors mediate the preferential release of somatostatin-28 in response to dopaminergic stimulation. Endocrinology., *119*:1712–1717, 1986.

105. Liao N., Bulant M., Nicolas P., Vaudry H., Pellitier G., Anatomical interactions of proopiomelanocortin (POMC)-related peptides, neuropeptide Y(NPY) and dopamine B-hydroxylase (DBH) fibers and thyrotropin-releasing hormone (TRH) neurons in the paraventricular nucleus of rat hypothalamus. Neuropeptides., *18*:63–67, 1991.

106. Lind R.W., Hoesen G.W.V., Johnson A.K. An HRP study of the connections of the subfornical organ of the rat. J. Comp. Neurol., *210*:265–277, 1982.

107. Lind R.W., Swanson L.W., Ganten D. Organization of angiotensin II immunoreactive cells and fibers in the rat central nervous system: an immunohistochemical study. Neuroendocrinology., *40*:1–24, 1985.

108. Lind R.W., Swanson L.W., Sawchenko P.E. Anatomical evidence that neural circuits related to the subfornical organ contain angiotensin II. Brain Res. Bull., *15*:79–82, 1985.

109. Liposits Z.S., Kallo I., Barkovics-Kallo M., Bohn M.C., Paull W.K. Innervatin of somatostatin neurons by adrenergic, phenylethanolamine-N-methyltransferase (PNMT)-immunoreactive axons in the anterior periventricular nucleus of the rat hypothalamus. Histochemistry., *94*:13–20, 1990.

110. Liposits Z.S., Merchenthaler I., Paull W.K., Flerko B. Synaptic communication between somatostatinergic axons and growth hormone-releasing factor (GRF) synthesizing neurons in the arcuate nucleus of the rat. Histochemistry., *89*:247–252, 1988.

111. Liposits Z.S., Paull W.K. Association of dopaminergic fibers with corticotropin releasing hormone (CRH)-synthesizing neurons in the paraventricular nucleus of the rat hypothalamus. Histochemistry., *93*:119–127, 1989.

112. Liposits Z.S., Paull W.K., Wu P., Jackson I.M.D., Lechan R.M. Hypophysiotropic thyrotropin releasing (TRH) synthesizing neurons: ultrastruc-

ture, adrenergic innervation and putative transmitter action. Histochemistry., *88*:1–10, 1987.

113. Liposits Z.S., Phelix C., Paull W.K. Electron microscopic analysis of tyrosine hydroxylase, dopamine-B-hydroxylase and phenylethanolamine-N-methyl-transferase immunoreactive innervation of the hypothalamic paraventricular nucleus in the rat. Histochemistry., *84*:105–120, 1986.

114. Liposits Z.S., Sievers L., Paull W.K. Neuropeptide-Y and ACTH- immunoreactive innervation of corticotropin releasing factor (CRF)- synthesizing neurons in the hypothalamus of the releasing factor (CRF)- synthesizing neurons in the hypothalamus of the rat. Histochemistry., *88*:227–234, 1988.

115. Mannisto P.T. Central regulation of thyrotropin secretion in rats: methodological aspects, problems and some progress. Medical Biology., *61*:92–100, 1983.

116. martin J.B. Brain mechanisms for integration of growth hormone secretion. Physiologist., *22*:23–29, 1979.

117. Mason W.T., Ho Y.W., Eckenstein F., Hatton G.I. Mapping of cholingeric neurons associated with rat supraoptic nucleus: combined immunocytochemical and histochemical identification. Brain Res., *11*:617–626, 1983.

118. Masotto C., Wisniewski G., Negro-Vilar A. Different gamma- aminobutyric acid receptor subtypes are involved in the regulation of opiate-dependent and independent luteinizing hormone-releasing hormone secretion. Endocrinology., *125*:548–553, 1989.

119. MCCann S.M., Rettori V. Gamma amino butyric acid (GABA) controls anterior pituitary hormone secretion. Adv. Biochem. Psychopharmacol., *42*:173–189, 1986.

120. McDonald J.K., Koenig J.I., Gibbs D.M., Collins P., Noe B. High concentrations of neuropeptide Y in pituitary portal blood of rats. Neuroendocrinology., *46*:538–541, 1987.

121. McDonald J.K. Role of neuropeptide Y in reproductive function. Ann. N.Y. Acad. Sci., *611*:258–272, 1990.

122. Medhamurthy R., Dichek H.L., Plant T.M., Bernardini I., Cutler G.B., Stimulation of gonadtropin secretion in prepubertal monkeys after hypothalamic excitation with aspartate and glutamate. J. Clin. Endocrinol. Metab., *71*:1390–1392, 1990

123. Meeker R.B., Swanson D.J., Hayward J.N. Local synaptic organization of cholinergic neurons in the basolateral hypothalamus. J. Comp. Neurol., *276*:157–168, 1988.

124. Meeker R.B., Swanson D.J., Hayward J.N. Light and electron microscopic localization of glutamate immunoreactivity in the supraoptic neclues of the rat hypothalamus. Neuroscience *33*:157–167, 1989.

125. Meister B., Hokfelt T., Geffard M., Oertel W. Glutamate Acid Decarboxylse-and gamma-aminobutytic acid-like immunoreactivities in corticotropin-releasing factor-containing parvocellular neurons of the hypothalamic paraventricular nucleus. Neuroendocrinology., *48*:516–526, 1988.

126. Merchenthaler I., Maderdrut J.L., Altschuler R.A., Petrusz P. Immunocytochemical localization of proenkephalin-derived peptides in the central nervous system of the rat. Neuroscience., *17(2):*325–348, 1986.

127. Michalkiewicz M., Suziki M., Kato M. Evidence for a synergistic effect of somatostatin on vasoactive intestinal polypeptide-induced prolactin release in the rat: comparison with its effect on thyrotropin (TSH)-releasing hormone-stimulated TSH release. Endocrinology., *121(1):*371–377, 1987.

128. Miki N., Ono M., Shizume K. Evidence that opiatergic and A-adrenergic mechanisms stimulate rat growth hormone-releasing factor (GRF). Endocrinology., *114(5):*1950–1952, 1984.

129. Millard W.J. Central regulation of growth hormone secretion. In: *Animal Growth Regulation.* Vol. XVIII. D.R. Crampton, G.J. Huusman and R.D. Martin. Ch. 11, pp. 237–255, New York, Plenum Press, 1989.

130. Miller R.J. PHI and GRF: Two new members of the glucagon/secretin family. Med. Biol., *61:*159–162, 1984.

131. Miselis R.R. The efferent projections of the subfornical organ of the rat: a circumventricular organ within a neural network subserving water balance. Brain Res., *230:*1–23, 1982.

132. Morel G., Pelletier G. Endorphinic neurons are contacting the tuberinfundibular dopaminergin neurons in the rat brain. Peptides., *7:*1197–1199, 1986.

133. Morello H., Caligaris L., Haymal B., Taleisnik S. Inhibition of proestrus LH surge and ovulation in rats evoked by stimulation of the medial raphe nucleus involves a GABA mediated mechanism. Neuroendocrinology., *50:*78–87, 1989.

134. Muller E.E. Neural control of somatotropic function. Physiol. Rev., *67:*962–1048, 1987.

135. Muller E.E. Some aspects of the neurotransmitter control of anterior pituitary function. Pharmacolo. Res., *21:*75–85, 1989.

136. Murakami K., Ganong W. Site at which angiotensin II acts to stimulate ACTH in vivo. Neuroendocrinology., *46:*231–235, 1987.

137. Mural I., Reichlin S., Ben-Jonathan N. The peak phase of the proestrous prolactin surge is blocked by either posterior pituitary lobectomy or antisera to vasoactive intestinal peptide. Endocrinology., *124(2):*1050–1055, 1989.

138. Nakagami Y., Suda T., Yajima F., Ushiyama T., Tomori N., Sumitomo T., Demura H., Shizume K. Effects of serotonin, cyproheptadine and reserpine on corticotropin-releasing factor release from the rat hypothalamus in vitro. Brain Res., *386:*232–236, 1986.

139. Navarra P., Tsagarakis S., Faria M.S., Rees L.H., Besser G.M., Grossman A.B. Interleukins-1 and -6 stimulate the release of corticotropin- releasing hormone-41 from rat hypothalamus in vitro via the eicosanoid cyclooxygenase pathway. Endocrinology., *128:*37–44, 1990.

140. Negoro H., Visessuwan S., Holland R.C. Inhibition and excitation of units in paraventricular nucleus after stimulation of the septum, amygdala and neurohypophysis. Brain Res., *57:*479–483, 1973.

141. Nikolarakis K.E., Loeffler J.P.H., Almeida O.F.X., Herz A. Pre- and postsynaptic actions of GABA on the release of hypothalamic gonadotropin-releasing hormone (GNRH). Brain Res. Bull., *21:*677–683, 1988.

142. Nimi M., Takahara J., Hashimoto K., Kawanishi K. Immunohistochemical identification of corticotropin releasing factor-containing neurons projecting to the stalk-median of the rat. Peptides., *9:*589–593, 1988.

143. Nimi M., Takahara J., Sato M., Kawanishi K. Sites of origin of growth hormone-releasing factor-containing neurons projecting to the stalk-median eminence of the rat. Peptides. *10:*605–608, 1989.

144. Ohtsuka S., Miyake A., Nishizaki T. Vasoactive intentinal peptide stimulates gonadotropin-releasing hormone release from rat hypothalamus in vitro. Acta Endocrinol., *117:*399–402, 1988.

145. Ondo J.G., Dom TR. The arcuate nucleus: a site fir gamma-aminobutyric acid regulation of prolactin secretion. Brain Res., *381:*43–48, 1986.

146. Page R.B. Directional Pituitary Blood Flow: a microcinephotographic study. Endocrinology., *112:*157–165, 1983.

147. Page R.B. The pituitary portal system. In: *Currrnt Topics in Neuroendocrinology: The Morphology of the Hypothalamus and its Connections,* Vol. 7, Editors D. Ganten and D. Pfaff, pp. 1–47, 1986.

148. Page R.B. The anatomy of the hypothalamo-hypophysial complex. In: *The Physiology of Reproduction.* Vol. 1, Chapter 27, Editors E. Knobil and J.D. Neill, pp. 1161–1234, New York, Raven Press, 1988.

149. Palkovits M. Neuropeptides in the Median eminence: their sources and destination. Peptides., *3:*299–303, 1982.

150. Palkovits M. Anatomy of neural pathways affecting CRH secretion. Ann. N.Y. Acad. Sci., *597:*139–148, 1990.

151. Palkovits M., Fekete M., Makara G.B., Herman J.P. Total and partial hypothalamic deafferentations for topographical identification of catecholaminergic innervations of certain preoptic and hypothalamic nuclei. Brain Res., *127:*127–136, 1977.

152. Palkovits M., Kakucska I., Makara G.B. Substance P-like immunoreactive neurons in the arcuate nucleus project to the median eminence in rat. Brain Res., *486:*364–368, 1989.

153. Pares-Herbute N., Diaz J., Astier H., Tapia-Arancibia L. Somatostatin Inhibition of VIP-induced somatostatin release, cyclic AMP accumulation and 45CA;+ uptake in diencephalic cells. Eur. J. Pharmacol., *161:*241–244, 1989.

154. Pelletier G., Leclerc R., Saavedra J.M., Brownstein M.J., Vaudry H., Ferland L., Labrie F. Distribution of B-lipotropin (B-LPH), adrenocorticotropin (ACTH) and A-melanocyte-stiumlating hormone (A- MSH) in the rat brain. I. Origin of the extrahypothalamic fibers. Brain Res., *192:*433–440, 1980.

155. Peterfreund R.A., Vale W.W. Muscarinic cholinergic stimulation of somatostatin secretion from

long term dispersed cell cultures of fetal rat hypothalamus: inhibition by γ-aminobutyric acid and serotonin. Endocrinology, *112*:526–534, 1983.

156. Petraglia F., Vale W., Rivier C. Opioids act centrally to modulate stress-induced decrease in luteinizing hormone in the rat. Endocrinology. *119(6)*:2445–2450, 1986.

157. Pfaff D., Keiner M. Atlas of estradiol-concentrating cells in the central nervous system of the female rat. J. Comp. Neurol. *151*:162–167, 1990.

158. Pittman Q.J., Blume H.W., Renaud L.P. Connections of the hypothalamic paraventricular nucleus with the neurohypophysis, median eminence, amygdala, lateral septum and midbrain periaqueductal gray: an electrophysiologic study. Brain Res., *215*:15–28, 1981.

159. Plotsky P.M. Facilitation of immunoreactive corticotropin-releasing factor secretion into the hypophysial-portal circulation after activation of catecholaminergic pathways or central norepinephrine injection. Endocrinology., *121*:924-930, 1987.

160. Plotsky P.M., Bruhn T.O., Vale W. Central modulation of immunoreactive corticotropin-releasing factor secretion by arginine vasopressin. Endocrinology., *115*:1639–1641, 1984.

161. Plotsky P.M., Cunningham E.T., Widmaier E.P. Catecholaminergic modulation of corticotropin-releasing factor and adrenocorticotropin secretion. Endocr. Rev., *10*:437–458, 1989.

162. Plotsky P.M., Otto S., Sutton S. Neurotransmitter modulation of corticotropin releasing factor secretion into the hypophysial-portal circulation. Life Sci., *41*:1311–1317, 1987.

163. Plotsky P.M., Sawchenko P.E. Hypophysial-portal plasma levels, median eminence content, and immunohistochemical staining of corticotropin-releasing factor, arginine vasopressin, and oxytocin after pharmacological adrenalectomy. Endocrinology., *120*:1361-n1369, 1987.

164. Plotsky P.M., Vale W. Hemorrhage-induced secretion of corticotropin-releasing factor-like immunoreactivity into the rat hypophysial portal circulation and its inhibition by glucocorticoids. Endocrinology, *114*:164–169, 1984.

165. Pretel S., Piekut D. Coexistence of Corticotropin-releasing factor and enkephalin in the paraventricular nucleus of the rat. J. Comp Neurol., *294*:192–201, 1990.

166. Pretel S., Piekut D.T. Coexistence of CRF peptide and oxytocin mRNA in the paraventricular nucleus. Peptides., *11*:621–624, 1990.

167. Racagni G., Apud J.A., Cocchi D., Locatelli V., Juliano E., Casanueva F. Regulation of the prolactin secretion during suckling: involvement of the hypothalamo-pituitary gabaergic system. J. Endocrinol. Invest., *7*:481–487, 1984.

168. Rasmussen D.D., Liu J.H., Worlf P.L., Yen S.S.C. Gonadotropin-releasing hormone neurosecretion in the human hypothalamus: in vitro regulation by dopamine. J. Clin. Endocrinol. Metab., *62*:479–483, 1986.

169. Rauhala P., Tuominen R.K. Opioid peptides in the regulation of TSH and prolactin secretion in the rat. Acta Endocrinol., *114*:383–388, 1987.

170. Rea M.A. VIP-stimulated cyclic AMP accumulation in the suprachiasmatic hypothalamus. Brain Res. Bull., *25*:843–847, 1990.

171. Reichlin S. Neuroendocrine significane of vasoactive intestinal polypeptide. Ann. N.Y. Acad. Sci., *527*:431–449, 1988.

172. Renaud L.P., Bourquet C.W. Neurophysiology and neuropharmacology of hypothalamic magnocellular neurons secreting vasopressin and oxytocin. Prog. Neurobiol., *36*:131–169, 1991.

173. Rettori V., Milenkovic L., Aguila M.C., McCann S.M. Physiologically significant effect of neuropeptide Y to suppress groth hormones release by stimulatin somatostatin discharge. Endocrinology., *126(2)*2296–2301, 1990.

174. Rho J-H., Swanson L.W. Neuroendocrine CRF motorneurons: intrahypothalamic axon terminals shown with a new retrograde- lucifer-immuno method. Brain Res., *436*:143–147, 1987.

175. Richardson S.B., Prasad J.A., Hollander C.S. Acetylcholine, melatonin, and potassium depolarization stimulate release of luteinizing hormone-releasing hormone from rat hypothalamus in vitro. Proc. Natl. Acad. Sci. USA., *79*:2686-2689, 1982.

176. Rivier C., Rivier J., Mormede P., Vale W. Studies of the nature of the interaction between vasopressin and corticotropin-releasing factor on adrenocorticotropin release in the rat. Endocrinology., *115*:882-886, 1984.

177. Roth K.A., Weber E., Barchas J.D. Immunoreactive corticotropin releasing factor (CRF) and vasopressin are colocalized in a subpopulation of the immunoreactive vasopressin cells in the paraventricular nucleus of the hypothalamus. Life Sci., *31*:1857–1860, 1982.

178. Sahu A., Crowley W.R., Kalra S.P. An opioid-neuropeptide-Y transmission line to luteinizing hormone (LH)-releasing hormone neurons: a role in the induction of LH surge. Endocrinology., *126*:876–838, 1990.

179. Saphier D., Feldman S. Effects of stimulation of the preoptic area on hypothalamic paraventricular nucleus unit activity and corticosterone secretion in freely moving rats. Neuroendocrinology., *42*:167–173, 1986.

180. Saphier D., Feldman S. Effects of septal and hippocampal stimulation on paraventricular nucleus neurons. Neuroscience., *20*:749–755, 1987.

181. Saphier D., Feldman S. Catecholaminergic projections to tuberinfundibular neurons of the paraventricular nucleus: II. Effects of stimulation of the ventral noradrenergic ascending bundle: evidence for cotransmission. Brain Res. Bull., *23*:397–404, 1989.

182. Saphier D. Catecholaminergic projections to tuberoinfundibular neurons of the paraventricular nucleus: I. Effects of stimulation of A1, A2, A6, and C2 cell groups. Brain Res. Bull., *23*:389–395, 1989.

183. Sapolsky R.M., Armanini M.P., Sutton S.W., Plotsky P.M. Elevation of hypophysial portal concentrations of adrenocorticotropin secretagogues after fornix transection. Endocrinology., *125*:2881-n2887, 1989.

184. Sato M., Kubota Y., Malbon C.G., Tohyama M.

Immunohistochemical evidence that most rat corticotrophs contain β-adrenergic receptors. Neuroendocrinology, *50:*5777–583, 1989.

185. Sawchenko P.E. Adrenalectomy-induced enhancement of CRF and vasopressin immunoreactivity in parvocellular neurosecretory neurons: anatomic, peptide, and steroid specificity. J. Neurosci., *7:*1093–1106, 1987.

186. Sawchenko P.E., Arias C., Bittencourt J.C. Inhibin β, somatostatin, and enkephalin immunoreactivities coexist in caudal medullary neurons that project to the paraventricular nucleus of the hypothalamus. J. Comp. Neurol., *291:*269–280, 1987.

187. Sawchenko P.E., Bohn M.C. Glucocorticoid receptor-immunoreactivity in C1, C2, and C3 adrenergic neurons that project to the hypothalamus or to the spinal cord in the rat. J. Comp. Neurol., *285:*107–116, 1989.

188. Sawchencko P.E., Swanson L.W. The organization and biochemical specificity of afferent projections to the paraventricular and supraoptic nuclei. In: *Progress in Brain Research. The Neurohypophysis: Structure, Function and Control.,* Vol 60, edited by B.A. Cross and G. Leng, pp. 19–29, Elsevier, 1983.

189. Sawchenko P.E., Swanson L.W. The organization of forebrain afferents to the paraventricular and supraoptic nuclei of the rat. J. Comp. Neurol., *218:*121–144, 1983.

190. Sawchenko P.E., Swanson L.W., Grzanna R., Howe P.R.C., Bloom S.R., Polak J.M. Colocalization of neuropeptide Y immunoreactivity in brainstem catecholaminergic neurons that project to the paraventricular nucleus. J. Comp. Neurol., *241:*138–153, 1985.

191. Sawchenko P.E., Swanson L.W., Jospeh S.A. The distribution and cells of origin of ACTH (1–39)-stained varicosities in the paraventricular and supraoptic nuclei. Brain Res., *232:*365–374, 1982.

192. Sawyer C.H., Everett J.W., Markee J.E., A neural factor in the mechanism by which estrogen induces the release of luteinizing hormone in the rat. Endocrinology., *44:*218–223, 1949.

193. Sawyer C.H., Markee J.E., Hollinshead W.H. Inhibition of ovulation in the rabbit by the adrenergic-blocking agent dibenamine. Endocrinology., *41:*395–402, 1947.

194. Shimatsu A., Kato Y., Matsushita N., Katakami H., Ohta H., Yanaihara N., Imura H. Serotonin stimulates vasactive intestinal polypeptide release from rat hypothalamus in vitro. Brain Res., *264:*148–151, 1983.

195. Shimatsu A., Kato Y., Matsushita N., Katakami H., Yanaiahara N., Imura H. Effects of glucagon, neurotensin, and vasoactive intestinal polypeptide on somatostatin release from perfused rat hypothalamus. Endocrinology., *110(6):*2113–2117, 1982.

196. Silverman A-J. The gonadotropin-releasing hormone (GnRH) neuronal systems: immunocytochemistry. In: *The Physiology of Reproduction.* Ch. 29. Editors E. Knobil and J. Neill, pp. 1283-1304, New York, Raven Press, 1988.

197. Silverman A-J., Hoffman D.L., Zimmerman E.A. The descending afferent connections of the para-

ventricular nucleus of the hypothalamus (PVN). Brain Res. Bull., *6:*47–61, 1981.

198. Silverman A-J., Oldfield B. Synaptic input to vasopressin neurons of the paraventricular nucleus (PVN). Peptides., *5:Suppl 1:*139–150, 1984.

199. Simerly R.B., McCall D., Watson S.J. Distribution of opioid peptides in the preoptic region. Immunohistochemical evidence for a steriod-sensitive enkephalin sexual dimorphism. J. Comp. Neurol. *276:*442–459, 1988.

200. Simerly R.B., Swanson L.W., Gorski R.A. Demonstration of a sexual dimorphism in the distribution of serotonin-immunoreactive fibers in the medial preoptic nucleus of the rat. J. Comp. Neurol., *225:*151–166, 1984.

201. Simerly R.B., Gorski R.A., Swanson L.W. Neurotransmitter specificity of cells and fibers in the medial preoptic nucleus: an immunohistochemical study in the rat. J. Comp. Neurol., *246:*343–363, 1986.

202. Simerly R.B., Swanson L.W. The organization of neural inputs to the medial preoptic nucleus of the rat. J. Comp. Neurol., *246:*312–342, 1986.

203. Sobel D.O. Characterization of angiotensis-mediated ACTH release. Neuroendocrinology., *36:*249–253, 1983.

204. Spinedi E., Negro-Vilar A. Angiotensin II and ACTH release: site of action and potency relative to corticotropin releasing factor and vasopressin. Neuroendocrinology., *37:*446–453, 1983.

205. Steele M.K., Gallo R.V., Ganong W.F. A possible role for the brain renin-angiotensis system in the regulation of LH secretion. Am. J. Physiol., *245(6):*R805–810, 1983.

206. Stobie K.M., Weick R.F. Vasoactive intestinal peptide inhibits luteinizing hormone secretion: the inhibition is not mediated by dopamine. Neuroendocrinology., *49:*597–603, 1989.

207. Suda T., Yajima F., Tomori N., Smuitomo T., Nakagami Y., Ushiyama T., Demura H., Shizume, K. Stimulatory effect acetylcholine on immunoreactive corticotropin-releasing factor release from the rat hypothalamus in vitro. Life Sci., *40:*673–677, 1987.

208. Suda T., Yajima F., Tomori N., Demura H., Shizume K. In vitro study of immunoreactive corticotropin-releasing factor release from the rat hypothalamus. Life Sci., *37:*1499–1505, 1985.

209. Swanson L.W. An autoradiographic study of the efferent connections of the preoptic region in the rat. J. Comp. Neurol., *167:*227–256, 1976.

210. Swanson L.W. The Hypothalamus. In: *Handbook of Chemical Neuroanatomy.* Ch. 5 Edited by A. Bjorkland, T. Hokfelt, and L.W. Swanson, pp. 5:1–124, Amsterdam-London-New York, Elsevier, 1987.

211. Swanson L.W., Cowan W.M. Hippocampal-hypothalamic connections: origin of subicular cortex, not Ammon's Horn. Science., *189:*303–304, 1975.

212. Swanson L.W., Cowan W.M. The connections of the septal region in the rat. J. Comp. Neurol., *186:*621–656, 1979.

213. Swanson L.W., Hartman B.K. The central aminergic system: an immunofluorescence study of

the location of cell bodies and their efferent connections in the rat utilizing dopamine-B-hydroxylase as a marker. J. Comp. Neurol., *163*:467–506, 1975.

214. Swanson L.W., Kuypers H.G.J.M. The paraventricular nucleus of the hypothalamus: cytoarchitectonic subdivisions and organization of projections to the pituitary, dorsal vagal complex, and spinal cord as demonstrated by retrograde fluorescence double-labeling methods. J. Comp. Neurol., *194*:555–570, 1980.

215. Swanson L.W., Sawchenko P.E. Hypothalamic integration: organizaiton of the paraventricular and supraoptic nuclei. Ann. Rev. Neurosci., *6*:269–324, 1983.

216. Swanson L.W., Simmons D.M. Differential steroid hormone and neural influences on peptide and mRNA levels in the CRH cells of the paraventricular nuclues: a hybridization histochemical study in the rat. J. Comp. Neurol., *285*:413–435, 1989.

217. Szentagothai J., Flerko B., Mess B., Halasz B. Hypothalamic control of anterior pituitary function. Akademiai Kiado, 1968.

218. Tago H., McGreer P.L., Bruce G., Hersh L.B. Distribution of choline acetyltransferase-containing neurons of the hypothalamus. Brain Res., *415*:49–62, 1987.

219. Takao T., Hashimoto K., Ota Z. Effect of atrial naturetic peptide on acetylcholone-induced release of corticotropin-releasing factor from rat hypothalamus in vitro. Life Sci., *42*:1199–1203, 1988.

220. Tanaka J., Saito H., Seto K. Involvement of the septum in the regulation of paraventricular vasopressin neurons bythe subfornical organ in the rat. Neurosci. Lett., *92*:187–191, 1988.

221. Tapia-Aranciba L., Astier H. Glutamate stimulates somatostatin release from diencephalic neurons in primary culture. Endocrinology., *123*:2360–2366, 1988.

222. Tapia-Arancibia, Reichlin S. Vasoactive Intestinal peptide and PHI stimulate somatostatin release from rat cerebral cortical and diencephalic cells in dispersed cell culture. Brain. Res., *336*:67–72, 1985.

223. Tapia-Arancibia L., Astier H. Opiate inhibition of K+-induced TRH release from superfused mediobasal hypothalami in rats. Neuroendocrinology., *37*:166–168, 1983.

224. Tappaz M.L., Aguera M., Belin M.F., Oertel W.H., Schmechel D.E., Kopin I.J., Pujol J.F. GABA markers in the hypothalamic median eminence. Adv. Biodhem. Psychopharc., *26*:229–236, 1981.

225. Tappaz M.L., Bosler O., Paut L., Berod A. Glutamate decarboxylase-immunoreactive boutons in synaptic contacts with hypothalamic dopaminergic cells: a light and electron microscopic study combining immunohistochemistry and radioautography. Neuroscience, *16*:112–122, 1985.

226. Tappaz M.L., Wassef M., Oertel W.H., Paut L., and Pujol J.F. Light- and electron-microscopic immunocytochemistry of glutamatic acid decarboxylase (GAD) in the basal hypothalamus: morphological evidence for neuroendocrine γ-amino-

butyrate (GABA). Neuroscience, *9(2)*:271–287, 1983.

227. Tasaka K., Miyake A., Sakumoto T., and Aono T. Dopamine decreases release of luteinizing hormone releasing hormone from superfused rat mediobasal hypothalamus. J. Endocrinol. Invest., *8*:373–376, 1985.

228. Taya K., and Sasamoto S. Inhibitory effects of corticotrophin-releasing factor and B-endorphin on LH and FSH secretion in the lactating rat. J. Endocrinol., *120*:509–515, 1989.

229. Ter Horst G.J., and Luiten P.G.M. Phaseolus vulgaris leuco-agglutinin tracing of intrahypothalamic connections of the lateral, ventromedial, dorsomedial and paraventricular hypothalamic nuclei in the rat. Brain Res. Bull., *18*:191–203, 1987.

230. Theodosis D.T., Paut L., and Tappaz M.L. Immunocytochemical analysis of the gabaergic innervation of oxytocin- and vasopressin-secreting neurons in the rat supraoptic nucleus. Neuroscience, *19*:207–222, 1986.

231. Thind K.K., and Goldsmith P.C. Gabaergic and catecholaminergic interactions in the macaque hypothalamus: double label immunostaining with perioxidase-antiperoxidase and colloidal gold. Brain Res., *383*:215–227, 1986.

232. Thind K.K., and Goldsmith P.C. Infundibular gonadotropin-releasing hormone neurons are inhibited by direct opioid and autoregulatory synapses in juvenile monkeys. Neuroendocrinology, *47*:203–216, 1988.

233. Thornton S.N., Jeulin A., Beaurepaire R., and Nocolaidis S. Iontophoretic application of angiotensin II, vasopressin and oxytocin in the region of the anterior hypothalamus in the rat. Brain Res. Bull., *14*:211–215, 1985.

234. Tinner B., Fuxe K., Kohler C., Hersh L., Anderson K., Jansson A., Goldstein M., and Agnati L.F. Evidence for the existence of a population of arcuate neurons costoring choline acetyltransferase and tyrosine hydroxylase immunoreactivities in the male rat. Neurosci. Lett., *99*:44–49, 1989.

235. Tojo K., Kato Y., Kabayama Y., Ohta H., Inoue T., and Imura H. Further evidence that central neurotensin inhibits pituitary prolactin secretion by stimulating dopamine release from the hypothalamus. Proceedings of the Society for Experimental Biology and Medicine, *181*:517–522, 1986.

236. Toni R., Jackson I.M.D., and Lechan R.M. Neuropeptide-Y-immunoreactive innervation of thyrotropin-releasing hormone-synthesizing neurons in the rat hypothalamic paraventricular nucleus. Endocrinology, *26*:2444–2453, 1990.

237. Tribollet E., Armstrong W.E., Dubois-Dauphin M., and Dreifuss J.J. Extra- ypothalamic afferent inputs to the supraoptic nucleus area of the rat as determined by retrograde and anterograde tracing techniques. Neuroscience, *15*:135–148, 1985.

238. Tsagarakis S., Holly J.M.P., Rees L.H., Besser G.M., and Grossman A. Acetylcholine and norepinephrine stimulate the release of corticotropin-releasing factor-41 from the rat hypothalamus in vitro. Endocrinology, *123*:1962–1969, 1988.

239. Tsagarakis S., Rees L.H., Besser G.M., and Gross-

man A. Neuropeptide-Y stimulates CRF-41 release from rat hypothalami in vitro. Brain Res., *502:*167–170, 1989.

240. Tsuda K., Yokoo H., and Goldstein M. Neuropeptide Y and galanin in norepinephrine release in hypothalamic slices. Hypertension, *14(1):*81–86, 1989.

241. Ungerstedt U. Stereotaxic mapping of the monoamine pathways in the rat brain. Acta Physiol. Scand., *Suppl.367:*1–48, 1971.

242. Van Den Pol A.N., Wuarin J.-P., and Dudek F.E. Glutamate, the dominant excitatory transmitter in neuroendocrine regulation. Science, *250:* 1276–1278, 1990.

243. Van Den Pol A.N. Dual ultrastructural localization of two neurotransmitter-related antigens: colloidal gold-labeled neurophysin-immunoreactive supraoptic neurons receive peroxidase-labeled glutamate decarboxylase- or gold-labeled gaba-immunoreactive synapses. J. Neurosci., *5:*2940–2954, 1985.

244. Van Den Pol A.N. Silver-intensified gold and peroxidase as dual ultrastructural immunolabels for pre- and postsynaptic neurotransmitters. Science, *228:*332–335, 1985.

245. Van Den Pol A.N. Tyrosine hydroxylase immunoreactive neurons throughout the hypothalamus receive glutamate decarboxylase immunoreactive synapses: a double pre-embedding immunocytochemical study with particulate silver and HRP. J. Neurosci., *6:*877–891, 1986.

246. Vincent S.R., Hokfelt T., and Wu J.-Y. Gaba neuron systems in hypothalamus and the pituitary gland. Neuroendocrinology, *34:*117–125, 1982.

247. Vivas L., Chiaraviglio, and Carrer H.F. Rat organum vasculosum laminae terminalis in vitro: responses to changes in sodium concentration. Brain Res., 294–300, 1990.

248. Wahlestedt C., Skagerberg G., Ekman R., Heilig M., Sundler F., and Hankanson R. Neuropeptide Y (NPY) in the area of the hypothalamic paraventricular nucleus activates the pituitary-adrenocortical axis in the rat. Brain Res., *417:*33–38, 1987.

249. Watson S.J., and Akil H. Anatomy of β-endorpin-containing structures in pituitary and brain. In: *Hormonal Proteins and Peptides.* Vol. 10, edited by C.H. Li, pp. 171–201, New York, Academic Press, 1981.

250. Weesner G.D., and Malven P.V. Intracerebral immunoneutralization of β-endorphin and met-enkephalin disinhibits release of pituitary luteinizing hormone in sheep. Neuroendocrinology, *52:*382–388, 1990.

251. Weindl A., and Joynt R.J. The median eminence as a circumventricular organ. In: *Brain Endocrine Interaction: Median Eminence Structure and Function.* edited by K.M. Knigge, D.E. Scott, and A. Weindl, pp. 280–297, Basel, Karger, 1972.

252. Weiner R.I., Findell P.R., and Kordon C. Role of classic and peptide neuromodulators in the neuroendocrine regulation of LH and prolactin. In: *The Physiology of Reproduction.* Ch. 28, edited by E. Knobil and J. Neill, pp. 1235–1281, New York, Raven Press, 1988.

253. Weiss M.L., and Hatton G.I. Collateral input to the paraventricular and supraoptic nuclei in the rat. II. Afferents from the ventral lateral medulla and nucleus tractus solitarius. Brain Res. Bull., *25:*561–567, 1990.

254. Whitnall M.H. Subpopulations of corticotropin-releasing hormone neurosecretory cells distinguished by presence or absence of vasopressin: confirmation with multiple corticotropin-releasing hormone antisera. Neuroscience, *36:*201–205, 1990.

255. Willoughby J.O., Brogan M., and Kapoor R. Hypothalamic interconnections of somatostatin and growth hormone releasing factor neurons. Neuroendocrinology, *50:*584–591, 1989.

256. Willoughby J.O., Beroukas D., and Blessing W.W. Ultrastructural evidence for γ aminobutyric acid-immunoreactive synapses on somatostatin-immunoreactive perikarya in the periventricular anterior hypothalamus. Neuroendocrinology, *46:*268–272, 1987.

257. Willoughby J.O., Jervois P.M., Menadue M.F., and Blessing W.W. Activation of GABA receptors in the hypothalamus stimulates secretion of growth hormone and prolactin. Brain Res., *374:*119–125, 1986.

258. Willoughby J.O., Menadue M.F., and Liebelt H.J. Activation of 5-HT 1 serotonin receptors in the medial basal hypothalamus stimulates prolactin secretion in the unanaesthetized rat. Neuroendocrinology, *47:*83–87, 1988.

259. Willoughby J.O., Menadue M.F., and Liebelt T.H. Activation of serotonin receptors in the medial basal hypothalamus stimulates growth hormone secretion in the unanesthetized rat. Brain Res., *404:*319–322, 1987.

260. Woodhams P.L., Roberts G.W., Polak J.M., and Crow T.J. Distribution of neuropeptides in the limbic system of the rat: the bed nucleus of the stria terminalis, septum and preoptic area. Neuroscience, *8:*677–703, 1983.

261. Yajima F., Suda T., Tomori N., Sumitomo T., Nakagami Y., Ushiyama T., Demura H., and Shizume K. Effects of opioid peptides on immunoreactive corticotropin-releasing factor release from the rat hypothalamus in vitro. Life Sci., *39:*181–186, 1986.

262. Yamada M., and Mori M. Alteration by thyroid hormones of TRH in the rat median eminence: role of the hypothalamic paraventricular nucleus. Exp. Clin. Endocrinol., *93:*104–110, 1989.

CHAPTER 4

The Molecular Biology of Pituitary Hormones

PETER McL. BLACK, M.D., Ph.D.

The molecular biology of hormone production in the pituitary gland is a fascinating story in neuroendocrinology that is still being written. This chapter will summarize information about hormone processing in both the anterior and posterior pituitary, with particular emphasis on the changes that may lead to neoplasia. It is divided into four sections: pituitary hormone processing in the normal anterior pituitary gland; pituitary hormone processing in the posterior pituitary; peptides produced by pituitary adenomas; and our present understanding of changes in the pituitary associated with tumor formation.

PITUITARY HORMONE PROCESSING IN THE ANTERIOR PITUITARY

William Chin has recently summarized the general steps that lead to hormone production in the pituitary as well as in other endocrine tissues (7). The sequence may be summarized as:

A **Gene** is transcribed to
Heteronuclear RNA, which, by
    processing, becomes
Messenger RNA, which is translated into
A **Protein Hormone Precursor,** which, by a
    series of post-translational events,
    becomes
The **Mature Protein Hormone**

The entire process begins in the nucleus with activation of a specific gene that is mediated by regulatory DNA sequences; "heteronuclear" RNA is thereby transcribed and processed in the nucleus to mature messen-

ger RNA (mRNA). This RNA is exported from nucleus to cytoplasm, where ribosomal RNA/protein complexes use it as a template to create a polypeptide precursor to the hormone being synthesized. This precursor differs from the final hormone in that it has a hydrophobic sequence (signal sequence) that guides its transfer to the appropriate cytoplasmic site and it contains fragments that may ultimately be cleaved to create the hormone. The final processing is usually done in the Golgi complex, where glycosylation, acetylation, sulfation, phosphorylation, and other post-translational processing steps may occur to create the final hormone in its definitive primary structure (peptide sequences), secondary structure, and tertiary structure (three-dimensional configuration).

There are three families of hormones in the normal anterior pituitary gland and one family in the posterior pituitary; their molecular biology will now be summarized.

The Prolactin and Growth Hormone Family

Prolactin (Prl), growth hormone (GH), and chorionic somatomammotropin (CS, also known as placental lactogen) comprise the first large family or "superfamily" of pituitary hormones. Their human forms are designated as hPrl, hGH, and hCS, respectively. They are similar in structure and ancestry and may have arisen by duplication of one common gene at an early stage of vertebrate development. It is generally believed that one of the daughter genes from this initial duplication evolved to the Prl gene and the other to the GH and CS genes; the latter genes have more homology with each other than with the prolactin gene (8). Because the CS gene is normally expressed primarily in the placenta, it will not be discussed further here.

Prolactin

The prolactin gene is found as a single sequence on chromosome 6 in humans. In other species, there is a complex family of prolactin genes that are expressed in differing phases of pregnancy and lactation (8).

The human prolactin molecule has 199 amino acids; 16% of these are homologous to hGH (Fig. 4.1). It exists in three immunoreactive forms: "little" prolactin, which has a molecular weight (mw) of 23 kilodaltons (kd), "big" prolactin, with an mw of 48–56 kd, and "void-volume prolactin" with a mw greater than 100 kd (9). These variants appear to be formed after the transcriptional phase of protein formation: "Big" prolactin appears to be a disulfide-bonded dimer of the "little" form. There are also other isohormone forms that represent variant processing.

Regulation of prolactin expression is complex. Dopamine inhibits both the synthesis and the release of prolactin; alpha-melanocyte-stimulating hormone is also an inhibitor of prolactin production at the DNA level. Stress of many kinds can stimulate the release of prolactin into serum; this release appears to be mediated by β-endorphin, which also stimulates transcription of prolactin mRNA. Prolactin expression also appears to be induced by estrogen at transcriptional and post-transcriptional levels (8).

Growth Hormone

There are five genes in the growth hormone family that, in the human, are found contiguously on a segment of chromosome 17, which stretches for 78 kilobases in positions q22–q24 (27). This set of five genes includes the "normal" GH gene, a variant GH gene, two genes that express CS, and a pseudogene for CS. In the normal nonpregnant adult only the "normal" GH gene is expressed.

HGH usually exists as a 20 kd peptide with 191 amino acids (Fig. 4.2), although there is also a 22 kd form created by aberrant processing. These are the two major forms found. There is also, however, "big" hGH, caused by interchain linking of the basic hormone units by disulfide dimers, and a "big-big" form, caused by aggregation of many units. Creation of these variant forms occurs at the post-translational level, that is, after the gene has coded for the polypeptide sequence (10).

HGH expression is regulated at the DNA level by growth hormone-releasing factor (somatocrinin or GRF), a 44-peptide hormone formed in the arcuate nucleus of the hypothalamus. It stimulates GH mRNA translation and transcription as well as cyclic AMP in somatotrope cells to allow secretion of GH. The presence of thyroid hormone and glucocorticoid response elements on the hGH gene suggest that thyroid hormone and corticosteroids may also directly stimulate hGH expression by a transcriptional mechanism. Somatostatin, on the other hand, acts as a growth hormone inhibitory factor by blocking hGH secretion and not transcription.

ACTH and the POMC Family

The second major family of pituitary hormones consists of ACTH and other products of the pro-opiomelanocortin (POMC) gene found on chromosome 6 (13). The POMC gene has 7667 base pairs (bp) in the human, with the following sequences from the 5′ end: exon 1, 86 bp; intron A, 3709 bp; exon 2, 152 bp; intron B, 2886 bp; exon 3, 833 bp. Among the other peptides encoded here are β-lipotropin, β-endorphin, and γ-melanocyte-stimulating hormone. α-Melanocyte-stimulating hormone, which has the same sequence as ACTH 1-13, and corticotropin-like intermediate peptide (CLIP), which has the same sequence as ACTH 18-39, are secreted only by the intermediate lobe and are not normally found in adult humans (17). Figure 4.3 summarizes these various gene products.

POMC is a very large molecule that may be processed in two ways: that used in the anterior pituitary, in which big gamma-MSH, ACTH, and β-LPH are major final products; and that of the neurointermediate pituitary, in which little gamma-MSH and β-endorphin are the end products (17). These prod-

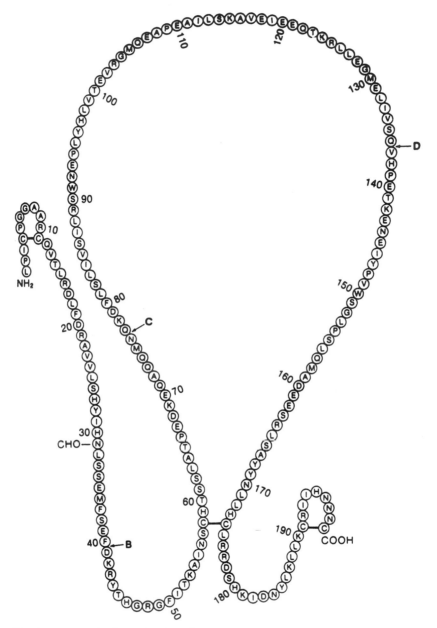

Figure 4.1. The human prolactin molecule. The human prolactin amino acid sequence is displayed in the single-letter amino acid code: A = alanine; R = arginine; N = asparagine; D = aspartic acid; C = cysteine; Q = glutamine; E = glutamic acid; G = glycine, H = histidine; I = isoleucine; L = leucine; K = lysine; M = methionine; F = phenylalanine; P = proline; S = serine; T = threonine; W = tryptophan; Y = tyrosine; V = valine. Disulfide bonds (C-C) are indicated. The bold-lettered arrows indicate the points at which the coding region of the prolactin gene is interrupted by introns. Intron A, which is located in the signal peptide, is not shown in this diagram of the secreted prolactin molecule. CHO indicates a potential N-linked glycosylation site at amino acid 31. (Reproduced with permission from Cooke N.E. Prolactin: normal synthesis, regulation, and actions. In: *Endocrinology,* 2nd ed. vol. 1, edited by L.J. Degroot, pp. 384–400, Philadelphia, W.B. Saunders, 1989.)

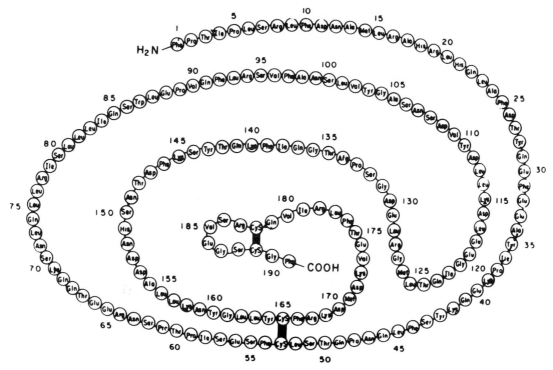

Figure 4.2. Covalent structure of GH. (Reproduced with permission from Chawla R.K., Parks J.S., Rudman D. Structural variants of human growth hormone: bio- chemical, genetic and clinical aspects. Annu. Rev. Med., *34*:519–547, 1983.)

ucts, including ACTH, are the result of cleavage from the longer POMC molecule (Fig. 4.4).

The Glycoprotein Hormones

The glycoprotein hormones comprise the third major family of pituitary hormones and include thyroid-stimulating hormone (TSH), follicle-stimulating hormone (FSH), luteinizing hormone (LH), and human chorionic gonadotropin (hCG). They differ significantly in their structure from the prolactin and POMC families in that they are dimeric, noncovalently associated molecules that share a common α subunit and depend on hormone-specific β subunits for their differential activity (6). The β subunits for TSH, FSH, and LH have a 40% homology with each other (Fig. 4.5). Each subunit contains multiple disulfide linkages and requires complex folding to interact with its receptor. Only a complete hormone of α and β subunits is biologically active, and its synthesis requires a number of events including gly-

cosylation, folding, and association of subunits as well as transcription of the subunits themselves (Fig. 4.6). Under normal conditions, the α subunit is produced in greater quantities than the β subunit.

In the human α subunit gene, the region between -178 and -111 is required for expression of the gene products. In the mouse, however, *cis*-acting promoter elements upstream of position -177 are important, demonstrating different elements than those acting in the human pituitary (28).

Other Peptides in the Normal Anterior Pituitary

Galanin

Galanin is a neuropeptide that is of increasing interest to neuroendocrinologists. It regulates prolactin and growth hormone secretion in animals and, in rats, is coexpressed with prolactin and growth hormone (15). In humans, galanin immunoactivity is found in corticotrophes but not in thyrotrophes or gonadotrophes (16). In one series of pituitary tumors, galanin was expressed in a number of adenomas of varying kinds, including 50% of 18 nonfunctioning pituitary adenomas, 2 of 14 prolactinomas, 19 of 22 patients with Cushing's disease, and 5 of 11 growth-hormone-secreting tumors (16). Most of the tumors that contained galanin also had ACTH immunoreactivity. It therefore appears that galanin is coexpressed with adrenocorticotropin in human pituitaries, in both normal and neoplastic states.

Other peptides, such as vasoactive interstitial polypeptide (VIP) and neuromedin B, are also found in anterior pituitary cells.

Posterior Pituitary Peptides

Peptides found in the posterior pituitary are not synthesized there; rather, they are transported from the magnocellular neurons of the supraoptic and paraventricular nuclei of the hypothalamus and stored in the nerve terminals of the posterior lobe. There are two peptides involved: arginine vasopressin (AVP, also called antidiuretic hormone or ADH) and oxytocin. Each carries with it a specific neurophysin, a large carrier molecule that is synthesized with it and accompanies it as it is released from the nerve terminal.

AVP is a small peptide with nine amino acids whose structure is as follows: **Cys. Tyr. Gln. Asn. Cys. Prl. Arg. Gly (NH2).** It is configured, in part, by a disulfide bond between the two cysteine residues (4). In the rat, arginine vasopressin is derived from a 145-amino acid precursor that contains AVP, a neurophysin, a glycosylated fragment, and a signal peptide. Over a period of 1.5 hours, the AVP precursor moves along axons to the posterior pituitary; some cleavage of "real"

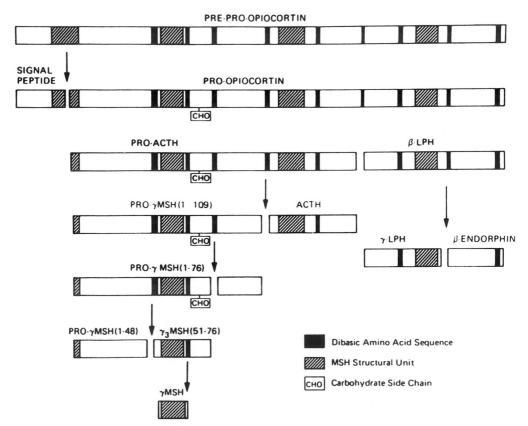

Figure 4.3. Pro-opiomelanocortin and derived proteins. (Reproduced with permission from Hale A.C., Rees L.H. ACTH and related peptides. In: *Endocrinol-* *ogy.* 2nd. ed., vol. 1., edited by L.J. Degroot, pp. 363–373, Philadelphia, W.B. Saunders, 1989.)

Anterior Pituitary

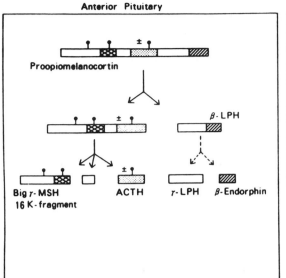

Neurointermediate Pituitary
Extrapituitary Tissues

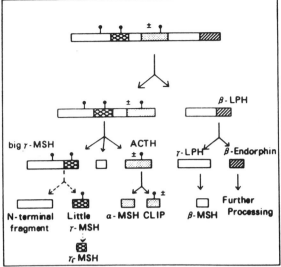

Figure 4.4. Processing of pro-ACTH/β-LPH in the anterior pituitary *(left)* and the neurointermediate pituitary *(right)*. (Reproduced with permission from Imura H.,

Nakai Y., Nakao K., *et al.* Biosynthesis and distribution of opioid peptides. J. Endocrinol. Invest. 6:139–149, 1983.)

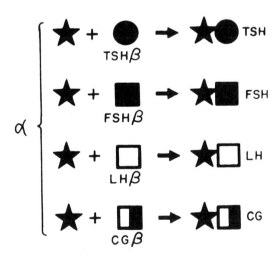

Figure 4.5. Subunit nature of the glycoprotein hormones. Each glycoprotein hormone is comprised of two different glycopeptide subunits called α and β, which are products of separate genes. The common α subunit *(star)* associates with a specific β subunit in a noncovalent fashion to yield the biologically active dimer. The four hormones in this family are TSH, FSH, LH, and CG. (Reproduced with permission from Chin W.W. Biosynthesis of the glycoprotein hormones. In: *Secretory tumors of the pituitary gland,* edited by P.McL. Black, N.T. Zervas, E.C. Ridgway, and J.B. Martin, pp. 327–342, New York, Raven Press, 1984.)

AVP occurs during the transport process. Most AVP is released into the blood stream along with its neurophysin. A similar set of events probably occurs in the release of human vasopressin.

Oxytocin is closely related to arginine vasopressin, with a structure as follows (19): **Cys. Tyr. Gln. Asn. Cys. Prol. Leu. Gly. (NH2).** Like AVP, it is synthesized in the magnocellular neurons of the supraoptic and paraventricular nucleus of the hypothalamus, but it is synthesized by individual cells in these groups that are different from those that synthesize AVP. The oxytocin gene has three exons and two introns. The peptide is synthesized as a precursor that has the following structure: **signal peptide-Oxytocin-Gly.Lys.Arg-neurophysin-His.** Like AVP, it is released from neuronal processes in the posterior lobe of the pituitary gland with a specific neurophysin from which it must be cleaved to have activity.

PEPTIDES PRODUCED BY PITUITARY ADENOMAS

Monoclonality

Pituitary tumors might arise from one aberrant cell or due to a "field" effect on a num-

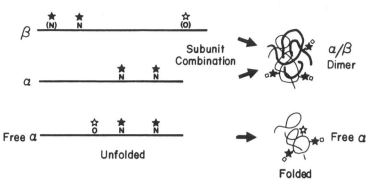

Figure 4.6. Complex structures of the subunits of the glycoprotein hormone. Subunits are glycosylated with carbohydrate moieties attached via either N- or O-glycosidic linkages. *Left,* structures of the subunits in the unfolded forms in schematic fashion. The *β* subunits may have one or two N-glycosidic linkages *(solid stars)* and hCGβ contains four O-glycosidic linkages *(open stars).* The common *α* subunit contains two N-linked oligosaccharides. The free or unassociated *α* subunit differs from the associated *α* subunit by an additional O- linked sugar group. This alteration prevents the free *α* subunit from combining with the *β* subunits. *Right,* the *β* and associated *α* subunits may combine after appropriate folding to yield the active *α/β* dimer. Finally, further modifications and additions to the oligosaccharides occur *(squares).* (Reproduced with permission from Chin W.W. Biosynthesis of the glycoprotein hormones. In: *Secretory tumors of the pituitary gland,* edited by P.McL. Black, N.T. Zervas, E.C. Ridgway, and J.B. Martin, pp. 327–342, New York, Raven Press, 1983.)

ber of cells. There has been controversy for some time about the possibility that pituitary adenomas may be the result of a generalized response of the pituitary to overstimulation by hypothalamic factors. One way of testing this possibility is to evaluate whether the daughter cells arise from one precursor (are monoclonal) or from many (are polyclonal). This assessment can be made with molecular biological techniques through an analysis of restriction fragment length polymorphisms and allelic X chromosome inactivation patterns based on the Lyons hypothesis of random X inactivation. The principle is to examine the differential expression of maternal and paternal genes on the X chromosome, if both the maternal and paternal genes are activated in the tissue, it is polyclonal; if only one or the other gene is activated, it is monoclonal. This can be compared with the pattern in leukocytes or other somatic cells.

Herman *et al.* applied this technique to different types of pituitary adenomas and found that all somatotroph and lactotroph adenomas and three of four corticotroph adenomas appeared to be monoclonal (14). Alexander *et al.* used methylation analysis of the phosphoglycerate kinase and hypoxanthine phosphoribosyltransferase (HPRT) genes in patients with nonfunctioning adenomas (1).

They compared the X-inactivation patterns in tumor cells with those from patients' control blood leukocytes and demonstrated that all six tumors in their series were monoclonal. Jacoby *et al.* examined three adenomas with similar results (18). These data suggest that, with the possible exception of some ACTH-producing adenomas, most pituitary adenomas arise from a single cell that becomes neoplastic rather than by stimulation of a number of cells by hypothalamic factors.

Peptides Produced in Cushing's Disease

Lloyd *et al.* looked at the distribution of pro-opiomelanocortin messenger RNA in 17 nonfunctional and 7 hypersecreting adenomas with corticotroph staining (24). In situ hybridization demonstrated that only a minority of the adenomas had expression of POMC messenger RNA. This suggests that the tumor cells overproduce ACTH selectively.

Peptides in Acromegaly

Lloyd *et al.* examined growth hormone and prolactin messenger RNA in 10 prolactinomas and 16 growth-hormone-secreting adenomas using in situ hybridization (25). Growth-hormone-secreting adenomas had both growth hormone and prolactin expression, indicating that the neoplastic process "turns on" both genes.

Hyperprolactinemia

Serum prolactin levels depend on estrogen levels in humans: Control occurs at the level of transcription of the prolactin gene, at mammotrope differentiation, and with neuroendocrine modulation (8). Transcriptional control occurs by enhancing the binding of estrogen nuclear receptors to 1.2-2.0 kilobases 5' to the start of transcription. There may also be a second sustaining mechanism through the hypothalamus, as it is known that estrogen induces an active suppression of hypothalamic dopamine secretion, inhibiting the short feedback loop on prolactin (3). Finally, estrogen increases the number of prolactin-secreting cells in the pituitary.

Glycoprotein Adenomas

Immunohistochemistry has shown that many "nonfunctional" pituitary tumors synthesize glycoprotein subunits (5). Scippo *et al.* used northern blot analysis to evaluate 10 "nonfunctional" pituitary adenomas and found that LH-β mRNA was detectable in three cases, FSH-β in five cases, and α subunit in one case (32). Oppenheim *et al.* used a new monoclonal antibody to the α subunit to evaluate its expression in nonfunctioning adenomas and in growth-hormone-producing adenomas; 22% of patients with nonfunctioning adenomas and 37% of acromegalic patients had elevated plasma levels of the α subunit (29). Jameson et al. have also demonstrated that nonfunctioning adenomas commonly expressed glycoprotein hormone genes (19).

Molecular biological techniques can be combined with more traditional regulation studies in tissue culture. Klibanski *et al.* noted that three out of four patients with α-secreting pituitary tumors had decreases of α subunit concentrations in serum with bromocriptine administration. Dopamine diminished the in vitro expression of the α subunit mRNA in a tissue culture preparation of the tumor from one such patient (20). A patient with an LH-secreting tumor showed an increase in LH with an LRH analogue; bromocriptine led to a reduction in serum LH (21).

Chromogranin-A

Chromogranin-A is a peptide associated with secretory granules in neuroendocrine cells. Pituitary tumors that produce chromogranin–A include glycoprotein hormone-producing tumors, null cell adenomas, and some others. Looking at the potential control of gonadotropin-releasing hormone on secretion of FSH and LH in these tumors, Song *et al.* found that gonadotropin-releasing hormone increased FSH and LH secretion in tumors that stained for chromogranin-A (34). Dexamethasone also increased chromogranin-A as well as FSH and LH secretion.

Activin

Activins are gonadal polypeptides that stimulate FSH release by pituitary gonadotrophins. They are formed by two inhibin subunits that are part of the TGF β gene family. In a series of glycoprotein-secreting adenomas studied in culture, Alexander et al. demonstrated that activin did not cause FSH release, which indicates the existence of an independent hormonal mechanism that uncouples secretion from activin stimulation (2).

ONCOGENESIS IN PITUITARY TUMORS

Prolactinoma

One of the most interesting models of pituitary tumor formation is the induction of prolactinomas in Fisher 344 rats by the implantation of subcutaneous estrogen. The Fisher 344 rat is prone to develop a number of tumors spontaneously, including pituitary adenomas, leukemia, mammary tumors, and testicular interstitial cell tumors (31). It is particularly susceptible to the induction of prolactinomas by estrogen implantation. The dysfunction in pituitary cells that leads to tumor formation has been examined by El-Azouzi *et al.,* who used an established model of hyperprolactinemia in Fisher 344 rats to demonstrate the importance of sustained receptor stimulation (11). Estrogen capsules were implanted subcutaneously for periods of time ranging from 30 to 120 days. If they were removed after time intervals of less than 60 days, hyperplastic changes in the pituitary regressed. Galanin immunoreactivity and kallikrein expression were induced during the time of estrogen stimulation (12, 15). If the implants were left longer than 60 days, however, there was autonomous tumor formation. This killed the animal despite subsequent removal of the capsule. This phenomenon was thought to be a result of two mechanisms: chemical induction of tumors by estrogen, and mechanical disinhibition caused by hypothalamic compression by the large tumor.

El-Azouzi et al. demonstrated that immunostaining for dopa decarboxylase in the hypothalamus was absent in animals with autonomous tumor formation, and hypothesized that it was the estrogen-mediated release from dopamine suppression that allowed tumors to develop. In analyzing the greater susceptibility of some strains to tumor formation, Shepel et al. suggested that a polymorphism of the rat prolactin gene may be important (33). They described an Alu-like allele whose absence leads to the formation of tumors that are larger than those of animals that have the insertion in the prolactin allele.

Growth-Hormone-Secreting Adenomas

Several hormones that act as growth factors use G proteins to transmit their signals as secondary messengers. An interesting discovery in growth-hormone-secreting tumors is that some carry mutations for the gene encoding the α chain of Gs. These inhibit the intrinsic GTP-ase that stabilizes the protein in its active confirmation, so that the adenyl cyclase is constitutively active as the putative oncogene "Gsp." Spada et al. found no clinical differences between tumors that bore this mutation and those that did not (35). A recent article looked at a number of other human tumors for mutations that might be placed out of these two amino acids. The first showed mutations that replaced arginine 179 with either cysteine or histidine. These were found primarily in the adrenal cortex. More interesting and relevant here, 18 out of 22 growth hormone-secreting pituitary tumors had Gs mutations, suggesting that the G protein α chain genes may have oncogenic mutations within them (23). No particular clinical pattern characterized this group of tumors (22).

New techniques in studying oncogenes in the pituitary are described by Windle et al.,

who directed SV-40 large T antigen into anterior pituitary of transgenic mice using the promoter enhancing region from the human glycoprotein hormone α subunit gene (36). These mice developed anterior pituitary tumors and expressed α subunit proteins, but not β subunit proteins. The α subunit was regulated by GnRH.

CONCLUSION

The application of molecular biology to the study of pituitary hormone regulation has allowed the recognition of important relationships between anterior and posterior pituitary hormones, and the characterization of factors that are important in the control of their synthesis and release. In addition, these techniques now promise to provide insight into the pathogenesis of pituitary tumors.

ACKNOWLEDGMENTS

I am grateful to Drs. Gary Richardson, Bill Chin, and Rona Carroll for their comments and suggestions for this chapter.

REFERENCES

1. Alexander J.M., Biller B.M., Bikkal H., et al. Clinically nonfunctioning pituitary tumors are monoclonal in origin. J. Clin. Invest., 86:336–340, 1990.
2. Alexander J.M., Jameson J.L., Bikkal H.A., et al. The effects of activin on follicle-stimulating hormone secretion and biosynthesis in human glycoprotein hormone-producing pituitary adenomas. J. Clin. Endocrinol. Metab. 72:1261–1267, 1991.
3. Azad N., Nayyar R., Tentler J., et al. Anatomical and functional effects of estrogen-induced prolactinomas in the rat hypothalamus. J. Exp. Pathol. 4:237–249, 1989.
4. Baylis P.H. Vasopressin and its neurophysin. In: Endocrinology, 2nd ed., vol. 1., edited by L. J. Degroot, pp. 213–225, Philadelphia, W.B. Saunders, 1989.
5. Black P.M., Hsu D.W., Klibanski A., et al. Hormone production in clinically nonfunctioning pituitary adenomas. J. Neurosurg. 66:244–250, 1987.
6. Chin W.W. Biosynthesis of the glycoprotein hormones. In: Secretory Tumors of the pituitary gland, edited by P.McL. Black, N.T. Zervas, E.C. Ridgway, and J.B. Martin, New York: Raven Press, 327-342, 1984.
7. Chin W.W. Hormonal regulation of gene expression. In: Endocrinology, 2nd ed., vol. 1., edited by L.J. Degroot, pp. 6–15, Philadelphia, W.B. Saunders, 1989.
8. Cooke N.E. Prolactin: normal synthesis, regulation, and actions. In: Endocrinology, 2nd ed., vol. 1., edited by L.J. Degroot, pp. 384–400, Philadelphia, W.B. Saunders, 1989.
9. Cooke N.E., Coit D., Chine J., et al. Human prolac-

tin: cDna structural analysis and evolutionary comparisons. J. Biol. Chem. *256*:4007–4016, 1981.

10. Daughaday W.H. Growth hormone: normal synthesis, secretion, control, and mechanisms of action. In: *Endocrinology,* 2nd ed. vol. 1., edited by L.J. Degroot, pp. 318–330, Philadelphia: W.B. Saunders, 1989.

11. El-Azouzi M., Hsu D.W., Black P.M., *et al.* The importance of dopamine in the pathogenesis of experimental prolactinomas. J. Neurosurg. *72*:273–281, 1990.

12. Fuller P.J., Matheson B.A., MacDonald R.J., *et al.* Kallikrein gene expression in estrogen-induced pituitary tumors. Mol. Cell. Endocrinol. *60*:225–232, 1988.

13. Hale A.C., Rees L.H. ACTH and related peptides. In: *Endocrinology,* 2nd. ed., vol. 1., edited by L.J. Degroot, pp. 363–373, Philadelphia, W.B. Saunders, 1989.

14. Herman V., Fagin J., Gonsky R., *et al.* Clonal origin of pituitary adenomas. J. Clin. Endocrinol. Metab. *71*:1427–1433, 1990.

15. Hsu D.W., El-Azouzi M., Black P.M., *et al.* Estrogen increases galanin immunoreactivity in hyperplastic prolactin-secreting cells in Fisher 344 rats. Endocrinology *126*:3159–3167, 1990.

16. Hsu D.W., Hooi S.C., Hedley-Whyte E.T., *et al.* Coexpression of galanin and adrenocorticotropic hormone in human pituitary and pituitary adenomas. Am. J. Pathol. *138*:897–909, 1991.

17. Imura H., Nakai Y., Nakao K., *et al.* Adrenocorticotropic hormone and related peptides in human tissue. In: *Secretory tumors of the pituitary gland,* edited by P.McL. Black, N.T. Zervas, E.C. Ridgway, and J.B. Martin, pp. 227–244, New York, Raven Press, 1984.

18. Jacoby L.B., Hedley-Whyte E.T., Pulaski K., *et al.* Clonal origin of pituitary adenomas. J. Neurosurg. *734*:731–735, 1990.

19. Jameson J.L., Klibanski A., Black P.M., *et al.* Glycoprotein hormone genes are expressed in clinically nonfunctioning pituitary adenomas. J. Clin. Invest *80*:1472–1478, 1987.

20. Klibanski A., Shunik M.A., Bikkal H.A., *et al.* Dopaminergic regulation of alpha-subunit secretion and messenger ribonucleic acid levels in alpha-secreting pituitary tumors. J. Clin. Endocrinol. Metab. *66*:96–102, 1988.

21. Klibanski A., Deutsch P.J., Jameson J.L., *et al.* Luteinizing hormone-secreting pituitary tumor: biosynthetic characterization and clinical studies. J. Clin. Endocrinol. Metab. *64*:536–542, 1987.

22. Landis C.A., Harsh G., Lyons J., *et al.* Clinical characteristics of acromegalic patients whose pituitary tumors contain mutant G_s protein. J. Clin. Endocrinol. Metab. *71*:1416–1420, 1990.

23. Landis C.A., Masters S.B., Spada A., *et al.* GTPase inhibiting mutations activate the α chain of G_s and stimulate adenylyl cyclase in human pituitary tumours. Nature *340*:692–696, 1989.

24. Lloyd R.V., Fields K., Jin. L., *et al.* Analysis of endocrine active and clinically silent corticotropic adenomas by in situ hybridization. Am. J. Pathol. *137*:479–488, 1990.

25. Lloyd R.V., Cano M., Chandler W.F., *et al.* Human growth hormone and prolactin secreting pituitary adenomas analyzed by in situ hybridization. Am. J. Pathol. *134*:604–613, 1989.

26. Lyons J., Landis C.A., Harsh G., *et al.* Two G protein oncogenes in human endocrine tumors. Science *249*:655–659, 1990.

27. Miller W.L., Eberhardt N.L., Baxter J.D. Growth hormone genes. In: Secretory tumors of the pituitary gland, edited by P.McL. Black, N.T. Zervas, E.C. Ridgway, and J.B. Martin, pp. 135–144, New York, Raven Press, 1984.

28. Ocran K.W., Sasrapura V.D., Wood W.M., *et al.* Identification of cis-acting promoter elements important for expression of the mouse glycoprotein hormone alpha-subunit gene in thyrotropes. Mol. Endocrinol. *4*:766–772, 1990.

29. Oppenheim D.S., Kana A.R., Sangha J.S., *et al.* Prevalennce of alpha-subunit hypersecretion in patients with pituitary tumors: clinically nonfunctioning and somatotroph adenomas. J. Clin. Endocrinol. Metab. *70*:859–864, 1990.

30. Pickering B.T. Oxytocin and its neurophysin. In: *Endocrinology,* 2nd. ed., vol. 1., edited by L.J. Degroot, pp. 230–237, Philadelphia, W.B. Saunders, 1989.

31. Sass B., Rabstein L.S., Madison R., *et al.* Incidence of spontaneous neoplasms in F344 rats throughout the natural life-span. J. Natl. Canc. Inst. *54*:1449–1456, 1975.

32. Scippo M.L., Beckers A., Frankenne F., *et al.* Adenohypophysis hormone gene products in 14 pituitary adenomas: analysis by immunohistochemistry and northern blotting. Arch. Int. Physiol. *99*:135–140, 1991.

33. Shepel L.A., Gorski J. Relationship of polymorphisms near the rat prolactin. N-ras, and retinoblastoma genes with susceptibility to estrogen-induced pituitary tumors. Cancer Res. *50*:7920–7925, 1990.

34. Song J.Y., Jin L., Chandler W.F., *et al.* Gonadotropin-releasing hormone regulates gonadotropin beta-subunit and chromogranin-B messenger ribonucleic acids in cultured chromogranin-A-positive pituitary adenomas. J. Clin. Endocrinol. Metab. *71*:622–630, 1990.

35. Spada A., Arosio M., Bochicchio D., *et al.* Clinical, biochemical, and morphological correlates in patients bearing growth hormone-secreting pituitary tumors with or without constitutively active adenylyl cyclase. J. Clin. Endocrinol. Metab. *71*:1421–1426, 1990.

36. Windle J.J., Weiner R.I., Mellon P.L. Cell lines of the pituitary gonadotrope lineage derived by targeted oncogenesis in transgenic mice. Mol. Endocrinol. *5*:597–603, 1990.

CHAPTER 5

Hormonal Effects on Brain Function

P. MURALI DORAISWAMY, M.D., K. RANGA KRISHNAN, M.D., CHARLES B. NEMEROFF, M.D., Ph.D.

INTRODUCTION

The brain is an exquisitely plastic organ that develops, grows, differentiates, and ages in response to environmental stimuli, behavior, and neural inputs. Hormones and neuromodulatory peptides arc the most important mediators of such neural plasticity, and their actions on the brain are mediated by specific- and often multiple-receptor proteins expressed by specific neuronal and non–neuronal brain cells. Hormonal influences on the brain can be broadly categorized into "organizational" and "activational (30)." Organizational effects are those produced during neuronal differentiation, growth, and development. These effects result in structural changes in the central nervous system and in the "permanent" organization of brain capacity and function. An example of this is the role of gonadal hormones in the sex–specific development of normal mating behavior (30). In contrast, "activational" influences are reversible effects produced by hormones to modify pre-established patterns of brain function. Several neuropeptides exert profound activational influences (42, 46). The effects of corticotropin–releasing factor (CRF) to regulate behavioral responses to acute stress as well as the ability of bombesin, a gastrin–releasing peptide homologue, to alter central thermoregulation in a state–dependent manner are examples of the latter.

An important evolving concept is that hormones and peptides often have effects on the brain that are harmonious with but independent of their peripheral effects. The (postulated) induction of maternal behavior by oxytocin, drinking behavior by angiotensin and related peptides, anxiety and arousal by CRF, hunger by insulin, and satiety by cholecystokinin are examples of how effects of hormones on the brain may complement and interact with their well–documented peripheral effects.

In the past few years, the primary structures of all the known steroid hormone receptors as well as those of two thyroid hormone receptors have been elucidated by the cloning and sequencing of their cDNAs (14). These studies have dramatically improved our understanding of how these hormones control gene expression in the brain. In addition, current evidence suggests that receptor proteins for steroidal and thyroidal hormones may in fact be part of a large family of receptors sharing a common mode of action (14). Combined with the recent development of highly selective pharmacological agonists and antagonists for glucocorticoid and gonadal hormone receptors, these discoveries promise potentially exciting therapeutic applications in neuroendocrinology. This chapter highlights our current knowledge of the pivotal role that adrenal, thyroid, gonadal, and neuropeptide hormones play in modulating central nervous system function.

ADRENAL STEROIDS

Adrenocortical steroids enjoy a unique interrelationship with the brain. CRF from the hypothalamus stimulates the release of

ACTH from the anterior pituitary, which, in turn, stimulates the release of glucocorticoids from the adrenal cortex. Stress, limbic signals, circadian rhythms, and glucocorticoid feedback are the most important mechanisms regulating the activity of the hypothalamo–pituitary–adrenal (HPA) axis. Cortisol is the major circulating glucocorticoid in man. Aldosterone, the major mineralocorticoid in man, is synthesized from corticosterone and secreted in response to angiotensin II, ACTH, and plasma concentrations of sodium and potassium.

Steroid Receptors: Structure and Function

Once released from the adrenal cortex, their lipophilic nature enables steroids to diffuse through the blood–brain barrier and through target neuronal (and non–neuronal) cell membranes in the brain (15). Here, their actions are believed to be mediated by specific intracellular nuclear receptors. However, certain steroid effects, such as fast–feedback, occur in minutes and are perhaps mediated by the recently characterized membrane receptors. For conceptual simplicity, the steroid receptor can be divided into three functional domains. The carboxy–terminus contains the hormone–binding domain. Binding of hormone to the carboxy-terminus induces various structural changes in the receptor that allow its central DNA-binding domain to position and bind with high affinity to specific DNA sequences in the chromatin. The amino–terminus of the receptor then stimulates the transcription of nearby target genes (15). Glucocorticoid regulation of gene expression has been recently reviewed (5).

Type 1 and Type 2 Glucocorticoid Receptor Classes

Pharmacological studies and molecular cloning have revealed that there are at least two classes of adrenosteroid receptors in the brain. The Type 1 glucocorticoid/mineralocorticoid receptor (GCR/MCR), in vitro, has a high affinity for glucocorticoids and mineralocorticoids and is similar to the renal mineralocorticoid receptor (2). However, in vivo, the presence of the enzyme 11-β-hydroxysteroid dehydrogenase in cells of peripheral tissues is believed to confer specificity by metabolizing glucocorticoids and allowing only aldosterone to activate the mineralocorticoid receptor (17). This enzyme is absent in the hippocampus (15), and, here, the Type 1 GCR/MCR is believed to respond to both glucocorticoids and mineralocorticoids. The Type 2 GCR has a low affinity for glucocorticoids and little or no affinity for mineralocorticoids.

The distribution of Type 1 GCR/MCR in the brain is not well known in man, although it is believed to be similar to that in the brains of rodents, where it is found in high densities in the hippocampus (CA1 > dentate > CA3 > ventral) and lateral septum. The Type 2 GCR in rodents exhibits a widespread distribution in the central nervous system (septum, dentate, amygdala, locus ceruleus, hypothalamus, CA3), pituitary, and adrenals. In humans, the Type 2 GCR is found in high densities in the pituitary, followed by the hypothalamus, hippocampus, and amygdala. The distributions of Type 1 and Type 2 GCR in the hippocampus are overlapping, and it is believed that some cells coexpress both receptor classes (5, 11, 12). Highly selective ligands have recently become available for the Type 2 GCR (RU 28362, RU 26988) and the Type 1 GCR/MCR (ZK 91587, RU28318, RU26752). Corticosterone and progesterone have also been shown to exhibit high affinities for the brain GCR. The presence of a Type 3 GCR is yet to be determined. Some types of glucocorticoids also bind to the barbiturate GABA receptor complex.

Binary Hormone Hypothesis of Steroid Action

The functional significance of Type 1 and 2 receptor classes in the brain is not known. In vitro, the Type 1 GCR/MCR is 10 times more "sensitive" to cortisol levels than the Type 2 GCR (5). Based on these differences, Evans and Arriza (5), have proposed the novel hypothesis that the Type 1 MCR is designed to respond to cortisol concentrations in the basal (0.5–50 nM) range, whereas the Type 2 GCR responds to cortisol concentrations in higher (50 nM–100 nM) ranges (such as those occurring during stress). Potentially, the two classes of glucocorticoids, with high and low affinity, could provide a continuum of control and expand the range of physiological responses. Thus, in this "binary hormone hypothesis," glucocorticoid responses in the brain are thought to result from the coordinate action of Type 1 and Type 2 GCR (5). Aldosterone is believed to act primarily on the Type 1 GCR/MCR (8). Further research, however, is needed to confirm this hypothesis.

Effects on Brain Function

In animal models, glucocorticoids affect a diverse number of brain functions, including electrical activity, neurotransmission, sexual behavior, aggression, conditioned behaviors, memory, brain development, oxygen consumption, sleep, sensory processes, mood and affect, and hippocampal mechanisms during stress and aging (Table 5.1) (2). Glucocorticoids also modulate the activity of tryptophan hydroxylase, glutamine synthetase, glycerolphosphate dehydrogenase, and spermidine acetylase as well as the levels of preproenkephalin and neurotransmitter–stimulated cAMP accumulation (11). The effects of glucocorticoids on the GABA complex is interesting in terms of its role in both anxiety and affective disorders. Glucocorticoid effects on development and mood as well as its neurotoxicity are briefly reviewed below.

Effects on Brain Development

It is difficult to demonstrate directly an absolute necessity for glucocorticoids in specific human developmental processes because steroid-deficient neonates do not often survive (13). However, laboratory animal studies have revealed some important findings. There does not seem to be a critical period for the actions of glucocorticoids, and they may exert many of their effects from the early stages of development. In rat pups, GCR have been detected in the brain on the first postnatal day. Large doses of glucocorticoids suppress brain growth and cell division, with those brain regions and cell types that normally show rapid growth (such as cerebellum and glial cells) being affected the most. Several behavioral milestones may also be delayed (13). Large doses of glucocorticoids inhibit synthesis of DNA, myelin, and gangliosides. In contrast, low doses of gluco-

TABLE 5.1.
Glucocorticoid Effects on Brain Function[a]

Neuroendocrine Function
  Feedback regulation of ACTH and CRF secretion
  Peripheral metabolic effects, stress hormone
Developmental Actions
  Inhibit growth in high doses
  Stimulate growth in low doses
  Regulation of myelination and enzyme levels
Brain Aging
  Age-related hippocampal degeneration
  Age-related loss of glucocorticoid receptors
  Age-related hypercortisolemia
Neurotransmitter Metabolism
  Modulate catecholamine metabolism
  Stimulate serotonin synthesis and metabolism
  Increase choline uptake (?)[b]
  Increase levels of amino acids (except GABA and
    glutamine)
  Modulate sensitivity to opiates
  Regulate brain renin-angiotension system (?)
  Electrical activity
  Dexamethasone decreases hippocampal activity
  Dexamethasone decreases hypothalamic activity
  Cortisol slows EEG activity, increases hippocampal
    firing (?)
Electrical Activity
  Dexamethasone decreases hippocampal activity
  Dexamethasone decreases hypothalamic activity
  Cortisol slows EEG activity, increases hippocampal
    firing (?)
Behavior
  Regulate perception of taste, odor, and auditory
    stimulii
  Feeding and drinking (?)
  Salt appetite (?)
  Mood and affect
  Avoidance and conditioned behaviors
  Maternal behaviors (?)
  Memory consolidation (?)
Sleep
  Reduce REM sleep
CNS metabolism
  Increase intracellular Na, reduce excitability (?)
  Cerebral blood flow and O_2 consumption (?)
  Inhibit oxidation of glucose (?)
  Induce GPDH (glial protein) (?), synapsin
  Regulate blood-brain barrier (?), reduce vasogenic
    edema
  Regulate neuroimmune mechanisms (?)

[a]Many of these effects are inferred from studies of intact or adrenalectomized animals. Some of these effects may be specific to the experimental paradigm used and hence used to be interpreted with caution.
[b](?) indicates precise role has not been proved.

corticoids have been shown to promote growth of cortical neurons and accelerate the synthesis of myelin and the activity of brain enzymes, such as Na/K-ATPase, ∂-GPD, glutamine synthetase, and tryptophan hydroxylase. Adrenalectomy prevents the normally observed developmental increase in tryptophan hydroxylase, the enzyme that converts tryptophan to 5-hydroxytryptophan, an integral step in serotonin synthesis (2, 13). These data suggest that physiological levels of glucocorticoids play an important role in normal brain maturation and that high levels of glucocorticoids may hamper brain development (13). Although it is well established that high levels of prenatal and neonatal stress can alter brain morphology, organization, and behavior, these deleterious effects have not been demonstrated unequivocally to be mediated via GCR.

Effects on Mood and Behavior

A large proportion of patients with Addison's disease (adrenocortical insufficiency) have psychiatric symptoms, including apathy, irritability, and negativity, all of which usually improve with glucocorticoid replacement (2). Further, approximately half of all patients with adrenal tumors or ACTH–dependent Cushing's syndrome (adrenal hypersecretion) exhibit depression. Other symptoms in these patients include insomnia, irritability, drowsiness, delusions, hallucinations, anxiety, REM sleep disturbances, impaired concentration, and fatigue (2). Of considerable interest is the fact that patients with adrenal insufficiency show dramatic increases in sensory detection abilities, such as a 100-fold increase in taste qualities and a 1000-fold increase in detecting odors (14). Patients with Cushing's syndrome reportedly have decreased taste sensation.

Approximately 50 to 70% of patients with major depression (melancholia) show sustained hypercortisolemia, which has been correlated with brain changes such as ventriculomegaly. A recent study (15) prospectively examined the effects of glucocorticoids on verbal memory tasks in three groups of subjects. Depressed patients who did not suppress cortisol (nonsuppressors) when given the synthetic glucocorticoid dexamethasone, were compared to dexamethasone suppressors; healthy volunteers given a single 1-mg dose of dexamethasone were compared to 19 given a placebo; 11 healthy volunteers given 80 mg/day of prednisone for five days were compared to placebo controls. Compared to their respective control groups, all three groups exposed to glucocorticoids made significantly more errors of commission in verbal memory tasks, with no significant change in the rates of errors of omission. These findings support the possibility of specific glucocorticoid–related cognitive impairment. However, it remains to be established whether hypercortisolemia follows or precedes depression and whether glucocorticoid–induced brain changes mediate the cognitive and behavioral symptomatology of depression and Cushing's syndrome. In this regard, it is of interest that, in the late stages of Alzheimer's disease, hypercortisolemia and dexamethasone nonsuppression are often present even in the absence of affective illness.

Neurotoxicity and Hippocampal Effects

The hippocampus, with a high concentration of both types of GCR, is extremely sensitive to the presence of glucocorticoids and is an important neural target for their actions (12, 16). Several, but not all, studies of laboratory animals have concluded that pharmacological or high physiological doses of glucocorticoids precipitate neuronal damage in the hippocampus and accelerate the rate of age–related pyramidal neuronal loss. In aging rats, a correlation has been demonstrated between the severity of age–related neuronal loss in the hippocampus and the severity of age–related glucocorticoid hypersecretion. Adrenalectomy at middle age and a glucocorticoid–free milieu prevented this hippocampal degeneration (16). Glucocorticoid neurotoxicity is accompanied by an increase in reactive microglia and a marked decrease in the densities of cells containing glucocorticoid receptors. Sapolsky (16) has proposed that glucocorticoids do not directly damage neurons, but act by disrupting various biochemical steps in energy metabolism (such as inhibiting glucose uptake), thereby impairing the ability of hippocampal neurons to survive insults. These effects are rapid, occur following as little as 24 hours of exposure to high levels of glucocorticoids, and are receptor-mediated (at least in part). Further, in specific hippocampal areas, glucocorticoids are believed to increase vulnerability to specific insults, including ischemia, excitotoxins, and aging. Sapolsky (16) has noted that dexamethasone binds only weakly to hippocampal glucocorticoid neurons, a finding that may explain why the administration of this steroid following ischemia does not enhance damage. It is difficult to reconcile this literature with the clinical literature describing the neuroprotective effects of high doses of glucocorticoids in head and spinal cord injury (i.e., Meinig and Deisenroth (17)).

Effects on Brain Electrolyte and Fluid Homeostasis

As noted above, glucocorticoids, such as dexamethasone and prednisone have been widely used clinically to reduce vasogenic brain edema and to treat increased intracranial pressure (ICP), although the physiological basis for these effects is not well understood. Many classes of steroids are probably capable of influencing ICP dynamics. This is exemplified by the fact that ICP fluctuates during the menstrual cycle, pregnancy, and during oral contraceptive use. In animal models, glucocorticoids have been shown to inhibit the activity of choroidal plexus Na/K-ATPase, lower K+ levels, reduce choline uptake in the lateral plexus, and reduce the rate of CSF formation (18). A recent study (18) examined the effects of five days of daily oral treatment with 2 mg/kg (with the addition of 0.5 mg/kg body weight subcutaneously on the last two days) of beclamethasone phosphate on CSF formation and choroid plexus transport in 25 rabbits, compared to 25 placebo–treated animals. The steroid-treated group showed a 43% reduction in CSF production rate (measured by ventriculocisternal perfusion with labeled insulin) and significant reductions in Na/K-ATPase activity and choroidal transport capacity (measured in vitro). Further studies are needed to determine whether these effects may be generalized to humans.

Mineralocorticoid Effects on Brain Function

The effects of mineralocorticoids on the central nervous system are poorly understood (2, 8). Mineralocorticoid effects on behaviors relating to food, salt, and water intake have been the subject of several studies with inconsistent results. It is well documented that adrenalectomized animals drink more sodium chloride than do intact animals, and that adrenalectomy alters the brain ratio of intracellular to extracellular sodium and potassium. These effects are sensitive to mineralocorticoid reversal, although it is not known whether they are mediated by neural or peripheral mechanisms. Further studies are also needed to determine the interactions between mineralocorticoids and the renin–angiotensin system in the brain.

Clinical Implications

Adrenocorticoid effects on brain function have far–reaching clinical applications. Glucocorticoid toxicity has been implicated in the normal age–related cognitive impairment, the dementia of Alzheimer's disease, the cerebralatrophy and psychopathology of Cushing's disease, and the cognitive dysfunction of major depressive illness. It is of interest that patients with Alzheimer's disease frequently exhibit hippocampal degeneration as well as hypercortisolemia. The development of selective GCR antagonists will offer potential therapeutic applications as well as investigative probes for these diseases. A further understanding of the effects of glucocorticoids and mineralocorticoids on fluid homeostasis in the brain, and the development of selective steroid agonists, may aid in the treatment of vasogenic edema and intracranial hypertension.

THYROID HORMONES

Thyroid hormones play an important role in the central nervous system, with their most prominent effects being those on the developing central nervous system. Transthyretin synthesis in the choroid plexus may have a role in the transport of thyroxine from the blood to the brain (19). Both thyroxine (T4) and triiodothyronine (T3) are active in the brain, with T3 being more potent than T4. There is now evidence that T4 is actively deiodinated to T3 within the brain, with the rate of conversion being regulated by thyroid state. Two enzymes are believed to be involved in this process and serve to stabilize T3 concentrations in the brain. One deiodinates T4 and is more active in the hypothyroid state, and the other deiodinates T3 and is less active in the hypothyroid state, thus raising T3 concentrations (1).

Thyroid Hormone Receptors

Thyroid hormone effects on the developing brain (and perhaps the adult brain) are believed to be mediated by a specific class or specific classes of intracellular nuclear receptors (4, 20). Such receptors are found on both neuronal and non–neuronal (glial) cells. Neurons contain nuclear receptors for both T3 and T4, and it is believed that about 80% of the T3 found attached to brain T3 receptors is derived from T4 (1). The structure of two thyroid hormone receptors has been elucidated (4). These studies have suggested that thyroid and steroid receptors may be part of a large family of nuclear receptors that, when occupied by a hormone, produce their effects by activating the synthesis of mRNAs that code for specific proteins (4, 21). The thyroid receptor, like the glucocorticoid receptor, is thought to consist of three functional domains that mediate hormone binding, DNA binding, and transcription. The affinity of receptors for T3 is approximately 10 times that for T4 and roughly parallels the biological potency in vivo. The affinity of T3 for neuronal receptors is believed to be higher than that for glial receptors (22). Neuronal T3 receptors are believed to be highly saturated under basal conditions due to local deiodination.

Relation to the Avian Erythroblastosis Virus

The avian erythroblastosis virus (AEV) induces sarcomas and neoplastic transformation of fibroblasts and erythroblasts in vivo; the v–erbA region of the AEV genome is involved in this transformation (20). The thyroid hormone receptor has been identified with multiple c–erbA genes in human chromosomes 3 and 17 and with the v–erbA oncogene product (4, 23). The evidence that dysthyroidism may be involved in neoplastic transformation in the brain has recently been reviewed (24). The presence of multiple c–erbA genes has also suggested the existence of multiple, as yet unidentified, thyroid receptor subtypes.

Effects on Brain Development

Thyroid hormones exert profound influences on brain maturation. Consequently, the ontogenic relationship between thyroid hormone secretion and brain development is of considerable clinical importance. Thyroid hormones exert their effects on CNS development primarily during the so–called critical periods that are characterized by accelerated growth and differentiation (23). In humans, the prenatal increase in circulating T3 levels and T3 receptor densities precedes the peak growth spurt in brain growth and glial replication (22). The source of circulating hormone is the fetal rather than the maternal thyroid gland, because sensitivity to thyroid hormone in the fetus appears almost simultaneously with the onset of fetal thyroid function (13).

Receptors for T3 are present in high concentrations at an early age in the developing brain (with regional differences) and appear to be found preferentially in neurons rather than glia (22). In the human fetus, high affinity T3–binding sites are barely detectable at 10 weeks gestation and increase 10-fold by week 16 (22). T3 receptor density peaks soon after birth (day nine in rats) and declines rapidly thereafter. This decline is associated with an increasing resistance to the actions of thyroid hormones (such as the inability of T4 to stimulate protein synthesis) as the animal matures (13). In humans, this is manifested by the inability to reverse the effects of cretinism if therapy is initiated too late. Further studies are needed to characterize ontogenic changes in distribution and sensitivity of T3 receptors in the human brain.

Thyroid hormones influence behavioral, morphological, and biochemical maturation of the brain (Table 5.2). At the cellular level, by affecting protein synthesis, they regulate growth, myelination, and enzymatic activities of many brain regions (13, 22, 23).

Hyperthyroidism

Exposure to excess concentrations of thyroid hormones initially stimulates DNA synthesis, ODC activity, myelination, and cell division, followed by a premature termina-

TABLE 5.2.
Thyroid Hormone Effects on Brain and Behavior[a]

Effects of Thyroid Excess

Developing Brain
  Premature and abnormal maturation of behavioral
    milestones
  Stimulation followed by premature termination of
    mitosis
  Dysmyelination
  Increase in numbers of glial cells
  Abnormal synaptic contacts in cerebellum
Adult Brain
  Organic delirium and encephalopathy in thyroid
    "storm"
  Apathy, irritability, and other behavioral symptoms

Effects of Thyroid Deficiency

Developing Brain
  Severe mental and skeletal retardation, low IQ
    (cretin)
  Impaired DNA and protein synthesis
  Myelination severely impaired
  Mitochondrial and ion transport enzymes do not
    mature
  Neurotransmitter (GAD, CHAT) metabolism
    impaired
  Region-specific loss of cell number or differentiation
  Reduced dendritic spines in cortical pyramidal
    neurons
  Reduced synaptic arborization in cerebellar
    Purkinje's cells
  Abnormal development of peripheral auditory
    system
Adult Brain
  Psychosis of myxedema, depression, anhedonia,
    hallucinations, delusions of persecution, amnesia,
    dementia (rare)

[a]It must be emphasized that the developing brain is maximally sensitive to thryoid actions during the so-called critical period.

tion of cell mitosis and myelination (13). This results in a large number of glial cells in the cortex. In the cerebellum, T4 administration accelerates the growth of axons and dendrites of Purkinje's cells and parallel fibers, but decreases the numbers of basket and granule cells (13, 21, 22). Exposure to an excess of thyroid hormone accelerates several developmental and behavioral landmarks, such as indices of cerebellar maturation. However, this apparent acceleration is only temporary and is later followed by the development of abnormal behaviors and neurochemical alterations (13).

Hypothyroidism

Hypothyroidism during development results in severe mental and skeletal retarda-

tion. DNA synthesis, myelination, and cellular growth (dendritic spines) are severely impaired. The normal maturational increase of several enzymes, such as those involved in mitochondrial reactions (SDH, NADPH), ion transport (Na/K-ATPase), neurotransmitter metabolism (GAD, CHAT), and myelination (galactosyl transferase) is impaired (13, 22). Specific morphological changes occur in rats thyroidectomized at early development. These include a region–specific reduction in cell number and/or a loss of ability for neuronal differentiation. For example, pyramidal cells in the visual cortex in hypothyroid rats show a reduction in the number of dendritic spines, which can be completely reversed by thyroxine replacement on day 12, partially reversed by treatment on day 15, and are irreversible after day 20 (22). In the olfactory mucosa, thyroid hormones appear to affect the olfactory mucosal surface area and density of neurons but not their ability to differentiate (23). In contrast, in the cerebellum, hypothyroidism retards differentiation and synaptic arborization of Purkinje's cells and does not seem to affect cell number (22, 23). Thyroid hormones also influence the development of the auditory system. Abnormalities in auditory brainstem responses, in thc onset of cvokcd cochlear activity, and in hearing/speech performances have been reported in hypothyroidism.

In human hypothyroidism, the failure to initiate treatment within the first few months after birth may result in a subnormal IQ. Thus, in man, there is a critical period of development, from approximately the end of the first trimester of gestation to six months after birth, when thyroid hormones are essential for normal anatomical, biochemical, and physiological maturation of the central nervous system (22). Further research is needed to elucidate these interactions and to understand the effects of thyroid hormones on the adult brain.

Effects on Adult Brain and Behavior

Thyroid hormone effects on adult brain remain poorly understood. Although the density of thyroid hormone receptors falls as development proceeds, the adult brain continues to exhibit relatively high concentrations of receptors for thyroid hormones.

However, in the adult brain, oxidative metabolism is not stimulated by thyroid hormones (1). Hence, the mechanism of action of T3 and T4 is obscure. In the adult, thyroid hormone dysfunction can sometimes be accompanied by prominent behavioral changes (25).

Profound behavioral changes occur in many patients with hyperthyroidism and include apathy, anxiety and panic attacks, irritability, and emotional lability (25). Organic delirium is one of the hallmarks of thyroid "storm," and, in some patients, deficits persist after treatment, suggesting irreversible brain damage (1). In general, the psychiatric manifestations of hyperthyroidism are reversible with antithyroid therapy (25).

In 1873, Gull (25) first reported that myxedema could result in psychosis. Subsequent studies have confirmed this observation and suggested, in addition, that depression, anhedonia, psychomotor retardation, amnesia, and apathy as well as delusions and hallucinations (persecutory) may accompany myxedema. In some patients, these symptoms may even precede the onset of recognizable myxedema. Thyroid replacement usually reverses these symptoms. Myxedematous "madness" or organic psychosis and dementia may occur in extreme cases. In depressions refractory to thyroxine replacement, electroconvulsive therapy has been reported to be effective (25). Interestingly, many patients with psychiatric illness (major depression, schizophrenia, alcoholism), exhibit subtle forms of thyroid dysfunction demonstrable by endocrine tests, such as elevated or blunted TSH responses to TRH or the presence of antithyroid antibodies. These data have been reviewed by Loosen and Prange (25) and by Nemeroff (26).

GONADAL STEROIDS

Gonadal steroids exert profound permanent and organizational effects on the central nervous system and influence the development of gender–specific patterns of gonadotropin secretion and sexual behavior. Gonadal steroids also exert well–documented activational influences on the adult brain and behavior. Although in some animal models gonadal steroids also appear to exert organizational changes in the adult brain, it is not known whether this is applicable to the adult human brain.

Estrogens, Progestins, and Androgens

Gonadal steroids are synthesized in the cytosol and mitochondria of hormone–producing cells in the testis and ovary, as well as in the adrenal cortex, via sequential enzymatic conversion from cholesterol. Estrogens, progestins, and androgens are the three classes of gonadal steroids, and their secretion in mammals is regulated by the pituitary gonadotropins, luteinizing hormone (LH), and follicle-stimulating hormone (FSH) (1). In humans, estradiol-17-β, progesterone, and testosterone are the principal members of these three classes, respectively, and all three are believed to enter the brain due to their lipophilic nature, although a role for carrier proteins has not been fully determined.

Mechanism of Action and Ontogeny

The actions of gonadal steroids on the brain and other tissues are mediated by specific classes of receptors. It has been suggested, on the basis of structure, that gonadal steroid receptors belong to the family of nuclear receptors (including thyroid and glucocorticoid receptors) that modulate protein synthesis by altering genomic transcription (4, 27). Sensitivity to gonadal steroids develops prenatally; male and female fetuses secrete significant quantities of testosterone and estrogen. The ontogeny of gonadal steroid receptors is not well understood in humans, although significant gonadal steroid binding is demonstrable in several parts of the developing brain. Estrogen receptors are distributed in the hypothalamus, preoptic area, amygdala, and anterior pituitary. Progesterone receptors in the hypothalamus apparently do not respond to corticosterone, whereas those in other parts of the brain do. The distribution of receptors for gonadal steroids matches very closely the areas that have been implicated in sexual behavior. Certain of the rapid effects of gonadal steroids may be mediated by membrane receptors, perhaps by stimulating intracellular cAMP production (28).

Effects of Gonadal Steroids on Brain Development and Dimorphism

Gonadal steroids are important for the development of gender–specific gonadotropin secretory patterns as well as for sexual behavior. Progesterone affects the brain directly. In the hypothalamus, it raises the set-point for body temperature, which is the basis for the postovulatory surge in basal body temperature. In other areas of the brain, it affects sexual behaviors and gonadotropin secretion synergistically with other sex steroids (1).

Estrogens and androgens secreted during critical periods in brain development are believed to determine neuronal gender, i.e., patterns of gonadotropin secretion, sexual orientation, and gender–specific social behavior (29). These effects are believed to begin in the fourth fetal month, after the somatic or genital gender is organized. Dorner (29) suggests that critical periods for the organization of gonadotropin secretory patterns, mating behavior, and gender–specific social behaviors overlap sequentially. In males, following the organization of genital gender, testosterone secreted by the developing testes is believed to affect specific morphological brain changes that result in "male" patterns of rhythms, behavior, and cognition. Androgenization of the female rat abolishes the normal cyclical gonadotropin secretory patterns and female mating behavior (lordosis). The absence of testosterone effects during development results in a female pattern of gonadotropin secretion and sexual behavior (30–33). Studies of testosterone implants in the central nervous system of rats have revealed that the sexual dimorphic nucleus of the preoptic area (SDN POA) and the spinal nucleus supplying the bulbocavernous muscle (SNB) are crucial to the induction of sexual behaviors by gonadal steroids. Testosterone stimulates the growth of neurons in both these areas, which in many species are larger in males than in females. Castration at birth results in a marked decrease in the size of the male SDN POA and SNB, and females treated at birth with gonadal steroids show male–sized nuclei. Transplantation of the SDN POA to the brains of castrated male rats restores mating and gonadotropin-regulating activity (1). In addition to the well–established gender differences in gross volume of the brain and cortex, sexual dimorphism has been reported, albeit inconsistently, in the planum temperale, corpus callosum, amygdala, and cerebellum (34). At the cellular level, studies have suggested gonadal, steroid–responsive gender differences in neuronal number as well as morphology and in neurotransmitter metabolism (35). Further studies are needed, however, to determine whether these differences arise from the effects of gonadal steroids. In addition to differences in brain anatomy, some studies have suggested small differences between males and females in physiological and intellectual functions. In-utero androgenization in the human female (raised as a female) does not affect the cyclic patterns of gonadotropin secretion and normal female mating behavior. However, these females reportedly show an increase in "tomboyish" behavior and in male stereotypic behaviors, a higher IQ, and greater mathematical ability, compared to "normal" females (1). Further studies are needed to confirm these findings.

Gonadal Steroid Metabolism in the Brain

Of great interest is evidence from dozens of studies in primates that has suggested a crucial role for aromatase enzyme in the differentiation of male patterns of cognition and behavior. Aromatization converts testosterone into estradiol and androstenedione into estrone. In primates, aromatase activity is high in the hypothalamus, preoptic area, hippocampus, cortex, and amygdala (36), corresponding to sites of androgen sensitivity and function. Ontogenically, the enzyme appears fairly early in gestation, peaks prenatally, and then declines. Blockade of aromatase or implants of nonaromatizable androgens (DHT) in early life interferes with the androgen–induced differentiation of hypothalamic mechanisms. In adults, it abolishes the expression of androgen–dependent mating behaviors (36). Thus, in androgen–sensitive areas of the brain, such as the hypothalamus, amygdala, and cortex, aromatases may convert, locally, testosterone and androstenedione into estrogens, which, in turn, may modulate the male pattern of neurogenesis, gonadotropin secretion, cognition, and sexual behavior (1, 36, 37). In females, the presence of the estrogen–binding protein α-fetoprotein in blood appears to exclude the local accumulation of high concentrations of estrogen. Additional research is needed to confirm and extend these findings.

Clinical Implications

Gonadal steroids have a critical role in the development of normal mating and social behaviors. It has been hypothesized that abnormalities in prenatal gonadal steroid–induced behavioral differentiation play a role in human heterosexual, homosexual, and transexual behaviors (29), although unequivocal evidence for the latter behaviors is lacking.

The neurodevelopmental effects of gonadal steroids have been linked to gender differences in the prevalence of various psychiatric disorders (35). For example, gonadal steroids are believed by many to play an important role in the pathophysiology of the premenstrual syndrome. Chemical hysterectomy, in which gonadotropin-releasing hormone (GnRH) agonists desensitize anterior pituitary GnRH receptors, which results in interference with gonadotropin secretion, has shown promise in the treatment of the premenstrual syndrome (Rubinow, NIMH personal communication). Estrogen increases plasma levels of fibrinogen and various clotting factors, enhances platelet aggregation, and suppresses antithrombin III and the fibrinolytic system (21). Gonadal steroids, such as oral contraceptives, may thus induce a state of hypercoagulability in the cerebral circulation. A series of retrospective and prospective studies has implicated oral contraceptives as a risk factor in thromoembolic cerebral infarction, subarachnoid hemorrhage, and cerebral venous thrombosis (21), and 60% to 85% of ischemic strokes in oral contraceptive users are in the carotid distribution. Gonadal steroids may also interact with anticonvulsant therapy and with the course of epilepsy. Estrogen and progestins have been shown in both human and animal studies to have epileptogenic and anticonvulsant properties, respectively (21, 38). Conversely, several anticonvulsants have been implicated in oral contraceptive failure (21).

Recent research suggests that estrogen may regulate the activity of dopamine–containing fibers in the nigrostriatal pathway. Consistent with these observations, estrogen has been found also to affect behaviors mediated by the basal ganglia (39). Chorea gravidarum is a rare complication of pregnancy in which gonadal steroids are believed to modulate the activity of basal ganglia previously damaged by rheumatic or hepatic encephalopathy (21). Dyskinesia is occasionally encountered in oral contraceptive users. It usually begins within four months of exposure and resolves upon stopping the medication. These data have been reviewed by Schipper (21). The psychotropic properties of ovarian estrogen have been reviewed by Arushanyan and Borovkova (40).

NEUROPEPTIDES

Over the past three decades, more than 50 peptides have been discovered to be present in the mammalian central nervous system. There is convincing evidence that most of these peptides are present in neurons and serve as chemical messengers modulating a diverse spectrum of brain functions (41, 42). The site of tissue identification has served as a convenient basis for classifying neuropeptides, although it is now clear that most, if not all, peptides have more than one native site. Table 5.3 presents a selected list of neuropeptides, including recent additions to this family, such as the growth factors, neuroleukins, and synapsins.

Neuropeptide Synthesis

There are several important features that serve to group neuropeptides into a single class of chemical messengers. First, neuropeptides are produced only in restrictive groups of neurons and endocrine cells that are derived from embryological precursors of nervous tissue, the so–called APUD cells. In these peptidergic neurons, neuropeptide synthesis is determined by the information stored in the DNA molecule in the nuclear genome. The DNA molecule is transcribed to a precursor mRNA molecule that is then

TABLE 5.3.
Neuropeptide Categories in Brain[a]

Hypothalamic Peptides Modulating Pituitary Function
Corticotropin-releasing hormone (CRF),
    Vasopressin (VP)
Growth hormone-releasing hormone (GHRH),
    Somatostatin (SRIF)
Thyrotropin-releasing hormone (TRH)
Gonadotropin-releasing hormone (GnRH, LHRH)
Neurotensin, Neuropeptide Y

Pituitary Peptides
Prolactin (Prl), Growth Hormone (GH)
Thyrotropin-stimulating hormone (TSH),
    Gonadotropins (follicle-stimulating hormone,
    luteinizing hormone)
Pro-opiomelanocrotin (POMC)
Corticotropin (ACTH)
Corticotropin-like immunoreactive peptides (CLIP)
β-endorphin, β-lipotropic hormone (β-LPH)
Melanocyte-stimulating hormone (α-MSH, γ-MSH)
Oxytocin, Vasopressin, Neurophysins

Brain-Gut Peptides
Vasoactive-Intestinal peptide (VIP)
Somatostatin (SRIF)
Insulin, Glucagon, Pancreatic Polypeptide, Gastrin
Cholecystokinin, Tachykinins (e.g., Substance-P)
Secretin, TRH, Glucagon, Bombesin

Growth Factors
Insulin-like growth factors (IGF-I, IFG-II,
    Somatomedins)
Nerve Growth Factors (NGF), Brain-derived growth
    factors

Opioid Family
Endorphins, Enkephalins (Met-, Leu-), Dynorphins,
    Kytorphin

Neuropeptides Modulating Immune Function
ACTH, Endorphins, Interferons, Neuroleukins,
    Thymosin, Thymopietin

Other Neuropeptides
Atrial natriuretic factors, Bradykinins, Angiotensin
Neurotensin, Galanin
Synapsins
Calcitonin Gene-Related Peptide (CGRP),
    Calcitonin
Sleep Peptides, Carnosine

Precursor Peptides
Pro-opiomelanocortin (POMC)
Pro-enkephalins (A and B)
Calcitonin gene product
VIP gene product
Pro-glucagon, pro-insulin

[a]This table lists only some of the representative members of each
category and is not a complete listing of all neuropeptides.

spliced and polyadenylated to the mature RNA. This RNA molecule is transported to the endoplasmic reticulum where it is translated to a large precursor protein, referred to as the prepropeptide. This precursor protein is then packaged into neurosecretory granules within the Golgi complex and transported by axonal transport to the release site. During transport, the precursor peptide is cleaved into both active and inactive peptide fragments that are intermittently released into the synaptic cleft (or into extracellular fluids), where they act at local (or distant) postsynaptic receptors to exert their actions. Active reuptake mechanisms (such as those for norepinephrine) do not appear to regulate the postsynaptic actions of neuropeptides, perhaps accounting for the prolonged and sustained actions of peptides on target tissues.

Neuropeptide Families

The second feature, is that most neuropeptides can be grouped into families, with members of each family often showing considerable structural homology (i.e., the tachykinin family, consisting of substance P and substance K), albeit with distinct anatomical distributions and functions. These differences arise from a tissue-specific modification of one or more steps involved in peptide synthesis. Tissue-specific alternate splicing of the same pre-mRNA produces calcitonin in the thyroid and calcitonin-gene-related peptide (CGRP) in the brain. Similar mechanisms of alternate translation, alternate post-translational processing, and alternate proteolysis have been described for other peptide families and account for the diversity of peptides.

In spite of rapid advances in the molecular and anatomical characterization of neuropeptides, elucidation of their precise function in the brain as well as their mechanism of action has proved elusive. Experiments using immunocytochemical methods have demonstrated unequivocally that neuropeptides often coexist with other peptides as well as with classical neurotransmitters, implying that, in some cases, they may be coreleased with classical neurotransmitters. For example, TRH and serotonin are colocalized in brainstem neurons, and CCK is found in mesolimbicocortical dopamine neurons. In such cases, the neuropeptide is almost always not responsible for fast depolarization, which is usually due to the classical neurotransmitter. Peptides may modulate the efficacy of the synapse by altering the amount of classical neurotransmitter released and the excitability (or refractory period) of the postsynaptic cell or by communicating the synaptic state to distant sites. As noted earlier, many neuropeptides, in addition to their classical functions, appear also to serve alternate roles in the central nervous system that often complement their classical actions (Table 5.4). For example, in addition to its well–described role in mediating the release of milk by the contraction of mammary gland tissue during lactation (milk-letdown reflex), oxytocin is capable of inducing maternal behavior and influencing placental and adenohypophyseal hormonal functions.

Neuropeptide Receptors and Second Messengers

The actions of neuropeptides on target tissues are mediated by specific receptors. Molecular characterization and cloning of peptide receptors has been achieved for substance K and the growth factors, and considerable progress has been made toward characterizing CRF, TRH, vasopressin, and somatostatin (SRIF) receptors. It is probable that multiple subtypes of receptors (perhaps tissue-specific) exist for each of the peptides, permitting the highly selective modulation of restricted populations of cells. For example, two SRIF receptor subtypes have been described.

The signal transduction mechanisms also are not well understood for most neuropeptide receptors. Vasopressin (V2 receptor subtype), oxytocin, ACTH, CRF, CCK, and GRH appear to act by stimulating the production of intracellular cyclic AMP, whereas the opioids and SRIF appear to decrease production of cyclic AMP. Vasopressin (V1 subtype), substance P, CCK, TRH, bradykinin, bombesin, and gastrin appear to act via the phosphoinositol second messenger systems. The growth factors as well as the oncogenes act via tyrosine kinase, which is the β subunit of the receptor; the α subunit of the receptor binds the peptide.

TABLE 5.4.
Neuropeptide Effects on Brain Function[a]

Peptide	CNS Function
CRF	Major regulator of ACTH secretion; integration of behavioral and biochemical responses to stress; hypersecreted in depression.
Vasopressin	Regulation of ACTH secretion learning and memory facilitation
Oxytocin	Memory processes; induction of maternal and sexual behaviors
Neurotensin	Endogenous neuroleptic regulates mesolimbic, mesocortical, and nigrostriatal dopamine neurons; thermoregulation
TRH	Regulates TSH secretion; may be involved in pathophysiology of depression, enhances neuromuscular function
Bombesin/gastrin-releasing peptide	Thermoregulation
Angiotensin	Thirst, drinking behavior, blood pressure regulation
Insulin	Feeding behavior (hunger)
Cholecystokinin	Feeding behavior (satiety); modulates dopamine neuron activity
Nerve growth factor	Axonal plasticity
Gonadotropin-releasing hormone	Regulates gonadotropin secretion; sexual receptivity
Opioids	Analgesic mechanisms/ feeding and temperature control; learning and memory
Sleep peptides	Regulation of sleep cycles
Substance P	Nociception; colocalized with serotonin

[a]Some of the functions listed here are species-specific and their generalizability to human brain function is not well understood.

Corticotropin-Releasing Factor (CRF)

CRF, a 41-amino-acid-containing-peptide, is the hypothalamic hypophysiotropic hormone that controls hypothalamic-pituitary-adrenal axis (HPA) activity and is the primary physiological regulator of ACTH release during stress (43, 44). There is convincing evidence that CRF also functions as a neurotransmitter in several extrahypothalamic brain regions (43, 44, 45). CRF perikarya (and terminal axons) are present in widespread regions of the CNS, including the limbic areas (amygdala), caudate–putamen, midbrain, pons (locus ceruleus), medulla (dorsal nucleus of vagus), and intrinsic neurons of the cerebral cortex (other than cingulate cortex). The highest concentrations of CRF, however, appear to be in the hypothalamic paraventricular nucleus and in the median eminence. In laboratory animals, CRF produces a variety of electrophysiological and behavioral responses (43, 44). These include increasing heart rate, arterial pressure, and oxygen consumption; producing locomotor activity alterations, anxiogenic behaviors, and hippocampal and EEG changes suggestive of arousal; and decreasing food intake and sexual receptivity. All of these effects appear to be independent of the CRF effects on HPA axis activity and may be mediated by noradrenergic neurons in the brainstem locus ceruleus and/or by increasing peripheral sympathetic outflow and catecholamine release. CRF abnormalities have been documented in neuropsychiatric disorders, such as major depression (increased CSF concentrations of CRF (46) and decreased CRF receptor number in suicide victims (43), and Alzheimer's dementia (decreased cortical CRF concentrations and increased cortical CRF receptor number (47). Based on these data, it has been hypothesized that CRF plays a pivotal physiological role in the central integration and coordination of multisystem responses following stress and emotional arousal (44) a pathophysiological role in depression and anxiety disorders, and Alzheimer's disease.

Oxytocin

Oxytocin is a nonapeptide synthesized in the hypothalamic magnocellular neurons and stored in the neurohypophysis. The best described roles for oxytocin are as a mediator of the milk-letdown reflex during lactation and of uterine contraction during parturition. Recent evidence supports a putative role for oxytocin as a central nervous system neurotransmitter. Immunocytochemical studies in rat brains have demonstrated that oxytocin-containing paraventricular neu-

rons project to widespread areas of the brain, such as the ventral hippocampus, entorhinal cortex, septal nuclei, amygdala, pineal gland, and brainstem. In humans, the distribution is poorly understood, although the locus ceruleus appears to be densely innervated with oxytocinergic terminals. Many of these regions also correspond to sites where high-affinity oxytocin (and vasopressin) receptors have been localized. Oxytocin has been reported to influence several brain functions, including hippocampal firing rates in rodents, memory (putative amnestic role antagonistic with vasopressin), osmoregulation, the regulation of prolactin secretion, and maternal and sexual behavior in rodents (possibly synergistic with estrogens). These data have been recently reviewed by Demitrack and Gold (48). Oxytocin's role in memory and dementia is supported by a study showing a 33% increase in oxytocin concentrations in the hippocampus and temporal cortex of patients with Alzheimer's disease (49). Further studies are warranted to examine the role of oxytocin in human memory and maternal behavior.

Vasopressin

Vasopressin is a posterior pituitary nonapeptide that is best known for its role as the major antidiuretic hormone. Evidence for a neurotransmitter role is supported by several findings (50). Vasopressin terminals are widely distributed in the brain and vasopressin is synthesized in several extra-hypothalamic sites. High-affinity vasopressin receptors have been found in several brain regions. Hypothalamic vasopressin appears to play a synergistic role with CRF in regulating the HPA activity. In animal models, vasopressin has been shown to release ACTH from the anterior pituitary following hemorrhagic stress and to potentiate CRF release. Vasopressin antagonism, with vasopressin antiserum, appears to partially block the HPA response to stress.

In animal models, vasopressin appears to facilitate certain types of learning and memory. The effects of exogenously administered vasopressin on human cognition have been evaluated in patients with head injury, dementia, Lesch–Nyhan syndrome, and age-related memory loss, with promising, albeit inconsistent, results. In addition, several investigators have implicated vasopressin in psychiatric disorders, such as affective illness, anorexia nervosa, and schizophrenia (51).

Neuropeptide Y

Neuropeptide Y, a 36-amino acid-containing-peptide contained in interneurons, is one of the most abundant and widely distributed peptides in the central nervous system. It is present in particularly high concentrations in the forebrain areas (limbic areas, striatum, all parts of the neocortex) and in lower concentrations in several subcortical areas. It is generally found colocalized with somatostatin (neocortex and striatum), GABA (cerebral cortex), galanin, or catecholamines (brainstem). High-affinity neuropeptide Y binding sites are present in several brain regions. It has been suggested to play a role in several brain functions, including neuroendocrine regulation and circadian rhythms; eating, drinking, sexual, and locomotor behaviors; as well as in the pathophysiology of Alzheimer's disease, Parkinson's dementia, Huntington's disease, and major depression. These data have been reviewed recently (52, 53).

Thyrotropin-Releasing Hormone (TRH)

TRH, a tripeptide, is the primary physiologic regulator of thyrotropin (TSH) from the anterior pituitary; it also releases prolactin. It is now well established that, although the concentrations of TRH are highest in the median eminence, a large majority of immunoreactive TRH resides in extrahypothalamic sites, including the brainstem, midbrain, preoptic area, septum, basal ganglia, and cerebral cortex (46, 54, 55).

TRH effects on the pituitary are mediated via the phosphoinositide hydrolysis second messenger system, although it is not certain whether this applies to the actions of the tripeptide in the brain (54). As other peptides, TRH affects a wide range of human behaviors and brain functions. Prominent among these are antagonism of sedation and hypothermia induced by CNS depressants (barbiturates, ethanol, and anesthetics), increases in body temperature, reductions in food consumption, and production of arousal and EEG activation (55, 56).

Neurotensin

Neurotensin is a tridecapeptide distributed heterogeneously throughout the mammalian central nervous system, gastrointestinal tract, CSF, adrenals, and pancreas (54, 55). In the human brain, it is found in high concentrations in the hypothalamus, substantia nigra (midbrain), striatum, and periaqueductal gray matter, and in relatively low concentrations in the cerebral cortex and cerebellum. Important purported neurotensin pathways include those from the central amygdaloid nucleus to the bed nucleus of stria terminalis and from the ventral tegmental area to the nucleus accumbens (57). Neurotensin receptors are found in high densities in the substantia nigra, amygdaloid nuclei, and cortex. Of considerable clinical interest is the fact that centrally administered neurotensin antagonizes mesolimbic dopamine–mediated behaviors in a fashion similar to that of clinically efficacious antipsychotic neuroleptic drugs (57). Based on these and other similarities between neurotensin and antipsychotic drugs, neurotensin has been proposed to be an endogenous neuroleptic (59).

In animal models, neurotensin enhances the depressant effects of barbiturates, antagonizes the actions of d–amphetamine and, unlike neuroleptics, produces analgesia that is more potent than morphine and not naloxone–reversible. It is particularly interesting that chronic treatment with antipsychotic drugs has been observed to produce a marked increase of neurotensin concentrations in the nucleus accumbens and caudate. Neurotensin's effects on the brain are summarized in Table 5.5.

CONCLUSION

It is apparent that hormones influence almost every aspect of brain function throughout development, adulthood, and aging. Ongoing preclinical and clinical research will undoubtedly reveal, in greater detail, the mechanisms, sites, interactions, and processes that are affected. Such an understanding will permit the development of better diagnostic tools and novel treatment strategies for the restoration of function following

TABLE 5.5.
Neurotensin Effects on Brain Function[a]

Neuroendocrine Effects
Decrease serum levels of TSH, GH, PRL
Decrease gastric acid secretion
Release somatostatin
Block TRH-induced TSH release in vivo

Neuropharmacologic Effects
Block amphetamine-induced locomotor activity
Enhance pentobarbital-induced sedation
Enhance ethanol-induced sedation and hypothermia

Neurophysiological Effects
Decrease firing in Nucleus Accumbens and locus
   ceruleus neurons
Excitability of spinal neurons
Excitation of neurons in frontal cortex, hippocampus,
   striatum, and lateral thalamus, and midbrain DA
   neurons

Neurobehavioral Effects
Altered performance in operant tasks
Diminished spontaneous locomotor activity
Analgesia, muscle relaxation, hypothermia, catalepsy

[a]Most of these effects are based on studies in laboratory rats or mice and may not be directly generalizable to humans. Adapted from Nemeroff, C. B., Kalivas, P. W., Golden, R. N., and Prange, A. T., Jr. Behavioral effects of hypothalamic hypophysiotropic hormones, neurotensin, substance P and other neuropeptides. Pharmacol. Ther., *24*:1–56, 1984; and Nemeroff, C. B., Prange, A. J. (eds.). *Neurotensin, a brain and gastrointestinal peptide.* Ann NY Acad Sci, vol. 400, 1982.

central nervous system dysfunction and damage.

ACKNOWLEDGMENTS

Supported by NIMH MH-42088, MH-40159, MH-39415, and MH-40524.

REFERENCES

1. Arushanyan E.B., and Borovkova G.K. Psychotropic properties of ovarian estrogens (review). Neurosci. Behav. Physiol., *19*:57–66, 1989.
2. Arriza J., and Evans R. The neuronal mineralocorticoid receptor as the mediator of the glucocorticoid response. Neuron, *1*:887–900, 1988.
3. Baum M. Gender dimorphism in the brain. Natl. Inst. Drug Abuse Res. Monogr. Ser., *65*:49–57, 1986.
4. Beyer C., and Feder H.H. Sex steroids and afferent input: their roles in brain sexual differentiation. Ann. Rev. Physiol. *49*:349–364, 1987.
5. Burnstein K.L., and Cidlowski J.A. Regulation of gene expression by glucocorticoids. Ann. Rev. Physiol., *51*:683–699, 1989.
6. Callard G.V., and Pasmanik M. The role of estrogen as a parahormone in brain and pituitary. Steroids, *50*:475–493, 1987.
7. Cohen R.S. Cell biology of the neural circuit for steroid-dependent female reproductive behavior. Prog. Brain Res., *72*:137–151, 1987.
8. Dallman M.F., Levin N., Cascio C.S., *et al.* Pharmacological evidence that the inhibition of diurnal adrenocorticotropin secretion by corticosteroids is mediated via Type I corticosterone-preferring receptors. Endocrinology. *124*:2844–2850, 1989.
9. Demitrack M.A., and Gold P.W. Oxytocin: Neurobiologic considerations and their implications for affective illness. Prog. Neuropsychopharmacol. Biol. Psychiatry, *12*:S 23–S 51, 1988.
10. DeSouza E.B., and Nemeroff C.B. *Corticotropin releasing factor: Basic and clinical studies of a neuropeptide.* Boca Raton, CRC Press Inc., 1990.
11. Doraiswamy P.M., Krishnan K.R.R., and Nemeroff C.B. Neuropeptides and neurotransmitters in Alzheimer's disease. In: *Psychoneuroendocrinology Vol 5,* Clinics in Endocrinology and Metabolism, edited by A. Grossman, Bailliere Tindall Press, London, pp. 59–77, 1991.
12. Dorner G. Neuroendocrine response to estrogen and brain differentiation in heterosexuals, homosexuals, and transsexuals. Arch. Sex. Behav. *17*:57–75, 1988.
13. Dussault J.H., and Ruel J. Thyroid hormones and brain development. Annu. Rev. Physiol. *49*:321–324, 1987.
14. Evans R.M. The steroid and thyroid hormone receptor superfamily. Science, *240*:889–895, 1988.
15. Evans R.M., and Arriza J.L. A molecular framework for the actions of glucocorticoid hormones in the nervous system. Neuron, *2*:1105–1112, 1989.
16. Funder J.W., and Sheppard K. Adrenocortical steroids and the brain. Annu. Rev. Physiol. *49*:397–411, 1987.
17. Funder J.W., Pearce P.T., Smith R., *et al.* Mineralocorticoid action: target tissue specificity is enzyme, not receptor, mediated. Science, *242*:583–585, 1988.
18. Gash D.M., and Boer G.J. (Eds). *Vasopressin: Principles and Properties.* New York, Plenum Press, 1987.
19. Henkin R.I. The role of adrenal corticosteroids in sensory processes. In *Handbook of Physiology-Endocrinology Vol 6,* edited by Blaschko, Sayers, and Smith. Williams and Wilkins, Baltimore, pp. 209–230, 1975.
20. Holmes G.L., Donaldson J.D. Effect of sexual hormones on the electroencephalogram and seizures. J. Clin. Neurophysiol. *4*:1–22, 1987.
21. Husain M.M., and Nemeroff C.B. Neuropeptides and Alzheimer's disease. J. Am. Geriatr. Soc. *38*:918–925, 1990.
22. Komisaruk B.R., Siegel H.I., Cheng M.F., and Feder H.H. (Eds). *Reproduction: a behavioral and neuroendocrine perspective.* Ann. N.Y. Acad. Sci. 474, 1986.
23. Kuhn C., and Schanberg S. Hormones and brain development. In: *Peptides, Hormones, and Behavior,* edited by C.B. Nemeroff and A.J. Dunn. New York, Spectrum Publications, pp. 775–822, 1984.
24. Levant B., and Nemeroff C.B. Psychobiology of neurotensin. In: *Neuroendocrinology of Mood,* edited by D. Ganlen and D. Pfaff. pp. 231–262, New York, Springer Verlag, 1988.

25. Lindvall-Axelsson M., Hedner P., and Owman C. Corticosteroid action on choroid plexus: reduction in Na^+-K^+-ATPase, choline transport capacity, and rate of CSF formation. Exp. Brain Research. 77:605–610, 1989.

26. Loosen P.T. TRH: Behavioral and endocrine effects in man. Prog. Neurophychopharmacol Biol. Psychiat. 12(Suppl):S87–S117, 1988.

27. Loosen P.T., and Prange A.J. Hormones of the thyroid axis and behavior. In: Peptides, Hormones, and Behavior, edited by C.B. Nemeroff and A.J. Dunn. pp. 533–577, New York, Spectrum Publications, 1984.

28. Luttge W.G. Cerebral effects of gonadal steroid hormones. In: Peptides, Hormones, and Behavior, edited by C.B. Nemeroff and A.J. Dunn. New York, Spectrum Publications, pp. 645–773, 1984.

29. MacLusky N.J., Clark A.S, Naftolin F. et al. Estrogen formation in the mammalian brain: possible role of aromatase in sexual differentiation of the hippocampus and neocortex. Steroids, 459–474, 1987.

30. Martin J.B., and Reichlin S. Clinical neuroendocrinology. 2nd edition Philadelphia, F.A. Davis Co. pp. 639–661, 1987.

31. McDonald J.K. NPY and related substances. Crit. Rev. Neurobiol., 4:97–135, 1988.

32. McDonald W.M., and Krishnan K.R.R. Vasopressin. In: Nemeroff C.B., Neuropeptides in Psychiatric Disorders, Washington. D.C., APA Press Inc. (in press).

33. Meinig G., and Deisenroth K. Dose-response relation for dexamenthasone in cold lesion-induced brain edema in rats. Adv. Neurol., 52:295–300, 1990.

34. Metcalf G., and Jackson I.M.D. (eds). Thyrotropin-releasing hormone. Biomedical significance. Ann. N.Y. Acad. Sci., 553:1–532, 1989.

35. Nemeroff C.B. Neurotensin: perchance an endogenous neuroleptic? Biol. Psychiatry., 15:283–302, 1980.

36. Nemeroff C.B.,and Bissette G. Neuropeptides in psychiatric disorders. In: American Handbook of Psychiatry, 2nd edition, edited by P.A. Berger and H.K. Brodie. pp. 64–110, New York, Basic Books, 1986.

36. Nemeroff C.B., and Cain S.T. Neurotensin dopamine interactions in the central nervous system. Trends Pharmacol. Sci., 6:201–205, 1985.

38. Nemeroff C.B., Bissette G., Manberg P.J., et al. Effects of hypothalamic peptides on the central nervous system. In: Peptides, Hormones, and Behavior. edited by C.B. Nemeroff and A.J. Dunn. New York, Spectrum Publications, pp. 217–272, 1984.

39. Nemeroff C.B., Kalivas P.W., Golden R.N., and Prange A.J., Jr. Behavioral effects of hypothalamic hypophysiotropic hormones, neurotensin, substance P and other neuropeptides. Pharmacol. Ther., 24:1–56, 1984.

40. Nemeroff C.B., and Prange A.J., Jr. (eds). Neurotensin, a Brain and Gastrointestinal Peptide. vol. 499, Ann. N.Y. Acad. Sci., 1982.

41. Nemeroff C.B., and Prage A.J. Peptides and psychoneuroendocrinology. A perspective. Arch. Gen. Psychiatry, 35:999–1010, 1978.

42. Nemeroff C.B. (ed). Neuropeptides in Psychiatric Disorders. Washington, D.C., APA Press, Inc., 1991.

43. Nemeroff C.B. Clincial significance of phychoneuroendocrinology in psychiatry: focus on the thyroid and adrenal. J. Clin. Phychiatry, 50 [suppl]:13–20, 1989.

44. Nemeroff C.B., Widerlov E., Bissette G., et al. Elevated concentrations of CSF corticotropin-releasing factor-like immunoreactivity in depressed patients. Science, 226:1342–1344, 1984.

45. Owens M.J., and Nemeroff C.B. The neurobiology of corticotropin-releasing factor: implications for affective disorders. In: The Hypothalamic-pituitary-adrenal Axis. Physiology, Pathophysiology and Psychiatric Implications. edited by A.F. Schatzberg and C.B. Nemeroff. New York, Raven Press, pp. 1–36, 1988.

46. Rees H., and Gray H. Glucocorticoids and mineralocorticoids: actions on brain and behavior. In: Peptides, Hormones and Behavior. edited by C.B. Nemeroff and A.J. Dunn. New York, Spectrum Publications, pp. 579–643, 1984.

47. Ritchie J.C., and Nemeroff C.B. Stress, the hypothalamic-pituitary-adrenal axis and depression. In: Stress Neuropeptides, and Systemic Disease. edited by J.A. McCubbin, P.G. Kaufman and C.B. Nemeroff. San Diego, Academic Press, pp. 181–197, 1991.

48. Rories C., and Spelsberg T.C. Ovarian steroid action on gene expression: mechanisms and models. Annu. Rev. Physiol., 51:653–681, 1989.

49. Samuels H.H., Forman B.B., Horowitz Z.C., and Ye, Z.S. Regulation of gene expression by thyroid hormone. Annu. Rev. Physiol., 51:623–639, 1989.

50. Sapolsky, R.M. Glucocorticoids and hippocampal damage. Trends. Neurosci., 10:346–349, 1987.

51. Schipper H.M. Sex hormones in stroke, chorea, and anticonvulsant therapy. Semin. Neurol., 8:181–186, 1988.

52. Schreiber G., Aldred A.R., Jaworowski A., et al. Thyroxine transport from the blood to brain via transthyretin synthesis in choriod plexus. Am. J. Physiol., 258:R338–R345, 1990.

53. Sikich L., and Todd R.D. Are the developmental effects of gonadal hormones related to sex differences in psychiatric illnesses? Psychiatr. Dev., 6:277–309, 1988.

54. Sousa R.J., Tannery N.H., and Lafer E.M. In situ hybridization mapping of glucocorticoid receptor messenger ribonucleic acid in rat brain. Mol. Endocrinol., 3:481–494, 1989.

55. Timiras P.S., and Nzekwe E.U. Thyroid homones and nervous system development. Biol. Neonate, 55(6):376–385, 1989.

56. Vaccari A. Teratogenic mechanisma of dysthyroidism in the central nervous system. Prog. Brain Res., 73:71–86, 1988.

57. Van Eekelne J.A.M., Jiang W., DeKloet E.R., and Bohn M.C. Distribution of the mineralocorticoid and the glucocorticoid receptor mRNAs in the rat hippocampus. J. Neurosci. Res., 21:88–94, 1988.

58. Van Hartesveldt C., and Joyce J.N. Effects of estrogen on the basal ganglia. Neurosci. and Bio. Behav. Rev., 10:1–14, 1986.

59. Wahlestedt C., Ekman R., and Widerlov E. Neuropeptide Y (NPY) and the central nervous system. Prog. Neuropsychopharmacol. Biol. Psychiatry, *13:*31–54, 1989.

60. Williams C.L. A reevaluation of the concept of separable periods of organizational and activational actions of estrogens in development of brain and behavior. In: *Reproduction: A Behavioral and Neuroendocrine Perspective.* edited by B.R. Komisaruk, H.I. Siegel, M.F. Cheng, and O.H. Feder. Ann. N.Y. Acad. Sci., *474:*282–292, 1986.

61. Wolkowitz O.M., Reus V.I., Weingartner H., *et al.* Cognitive effects of corticosteroids. Am. J. Psychiatry, *147(10):*1297–1303, 1990.

PART 2

Clinical Neuroendocrinology

CHAPTER 6

Physiology and Pathophysiology of Prolactin Secretion

BAHA M. ARAFAH, M.D., SAMIR KAILANI, M.D., AND WARREN R. SELMAN, M.D.

INTRODUCTION

Prolactin (Prl) is one of the lactogenic hormones that was known to exist in animals for several decades (126). However, it was not until 1970 that, in humans, Prl was documented to be distinct from growth hormone (50). The development of radioimmunoassay for its measurement by Hwang et al. (65) was followed by an intensive research effort into the physiology and pathophysiology of Prl secretion.

Since its discovery, Prl was known primarily for its lactogenic properties. However, over the years it became apparent that, in many mammals, Prl has other properties in addition to its known lactogenic activity. These include: osmoregulation (23, 76), steroid biosynthesis (10, 31, 101), tumor cell growth (9, 11, 21, 91, 111) modulation of the immune system (130, 131), and blood pressure regulation (10, 103, 104). Although the degree of modulation of these functions by Prl varies from one species to another, it is reasonable to assume that, within each species, the biological effects of Prl are not limited to its lactogenic properties.

Prl is secreted by the anterior pituitary lactotrophs. These cells represent approximately 20% of the hypophysis and are predominantly localized in the lateral wings of the gland. Like other cells in the anterior pituitary, lactotrophs originate from ectodermal cells of Rathke's Pouch. Acidophilic stem cells are considered to be common precursor cells for lactotrophs and somatotrophs. The recent documentation of the existence of acidophil stem cell pituitary adenomas that secrete growth hormone and Prl is consistent with this view. Marked lactotroph hyperplasia is seen in states where excessive estrogen levels prevail, such as in the fetal pituitary gland and in the pituitary of women during the second and third trimesters of pregnancy. Lactotroph cell hyperplasia accounts for the increase in the weight and size of the pituitary gland that occurs during pregnancy and resolves in the course of a few weeks after delivery.

In this report, we will review available data on prolactin secretion under physiologic and pathologic conditions. Whereas most of the mechanisms controlling normal prolactin secretion are well defined, others are still being investigated. Significant progress has been made in our understanding of prolactin secretion by adenomatous lactotrophs. The natural history, complications, and management of these adenomas are now well recognized and appreciated.

PRL SECRETION

Synthesis, Storage, and Size Heterogeneity

Prl synthesis occurs on polyribosomes in the rough endoplasmic reticulum of the lactotrophs. The hormone is initially synthesized as a precursor and is cleaved before the native peptide is completed. Synthesized hormone is transferred to the Golgi apparatus, where it is packaged into secretory granules. The granules are stored within cytoplasmic vesicles that appear on immunoelectron microscopy as granules. It is subsequently released into the perivascular space, by exocytosis, or into intracellular compartments, by lysis (46).

The molecular structure of human Prl (hPrl) was determined in 1977 (142) and found to consist of 198 amino acid residues with a molecular weight of 21.5 kilodalton (kd). It was found to have 77% and 73% sequence identity with porcine and ovine Prl, respectively, and only 16% with human growth hormone (142).

Different molecular forms of Prl have been confirmed by radioreceptor and radioimmunoassays of the circulating or the intrapituitary pool (14, 45, 51, 151, 164). The monomeric form of Prl normally accounts for 80–90% of the circulating hormone. At least two other molecular forms of Prl have been characterized in the serum: A "big" form, with a molecular weight of approximately 45–50 kd, is thought to represent two peptide chains linked by a disulfide bond (51, 151, 164); the "big-big" molecular form has a molecular weight of more than 100 kd and apparently represents aggregates of the monomeric form of the peptide (51, 151, 164). The polymeric forms of the hormone have substantially less biological activity than the monomeric variant (45, 59). Little is known about factors or disorders that influence the secretion of polymeric forms of Prl.

Recent reports describe a small number of patients who have sustained hyperprolactinemia, normal menses, and minimal galactorrhea and in whom the predominant circulating molecular form of Prl was the one with the large molecular weight (macroprolactin), having a molecular weight of more than 100 kd (51, 68, 69). Although Prl-secreting adenomas sometimes are capable of secreting these forms, most of the recently reported cases did not have demonstrable pituitary tumors. There was no evidence for the existence of circulating Prl-binding protein in the sera of these patients. Macroprolactin levels in these patients increase throughout pregnancy during normal gestation (28), although to a lesser degree than the expected rise of monomeric Prl. Since practically all of these patients have no significant symptoms

related to hyperprolactinemia, they are discovered by chance, and the incidence or prevalence of this abnormality is hard to define. The lack of symptoms, despite significant elevation in the circulating hormone level in these patients, is consistent with other observations demonstrating reduced biological effects (receptor binding, mitogenic activity in Nb_2 rat lymphoma bioassay) of macroprolactin.

Glycosylated forms of Prl have also been identified in various mammalian pituitary glands, including that of humans (85, 86, 94, 95). It is also reported to be present in small quantities in the serum of normal men and women (94). The significance of glycosylated Prl in humans is uncertain. As was reported for macroprolactin, the glycosylated form of the peptide is reported to have reduced potency in the sheep, as determined by receptor binding (95).

CONTROL OF PRL SECRETION

Prl is unique among pituitary hormones in that its secretion is spontaneous in the absence of hypothalamic or hypophysiotropic influences. The primary mechanism controlling Prl secretion is tonic inhibition by hypothalamic dopamine secretion. However, as will be discussed, other factors can influence Prl synthesis and release. In addition to regulation by hypothalamic and pituitary factors, Prl secretion is modulated by the peptide itself and by other peripheral hormones, such as estrogens, glucocorticoids, and thyroxine (Table 6.1).

Inhibitory

Dopamine

The tuberoinfundibular dopaminergic system has its cell bodies in the arcuate nucleus and short axons that terminate in the median eminence. Secreted dopamine is transported to the anterior pituitary gland via the portal vessels. Recent evidence indicates that, in addition to the axons terminating in the median eminence, other dopaminergic neurons terminate in the posterior pituitary (15, 109). Dopamine can then be transported to the anterior pituitary through short portal vessels. Thus, dopamine can

TABLE 6.1.
Hormones and Factors Controlling Prolactin Secretion

Inhibitory	Stimulatory	Modulators
Dopamine	TRH[c]	Autocrine/paracrine
GABA[a]	VIP[d]	Peripheral hormones
GnRH[b]-related peptide	Serotonin	Estrogens
Somatostatin		Glucocorticoids
		Thyroid hormones

[a]GABA: gamma-amino butyric acid.
[b]GNRH: gonadotropin-releasing hormone.
[c]TRH: thyrotropin-releasing hormone.
[d]VIP: vasoactive intestinal peptide.

reach the anterior pituitary lactotrophs from the posterior pituitary via short portal vessels (15, 109, 110) as well as from the median eminence by transportation through long portal vessels running along the pituitary stalk. Stimulation of the tuberoinfundibular dopaminergic neurons results in the secretion of dopamine into the portal vessels, where its concentration is much greater than that of the systemic circulation (53, 113, 119). Several studies have shown that stalk dopamine concentrations are inversely correlated to circulating serum Prl levels (15, 16, 119).

Unlike other dopaminergic mechanisms in the brain, the tuberoinfundibular system is not directly regulated by dopamine receptors, but, instead, is stimulated by implanted, systemically or intracisternally administered Prl (5, 71). This provides another mechanism by which Prl regulates its own secretion. Other hormones, neurotransmitters, and neuropeptides modulate dopamine secretion by the tuberoinfundibular system. For example, estrogen administration results in a several-fold increase in the dopamine concentration in the portal vessels, and this effect is more pronounced in females than in males (15, 16, 40, 58). Similarly, opiates modulate Prl secretion through their inhibitory effects on the release of dopamine by the tuberoinfundibular system (125, 155).

Dopamine receptors (D_2 receptors) have been identified on lactotrophs (24, 30, 54) and mediate the effects of dopamine on Prl secretion. It is generally believed that dopamine exerts inhibitory action on lactotrophs by activating a guanine nucleotide-sensitive, high-affinity D_2 receptor, resulting in decreased cAMP (36). However, it is also recognized that the dopamine-induced changes in lactotroph cAMP levels are secondary and

are not primarily associated with the early inhibitory events that lower Prl secretion. Although initial studies suggested involvement of phospholipid metabolism in the signal transduction of dopamine, recent studies indicate that activation of pituitary D_2 receptors is unlikely to be coupled with phospholipase-C (154). Thus, although dopamine affects several metabolic processes, the exact mechanisms through which this transmitter exerts its inhibitory effects on Prl release were unknown until recently. More current studies demonstrate a primary role for Ca^{2+} in dopamine-mediated lactotroph inhibition of Prl release (90, 92, 137). The studies support the hypothesis that dopamine causes hyperpolarization of lactotrophs' plasma membrane through activation of D_2 receptors and reduces spontaneous action potential, resulting in decreased Ca^{2+} influx and inhibition of intracellular Ca^{2+} redistribution. Dopamine has additional inhibitory effects on Prl gene expression: It is known to inhibit mRNA at the transcriptional level (98, 99).

γ-Aminobutyric Acid (GABA)

This neurotransmitter appears to have an inhibitory role on Prl secretion and gene expression when given at high concentrations (56, 89, 135). Although GABA receptors have been described on pituitary membranes, the high concentrations of GABA necessary to inhibit Prl secretion suggested a limited physiologic significance for this mechanism.

GnRH-Associated Peptide

This 56-amino acid-peptide has been characterized as part of the human GnRH precursor molecule that can inhibit Prl secretion and simultaneously stimulate gonadotropin release (114). Recent studies suggest that this peptide inhibits Prl secretion when administered in vivo to lactating or ether-stressed rats (167). The physiologic significance of this inhibitory peptide remains unclear.

Somatostatin

This peptide has been shown to inhibit Prl secretion in cultured pituitary cells (47, 60). Recent studies have demonstrated that the inhibitory action of somatostatin required the presence of estradiol (35, 66). The latter steroid influences lactotroph sensitivity to somatostatin by regulating its receptor on these cells (66). In humans, somatostatin and its long-acting analogue (sandostatin) do not significantly affect the basal or TRH-stimulated serum Prl levels (87). However, when given to estrogen-treated agonadal subjects, somatostatin infusion inhibits Prl secretion (55).

Autoregulation by Prl Itself

Extensive evidence from tumor-bearing animals (34, 81) or from animals treated with exogenous Prl (133, 144) indicates a negative autoregulatory effect of this peptide on its own secretion. However, the site of action of this autoregulatory mechanism remains controversial. While some studies have suggested the hypothalamus (132, 138), others demonstrated the pituitary to be the site of autoregulation (2, 52, 157). Alterations in hypothalamic dopamine turnover and secretion mediate the hypothalamic autoregulation of Prl secretion. Although it is difficult to provide convincing data to document autoregulation of Prl secretion in humans, published data in patients with microprolactinomas are consistent with this concept (7, 8,

12). Immediately after surgical adenomectomy, serum Prl levels decrease to very low levels (Fig. 6.1) and gradually increase to the normal range over several weeks (7, 12). Other pituitary functions remain normal throughout this period, especially in the immediate postoperative time (7, 63). Furthermore, lactotroph responsiveness to dynamic stimulation using TRH, hypoglycemia, and phenothiazines improves gradually after adenomectomy, such that by one year it becomes indistinguishable from normal responsiveness (7, 8). These data support the existence of an autoregulatory mechanism controlling Prl secretion in humans.

Stimulatory

Although the predominant mechanism controlling Prl secretion is inhibitory in nature, the existence of Prl-releasing factors is well documented. Three physiologically active compounds, TRH, VIP, and serotonin, are known Prl-stimulating factors that act through distinctly different mechanisms.

TRH

This hypothalamic hormone is present at high concentrations in the hypophyseal stalk blood and directly stimulates Prl release. In

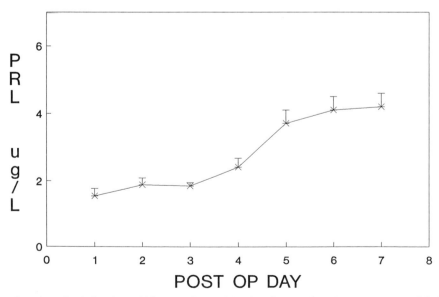

Figure 6.1. Serum prolactin levels (μg/L) in 75 patients with prolactin-secreting adenomas measured during the first week after transsphenoidal adenomectomy. All patients had immunocytochemical documentation of prolactin secretion by the resected adenoma. Mean ($\pm$SE) preoperative serum prolactin level was 152 ± 25 μg/L.

addition to its effect on lactotrophs, TRH primarily regulates TSH secretion. During states of physiologic hyperprolactinemia (i.e., lactation), no associated changes in TSH secretion occur. Because of this dissociation of Prl and TSH secretion, the physiologic role of TRH as a Prl-releasing hormone is still not clear. Studies in rats indicate that TRH is involved in suckling-induced Prl secretion (38). No such association was documented in humans. TRH is known to stimulate Prl-gene expression (37).

Vasoactive Intestinal Peptide (VIP)

The ability of this peptide to stimulate Prl-gene expression as well as hormone release has been well documented by in vivo as well as in vitro studies (1, 44). VIP is present in hypophyseal venous blood (130) and also in the pituitary gland (14). Specific receptors for VIP have been demonstrated on pituitary lactotrophs. Peptide histidine isoleucine (PHI) is a protein that is analogous to VIP and is cosecreted with it as part of a VIP prohormone (67). Both VIP and PHI stimulate Prl release (72, 161). VIP appears to act as a modulator of other Prl-regulating factors. For example, serotonin stimulates the release of VIP into the portal stalk blood (141). Similarly, treatment of rats with estrogen increased VIP concentration in the pituitary gland (120).

VIP is synthesized and secreted by pituitary lactotrophs (14, 107). Locally synthesized VIP can therefore modulate Prl release through its autocrine effects (112). This contention has been used to argue for the existence of autocrine mechanisms controlling Prl secretion.

Serotonin

Administration of large doses of this biogenic amine or its precursor stimulate Prl release (163). Serotonin may stimulate Prl secretion through its modulating effect on VIP or, alternatively, as a neurotransmitter interacting with receptors in the arcuate nucleus. Modulation of specific mechanisms (i.e., dopamine, VIP) involved in Prl secretion appear to mediate most of the effects of serotonin on the secretion of this peptide. For example, the intraventricular administration of serotonin results in an increase in TRH

and VIP levels and a decrease in dopamine concentration in the portal blood (118, 141).

Cyproheptadine, a known antiserotoninergic drug, was used with moderate success in the treatment of hyperprolactinemia (165). The doses required were high and often associated with side effects. It is difficult to discern from these studies whether the Prl-lowering effects of the drug were mediated through its antiserotonin effects or through the anticholinergic, antihistaminic, or the mild dopaminergic properties of this drug (165).

Autocrine/Paracrine Regulation

It has become evident over the past few years that many cell types, including endocrine cells, produce substances or growth factors that potentially modulate their own function (autocrine regulation) or that of neighboring cells (paracrine regulation). Evidence supporting the existence of such mechanisms in the control of Prl secretion is increasing. One such piece of evidence is the demonstration that VIP is synthesized by pituitary lactotrophs (14) and that, through this unique location, it can regulate Prl secretion. The finding of a stimulatory effect by GnRH on Prl release from lactotrophs cocultured with gonadotroph-enriched cell population (41, 42) but not from isolated lactotrophs, has been used as evidence supporting the existence of paracrine mechanisms controlling Prl secretion. Recent studies support the view that anterior pituitary cells, including lactotrophs, synthesize and probably secrete multiple growth factors, such as insulin-like growth factor I (IGF-I). These growth factors can modulate lactotroph function and regulate Prl secretion.

Influence of Peripheral Hormones

Estrogens

Endogenous and exogenous estrogens modulate basal and stimulated Prl levels in most mammalian species, including humans (49). The difference between men and women is that the basal Prl levels are related to endogenous estrogen production. The reported elevations in serum Prl levels and the associated increase in lactotroph size, as well as that of the pituitary gland in pregnant women, are related to excessive estrogen production during pregnancy. Cytoplasmic and nuclear receptors for estrogens are well documented on lactotrophs (117). Estrogens exert direct mitotic action on lactotrophs and induce transcription of the Prl gene, resulting in increased Prl synthesis (3, 70). Despite these effects, no firm causal relationship was established between estrogens and the development of prolactinomas in humans. The demonstrable antiproliferative effects of antiestrogens on lactotroph cell growth in vivo and in vitro (13, 82) support a modulating role for estrogens on tumor cell growth. Estrogens can also regulate Prl secretion by their ability to modulate known Prl inhibitory and stimulatory factors. The reported decrease in the concentration of dopamine in the hypophyseal blood of animals after chronic estrogen therapy (16) is consistent with this hypothesis. Similarly, the reported increase in VIP concentration in the pituitary gland of estrogen-treated animals (120) provides further support for the existence of this mechanism. Estrogens can influence Prl secretion by their ability to modulate lactotroph responsiveness to Prl-regulating factors such as dopamine. For example, estrogen administration results in decreased responsiveness to dopamine and increased response to TRH (28, 124). These dual effects have been ascribed to the effects of estrogens on dopamine and on TRH receptors in the pituitary (39, 124). Recent evidence indicates that locally-produced growth factors (i.e., galanin) might mediate at least some of the estrogen-induced changes (158). However, the extent to which this mechanism explains estrogen-induced effects remains unknown.

Glucocorticoids

Minimal alterations in the basal levels of Prl are reported in patients receiving exogenous glucocorticoid therapy. However, the rise in serum Prl level in response to TRH stimulation is blunted during glucocorticoid therapy (147, 149). The mechanisms mediating this alteration in prolactin secretion are not known.

Thyroid Hormone

T3 suppresses Prl gene expression and inhibits Prl synthesis (100, 163). Although the basal Prl level is normal in thyrotoxic patients, TRH-stimulated levels in these subjects are often blunted (146). Primary hypothyroidism, on the other hand, is associated with moderate elevation in the basal and TRH-stimulated serum Prl levels in 20–30% of the patients (20, 43, 62, 166). It is postulated that, as one of the consequences of primary hypothyroidism, the rise in TRH contributes to the development of hyperprolactinemia in subjects with this disease (20, 62, 166). In addition, recent studies show that an increase in pituitary VIP was noted during primary hypothyroidism (80).

PHYSIOLOGICAL FACTORS REGULATING SERUM PRL LEVELS

Serum Prl levels vary only slightly from one laboratory to another, depending on the assay used. Serum levels range from 4–20, with a mean of about 10 μg/L in normal premenopausal, nonlactating women. The levels are 20–30% lower in normal men and postmenopausal women. During the first 20 weeks of fetal development, serum Prl levels are slightly higher than adult values. However, during the third trimester of pregnancy, fetal Prl levels increase progressively to values similar to those in the maternal circulation (150–200 μg/L). After birth, serum Prl levels decrease to approximately 50–75 μg/L in the newborn and gradually stabilize by 5–6 weeks to the prepubertal range of 2–12 μg/L. During puberty, the levels increase more noticeably in females and stabilize around adult values.

Recent studies (106) estimated the production rate of Prl in adults to be 802 ± 377 μg/m^2/day, and the metabolic clearance rate to be 71 ± 19 ml/m^2/min. The same in vivo study (107) determined the circulating half life (t1/2) of Prl to be 26–49, with a mean $\pm$ SD of 37 ± 10 minutes.

Prl levels vary significantly throughout the day, with the highest levels noted during sleep (Fig. 6.2). Frequent blood sampling (at 10–20 minute intervals) throughout a 24-hour period provided data (Fig. 6.2) to demonstrate the circadian rhythm in serum Prl concentration (134, 156). The circadian rhythm in Prl secretion persists during the physiological hyperprolactinemia seen throughout lactation (150). In addition to the

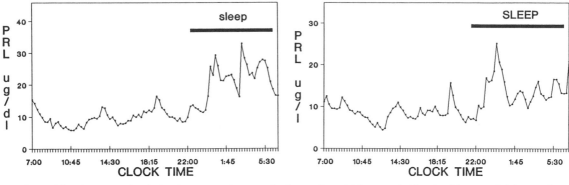

Figure 6.2. Serum prolactin levels measured every 15 minutes for a 24-hour period in a healthy man (*right panel*) and a normal premenopausal woman (*left panel*). The x-axis shows the actual clock time throughout the day. Subjects slept between 10:30 pm and 6:30 am. Standard meals were provided at 8:00 am, 1:00 pm, and 6:00 pm.

circadium rhythm, multiple ultradian Prl rhythms could be detected. There were approximately 14 Prl peaks/24 hours, each with an amplitude of 4 μg/L. These data are helpful in the interpretation of single-serum Prl-level measurements in the clinical setting.

Stress is another variable that is known to increase serum Prl levels (116). This is commonly seen during increased physical activity, general anesthesia, surgery, and myocardial infarction. It is not known why the serum Prl level increases after certain types of seizures. Nipple and/or chest wall stimulation are known to result in stimulation of Prl release (78, 108, 115, 123). Sexual intercourse is also known to stimulate Prl release in some women, but not in men. Ingestion of proteins was also reported to stimulate Prl release (29, 121). Recent studies suggest that the ingestion of certain amino acids (phenylalanine and tyrosine) can account for most of the Prl-releasing activity of food (26).

In humans, Prl levels increase during pregnancy and lactation, reaching 200–300 μg/L by the third trimester. The increase can be accounted for by the stimulatory effects of elevated estrogen levels occurring during pregnancy. Serum Prl levels fall rapidly after delivery and reach nonpregnant levels within 2–3 weeks if breast-feeding does not occur (115). If, on the other hand, breast-feeding is started, serum Prl levels remain elevated and decline gradually over 2–6 months to nonpregnant values. Surges in serum Prl levels associated with suckling are noted through-

out the lactation period (115). As breast-feeding decreases, a gradual drop in serum Prl is noted.

DYNAMIC TESTING OF PRL SECRETION

Although many factors can influence Prl levels, the best single parameter to determine its overall secretion is a determination of the basal serum concentration. Because of the relative stability of the serum Prl level during the day within the physiologic range, dynamic evaluation of the level using stimulation and suppression tests is not routinely necessary. Such tests are, however, useful in the clinical research setting where more detailed information on Prl secretion and lactotroph responsiveness can be generated. One of earlier indications for the evaluation of Prl dynamics was the identification of patients with prolactinomas (97). Being autonomous, Prl secretion in these individuals is usually (but not always) unresponsive to standard physiologic stimuli, such as TRH and phenothiazines (Fig. 6.3). In contrast, patients with hyperprolactinemia associated with pregnancy or primary hypothyroidism have exaggerated responses. However, "normal" responsiveness to stimuli has been reported in about 10–20% of patients with documented prolactinomas. These data limit the usefulness of dynamic tests in such patients. Furthermore, the remarkable advances in imaging the contents of the sella turcica during the past few years have resulted in the early detection and easier recognition of pituitary microadenomas. Dynamic studies

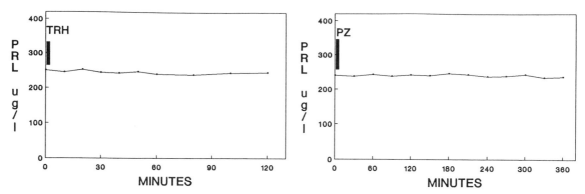

Figure 6.3. Prolactin levels measured after the administration of TRH (500 µg,IV) or perphenazine (PZ, 8 mg by mouth) to a patient with documented prolactin-secreting pituitary adenoma. There was no change in prolactin levels during either test.

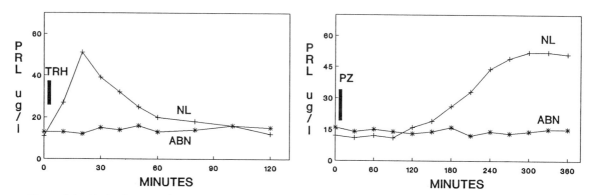

Figure 6.4. Prolactin dynamic studies 6 months after transsphenoidal resection of immunocytochemically documented prolactin-secreting adenomas in two subjects. Prolactin levels were measured after the administration of TRH (500 µg IV) or perphenazine (PZ, 8 mg by mouth) to these subjects. Although basal prolactin levels were normal in both subjects, responses to stimuli were distinctly different. In one subject, the response to either stimulus was normal (NL) and she continues to do well 10 years after surgery. Despite a normal basal level, the response to either stimulus was abnormal (ABN) in the other subject, where no changes in serum prolactin level could be appreciated during the study. The latter subject showed biochemical and clinical signs of recurrence 3 years after surgery. No demonstrable tumor mass could be seen on a CT scan of the sella turcica at the time of documented recurrence.

are, however, very valuable in the research setting, especially in the evaluation of patients after adenomectomy (7, 8, 12). In this regard, dynamic studies can identify subjects with normal basal Prl levels who are at risk for recurrence in the future (7, 12). These individuals have abnormal responsiveness to stimuli despite their normal basal level (Fig. 6.4).

DISORDERS OF PRL SECRETION

Excessive Prl secretion is a common clinical disorder. In contrast, Prl deficiency is less common and, with a few exceptions, it is always associated with panhypopituitarism. The clinical manifestations depend primarily on the degree of abnormality, the associated illness, and the etiology of hyper- or hypoprolactinemia.

Hypoprolactinemia

Deficiency in Prl secretion is commonly seen in patients with panhypopituitarism and is often associated with intrinsic pituitary diseases, such as ischemic necrosis, infiltrative and destructive processes, surgical hypophysectomy, and also as a late manifestation of large intrasellar tumors. Symptoms of hypopituitarism predominate in these patients, although failure to lactate can be a presenting symptom in women with postpartum ischemic necrosis of the pituitary (Sheehan's syndrome).

Isolated deficiency of Prl is extremely rare, as only a few cases have been reported (27, 153). In one of these reports, Prl deficiency was found in six subjects from two families with pseudohypoparathyroidism (27). The basal and stimulated (TRH, chlorpromazine, hypoglycemia) Prl levels remained low and did not change appreciably after estrogen therapy. No associated clinical abnormalities related to Prl were reported in these individuals.

We evaluated a young woman with well-documented isolated Prl deficiency that occurred after surgical removal of a suprasellar eosinophilic granuloma. The patient presented at age 18 with headaches and a suprasellar mass. Endocrine studies at that time demonstrated an elevated serum Prl level (30–40 μg/L), associated with growth hormone, and ACTH, TSH, FSH, and LH deficiencies. Following surgical resection of the granuloma, she recovered normal pituitary function (ACTH, TSH, FSH, and LH secretion) but developed very low serum Prl levels ($<$0.5–1 μg/L). Minimal changes in serum Prl levels were noted 3 months postoperatively, even after stimulation with insulin-induced hypoglycemia, TRH, and phenothiazines. During a 6-year follow-up period, she maintained normal pituitary function, but continued to have low-to-undetectable Prl levels. She got pregnant on two occasions during the 6-year follow-up period and, during both instances, serum Prl levels remained low ($<$2 μg/L). However, despite low serum Prl levels, she was noted to have clear and/or milky discharge during pregnancy. Normal imaging studies (MRI) of the sellar region were documented on repeat testing. Although the pathophysiology of Prl deficiency in this patient is not known, the case illustrates the absence of any clinical manifestations associated with this disorder and the development of galactorrhea during pregnancy despite low serum Prl levels.

Hyperprolactinemia

Serum prolactin levels may be elevated in a variety of medical conditions and through different pathophysiologic mechanisms. The major causes of hyperprolactinemia are listed in Table 6.2.

Of all functioning pituitary adenomas, those secreting prolactin account for about 60%. While most of these tumors secrete prolactin alone, some cosecrete other pituitary hormones, such as growth hormone and ACTH. Secreting and nonsecreting pituitary tumors can also cause hyperprolactinemia if the adenoma is large enough ($>$ 1cm) to impinge on the pituitary stalk and/or portal circulation and thus result in decreased delivery of dopamine, the major prolactin inhibitory factor, to pituitary lactotrophs (6). In these instances, at least partial hypopituitarism is commonly seen (6). Likewise, hypothalamic involvement by primary or metastatic tumors, infiltrative diseases, or granuloma can cause hyperprolactinemia (and often hypopituitarism) through similar mechanisms. Medications known to block dopamine receptors (i.e., phenothiazines, haldol) and those that result in decreased dopamine synthesis and release (i.e., reserpine) can cause Prl levels to increase. Endogenous (i.e., pregnancy) or exogenous hyperestrogenemia (i.e., medications) result in variable degrees of hyperprolactinemia. About 20–30% of patients with primary hypothyroidism have an associated elevation in serum Prl levels (18,

TABLE 6.2.
Causes of Hyperprolactinemia

Pituitary Diseases	Drugs
* Functioning adenomas	* DA receptor antagonist
Prolactin	* Inhibitors of DA synthesis and release
Growth hormone	* Estrogens
Others	Neurogenic
* Nonfunction adenomas	* Chest wall/spinal cord lesions
* Stalk section	* Breast stimulation
Hypothalamic Diseases	* Suckling
* Tumors, granulomas, irradiation	Others
	* Primary hypothyroidism
	* Renal Failure
	* Idiopathic

20, 43, 62, 166) resulting from the TRH levels in the portal circulation.

Hyperprolactinemia occurs frequently in patients with chronic renal failure, with a reported incidence of between 20–70%, especially among patients maintained on hemodialysis (143). Multiple factors appear to contribute to the development of hyperprolactinemia in this setting. These include reduced metabolic clearance rate, increased secretion rate, and lactotroph resistance to dopamine (143).

The clinical manifestations of hyperprolactinemia may vary from one individual to another, depending on many factors that include the patient's age, sex, duration, and degree of increase in serum Prl level. Major symptoms in men and women are related to gonadal dysfunction. In women, these include oligomenorrhea/amenorrhea, infertility, diminished libido, and hypoestrogenemia. The latter can often lead to decreased bone density and possible osteoporosis (57, 76, 77). Symptoms of hypogonadism in men with hyperprolactinemia include diminished libido, impotence, oligospermia, and infertility. The chronic state of hypogonadism in men and women often leads to decreased bone density and possible premature osteoporosis (57, 76, 77). Some men also develop gynecomastia as a result of the chronic hypogonadism. While galactorrhea is seen in the majority of women, it is not commonly seen in men with this disorder (32). It is important to point out that minimal expressible galactorrhea can be seen in up to 20% of women with normal gonadal function and normal prolactin secretion. Thus, galactorrhea cannot be used by itself as a biological marker for hyperprolactinemia. As discussed earlier, polymeric forms of prolactin ("big" and "big-big" prolactin, which are macroprolactins) have diminished biological activities. Recent reports have described a few patients with an apparent elevation of serum prolactin level who have little, if any, associated symptoms. In these patients, excess circulating levels of macroprolactins ("big" and "big-big" prolactins) were reported. These patients do not require any treatment since they have no significant clinical symptoms.

As can be seen from the table and the previous discussion, the differential diagnosis of hyperprolactinemia is extensive. However, the clinical history is extremely important in narrowing the differential diagnosis and pursuing the appropriate work-up. Thus, careful review of medications, in addition to history for thyroid disorder, headaches, visual symptoms, and symptoms of hypopituitarism, are important in defining the etiology. These symptoms should be integrated with the original presentation of the patient that prompted the measurement of the patient's serum prolactin. The extent of the work-up depends on the presence or absence of associated symptoms listed above. The degree of elevation in serum prolactin level can often, but not always, help in defining the etiology of hyperprolactinemia. In the absence of a history of drugs known to elevate serum Prl concentration, (i.e., antipsychotics) a level > 150 μg/L is highly suggestive of a prolactinoma. It is important to keep in mind that patients with documented prolactinomas can have serum levels that are as low as 40 μg/L and as high as several thousands (7).

Large pituitary tumors and other mass lesions in the sella or suprasellar region (i.e., meningiomas, craniopharyngiomas, granulomas, etc.) can cause mild to moderate hyperprolactinemia (25–100 μg/L) by compression of the pituitary stalk and/or portal circulation (6, 73, 74, 122, 140). In these instances, partial hypopituitarism is commonly encountered and visual abnormalities can often be detected. Imaging procedures are indicated in patients with marked elevations in serum Prl levels and in those with significant headaches, visual disturbances, or signs or symptoms that are suggestive of hypopituitarism. The imaging procedure of choice is MRI scan of the sella. Additional studies (i.e., angiograms) are rarely needed in patients who have had MRI scans. Despite extensive evaluation, including MRI scanning, the etiology of hyperprolactinemia in some patients may not be defined and is therefore labelled as idiopathic or essential.

Prl-Secreting Adenomas

Prolactin-secreting tumors are the most common pituitary adenomas in humans. Autopsy studies have demonstrated that 8–20% of humans have pituitary adenomas, most of which were unrecognized antemortem (22). Of all pituitary adenomas, those secreting Prl represent about 40–50%. It is important to point out that the definition of prolactinomas should include the presence of hyperprolactinemia in addition to documented immunocytochemical evidence for Prl secretion or storage by adenomatous cells (7, 122, 131). The distinction is important, since large tumors of any cell type can compress the portal circulation and/or the pituitary stalk and result in hyperprolactinemia (6, 122). Thus, the presence of hyperprolactinemia in association with a pituitary adenoma need not imply the existence of a prolactinoma (7, 122). These issues are important not only in defining the pathophysiology of hyperprolactinemia, but also in choosing appropriate treatments.

Lactotroph cell adenomas typically originate in the lateral wings of the anterior pituitary gland. Most of these tumors are soft and are surrounded by a pseudocapsule. The structural features of tumor cells are similar to those seen in nontumorous lactotrophs, including the well-developed endoplasmic reticulum and Golgi apparatus. On electron microscopy, both the densely granulated and the more common sparsely granulated forms of adenomatous lactotrophs can be seen (79). Although most prolactinomas contain uniform Prl-staining cells, others can, in addition, stain for other pituitary hormones, such as growth hormone (79). Such adenomas may be composed of a one-cell population that produces two or more hormones (monomorphous adenomas). Alternatively, they can be composed of multiple cell types (79), each producing one hormone (pleurimorphous adenomas).

The pathogenesis of Prl-secreting adenomas has been extensively debated in the course of the past decade (25, 102, 105). While some postulate that these tumors arise as a result of disordered hypothalamic secretion (19, 48, 148), others believe adenomas arise de novo, independent of hypothalamic stimulation (7, 61, 88, 105, 127). The former view is supported by some reports demonstrating decreased sensitivity of adenomatous cells to dopamine (149) and others showing decreased dopamine receptors on these cells (21). Several observations support the alternative hypothesis suggesting a primary pituitary origin of these adenomas (7, 61, 105, 127). Pituitary tissue surrounding the adenoma is not usually hyperplastic, implying that there is no hypothalamic stimulation of nonadenomatous cells. Surgical resection of adenomas cures most patients of the disorder (7, 127). The drop in serum Prl levels to very low levels immediately after adenomectomy (Fig. 6.1), followed by the gradual recovery of lactotroph responsiveness to stimuli over months (7, 8, 33) is consistent with a primary pituitary origin of these adenomas. Recurrence of hyperprolactinemia after successful surgery varies from one series to another and generally is less than 20% (7, 127, 139).

We have utilized normalization of Prl dynamics (response to TRH, phenothiazines, and insulin-hypoglycemia) rather than the basal Prl level as the standard for defining successful outcome of surgery (7, 8). The recurrence rate after an average of 6 years of follow-up for subjects who had normal basal and stimulated Prl levels following adenomectomy is only 3% (7). In contrast, patients who continued to have blunted responses to stimulation despite normal basal levels, have a high recurrence rate approaching 70% over 5 years (7). We postulated that incomplete resection of the adenoma caused the observed differences in Prl dynamics, although this could not be documented with imaging studies.

Recent studies investigating the clonal origin of pituitary adenomas (61), demonstrated that prolactinomas are monoclonal in nature and suggested that somatic cell mutations precede clonal expansion of these cells and play a major role in pituitary tumorigenesis. The current view is that pituitary adenomas arise de novo because of a primary pituitary cell abnormality. However, a facilitating role for the hypothalamus in pituitary tumorigenesis can not be totally excluded.

The clinical manifestations of Prl-secreting pituitary tumors can be conveniently divided into three categories. These include: a) Symptoms related to hyperprolactinemia: oligolamenorrhea, galactorrhea, infertility, and hypoestrogenemia in women; diminished libido, impotence, oligolazospermia and, less commonly, gynecomastia and galactorrhea in men. In both men and women, the prolonged state of hypogonadism can potentially lead to the development of premature osteoporosis (57, 76, 77). b) Symptoms caused by mechanical pressure by the adenoma on surrounding structures. These are only seen with large tumors that are > 1 cm in diameter and often associated with headaches. Extension of the adenoma into the suprasellar region will result in pressure on the optic apparatus, whereas extension medially results in the invasion of the cavernous sinus and potential disruption of the function of cranial nerves III, IV, V, and VI. c) Symptoms due to impairment of normal pituitary function by the expanding adenoma, resulting in partial or complete loss of pituitary function. These effects are expected only in patients with large adenomas. Recent studies have demonstrated that, following surgical (6) or medical (159) treatment of the adenoma, pituitary function can be restored to normal in most subjects. Based on dynamic studies of pituitary function before and after surgery, we postulated that hypopituitarism in this setting is primarily caused by the compression of the portal vessels and/or pituitary stalk and that, once this is relieved, normal pituitary function can be restored in most subjects (6).

Recent studies on the natural history of untreated hyperprolactinemia have raised questions on the indications for treatment in subjects with prolactinomas. It is currently believed that if untreated, most patients with Prl-secreting adenomas follow a benign course and that hyperprolactinemia and continued tumor growth can be documented in only a small percentage of patients (93, 96). Most others showed either no change in tumor size, or reduction or stabilization of serum Prl level in the course of years (136, 145). Clinical symptoms often, but not always, follow the associated change in serum Prl level (161). Despite tumor-size stability in the majority of patients, therapy may be necessary for a variety of reasons. These include menstrual abnormalities and infertility as well as excessive galactorrhea in women and sexual dysfunction in men. In both men and women, Prl-induced hypogonadism is associated with premature osteoporosis and can be partly reversed after therapy (57, 76, 77).

Since therapeutic options will be discussed in great detail in a different chapter, they will be mentioned only briefly. The two major options for treating patients with prolactinomas include medical treatment with dopamine agonists or surgical adenomectomy. Either option is effective, and the choice between the two depends on many factors that include: tumor size and extension outside the sell turcica, the patient's preference for and commitment to prolonged therapy, the availability of an experienced surgeon, side effects from medications, response to medication, and the financial impact of the treatment.

Our approach is to discuss all of these issues with the patient and make a joint decision on the management plan. In patients with large tumors, some advocate the use of a dopamine agonist for a limited period of time (2–3 months) to attempt to decrease the size and extension of the adenoma and thereby improve surgical outcome (17, 64, 83, 84, 152). While this approach seems reasonable, there are no available studies demonstrating its superiority to the use of either medical or surgical treatment alone.

ACKNOWLEDGMENTS

This work was supported by an NIH Grant to the Clinical Research Center from the General CRC Branch. The authors wish to thank the staff of the Clinical Research Center for conducting the studies and Michelle E. Hall for preparing the manuscript.

REFERENCES

1. Abe H., Engler D., Molitch M., Bollinger-Gruber J., and Reichlin S. Vasoactive intestinal peptide is a physiological mediator of Prl release in the rat. Endocrinology, 116:1383–1390, 1985.
2. Advis J.P., Hall T.R., Hodson C.A., Mueller G.P., and Meites J. Temporal relationship and role of dopamine in "short-loop" of prolactin. Proc. Soc. Exp. Biol. Med., 155:567–570, 1977.
3. Amara J.F., Van Itallie C., and Dannies P.S. Regulation of prolactin production and cell growth by estradiol: difference in sensitivity to estradiol occurs at level of messenger ribonucleic acid accumulation. Endocrinology, 120:264–271, 1987.
4. Anderson A.N., Pederson H., Djursing H., Andersen B.N., and Friesen H.G. Bioactivity of prolactin in a woman with an excess of large molecular size prolactin, persistent hyperprolactinemia and spontaneous conception. Fertil. Steril., 38:625–628, 1982.

5. Annunziato L., and Moore K.E. Prolactin in CSF selectively incrases dopamine turnover in the median eminence. Life Sci. *22*:2037–2042, 1978.

6. Arafah B.M. Reversible hypopituitarism in patients with large nonfunctioning pituitary adenomas. J. Clin. Endocrinol. Metab. *62*:1173, 1986.

6. Arafah B.M., Brodkey J.S., and Pearson O.H. Gradual recovery of lactotroph responsiveness to dynamic stimulation following surgical removal of prolactinomas: long-term follow-up studies. Metabolism, *35*:905–912, 1986.

8. Arafah B.M., Brodkey J.S., and Pearson O.H. Prolactin secreting pituitary adenomas in women. In: *Diagnosis and management of endocrine-related tumors,* pp. 63, edited by R.J. Santen and A. Manni. Boston, Martinus Nijhoff Publishers, 1984.

9. Arafah B.M., Finegan H.M., Roe J., Manni A., and Pearson O.H. Hormone dependency in N-nitrosomethyurea-induced rat mammary tumors. Endocrinology, *111*:584, 1982.

10. Arafah B.M., Gordon N.H., Salazar R., and Douglas J.G. Modulation of tissue responsiveness to angiotensin-II in hyperprolactinemic subjects. J. Clin. Endocrinol. Metab., *71*:60–66, 1990.

11. Arafah B.M., Griffin P., Gordon N.H., and Pearson O.H. Growth enhancement of N-nitrosomethyleurea-induced rat mammary tumor cells in soft agar by estrogen or prolactin. Cancer Res., *44*:5506–5608, 1984.

12. Arafah B.M., Manni A., Brodkey J.S., *et al.* Cure of hypogonadism after removal of prolactin-secreting adenomas in men. J. Clin. Endocrinol. Metab., *52*:91–94, 1981.

13. Arafah B.M., Wilhite B.L., Rainieri J., Brodkey J.S., Pearson O.H. Inhibitory action of bromocriptine and tamoxifen on the growth of human pituitary tumors in soft agar. J. Clin. Endocrinol. Metab., *57*:986–992, 1983.

14. Arnaout M.A., Garthwaite T.L., Martinson D.R., and Hagen T.C. Basoactive intestinal peptide is synthesized in anterior pituitary tissue. Endocrinology, *119*:2052–2057, 1986.

15. Ben-Jonathan N. Dopamine: a prolactin-inhibiting hormone. Endocr. Rev., *6*:564–589, 1985.

16. Ben-Jonathan N., Oliver C., Weiner H.J., Mical R., and Porter J.C. Dopamine in hypophyseal portal plasma of the rat during the estrus cycle and throughout pregnancy. Endocrinology, *100*:452–458, 1977.

17. Bevan J.S., Adams C.B.T., Burke C.W., *et al.* Factors in the outcome of transsphenoidal surgery for prolactinoma and non-functioning pituitary tumor, including pre-operative bromocriptine therapy. Clin. Endocrinol. (Oxf), *26*:541–56, 1987.

18. Bigos S.T., Ridgway E.C., Kourides I.A., and Maloof F. Spectrum of pituitary alterations with mild and severe thyroid impairment. J. Clin. Endocrinol., *46*:317–325, 1978.

19. Bression D., Brandi A.M., Martes M.P., *et al.* Dopaminergic receptors in human prolactin-secreting adenomas: A quantitative study. J. Clinic. Endocrinol. Metab., *51*:1037–1048, 1980.

20. Buchanan C.R., Stanhope R., Adlard P., Jones J.,

Grant D.B., and Preece M.A. Gonadotropin, growth hormone and prolactin secretion in children with primary hypothyroidism. Clin. Endocrinol. (Oxf), *29*:427–436, 1988.

21. Buckley A.R., Putnam C.W., Montgomery D.W., and Russell D.H. Prolactin administration stimulates rat hepatic DNA synthesis. Biochem. Biophys. Res. Commun., *138*:1138–1145, 1986.

22. Burrow G.N., Wortzmann G., Rewcastle N.B., Holtgate R.C., and Kovacs K. Microadenomas of the pituitary and abnormal sellar tomograms in an unselected autopsy series. N. Engl. J. Med., *304*:156, 1981.

23. Burstyn P.G.R. Sodium and water metabolism under the influence of prolactin, aldosterone and antidiuretic hormone. J. Physiol. (London), *275*:39, 1978.

24. Calabro M.A., and Macleod R.M. Binding of dopamine to bovine anterior pituitary gland membrane. Neuroendocrinology, *25*:32–46, 1978.

25. Camanni F., Ciccarelli E., Ghigo E., and Muller E.E. Hyperprolactinemia: Neuroendocrine and diagnostic aspects. J. Endocrinol. Invest., *12*:653–668, 1989.

26. Carlson H.E. Prolactin stimulation by protein is mediated by amino acids in humans. J. Clin. Endocrinol. Metab., *69*:7–14, 1989.

27. Carlson H.E., Brickman A.S., and Bottazzo G.F. Prolactin deficiency in pseudohypoparathyroidism. N. Engl. J. Med., *296*:140–144, 1977.

28. Carlson H.E., Jacobs L.S., and Daughaday W.H. Growth hormone, thyrotropin and prolactin responses to thyrotropin releasing hormone following diethylstilbestrol pre-treatment. J. Clin. Endocrinol. Metab., *37*:488–494, 1973.

29. Carlson H.E., Wasser H.L., Levin S.R., and Wilkins J.N. Prolactin stimulation by meals is related to protein content. J. Clin. Endocrinol. Metab., *57*:334–338, 1983.

30. Caron M.G., Beaulieu M., Raymond V., Gagne B., Drouin J., and Lefkowitz R.L. Dopaminergic receptors on the anterior pituitary gland. J. Biol. Chem., *253*:2244–2253, 1978.

31. Carrol J.E., Campanile C.P., and Goodfriend T.L. The effect of prolactin on human aldosterone-producing adenoma in vitro. J. Clin. Endocrinol. Metab., *54*:689, 1982.

32. Carter J.N., Tryson J.E., Tolis G., Van Vliet S., Faiman C., and Freisen H.G. Prolactin secreting tumors and hypogonadism in 22 men. N. Engl. J. Med., *299*:847–855, 1978.

33. Casper R.F., Rakoff J.S., Quigley M.E., Gilliland B., Alksne J., and Yen S.S.C. Changes in pituitary hormones during and following transsphenoidal removal of prolactinomas. Am. J. Obstet. Gynecol., *136*:518, 1980.

34. Chen C.L., Minaguchi H., and Meites J. Effects of transplanted pituitary tumors on host pituitary prolactin secretion. Proc. Soc. Exp. Biol. Med., *126*:317–325, 1967.

35. Cooper G.R., and Shin S.H. Somatostatin inhibits prolactin secretion in the estradiol primed male rat. Can. J. Physiol. Pharmacol., *59*:1082–1088, 1981.

36. Cronin M.J., Myers G.A., Macleod R.M., and Hewlett E.L. Pertussis toxin uncouples dopamine agonist inhibition of prolactin release. Am. J. Physiol., *244 (Endocrinol. Metab.)*:E499–E504, 1983.

37. Dannies P.S., and Tashijan A.H. Thyrotropin-releasing hormone increases prolactin mRNA activity in the cytoplasm of GH-cells as measured by translation in a wheat germ cell-free system. Biochem. Biophys. Res. Commun., *70:*1180–1189, 1975.

38. De Greef W.J., and Visser T.J. Evidence for the involvement of hypothalamic dopamine and thyrotrophin-releasing hormone in suckling-induced release of prolactin. J. Endocrinol., *91:*213–223, 1981.

39. De Lean A., Ferland L., Drouin J., Kelly P., and Labrie F. Modulation of pituitary thyrotrophin releasing hormone receptor levels by estrogens and thyroid hormone. Endocrinology, *100:*1486–1501, 1977.

40. Demarest K.T., and Moore K.E. Sexual differences in the sensitivity of tuberinfundibular dopamine neurons to the actions of prolactin. Neuroendocrinology, *33:*230–234, 1981.

41. Denef C. LHRH stimulates prolactin release from rat pituitary lactotrophs cocultured with a highly purified population of gonadotrophs. Ann. Endocrinol. (Paris), *42:*65–67, 1981.

42. Denef C., and Andries M. Evidence for paracrine interaction between gonadotrophs and lactotrophs in pituitary cell aggregates. Endocrinology, *112:*813–822, 1983.

43. Edwards C.R.W., Forsyth I.A., and Besser G.M. Amenorrhoea, galactorrhoea, and primary hypothyroidism with high circulating levels of prolactin. B.M.J., *3:*462–464, 1971.

44. Enjalbert A., Arancibia S., Ruberg M., et al. Stimulation of in vitro prolactin release by vasoactive intestinal peptide. Neuroendocrinology, *31:*200–204, 1980.

45. Farkouh N.H., Packer M.G., and Frantz A.G. Large molecular size prolactin with reduced receptor activity in human serum: High proportion in basal state and reduction after thyrotropin-releasing hormone. J. Clin. Endocrinol. Metab., *48:*1026–1032, 1979.

46. Farquhar M.G., Reid J.J., and Daniell L.W. Intracellular transport and packaging of prolactin: A quantitative electron microscope autoradiographic study of mammotrophs dissociated from rat pituitaries. Endocrinology, *102:*296–311, 1978.

47. Ferland L., Labrie F., Jobin M., Arimura A., and Schally A.V. Physiological role of somatostatin in the control of growth hormone and thyrotropin secretion. Biochem. Biophys. Res. Commun., *68:*149–156, 1976.

48. Fine S.A., Frohman L.A. Loss of central nervous system component of dopaminergic inhibition of prolactin-secretion in patients with prolactin-secreting pituitary tumors. J. Clin. Invest., *61:*973–980, 1978.

49. Franks S. Regulation of prolactin secretion by oestrogens: physiological and pathological significance. Clin. Sci., *65:*457–462, 1983.

50. Frantz G., and Likeinberg D.L. Prolactin: Evidence that it is separate from growth hormone in human blood. Science, *170:*745–746, 1970.

51. Fraser I.S., Lun Z.G., Zhou J.P., et al. Detailed assessment of big-big prolactin in women with hyperprolactinemia and normal ovarian function. J. Clin. Endocrinol. Metab., *69:*585–592, 1989.

52. Frawley L.S., and Clark C.L. Ovine prolactin (Prl) and dopamine preferentially inhibit Prl release from the same subpopulation of rat mammotrophs. Endocrinology, *119:*1462–1466, 1986.

53. Gibbs D.M., and Neill J.D. Dopamine levels in hypophysial stalk blood in the rat are sufficient to inhibit prolactin secretion in vivo. Endocrinology, *102:*1895–1900, 1978.

54. Goldsmith P.C., Cronin M.J., and Weiner R.I. Dopamine receptor sites in the anterior pituitary. J. Histochem. Cytochem., *27:*1205–1207, 1979.

55. Gooren L.J.G., Harmsen-Louman W., Van Kessel H. Somatostatin inhibits prolactin release from the lactotroph primed with oestrogen and cyproterone acetate in man. J. Endocrinol., *102:*333–335, 1984.

56. Grandison L., and Guiddotti A. Gamma-aminobutyric acid receptor function in rat anterior-pituitary: evidence for control of prolactin release. Endocrinology, *105:*745–759, 1979.

57. Greenspan S.L., Oppenheim D.O., and Klibanski A. Importance of gonadal steroids to bone mass in men with hyperprolactinemic hypogonadism. Ann. Intern. Med., *110:*526–531, 1989.

58. Gudelsky G.A., and Porter J.C. Sex related difference in the release of dopamine into hypophysial portal blood. Endocrinology, *109:*1394–1398, 1981.

59. Guyda H.J. Heterogeneity of human growth hormone and prolactin secreted in vitro: Immunoassay and radioreceptor assay correlation. J. Clin. Endocrinol. Metab., *41:*953, 1975.

60. Hanew K., and Rennels E.G. Effects of culture age on Prl and GH responses to bromocriptine and somatostatin from pituitary cultures of rat anterior pituitary cells. Proc. Soc. Exp. Biol. Med., *171:*112–118, 1982.

61. Herman V., Fagin J., Gonsky R., Kovacs K., and Melmed S. Clonal origin of pituitary adenomas. J. Clin. Endocrinol. Metab., *71:*1427–1433, 1990.

62. Honbo K.S., Vantterle A.J., and Kellett K.A. Serum prolactin levels in untreated primary hypothyroidism. Am. J. Med., *64:*782–787, 1978.

63. Hout W.M., Arafah B.M., Salazar R., and Selman W. Elevation of the hypothalamic-pituitary-adrenal axis immediately after pituitary adenomectomy: is perioperative steroid therapy necessary? J. Clin. Endocrinol. Metab., *66:*1208–1212, 1988.

64. Hubbard J.L., Scheithauer B.W., Abboud C.F., and Laws E.R. Jr. Prolactin-secreting adenomas: the preoperative response to bromocriptine treatment and surgical outcome. J. Neurosurg., *67:*816–821, 1987.

65. Hwang P., Guyda H., and Friesen H. A radio-immunoassay for human prolactin. Proc. Natl. Acad. Sci. USA, *68:*1902–1906, 1971.

66. Kimura N., Hayafuji C., Konagaya H., and Takahashi K. 17β-Estradiol induces somatostatin

(SRIF) inhibition of prolactin release and regulates SRIF receptors in rat anterior pituitary cells. Endocrinology, *119:*1028–1036, 1986.

67. Itoh N., Obata K., Yanaihara N., and Okamoto H. Human preprovasoactive intestinal polypeptide contains a novel PHI-27-like peptide, PHM-27. Nature, *304:*547–549, 1973.

68. Jackson R.D., Worstman J., and Malarkey W.B. Characterization of a large molecular weight prolactin in women with idiopathic hyperprolactinemia and normal menses. J. Clin. Endocrinol. Metab., *61:*258–264, 1985.

69. Jackson R.D., Wortsman J., and Malarkey W.B. Persistence of large molecular weight prolactin secretion during pregnancy in women with macroprolactinemia and its presence in fetal cord blood. J. Clin. Endocrinol. Metab., *68:*1046–1050, 1989.

70. Jacobi J., Lloyd H.M., and Meares J.D. Onset of oestrogen-induced prolactin secretion and DNA synthesis by the rat pituitary gland. J. Endocrinol., *72:*35–40, 1977.

71. Johnston C.A., Demarest K.T., and Moore K.E. Cycloheximide disrupts the prolactin-mediated stimulation of dopamine synthesis in tuberoinfundibular neurons. Brain Res., *195:*236–240, 1980.

72. Kaji H., Chihara K., Abe H., *et al.* Stimulatory effect of peptide histidine isoleucine amide 1–27 on prolactin release in the rat. Life Sci., *35:*641–647, 1984.

73. Kapacala L.P., Molitch M.E., Arno J., King L.W., Reichlin S., and Wolpert S.M. Twenty-four-hour prolactin secretory patterns in women with galactorrhea, normal menses, normal random prolactin levels and abnormal sellar tomograms. J. Endocrinol. Invest., *7:*455, 1984.

74. Kapcala M.T., Molitch M.E., Post K.T., Miller B.J., Jackson J.M.D., and Reichlin S. Galactorrhea, oligo-amenorrhea and hyperprolactinemia in patients with craniopharyngioma. J. Clin. Endocrinol. Metab., *53:*798, 1980.

75. Kaufman S. The dipsogenic activity of prolactin in male and female rats. J. Physiol. (Lond.), *310:*435–444, 1981.

76. Klibanski A., Biller B.M.K., Rosenthal D.I., Schoenfeld D.A., and Saxe V. Effects of prolactin and estrogen deficiency in amenorrheic bone loss. J. Clin. Endocrinol. Metab., *67:*124–130, 1988.

77. Klibanski A., and Greenspan S.L. Increase in bone mass after treatment of hyperprolactinemic amenorrhea. N. Engl. J. Med., *315:*542, 1986.

78. Kolodny R.C., Jacobs L.S., and Daughaday W.H. Mammary stimulation causes prolactin secretion in non-lactating women. Nature, *238:*284, 1972.

79. Kovacs K., and Horvath E. Pathology of pituitary tumors. Endocrinol. Metab. Clin. North Am., *16:*529–551, 1987.

80. Lam K.S.L., Lechan R.M., Minamitani N., Segerson T.P., and Reichlin S. Vasoactive intestinal peptide in the anterior pituitary is increased in hypothyroidism. Endocrinology, *124:*1077–1084, 1989.

81. Lamberts S.W.J., and MacLeod R.M. The inability of bromocriptine to inhibit prolactin secretion by transplantable rat pituitary tumors: observations on the mechanism and dynamics of the au-

tofeedback regulation of prolactin secretion. Endocrinology, *104:*65–70, 1979.

82. Lamberts S.W.J., Verleun T., and Oosterom R. Effect of tamoxifen administration on prolactin release by invasive prolactin-secreting pituitary adenomas. Neuroendocrinology, *34:*339–342, 1982.

83. Landolt A.M., Keller P.J., Froesch E.R., and Mueller J. Bromocriptine: does it jeopardize the result of later surgery for prolactinomas? Lancet, *2:*657, 1982.

84. Landolt A.M., and Osterwalter V. Perivascular fibrosis in prolactinomas: is it increased by bromocriptine? J. Clin. Endocrinol. Metab., *58:*1179, 1984.

85. Lewis U.J., Singh R.N.P., Lewis L.J., Saevey B.K., and Sinha Y.N. Glycosylated ovine prolactin. Proc. Natl. Acad. Sci. USA, *81:*385–391, 1984.

86. Lewis U.J., Singh R.N.P., Sinha Y.N., and Vanderlaan W.P. Glycosylated human prolactin. Endocrinology, *116:*359–363, 1985.

87. Lightman S.L., Fox P., and Dunne M.J. The effect of SMS 201–995, a long-acting somatostatin analogue, on anterior pituitary function in healthy male volunteers. Scand. J. Gastroenterol. Suppl., *119:*84–95, 1986.

88. Lloyd R.V., Cano M., Chandler W.F., Barkan A., Horvath E., and Kovacs K. Human growth hormone and prolactin secreting pituitary adenomas analyzed by in situ hybridization. Am. J. Pathol., *134:*605–13, 1989.

89. Loeffler J.P., Kley N., Pittius C.W., Almeida O.F., and Holt V. In vivo and in vitro studies of GABAergic inhibition of prolactin biosynthesis. Neuroendocrinology, *43:*504–510, 1986.

90. Login I.S., Judd A.M., and MacLeod R.M. Dopamine inhibits calcium flux in the 7315a prolactin-secreting pituitary tumor. Cell Calcium, *9:*27–31, 1988.

91. Malarkey W.B., Kennedy M., Allred L.E., and Milo G. Physiological concentrations of prolactin can promote the growth of human breast tumor cells in culture. J. Clin. Endocrinol. Metab., *56:*673–677, 1983.

92. Malgaroli A., Vallar L., Elahi F.R., Tozann T., and Spada A. Dopamine inhibits cytosolic Ca^{2+} increases in rat lactotroph cells. J. Biol. Chem., *262:*13920–13927, 1987.

93. March C.M., Kletzky O.A., Davajan V., *et al.* Longitudinal evaluation of patients with untreated prolactin-secreting pituitary adenomas. Am. J. Obstet. Gynecol., *139:*835, 1981.

94. Markoff E., and Lee D.W. Glycosylated prolactin is a major circulating variant in human serum. J. Clin. Endocrinol. Metab., *65:*1102–1106, 1978.

95. Markoff E., Sigel M.B., Lacour N., Seavey B.K., Friesen H.G., and Lewis U.J. Glycosylation selectively alters the biological activity of prolactin. Endocrinology, *123:*1303–1306, 1988.

96. Martin T.L., Kim M., and Malarkey W.B. The natural history of idiopathic hyperprolactinemia. J. Clin. Endocrinol. Metab., *60:*855, 1985.

97. Mattox J.H., and Fortunato S.J. Prolactin response to perphenazine. A sensitive and specific test for pituitary tumor in hyperprolactinemic

women. J. Reproductive Med., *31*:1089–1101, 1986.

98. Maurer R.A. Transcriptional regulation of the prolactin gene by erocryptine and cyclic AMP. Nature, *294*:94–97, 1981.

99. Maurer R.A. Dopaminergic inhibition of prolactin synthesis and prolactin messenger RNA accumulation in cultured pituitary cells. J. Biol. Chem., *255*:8092–8099, 1980.

100. Maurer R.A. Thyroid hormone specifically inhibits prolactin synthesis and decreases prolactin messenger ribonucleic acid levels in cultured pituitary cells. Endocrinology, *110*:1507–1514, 1982.

101. Mazzocchi G., Robba C., Rebuffat P., and Nussedorfer G.G. Effects of prolactin administration on the zona glomerulosa of the rat adrenal cortex: Stereology and plasma hormone concentrations. Acta Endocrinol. (Copenh.), *111*:101–105, 1986.

102. Melmed S., Braunstein G.D., Chang R.J., and Becker D.P. Pituitary tumors secreting growth hormone and prolactin. Ann. Intern. Med., *105*:238–253, 1986.

103. Mills D.E., and Ward R.P. Effect of prolactin on blood pressure and cardiovascular responsiveness in the rat (42217). Proc. Soc. Exp. Biol. Med., *181*:3–8, 1986.

104. Mills D.E., and Woods R.B. Interaction of prolactin with adrenal hormones in blood pressure regulation in rats. Am. J. Physiology (Endocrinol. Metab. 12), *249*:E614–E618, 1985.

105. Molitch M. Pathogenesis of pituitary tumors. Endocrinol. Metab. Clin. North Am., *16*:503–527, 1987.

106. Molitch M.E., Raiti S., Baumann G., Belknap S., and Reichlin S. Pharmacokinetic studies of highly purified human prolactin in normal human subjects. J. Clin. Endocrinol. Metab., *65*:299–304, 1987.

107. Morel G., Besson J., Rosselin G., and Dubois P.M. Ultrastructural evidence for endogenous vasoactive intestinal peptide-like immunoreactivity in the pituitary gland. Neuroendocrinology, *34*:85–89, 1982.

108. Morely J.E., Dawson M., Hodgkinson H., and Kalk W.J. Galactorrhea and hyperprolactinemia associated with chest wall injury. J. Clin. Endocrinol. Metab., *45*:931, 1977.

109. Murai I., and Ben-Jonathan N. Chronic posterior pituitary lobectomy: prolonged elevation of plasma prolactin and interruption of cyclicity. Neuroendocrinology, *43*:453–461, 1986.

110. Murai I., Garris P.A., and Ben-Jonathan N. Time-dependent increase in plasma prolactin after pituitary stalk section: role of posterior pituitary dopamine. Endocrinology, *124*:2343–2349, 1989.

111. Murphy P.R., Dimattia G.E., and Freisen H.G. Role of calcium in prolactin-stimulated c-myc gene expression and mitogenesis in NB2 lymphoma cells. Endocrinology, *122*:2476–2485, 1988.

112. Nagy G., Mulchahey J.J., and Neill J.D. Autocrine control of prolactin secretion by vasoactive intestinal peptide. Endocrinology, *122*:364–366, 1988.

113. Neill J.D., Frawley L.S., Plotsky P.M., and Tindall G.T. Dopamine in hypophysial stalk blood of the rhesus monkey and its role in regulating prolactin secretion. Endocrinology, *108*:489–494, 1981.

114. Nikolics K., Mason A.J., Szonyi E., Ramachandran J., and Seeburg P.H. A prolactin-inhibiting factor within the precursor for human gonadotropin-releasing hormone. Nature, *316*:511–517, 1985.

115. Noel G.L., Suh H.K., and Frantz A.G. Prolactin release during nursing and hormone stimulation in postpartum and nonpostpartum subjects. J. Clin. Endocrinol. Metab., *38*:413, 1974.

116. Noel G.L., Suh H.K., Stone J.G., and Frantz A.G. Human prolactin and growth hormone release during surgery and other conditions of stress. J. Clin. Endocrinol. Metab., *35*:840, 1972.

117. Pichon M.F., Bression D., Peillon F., and Milgrom E. Estrogen receptors in human pituitary adenomas. J. Clin. Endocrinol. Metab., *51*:897, 1980.

118. Pilotte N.J., and Porter J.C. Dopamine in hypophysial portal plasma and prolactin in systemic plasma of rats treated with 5-hydroxytryptamine. Endocrinology, *108*:2137–2141, 1981.

119. Plotsky P.M., Gibbs D.M., and Neill J.D. Liquid chromatographic and electrochemical measurement of dopamine in hypophyseal stalk blood of rats. Endocrinology, *102*:1887–1894, 1978.

120. Prysor-Jones R.A., Sliverlight J.J., Jenkins J.S., and Merry B.J. Vasoactive intestinal polypeptide and dopamine in the hypothalamus and pituitary of ageing rats with prolactinomas. Acta Endocrinol. (Copenh.), *116*:150–154, 1987.

121. Quigley M.E., Roper J.F., and Yen S.S.C. Acute prolactin release triggered by feeding. J. Clin. Endocrinol. Metab., *52*:1043–1045, 1981.

122. Randall R.V., Scheithauer R.W., Laws E.R., Abboud C.F., Ebersold M.J., and Koa P.C. Pituitary adenomas associated with hyperprolactinemia: A clinical and immunohistochemical study on 97 patients operated on transsphenoidally. Mayo Clin. Proc., *60*:753, 1985.

123. Ratner R.E., Sherry S.H., and Guay A.T. Secretion of prolactin after acute and chronic stimulation of the breast: effect of timing during the menstrual cycle. Fertil Steril., *38*:410, 1982.

124. Raymond V., Beaulieu M., and Labrie F. Potent antidopaminergic activity of estradiol at the pituitary level on prolactin release. Science, *200*:1173, 1978.

125. Reymond M.J., Kaur C., and Porter J.C. An inhibitory role for morphine on the release of dopamine into hypophysial portal blood and on the synthesis of dopamine in tuberoinfundibular neurons. Brain Res., *262*:252–258, 1983.

126. Riddle O., Bates R.W., and Dykshorn S. The preparation, identification and assay of prolactin. A hormone of the anterior pituitary. Am. J. Physiol., *105*:191, 1933.

127. Rodman E.F., Molitch M.E., Post K.E., biller B.J., and Reichlin S. Long-term follow-up of transsphenoidal selective adenomectomy for prolactinoma. JAMA, *252*:921–924, 1984.

128. Russel D.H., Kibler R., Matrisian L., Larson D.F., Poulos B., and Magun B.F. Prolactin receptors on

human T and B lymphocytes: Antagonism of prolactin binding by cyclosporine. J. Immuno., *134*:3027–2031, 1985.

129. Russell D.H., and Larson D.F. Prolactin-induced polyamine biosynthesis in spleen and thymus: specific inhibition by cyclosporine. Immunopharmacology, *9*:165–174, 1985.

130. Said S.I., and Porter J.C. Vasoactive intestinal polypeptide release into hypophysial portal blood. Life Sci., *24*:227–230, 1979.

131. Sakurai T., Seo H., Yamamoto N., *et al.* Detection of mRNA of prolactin and ACTH in clinically nonfunctioning pituitary adenomas. J. Neurosurg., *69*:653–659, 1988.

132. Sarkar D.K. Evidence for prolactin feedback actions on hypothalamic oxytocin, vasoactive intestinal peptide and dopamine secretion. Neuroendocrinology, *49*:520–524, 1989.

133. Sarkar D.K., Miki N., and Meites J. Failure of prolactin short loop feedback mechanism to operate in old as compared to young female rats. Endocrinology, *113*:1452–1458, 1983.

134. Sassin J.F., Frantz A.G., Weitzman E.D., and Kapen S. Human prolactin: 24 hr pattern with increased release during sleep. Science, *177*:1205–1207, 1972.

135. Schally A.V., Redding T., Armura A., Dupont A., and Linthicum G.L. Isolation of gamma-amino butyric acid from pig hypothalamin and demonstration of its prolactin releasing-inhibiting (PIF) activity in vivo and in vitro. Endocrinology, *100*:681–691, 1977.

136. Schlechte J., Dolan K., Sherman B., Chapler F., and Luciano A. The natural history of untreated hyperprolactinemia: a prospective analysis. J. Clin. Endocrinol. Metab., *68*:412–418, 1989.

137. Schrey M.P., Clark H.J., and Franks S. The dopaminergic regulation of anterior pituitary ^{45}Ca homeostasis and prolactin secretion. J. Endocrinol., *108*:423–429, 1986.

138. Selmanoff M. Rapid effects of hyperprolactinemia on basal prolactin secretion and dopamine turnover in the medial and lateral median eminence. Endocrinology, *116*:1943–1952, 1985.

139. Serri O., Rasio E., Beauregard H., Hardy J., and Somma M. Recurrence of hyperprolactinemia after selective transsphenoidal adenomectomy in women with prolactinoma. N. Engl. J. Med., *309*:280–283, 1983.

140. Shas R.P., Leavens M.E., and Samaan N.A. Galactorrhea, amenorrhea and hyperprolactinemia as manifestations of parasellar meningioma. Arch. Intern. Med., *140*:1608, 1980.

141. Shimatsu A., Kato Y., Matsushita N., Katakami H., Yanaihara N., and Imura H. Stimulation by serotonin of vasoactive intestinal polypeptide release into rat hypophysial-portal blood. Endocrinology, *111*:338–340, 1982.

142. Shome B., and Parlow A.R. Human pituitary prolactin (hPrl): The entire linear amino acid sequence. J. Clin. Endocrinol. Metab., *45*:112, 1977.

143. Sievertsen G., Lim V.S., Nakawatase C., and Frohman L.A. Metabolic clearance and secretion rates of human prolactin in normal subjects and in patients with chronic renal failure. J. Clin. Endocrinol. Metab., *50*:846–852, 1980.

144. Sinha Y.N., and Tucker H.A. Pituitary prolactin content and mammary development after chronic administration of prolactin. Proc. Soc. Exp. Biol. Med., *128*:84–88, 1968.

145. Sisam D.A., Sheehan J.P., and Sheeler L.R. The natural history of untreated microprolactinomas. Fertil. Steril., *48*:67, 1987.

146. Snyder P.J., Jacobs L.S., Utiger R.D., and Daughaday W.H. Thyroid hormone inhibition of the prolactin response to thyrotropin-releasing hormone. J. Clin. Invest., *52*:2324, 1973.

147. Sowers J.E., Carlson H.E., Brautbar N., and Hershaman J.M. Effects of dexamethasone on prolactin and TSH response to TRH and metocloprimide in man. J. Clin. Endocrinol. Metab., *45*:44–50, 1977.

148. Spada A., Nicosia S., Cortelazz L., *et al.* In vitro studies on prolactin release and adenylate cyclase activity in human prolactin secreting adenomas. Different sensitivity of macro- and microadenomas to dopamine and vasoactive intestinal polypeptide. J. Clin. Endocrinol. Metab., *56*:1–10, 1983.

149. Steger R.W., Silverman A.Y., and Asch R.H. Glucocorticoid suppression of pituitary prolactin release in the nonhuman primate. J. Clin. Endocrinol. Metab., *53*:1167–1170, 1981.

150. Stern J.M., and Reichlin S. Prolactin circadian rhythm persists throughout lactation in women. Neuroendocrinology, *51*:31–37, 1990.

151. Suh H.R., and Frantz A.G. Heterogeneity of human prolactin in plasma and pituitary extract. J. Clin. Endocrinol. Metab., *39*:928, 1974.

152. Tindall G.T., Kovacs K., Horvath E., and Thorner M.O. Human prolactin-producing adenomas and bromocriptine: a histological, immunocytochemical, ultrastructural, and morphometric study. J. Clin. Endocrinol. Metab., *55*:1178, 1982.

153. Turkington R.W. Phenothiazine stimulation test for prolactin reserve: the syndrome of isolated prolactin deficiency. J. Clin. Endocrinol. Metab., *34*:247–249, 1972.

154. Vallar L., Vicentini L.M., Mendolesi J. Inhibition of inositol phosphate production is a late, Ca^{2+}-dependent effect of D_2 dopaminergic receptor activation in rat lactotroph cells. J. Biol. Chem., *263*:10127–10134, 1988.

155. Van Vugt D.A., Bruni J.F., Sylvester P.W., Chen H.T., Ieri T., and Meites J. Interaction between opiates and hypothalamic dopamine on prolactin release. Life Sci., *24*:2361–2368, 1979.

156. Veldhuis J.D., and Johnson M.L. Operating characteristics of the hypothalamic-pituitary-gonadal axis in men: circadian, ultradian and pulsatile release of prolactin and its temporal coupling with luteinizing hormone. J. Clin. Endocrinol. Metab., *67*:116–123, 1988.

157. Vician L., Lieberman M.E., and Gorski J. Evidence that autoregulation of prolactin production does not occur at the pituitary level. Endocrinology, *110*:722–726, 1982.

158. Vrontakis M.E., Peden L.M., Duckworth M.L.,

and Friesen H.G. Isolation and characterization of a complementary DNA (galanin) clone from estrogen-induced pituitary tumor messenger RNA. J. Biol. Chem., *262:*16755–16758, 1987.

159. Warfield A., Finkel D.M., Schatz N.J., Savino P.J., and Snyder P.J. Bromocriptine treatment of prolactin-secreting pituitary adenomas may restore pituitary function. Ann. Intern. Med., *101:*783–785, 1984.

160. Weiss M.H., Teal J., Gott P., *et al.* Natural history of microprolactinomas: six year follow-up. Neurosurgery, *12:*180, 1983.

161. Werner S., Hulting A.L., Hokfelt T., *et al.* Effect of peptide PHI-27 on prolactin release in vitro. Neuroendocrinology, *37:*476–478, 1983.

162. Wood D.F., Docherty K., Ramsden B.D., Shennan K.I.J., and Sheppard M.C. Thyroid status affects the regulation of prolactin mRNA accumulation by triiodothyroinine and thyrotrophin-releasing hormone in cultured rat anterior pituitary cells. J. Endocrinol., *115:*497–503, 1987.

163. Woolf P.D., and Lee L. Effect of the serotonin precursor, tryptophan, on pituitary hormone secretion. J. Clin. Endocrinol. Metab., *45:*123–126, 1977.

164. Wortsman J., Carlson H.E., and Malarkey W.B. Macroprolactinemia as the cause of elevated serum prolactin in men. Am. J. Med., *86:*704–706, 1989.

165. Wortsman J., Soler N.G., and Hirschowitz J. Cyproheptadine in the management of the galactorrhea-amenorrhea syndrome. Ann. Intern. Med., *90:*923–925, 1979.

166. Yamamoto K., Saito K., Takai T., Naito M., and Yoshida S. Visual field defects and pituitary enlargement in primary hypothyroidism. J. Clin. Endocrinol. Metab., *57:*283–287, 1983.

167. Yu W.H., Seeburg P.H., Nikolics K., and McCann S.M. Gonadotropin-releasing hormone-associated peptide exerts a prolactin-inhibiting and weak gonadotropin-releasing activity in vivo. Endocrinology, *123:*390–395, 1988.

CHAPTER 7

Growth Hormone: An Overview of Its Regulation, Associated Disorders, and Clinical Evaluation

WILLIAM F. CHANDLER, M.D.

Advances in biochemistry, molecular biology, and human genetics have provided a substantial though incomplete picture of the complex physiology of growth hormone regulation and influence. Excess growth hormone release creates an insidious and life-shortening process that is critical to recognize and eliminate. Deficient growth hormone production in a child produces a tragic loss of growth potential that can be treated only if recognized in a timely fashion. Although much is known about the regulation of growth hormone in the normal pituitary, little is known about the etiology and control of neoplastic disorders associated with this hormone.

REGULATION

Growth hormone (GH) is a 191-amino acid polypeptide that is secreted in a pulsatile fashion from anatomically distinct somatotrophs located in abundance in the anterior pituitary (7). These cells contain numerous secretory granules that store GH and release it by exocytosis. Messenger RNA for GH (mRNA-GH) is formed by transcription at the GH gene cluster located on chromosome 17. The mRNA-GH travels to the Golgi region, where GH is generated and stored in granules.

Regulation of mRNA-GH formation and, ultimately, GH release comes mainly from dual and opposing polypeptides secreted by the hypothalamus. Growth hormone releasing hormone (GHRH) induces transcription of the GH gene and stimulates secretion of GH; the second hypothalamic polypeptide, somatostatin (SRIF), suppresses GH secretion but does not decrease mRNA-GH levels (6). Both of these hypothalamic hormones are secreted into the hypothalamic-hypophyseal portal system and bind to receptors in the anterior pituitary. The pulsatile secretion of GH is regulated more by changes in somatostatin than by changes in GHRH (10). Hypothalamic release of GHRH and SRIF is ultimately regulated by neural connections from the brainstem and limbic system. Thus, many neurotransmitters are involved in the regulation of GH secretion. There are normal increases in GH pulse frequency associated with obesity, sleep, and fasting (7). Estrogens, thyroid hormone, and insulin-like growth factor 1 (IGF-1) also have lesser roles in the regulation of GH release (3). The highest levels of GH per day, not surprisingly, occur during adolescence.

GH circulates in an unbound state in plasma and has a half-life of between 17 and 45 minutes. Most of the growth-related effects of GH occur not by GH itself, but by its stimulation of IGF-1, also known as somatomedin C. This polypeptide is synthesized primarily in the liver, but also in the kidney, muscle, chondrocytes, gastrointestinal tract, and the pituitary itself. IGF-1 causes growth by directly stimulating chondrocytes and inducing replication of epithelial cells. IGF-1 also suppresses the production of mRNA-GH and the secretion of GH and, thus, is part of a negative feedback loop (1).

DISORDERS

Disorders of growth hormone synthesis and secretion ultimately result in either an excess or a shortage of this important pituitary hormone. Etiologies of the various disorders range from true neoplasia to alterations in the normal regulation process discussed above.

Hypersecretion of Growth Hormone

Most clinical problems in adults arise from an oversecretion of GH, since hyposecretion is noticed only during the years of physical growth and development. The discussion of hypersecretion of GH will be divided into primary excess secretion and those situations in which GH excess is secondary to an increase in GHRH.

Primary Hypersecretion of GH

The most common cause of excess GH is hypersecretion by a pituitary adenoma composed primarily or exclusively of somatotrophs. Of adenomas that secrete GH, 80% are exclusively somatotrophs and 20% are composed of mammosomatotrophs, containing some excess prolactin secretion as well (7). Current evidence would suggest that GH-adenomas are a nest of clonogenic cells arising from a simple mutation, since these tumors are monoclonal (4). If the neoplasia were a response to external stimulation, the cell population would be expected to be polyclonal. Another factor favoring de novo mutation is that the surrounding cells do not show hyperplasia. Somatostatin does not appear to play a role, since the serum levels of somatostatin remain normal in cases of GH-adenomas.

Primary adenomas are benign histologically, with only very rare reported cases of a pituitary carcinoma secreting GH. True hyperplasia of pituitary somatotrophs without an underlining increase in GHRH may exist but is very rare. Growth hormone may be secreted ectopically by malignant tumors of the lung, breast, ovaries, or pancreas. In rare cases, a true benign pituitary adenoma may arise ectopically in the "sphenoidal" pituitary tissue located in the sphenoid sinus of many normal individuals (9).

Secondary Hypersecretion of GH

Growth hormone production may rise following an increase in GHRH. The hypothalamic hormone GHRH may be primarily increased eutopically in the presence of a hypothalamic hamartoma, glioma, ganglioglioma, or chorestoma. It may be secreted ectopically by a variety of tumors. Carcinoids of the lung, gastrointestinal tract, or pancreas may secrete GHRH, as may lung carcinomas, Islet cell tumors, pheochromocytomas, and adrenal adenomas (7). As would be expected, ectopic GHRH-secreting tumors result in elevated circulating levels of GHRH.

Growth Hormone Deficiency

Deficiency of growth hormone is clinically relevant only during growth and development and, therefore, will be discussed as a problem of childhood and adolescence. Growth hormone deficiency may occur as an isolated hormone deficiency or as part of a multiple pituitary hormone deficiency. The majority of patients with growth hormone deficiency remain in the category of idiopathic pituitary deficiency. This group is divided equally into isolated growth hormone deficiency and multiple pituitary hormone deficiency and is more common in men than in women (8). In prepubertal patients with multiple hormones involved, GH and thyrotropin (TSH) are the most commonly deficient hormones, with ACTH being the next most commonly deficient hormone. In the pubertal years, patients are most commonly deficient in GH, TSH, ACTH, and the gonadotropins FSH and LH. It is not possible to document gonadotropin deficiency until a child has reached a bone age of 12. Patients with isolated growth hormone deficiency may have only a partial rather than a complete deficiency of growth hormone. Although a small percentage of congenital growth hormone deficiency patients have an inherited disorder, many are suspected to be related to birth trauma. There is also a group of young prepubertal adolescents who have a transient deficiency of GH that delays, but does not eliminate, normal growth potential.

A second group of patients will have growth hormone deficiency related to a mass lesion, such as a craniopharyngioma, optic nerve glioma, or hypothalamic glioma. These mass lesions generally result in a multiple hormone deficiency that presents later in childhood than idiopathic growth hormone deficiency. Histiocytosis-X may also cause growth hormone deficiency and is often associated with diabetes insipidus.

Cleft lip and palate are occasionally associated with growth hormone deficiency as is septo-optic dysplasia (2). Turner's syndrome and rubella may also have associated growth hormone deficiency.

CLINICAL EVALUATION

Hypersecretion

The clinical manifestations of excessive GH and, concomitantly, IGF-1 are collectively known as acromegaly. The outward signs include the insidious enlargement of facial features (tongue, nose, lips, and supraorbital ridge) and enlargement of the hands and feet. More threatening to normal survival is the increased incidence of hypertension and coronary artery disease. Patients also suffer from carpal tunnel syndrome, goiter, osteoarthritis, hyperhidrosis, glucose intolerance, colonic polyps, and sleep apnea. Local growth of a pituitary adenoma can cause headache, decreased vision, and hypopituitarism. Untreated acromegaly causes a marked decrease in life expectancy, doubling the expected death rate at any age. The younger the patient is at the onset of the hypersecretion of GH, the more rapid and dramatic will be the onset of the clinical manifestations.

The endocrine evaluation of patients with suspected acromegaly centers around the fasting morning levels of growth hormone (normally less than 5 ng/ml). If this level is clearly elevated in a patient with classic clinical features, the diagnosis may be secure. A serum IGF-1 level should also be obtained and would be expected to be correspondingly elevated. If the GH is normal or marginally elevated, then provocative tests may be useful. Normally, a glucose load of 75 gm will drive the GH down to less than 2 ng/ml. This test does not provide normal suppression in 93% of acromegalics (11). Thyrotropin-releasing hormone (TRH) normally suppresses GH but will cause a paradoxical rise in 80% of acromegalic patients (11). Dopaminergic agents, such as levodopa or bromocriptine, normally cause a rise in GH, but they cause a decrease in GH in 66% of acromegalics. Growth hormone-releasing hormone would only be elevated if there were an ectopic source.

Imaging of the pituitary and parasellar region is best done with magnetic resonance imaging (MRI). It is superior to computerized tomography (CT) and will image microadenomas down to 5 mm in size. Skull x-rays will show the bony changes of acromegaly and, often, an enlarged sella related to tumor growth. These changes include calvarial thickening, enlarged frontal sinuses, and mandibular enlargement. X-rays of the hands show the classic changes associated with acromegaly.

Hyposecretion

Most children with growth hormone deficiency present with stature below the third percentile, growth velocity below the 25th percentile for 1 year, decreased bone age (average 2–3 years), and increased subcutaneous fat (8). Patients also tend to have a decrease in muscle mass. Even with an isolated growth hormone deficiency there is a significant delay in the onset of puberty, particularly in males. Most infants born with growth hormone deficiency will have a normal birth weight, but males may have underdeveloped genitalia. Infants and young children with multiple pituitary hormone deficiencies may have significant hypoglycemia.

The differential diagnosis in patients with growth hormone deficiency includes primary hypothyroidism and Cushing's disease, both of which result in a child who is short, obese, and has a decreased bone age. Patients with isolated gonadotropin deficiency may look similar in adolescent years. Children with significant gastrointestinal diseases, such as Crohn's disease or celiac disease, may have delayed growth and bone age but will have a decrease in subcutaneous fat. Patients with chronic renal or cardiac disease will also have short stature. A syndrome of deficiency of IGF-1 also exists but would be associated with elevated levels of GH (5). Situations have also been reported in which GH levels are normal but the GH appears to be biologically inactive. Short stature may also exist related to psychosocial deprivation.

The clinical, radiographic, and endocrine evaluation of a child with growth delay is best managed by a pediatric endocrinologist and should include a bone age study and complete pituitary function testing, including an IGF-1 level. Likewise, the treatment, including GH replacement, is best managed by a pediatric endocrinologist specializing in this area.

REFERENCES

1. Berelowitz M., Szabo M., Frohman L.A., Firestone S., Chu L., and Hintz R.L. Somatomedin-C mediates growth hormone negative feedback by effects on both the hypothalamus and the pituitary. Science, *212*:1279–1281, 1981.
2. Brook C.G.D., Sanders M.D., and Hoare R.D. Septo-optic dysplasia. BMJ, *3*:811–813, 1972.
3. Frohman L.A., and Jansson J.O. Growth hormone-releasing hormone. Endocr. Rev., *7*:223–253, 1986.
4. Herman V., Fagin J.A., Gonsky R., Riordan-Mita M.A., Kovacs K., and Melmed S. Heterogeneous clonal origin of functional anterior pituitary tumors [abstract]. Clin. Res., *38*:97A, 1990.
5. Laron Z. Syndrome of familial dwarfism and high plasma immunoreactive growth hormone. Israel J. Med. Sci. *10*:1247–1253, 1974.
6. Martin J.B. Hypothalamic regulation of growth hormone secretion. In: *Secretory Tumors of the Pituitary Gland,* edited by P.M. Black, N.T. Zervas, E.C. Ridgway, and J.B. Martin, pp. 109–133, New York: Raven Press, 1984.
7. Melmed S. Acromegaly. New Eng. J. Med. *322*:966–977, 1990.
8. Preece M.A. Diagnosis and treatment of children with growth hormone deficiency. In Bailey J.D., Ed., *Clinics in Endocrinology and Metabolism,* London: W.B. Saunders, Ltd., 1982:1–24.
9. Schteingart D.E., Chandler W.F., Lloyd R.V., and Ibarra-Perez G.: Cushing's syndrome caused by an ectopic pituitary adenoma. Neurosurgery, *21*:223–227, 1987.
10. Thorner M.O., and Vance M.L. Growth hormone, 1988. J. Clin. Invest., *82*:745–747, 1988.
11. Tolis G., Koutsilieris M., and Bertrand G. Endocrine diagnosis of growth hormone secreting pituitary tumors. In: Black P.M., Zervas N.T., Ridgway E.C., and Martin J.B., ed. *Secretory Tumors of the Pituitary Gland.* New York: Raven Press, 145–154, 1984.

CHAPTER 8

Cortisol: Regulation, Disorders, and Clinical Evaluation

IAN E. MCCUTCHEON, M.D., AND EDWARD H. OLDFIELD, M.D.

Cortisol is essential for homeostasis and for the physiological and biochemical adaptive response to stress. Thus, it occupies a central position in the mammalian response to exogenous or endogenous stress. It also affects the secretion and activity of many other hormones. Synthesis and release of cortisol from the adrenal cortex is controlled by the pituitary gland. Patients with disordered cortisol regulation often harbor pituitary neoplasms that can cause hypercortisolism, via excess ACTH secretion by the tumor, or hypopituitarism, by the mass effects of the tumor on the infundibulum or the pituitary gland. Furthermore, cortisol is of vital interest to all physicians in a general sense because of its essential role in the adaptive response to medical and surgical insults.

The first suggestion that the adrenal gland was essential for life came from Brown-Séquard, who showed, in the 1850s that bilateral adrenalectomy in animals caused death within a few days. It was not, however, until Cushing linked adrenal hypersecretion of cortisol with the presence of pituitary tumors, and Selye promulgated the concept that the adrenal cortex (through control by the central nervous system) responded to stress, that the current concepts of a hypothalamic-pituitary–adrenal axis began to take shape.

REGULATION OF CORTISOL SECRETION

Anatomy

Pituitary

The anterior lobe of the pituitary gland (the adenohypophysis) contains at least five types of parenchymal cells distinguished by immunohistochemical labeling of their hormonal contents (125, 158, 159). The five types comprise cells that secrete growth hormone, prolactin, thyrotropin (TSH), gonadotropins, or adrenocorticotropin (corticotropin, ACTH). The cells that produce ACTH, the corticotrophs, comprise 10-20% of the pituitary cells. They are concentrated in the central third of the adenohypophysis, but are also distributed over the lateral wings of the adenohypophysis and in the pars intermedia (11).

Adrenal

Cortisol is produced only by the adrenal cortex. The outer layer of cells of the adrenal cortex comprise the zona glomerulosa, which secretes aldosterone. Beneath the outer layer is the cortisol–secreting zona fasciculata, which forms the majority of the cortex and which is so named because its cells lie in parallel cords. The zona reticularis, the innermost of the three layers, contains eosinophilic cells, which seem to be the source of adrenal androgen production.

Physiology

Regulation and Biochemistry of Corticotropin-Releasing Hormone (CRH)

Several endogenous hormones, particularly corticotropin-releasing hormone (CRH) and antidiuretic hormone (ADH, vasopressin), stimulate the release of adrenocorticotropin hormone from the pituitary corticotrophs (Fig. 8.1.). However, physiological release appears to be principally controlled by CRH (278). This 41-amino acid peptide, first isolated and sequenced by Vale

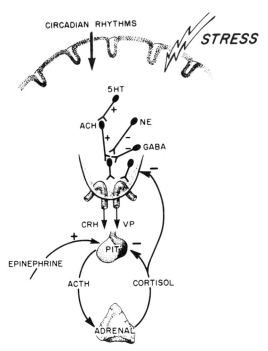

Figure 8.1. Functional relationships of the elements of the hypothalamic-pituitary-adrenal axis. Secretion of adrenocorticotropic hormone (ACTH) from the pituitary is stimulated by corticotropin-releasing hormone (CRH) from the hypothalamus. ACTH secretion regulates cortisol production and secretion by the adrenals. CRH secretion is regulated by cholinergic (ACH) and serotonergic (5HT) stimulatory components and by an adrenergic inhibitory pathway, all of which mediate stress-induced and circadian ACTH secretion. Cortisol exerts negative feedback at the pituitary and the hypothalamus. (Reprinted with permission from Martin J.B. and Reichlin S. *Clinical Neuroendocrinology,* Philadelphia, F.A. Davis Co., 1987.)

and his coworkers in 1981 (344), is produced in the paraventricular nuclei of the hypothalamus. Rhythmic release of CRH into the hypothalamo-hypophyseal portal system probably underlies the circadian rhythms of the peripheral plasma levels of ACTH and cortisol (182).

The existence of ACTH-releasing factor was proposed as long ago as 1955 by Saffron and Schalley (288), who demonstrated ACTH-releasing activity in extracts from the posterior lobe of the pituitary gland. In the same year, Guillemin and Rosenberg suggested the existence of a CRH-like substance after they coincubated fragments of anterior pituitary gland and hypothalamus and found secretion of ACTH (120). Not until the isolation of the first pure preparation of CRH from 490,000 sheep hypothalami was it possible to study its metabolism and action in detail (344). In addition to its role as the specific stimulus for phasic ACTH release, CRH mediates stress-induced ACTH secretion, as such secretion is blocked in animals given anti-CRH antibodies (258). CRH also stimulates the release of growth hormone and prolactin from the isolated pituitary gland in primates (305) and elicits release of growth hormone in some acromegalic patients and in patients with depression (257).

Secretion of CRH by the hypothalamus is modulated by positive influences from other sites in the brain and by negative feedback from glucocorticoids. Receptors for glucocorticoids in the brain cluster particularly in the distribution of the CRH-containing neurons in the paraventricular nuclei (99). The rise in CRH concentration in the median eminence and in the hypophyseal portal blood after adrenalectomy, and the fall that occurs after the administration of glucocorticoids, also indicate negative feedback by glucocorticoids at the level of the hypothalamus (154, 260). Human CRH is cleared from the plasma quite rapidly (half-life of 4 min) (231), permitting rapid fluctuations of plasma ACTH and cortisol concentrations during endogenous regulation of ACTH secretion. After systemic injection, synthetic ovine CRH is cleared slowly from the blood, with a half-life of 60 to 80 min (52, 68, 231, 304). ACTH and cortisol concentrations peak at 10 to 20 and at 30 to 60 min, respectively, and remain elevated for as long as three hours after the introduction of synthetic CRH (50, 51, 52, 68, 248, 306).

Although direct proof is lacking, it has been suggested that the rhythmic secretion of CRH is mediated through serotoninergic neural pathways (98, 331). Adrenergic and cholinergic inputs to the hypothalamus also influence CRH release (33, 123). After administration into the cerebral ventricles, acetycholine, epinephrine, and serotonin provoke, and α-aminobutyric acid (GABA) inhibits CRH secretion (34, 332).

The pathways that impinge on the neurons of the paraventricular nuclei that release CRH are complex and bring neural input to the hypothalamus from many areas of the nervous system (182). Isolation of the hypothalamus from the remaining brain activates sustained increases in corticosterone levels in rats and suggests that extrahypothalamic areas provide tonic inhibitory effects on hypothalamic CRH secretion (95, 133). The origin of afferents to the paraventricular nucleus include the nucleus of the tractus solitarius (fed by vagal and glossopharyngeal afferents), the hypothalamus, the nucleus of the subforniceal region, the medullary reticular formation, the locus ceruleus, and various parts of the limbic system, particularly the hippocampus (132) and the lateral septal region (71).

These provide routes through which stress influences the secretion of CRH and, thus, the production and secretion of ACTH and cortisol (37, 88, 104, 197). The fact that different types of stress have different sensitivity to inhibition by glucocorticoids suggests that the varied types of stress exert their effects by separate neural pathways. For instance, in rats, stimulation of the amygdala facilitates pituitary ACTH release (203) and the amygdaloid complex is required for ACTH release in response to neurogenic stress (trauma), but the amygdala is not required for the ACTH–cortisol response after systemic stress (anesthesia) (3).

Regulation of Adrenocorticotropin Synthesis and Secretion

The most important physiological releasing factors for ACTH release are CRH and vasopressin (278). These two molecules are coexpressed in a subset of parvocellular neurons in the paraventricular nucleus, an anatomic link that implies coordinated synthesis and release. In addition, vasopressin potentiates the positive effects of CRH on ACTH synthesis and release (69, 360) and both CRH and vasopressin mediate ACTH secretion provoked by hypoglycemia (84).

The periodicity of ACTH release mirrors that of CRH release. This rhythmicity is impaired in patients with hypothalamic lesions, Wernicke's encephalopathy, and impairment of consciousness (161, 287). In healthy humans, secretory bursts of ACTH and cortisol occur throughout the day, on average about 15 times in a 24-hour period (Fig. 8.2.) (347). As a result, plasma levels of ACTH vary as much as 10-fold throughout the day, and most normal individuals actively secrete cortisol only about one-quarter of the time. Each major quantum of cortisol release follows a burst of ACTH secretion (356), and integration of the amplitude and frequency of the cortisol pulses produces a circadian rhythm of plasma cortisol concentration. However, it should be noted that these concepts are still evolving: Recent work suggests that CRH acts mainly by increasing the amplitude of an intrinsic, high-frequency rhythm of ACTH secretion by the pituitary gland (38) and that cortisol levels are a result of variation in amplitude of ACTH secretion, instead of a result of frequency modulation (350).

Glucocorticoids inhibit the stimulatory effects of CRH on the corticotrophs. Increased cortisol levels also inhibit basal secretion of ACTH, whereas the elimination of cortisol by adrenalectomy markedly increases plasma ACTH concentrations (135, 148, 154). In the corticotrophs of the normal pituitary gland, glucocorticoids also suppress ACTH synthesis by suppressing transcription of the mRNA for its prohormone, proopiomelanocortin (POMC)(8, 21), by inhibiting production of cAMP (20), and by reducing the expression of CRH receptors (365). The presence of glucocorticoid receptors in the pituitary, the hypothalamus, and the extrahypothalamic areas of the brain makes it difficult to establish which, if any, of these sites serves as the principal target for feedback control (99), but all are undoubt-

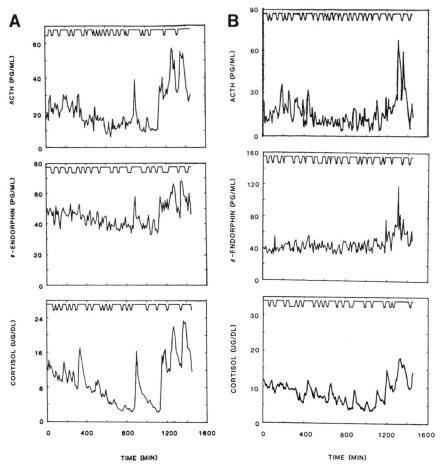

Figure 8.2. Diurnal rhythms of ACTH and cortisol in normal subjects. Plasma ACTH, β-endorphin, and cortisol concentrations in each of two (A and B) normal men who received blood sampling every 10 minutes for 24 hours. (Reprinted with permission from Veldhuis J.D., Iranmanesh A., Johnson M.L., and Lizarralde G. Amplitude, but not frequency, modulation of adrenocorticotropin secretory bursts gives rise to the nyctohemeral rhythm of the corticotropic axis in man. J. Clin. Endocrinol. Metab., *71*:452–463, 1990).

edly involved in regulating the function of the hypothalamic–pituitary-adrenal axis.

ACTH secretion is also influenced (directly and via CRH) by several neurotransmitters (173,278,341). Acetylcholine and serotonin stimulate, whereas the catecholamines inhibit, ACTH secretion (337). The opioid peptides also affect ACTH secretion. Most importantly, β-endorphin lowers ACTH and cortisol levels (335). This is not surprising, given its derivation from β-lipotropin (β-LPH) and, ultimately, from POMC, the precursor of ACTH. Dopamine may also inhibit ACTH release, as it de-

creases ACTH levels in some patients with corticotroph hyperplasia (61).

The capacity of lymphokines and other immune molecules to modify the activities of the hypothalamus and pituitary has recently become evident and provides another link between systemic homeostasis and the function of the hypothalamic-pituitary-adrenal axis (12). The best-studied compound, interleukin-1 (IL-1), stimulates secretion of CRH and ACTH (292). Although it has been suggested that it acts directly on CRH-producing neurons in the hypothalamus (339) and on corticotrophs in the adenohypophysis

(190), IL-1 does not enhance the secretion of glucocorticoids by animals that have undergone hypophysectomy or hypothalamic deafferentation (122, 251). This suggests that the action of IL-1 lies outside the hypothalamic–pituitary-adrenal axis, but that its effects channel through the axis, perhaps from receptors elsewhere in the central nervous system. IL-1 may also directly effect secretory activity from the adrenal cortex (4).

Biochemistry and Synthesis of ACTH

Within the corticotrophs in the anterior pituitary lobe, ACTH is synthesized from POMC, a large molecular weight polypeptide prohormone that gives rise to a variety of molecular species (Fig. 8.3.). Processing of POMC by enzymatic cleavage at specific sites takes place within specialized secretory vesicles, where the two primary products of cleavage, ACTH and β-LPH, are made in equimolar quantities. ACTH and β-LPH each contain smaller peptides of debatable important function (320). Cells containing POMC are also found in the intermediate lobe of the pituitary, where the predominant cleavage products are α-MSH, γ-MSH, corticotropin-like intermediate lobe peptide (CLIP), γ-LPH, and β-endorphin.

The bioactivity of ACTH resides within the N-terminal 24 amino acids of the molecule in all mammalian species; this fragment, in synthetic form, is used in screening tests of the hypothalamic–pituitary-adrenal. The carboxyl terminal fragment of ACTH prolongs the hormone's duration of action within the adrenal cortex. Synthesis of ACTH by ectopic ACTH-secreting tumors may be disordered and result in the secretion of larger forms of ACTH with impaired, or even absent, bioactivity, a phenomenon that does not occur in normal corticotrophs or in the ACTH-secreting pituitary adenomas (276).

Effects of ACTH on the Adrenal Gland

ACTH acts on the adrenal cortex via specific receptors on cell surfaces. Hormone-receptor interaction activates adenylate cyclase within the plasma membrane, which provokes synthesis of cAMP (283). Cyclic AMP stimulates cAMP-dependent protein kinase (protein kinase A) and phosphorylation of a number of proteins and initiates a sequence of events that leads to increased production of glucocorticoids (268). Since inhibitors of protein synthesis block the steroidogenic action of ACTH (263), synthesis of new proteins also appears to be a part of the chain of intracellular events provoked by this hormone.

ACTH is essential for the maintenance of the enzymes of the steroidogenic pathway and for trophic maintenance of the adrenal cortex. Acutely, ACTH increases conversion of cholesterol to pregnenolone (Fig. 8.4.). It

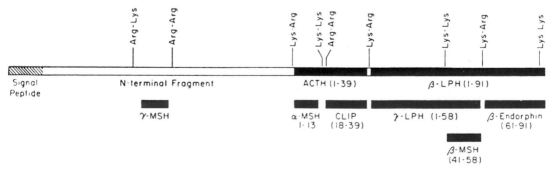

Figure 8.3. Diagrammatic representation of bovine pro-opiomelanocortin (POMC). POMC undergoes extensive post-translational processing to produce multiple peptides, including ACTH. The pattern of cleavage is tissue-specific. In the anterior lobe (upper bar), the principal products are the NH_2-terminal peptide, ACTH, β-lipotropin hormone (β-LPH) and, to a lesser extent, β-endorphin. In the intermediate lobe (middle bar)—which is not functional in adult humans—and in other tissues, ACTH is further processed to γ-MSH and corticotropin-like intermediate lobe peptide (CLIP), and β-LPH is further cleaved and processed to yield γ-LPH and β-endorphin. (Reprinted with permission from Krieger D.T., Liota A.S., Brownstein M.J., *et al.* ACTH, lipotropin, and related peptides in brain, pituitary, and blood. Recent Prog. Horm. Res., *36*:272–344, 1980.)

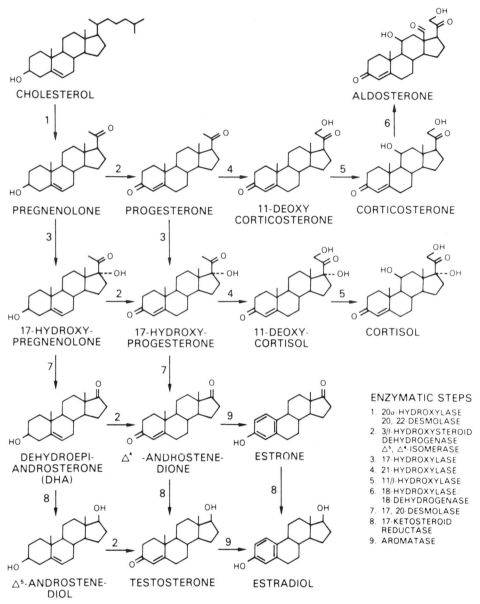

Figure 8.4. Major pathways of adrenal steroid synthesis. (From Loriaux D.L. and Cutler G.B. Jr. Diseases of the adrenal glands. In: *Clinical Endocrinology,* edited by Peter O. Kohler, M.D., pp. 167–238, John Wiley and Sons, Inc., 1986).

also stimulates uptake of cholesterol into the adrenal cortex from plasma lipoproteins (263). Thus, it primes the gland to respond maximally to further stimulation. A maximal response requires prior adrenal exposure to ACTH, which underlies the basis of the ACTH stimulation test. ACTH also stimulates melanocytes by cross-reacting with MSH receptors, and, when present in excess, causes the characteristic hyperpigmentation of patients with primary adrenal insufficiency (Addison's disease) and the hyperpigmentation associated with ACTH-secreting pituitary tumors after adrenal ablation (Nelson's syndrome) (24).

Pathways of Cortisol Synthesis

The products of the adrenal cortex are classified into three categories: mineralocorticoids, androcorticoids, and glucocorticoids (Fig. 8.4.). Of the latter, cortisol (hydrocortisone) is the most important in man. As a glucocorticoid, it acts broadly to influence the metabolism of carbohydrates (depletion of hepatic glycogen stores, increase of hepatic gluconeogenesis), fats (lipolysis), and protein (release of glucogenic amino-acids from the peripheral tissues, such as skeletal muscle). Mineralocorticoid activity (the promotion of potassium excretion and sodium retention) and androgen activity (masculinization) also reside weakly in the endogenous glucocorticoid hormones.

The adrenal steroids are synthesized from cholesterol along three pathways: the mineralocorticoid in the zona glomerulosa, the glucocorticoid in the zona fasciculata, and the adrenal androgens in the zona reticularis. Each pathway requires five steps for the conversion of cholesterol to its final product, and each intermediate product is secreted by the adrenal gland and is measureable in peripheral plasma. Compounds containing an oxygen moiety at positions 11, 18, or 21 (cortisol and aldosterone, for example) are produced solely by the adrenal glands. Other steroids are produced partially by the adrenals and partially by conversion of the adrenal precursors in the gonads.

Regulation of Cortisol Secretion

Cortisol is secreted in a pulsatile and circadian pattern that follows the pattern of secretion of ACTH, its primary controlling factor. Negative feedback by glucocorticoids restrains the hypothalamic-pituitary-adrenal axis at the level of the pituitary gland and the hypothalamus (Fig. 8.1.). In addition, poorly specified mechanisms that originate outside the pituitary-adrenal axis, and that circumvent the actions of ACTH, have been suggested to influence the regulation of the circadian rhythm of plasma cortisol (87). However, these have not been confirmed by other investigators and their importance, if they exist, is unclear. CRH can also stimulate cortisol secretion by a direct action on the adrenals, but the physiological importance of this is unclear (67). The amount of cortisol synthesized daily in healthy humans is 5 to 7 mg/m^2/day.

Diurnal variation in cortisol secretion produces low plasma cortisol levels at around midnight and the highest levels at about 6 to 8 a.m. in individuals with a normal sleep-wake cycle (Fig. 8.2.) (103). Thus, the pattern of plasma cortisol concentrations depends on the individual's cycle of sleep and wakefulness. The periodicity of the rhythm is not of necessity a 24-hour cycle, as experimental sleep-wake cycles lasting 12 or 33 hrs lead to a similar cortisol rhythm (249). If the time of sleeping changes, the cortisol rhythm also changes after a lag time of several days. Although the rhythms of CRH, ACTH, and cortisol secretion can be altered by hypothalamic dysfunction, they cannot be abolished altogether (160, 161, 287): The rhythms persist even during such derangements of wakefulness as coma and narcolepsy (136). The daily pattern of cortisol secretion is not caused by environmental cues or by the sleep cycle of the individual, but it adapts to them. An unexplained seasonal variation in the amplitude of the cortisol rhythm causes higher levels of cortisol secretion in winter in people living in the northern hemisphere (347). In males, ACTH pulses are released more frequently and in higher amplitude than in females, but cortisol secretion is similar in males and females (140).

The circadian cortisol rhythm is not present at birth but becomes manifest by the age of one year (96, 318). It depends neither on negative feedback from cortisol, as the ACTH rhythm is present in patients with primary adrenal insufficiency, nor on obvious metabolic factors, for it persists during fasting and during continuous feeding (162). Changes through the day in the sensitivity of the hypothalamus and pituitary to glucocorticoids keep cortisol levels from varying too much; these tissues are most sensitive to negative feedback at midnight, when plasma cortisol is at its lowest, and least sensitive in the morning, when plasma cortisol is highest

(230). Furthermore, cycling of the sensitivity of the adrenal gland to ACTH provides an additional check on cortisol production and is influenced by the light-dark cycle and by feeding times (363). Due to its circadian pattern, measurement of plasma cortisol in the morning is a more sensitive indicator of adrenal insufficiency, whereas late evening measurements are more valuable for detecting adrenal hyperfunction.

Stress stimulates the secretion of glucocorticoids. A wide variety of physiological and psychological stresses increase cortisol levels. These include the malnutrition of anorexia nervosa (86, 355), the normal fasting state (348), insulin-induced hypoglycemia (73, 117), trauma (127), surgery (49, 56, 85, 127), and psychiatric depression (41-43). After surgery, mean plasma cortisol levels are increased for 48 hrs or more. Such changes are erratic and are caused by alterations in the magnitude and duration of secretory pulses rather than by a fundamental recalibration of the rhythm of release (207). During severe stress, increased cortisol secretion can increase the plasma cortisol concentration over basal values by as much as 10-fold. The overall effect of prolonged stress is to blunt the excursion of the circadian rhythm by increasing the noctural plasma cortisol levels, whereas morning levels change much less. The effects of stress on cortisol secretion are mediated through pituitary ACTH release.

Most circulating cortisol is bound by a plasma protein, transcortin, and is biologically inactive. However, bound and unbound cortisol are measured with most assays of plasma cortisol levels. Because they increase transcortin levels, and thus increase cortisol binding capacity, oral contraceptive agents increase the amplitude of the circadian rhythm of cortisol secretion (345). In pregnancy, levels of cortisol in the bound and, to a much lesser extent, the free forms are elevated (309). The circadian pattern of the plasma cortisol level persists, but it is at a higher set-point (236). In hyperthyroidism, the amplitude of the circadian rhythm is enhanced by increased production and decreased clearance of cortisol (102, 146), but the majority of hyperthyroid patients have normal plasma cortisol levels (255). Liver disease blunts the range of excursion of cor-tisol levels during the circadian cycle because of a decrease in the rate of cortisol degradation (281). Alcoholics may have elevation of plasma cortisol levels that should not be confused with true Cushing's syndrome (156).

Psychiatric depression may induce moderate hypercortisolemia, in which the circadian rhythm persists and ACTH and cortisol pulse more frequently. For unknown reasons, the excess cortisol does not produce the physical manifestations of Cushing's syndrome, and hypercortisolism is more consistently seen with unipolar than with bipolar affective disorders. As the alteration in mood clears in patients who undergo successful treatment, normal cortisol dynamics reappear (105, 106). The increased activity of the hypothalamic-pituitary-adrenal axis in depression probably results from hypersecretion of CRH, although the mechanism underlying excess CRH secretion is unknown (109, 286).

Cortisol Action

The mechanism of interaction of steroid hormones with target cells differs from that of the peptide hormones, which initially bind receptors on the external surface of the cell membrane. In the "two-step" model, the lipophilic steroid hormone crosses the cell membrane and binds to a specific cytosolic receptor, which then becomes activated and gains affinity for acceptor sites within the nucleus. In the "one-step" model of steroid action, the unbound receptor is already within the nucleus near its acceptor site. As immunohistochemical studies have shown glucocorticoid receptors in the nucleus and in the cytoplasm, both models may be valid (121). Binding of the hormone-receptor complex to the acceptor sites alters the transcription rate of certain genes, which, in turn, alters the rate of protein synthesis from those genes (284). The specific genes affected by the steroid-receptor interaction depend on the tissue type. Steroids of one of the three main classes may show some biological activity most associated with one of the other classes because of the capacity to interact, albeit less strongly, with several classes of receptor. Depending on the specificity, steroid hormones bind receptors and act as optimal agonists, suboptimal agonists, or antagonists.

The glucocorticoid hormones allow integrated metabolic homeostasis within the organism that maintains it against forces of disorganization and decay (13, 32, 118, 210). The term "glucocorticoid" was orginally applied because of early discoveries of the effects of such substances on glucose metabolism. However, glucocorticoids are now known to influence several other hormones (including insulin, growth hormone, glucagon, and catecholamines) in a permissive sense, allowing each to exert its specific actions. Because of the ability of the hypothalamic-pituitary–adrenal axis to respond rapidly during stress, the glucocorticoids allow adaptation of the other endocrine pathways to changing conditions. In general, they are catabolic and anti-inflammatory. Increased cortisol levels stimulate protein breakdown in many tissues to provide amino-acids for gluconeogenesis, although essential muscles, such as the heart, are spared. In contrast, in the liver, where cortisol induces synthesis of the enzymes involved in gluconeogenesis, the effects of glucocorticoids are anabolic. Through their interaction with epinephrine, the glucocorticoids increase cardiac contractility and cardiac output and increase the efficiency of skeletal muscle contraction.

It is the anti-inflammatory effects of glucocorticoids, however, that provide the basis of many therapeutic pharmacological analogues. Many of the anti-inflammatory effects, such as the stabilization of cell membranes, do not occur at physiological levels of glucocorticoids, but appear only when higher, pharmacological, doses are given. Thus, some of the pharmacological effects of glucocorticoids occur through mechanisms that are not receptor-mediated (13, 14).

Excess cortisol secretion might be expected to have grave consequences for the metabolic function of the organism. Sustained hypercortisolism does produce metabolic imbalance, but one that is tempered in many aspects by the opposing actions of insulin. It is the clinical effects of this imbalance that lead to the gradual evolution of the syndrome first described by Harvey Cushing in 1912 (63, 64).

In Cushing's syndrome, derangements occur in the metabolism of proteins, fats, and carbohydrates. Patients become hyperglyce-mic, with secondary hyperinsulinemia and insulin resistance (237). Normal utilization of carbohydrate continues despite hypercortisolism, because secondary hyperinsulinemia impedes gluconeogenesis and enhances the peripheral uptake of glucose, in both respects directly opposing the effects of cortisol. Thus, production and consumption of carbohydrates are maintained despite high plasma levels of glucose and insulin. Because hypercortisolism increases the hepatic production of very-low-density lipoproteins (VLDL), but does not change their clearance, VLDL levels rise, as do the levels of cholesterol and triglyceride. The hyperinsulinemia (which inhibits glycolysis) predominates over the lipolytic effects of cortisol and elicits a gain in body fat. The well-known truncal obesity of Cushing's syndrome, the redistribution of fat from the extremities to the central portions of the body, may reflect differential sensitivity of adipose tissues in different locations to the increased levels of glucocorticoids and insulin. In contrast, in protein metabolism, catabolism predominates and chronic progressive atrophy of muscle and connective tissue occurs (187).

Hypocortisolism also alters metabolism and, by the absence of the usual action of cortisol to enhance the effects of epinephrine, is associated with reduced cardiac output, which, if severe, may lead to cardiogenic shock. Impairment of gluconeogenesis decreases the supply of glucose. Lipolysis is also impaired, increasing the reliance of the organism on glucose. The combination of the low glucose supply in the face of high demand underlies the symptomatic hypoglycemia and chronic fatigue in patients with cortisol deficiency.

Metabolism and Inactivation of Cortisol

Most of the metabolism of steroids occurs in the liver. The rapid hepatic clearance of many steroids results in a plasma half-life of 20 min or less in most people. The kidneys also degrade cortisol in small amounts (361). Because clearance is rapid and adrenal secretion is intermittent, plasma steroid concentrations can change quickly. The half-life of cortisol in plasma is longer (60 to 80 min) than the half-life of most other steroids because most plasma cortisol is reversibly bound by transcortin and albumin and is protected from metabolic inactivation (291).

At least seven enzymatic steps participate in the metabolism of cortisol. These steps occur in various combinations that produce several metabolites that are ultimately excreted in the urine. One-quarter exits in the form of tetrahydrocortisol or its isomer. Only 1% or less of the cortisol that is secreted escapes into the urine without enzymatic breakdown. The plasma half-life and clearance of cortisol are quite similar among normal subjects, possibly due to the variety of pathways available for its degradation. Thus, since the variation in the metabolism of synthetic steroids (e.g., dexamethasone) varies considerably from patient to patient, iatrogenic Cushing's syndrome occurs more sporadically and unpredictably in patients receiving synthetic steroids than in patients receiving hydrocortisone.

The adult pattern of cortisol metabolism is established within a few days after birth. In the fetus and neonate, the predominant glucocorticoid is cortisone, not cortisol, and some of the enzymatic systems are not yet fully developed. As a result, the steroid metabolites are different in quantity and quality from those of adults. Assessment of the pituitary-adrenal axis in the neonate can lead to an incorrect diagnosis of adrenal insufficiency if these differences are not considered in the interpretation of the steroid profile in the blood and urine, which contain large amounts of the C–6 hydroxylated steroids (137, 277).

HYPOSECRETION OF CORTISOL

Etiology

Hyposecretion of cortisol implies a diminution of adrenal activity. This may be primary, in which there is a defect intrinsic to the adrenal gland, or occur secondarily, when pituitary or hypothalamic dysfunction causes decreased secretion of CRH and/or ACTH (Table 8.1.). Hypoadrenalism from any cause may be life-threatening, particularly in circumstances that require increased glucocorticoid secretion for the physiological response to stress.

TABLE 8.1.
Causes of Adrenal Insufficiency

I. Primary adrenal insufficiency
  A. Idiopathic (autoimmune)
  B. Infection
    1. Tuberculosis
    2. Acquired immunodeficiency syndrome
    3. Fungal infections
  C. Metastatic tumor
  D. Genetic
    1. Adrenoleukodystrophy
    2. Adrenomyeloneuropathy
    3. Congenital adrenal hypoplasia
  E. Other
    1. Adrenal hemorrhage (shock, trauma)
    2. Sarcoidosis
II. Secondary adrenal insufficiency
  A. Exogenous
    1. Glucocorticoid (or ACTH) therapy
    2. Pituitary or hypothalamic surgery
    3. Irradiation therapy of sellar region
    4. Trauma with injury of pituitary stalk
  B. Endogenous
    1. Hypothalamic-pituitary suppression in Cushing's syndrome
    2. Neoplasms
      a) Pituitary tumor
      b) Pituitary apoplexy
      c) Craniopharyngioma
      d) Metastatic tumor
    3. Vascular disorders
      a) Pituitary infarction (Sheehan's syndrome)
      b) Arterial aneurysm
    4. Lymphocytic hypophysitis
    5. Sarcoidosis

Primary Adrenal Insufficiency

In 1855, Thomas Addison described 11 patients with what are still recognized as the typical and important clinical and pathological features of adrenal insufficiency (2). The ailment that bears his name results from the chronic hypofunction of the adrenal glands and encompasses multiple etiologies. Since in Addison's disease hypothalamic and pituitary function are normal, ACTH levels are high in response to the low plasma levels of glucocorticoids. Despite the overall elevation of circulating plasma ACTH levels, the circadian periodicity is maintained.

Although in Addison's time the most common cause of primary adrenal insufficiency was tuberculosis, most cases now represent an apparent autoimmune disorder (186, 227, 247). In this "idiopathic" adrenal atrophy, most patients have adrenal autoantibodies and often have associated autoimmune disorders of other endocrine organs. The combination of Addison's disease, hypoparathyroidism, and mucocutaneous candidiasis is known as autoimmune polyglandular syndrome type I. More common is the combination of Hashimoto's thyroiditis and diabetes mellitus, which, with adrenal insufficiency, form a triad known as Schmidt's syndrome or autoimmune polyglandular syndrome type II. Hypoparathyroidism, hypogonadism, and adrenal insufficiency, together with pernicious anemia, form another autoimmune constellation that usually has its onset in childhood. Autoimmune adrenal insufficiency is often familial.

The pathological findings are specific to the etiology. To produce clinically evident adrenal insufficiency, the offending process must be bilateral and extensive enough to destroy greater than 90% of the adrenal cortex (312). In tuberculosis, a caseating mass enlarges and replaces the entire gland; calcification occurs in about half of chronic cases. In the autoimmune disorders the glands are small, with loss of cells in all zones of the cortex, diffuse lymphocytic infiltration, and fibrosis (147). Some studies suggest that the circulating antiadrenal antibodies associated with these endocrine disorders (227) are not sufficient in and of themselves to produce the disease and that they may be an epiphenomenon of organ destruction, rather than its cause.

The acquired immunodeficiency syndrome (AIDS), a more recent addition to the differential diagnosis of Addison's disease, can produce profound adrenocortical hypofunction (116). Infectious agents that attack the adrenal glands of the immunocompromised host include *Cryptococcus neoformans* and *Mycobacterium avium intracellulare.* Pathological evidence of infection by cytomegalovirus occurs more frequently in the adrenal glands of patients with AIDS than in any other organ, but fulminant necrotizing adrenalitis is uncommon (108, 139, 266). Kaposi's sarcoma can also involve the adrenals to a degree sufficient to cause symptoms in a few patients.

Less common causes of adrenal insufficiency are fungal infections, most promi-nently histoplasmosis (59, 110). Other fungal infections that involve the adrenal glands include cryptococcosis (353) and coccioidomycosis (94). The most common metastatic tumors of the adrenal are lymphomas (144) and carcinomas from the lung and breast.

Other entities in the differential diagnosis of primary adrenal insufficiency are sarcoidosis and adrenoleukodystrophy (220,2295). Adrenoleukodystrophy is an X-linked recessive trait that first becomes apparent in childhood. It is characterized by diffuse demyelination of the central nervous system, resulting in seizures, dementia, coma, and death (220). The demyelination seems to be due to an enzymatic defect in myelin synthesis, but it has not yet been precisely identified. The adrenal glands accumulate pathological levels of long-chain fatty acids, as does the myelin of the CNS. The increased secretion of such fatty acids in the urine provides diagnostic confirmation of the disorder.

Secondary Adrenal Insufficiency

Secondary adrenal insufficiency is produced either by the suppression of hypothalamic-pituitary function via the chronic administration of exogenous glucocorticoids, or by hypothalamic or pituitary disorders that impair secretion of ACTH. Although an occasional patient presents with adrenal failure from primary deficiency of ACTH synthesis (327), in the current age of glucocorticoid treatment for various medical disorders, chronic steroid therapy is the most common cause of adrenal insufficiency. The sensitivity of individuals to hypothalamic-pituitary suppression by exogenous glucocorticoids is highly variable (297). Some patients, treated for as long as a year with replacement doses, have safely undergone surgery without steroid supplementation (66). Although patients treated for 14 days with high doses of glucocorticoids will generally normalize their hypothalamic-pituitary-adrenal axis within a week after terminating therapy (325), complete recovery from long-term adrenal suppression usually requires a year (Fig. 8.5) (113). The last site of the hypothalamic-pituitary-adrenal axis to recover after chronic glucocorticoid suppression is hypothalamic secretion of CRH (9, 10, 50, 51,

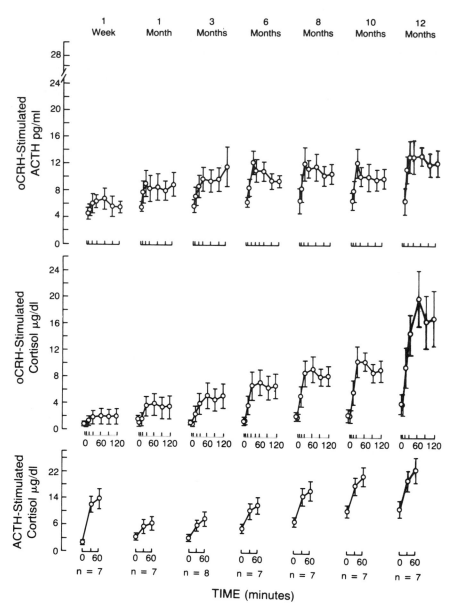

Figure 8.5. Recovery of the hypothalamic-pituitary-adrenal axis from chronic hypercortisolism. Nine patients with Cushing's syndrome (six patients with Cushing's disease, two with adrenal adenomas, and one with ectopic ACTH syndrome) were tested longitudinally for 12 months after surgical correction of Cushing's syndrome with the 1-hour ACTH test (lower panel) and the oCRH test (upper and middle panels). The times at the top of the figure indicate the intervals between the testing and surgery and the number of patients studied at each time point is shown at the bottom. The shaded areas represent the mean (± SD) responses in normal subjects. (From Avgerinos P.C., Chrousos G.P., Nieman L.K., Oldfield E.H., Loriaux D.L., Cutler G.B. Jr. The corticotropin-releasing hormone test in the postoperative evaluation of patients with Cushing's syndrome. J. Clin. Endocrinol. Metab., 65:906–913, 1987.)

113). Patients with Cushing's disease who have undergone successful pituitary surgery have impaired ACTH and cortisol responses to CRH stimulation for at least a month after the operation (9, 10, 51, 142), and hypercortisolemic patients who have undergone the excision of a pituitary adenoma, a source of ectopic ACTH secretion, or of an adrenal adenoma have an adrenocortical insufficiency that lasts as long as 6 to 18 months (112, 142). Patients who have received glucocorticoid therapy for two weeks or more, or who have undergone successful treatment of Cushing's syndrome—such as removal of an ACTH-secreting pituitary adenoma—should be considered to have an impaired adrenal response to stress until recovery of the hypothalamic-pituitary-adrenal axis has been demonstrated with endocrine assessment.

Pituitary disorders, such as tumor, infarction, or granuloma can also produce adrenal insufficiency by causing hypopituitarism—usually panhypopituitarism. Hypothalamic lesions that produce secondary adrenal insufficiency may be intrinsic to the hypothalamus or arise from the skull base. Hypothalamic disturbance, however, more frequently alters other pituitary functions long before it affects ACTH regulation and, although structural lesions of the hypothalamus can alter the secretory pattern of corticosteroids, they rarely produce severe adrenal insufficiency (163). Nevertheless, disturbances in the diurnal rhythm of ACTH and cortisol secretion commonly occur with intracranial disease (161, 287).

Clinical Presentation of Hypocortisolism

Clinical syndromes associated with adrenal insufficiency include weakness, fatigue, and anorexia in all instances. About half of affected patients have nausea and diarrhea and most patients lose weight. Postural hypotension is common. Many patients with primary adrenal insufficiency have hyperpigmentation, which can best be detected by examining the buccal mucosa. Only 10% have vitiligo (227). The clinical pictures of a secondary and a primary adrenal insufficiency are similar, except that patients with secondary insufficiency do not have hyperpigmentation, vitiligo, or adrenal calcification and

they are less vulnerable to acute adrenal insufficiency (adrenal crisis).

The mineralocorticoid insufficiency that accompanies glucocorticoid insufficiency accounts for the electrolyte abnormalities and anemia that are usually present. About 90% of patients with adrenal insufficiency have hyponatremia and 65% have hyperkalemia (181, 227). Patients with isolated glucocorticoid deficiency have decreased ability to excrete water, and hyponatremia with normokalemia results. The basis of inefficient clearance of free water is unclear, but it may reflect interference with regulation of the concentrating function of the distal nephron by ADH.

Evaluation of Hypocortisolism (Table 8.2.)

Adrenal insufficiency is detected biochemically by measuring the plasma cortisol. It is suggested by morning plasma levels of cortisol of less than 10 μg/dl and confirmed by levels that are <5 μg/dl. However, the AM cortisol level must be assessed in light of the circumstances in which it was drawn. The time of day is important, as is the presence of stress. Normal plasma cortisol levels in patients undergoing abdominal surgery (153) and in patients in shock (204) range between 20 and 120 μg/dl. In stressed patients, therefore, plasma cortisol levels that are <20 μg/dl suggest adrenal insufficiency. To avoid inappropriate treatment of patients who do not

TABLE 8.2.
Diagnostic Approach to Patients Suspected of Having Adrenal Insufficiency

I. Establish presence of adrenal insufficiency
  A. Establish presence of adrenal insufficiency
    1. Plasma cortisol at 6–8 AM
    2. 24-hour urine for:
      a. Urine-free cortisol
      b. 17-Hydroxysteroid/gm of urinary creatinine
  B. Short ACTH stimulation test
II. Distinguish adrenal, pituitary, and hypothalamic disorders
  A. Plasma ACTH
  B. 48-hour ACTH stimulation test
  C. CRH stimulation test
III. Establish etiology
  A. Radiographic imaging
    1. Adrenal CT
    2. Pituitary and cerebral MRI
  B. Additional special testing as indicated by results of endocrine and radiologic testing

have hypocortisolism, and iatrogenic production of secondary adrenal insufficiency by exogenous glucocorticoid administration, the presence of adrenal insufficiency should be confirmed by measurement of 24-hr urinary-free cortisol and 17-hydroxycorticosteroids (17-OHCS). In severe adrenal insufficiency, 24-hr urinary-free cortisol and daily urine 17-OHCS are low. However, basal plasma cortisol levels and urinary measurements of cortisol secretion may be in the low normal range in even moderately severe hypoadrenalism. Thus, dynamic testing is usually required to establish the presence of adrenal insufficiency and the differential diagnosis of its etiology.

Since without normal ACTH stimulation the adrenal cortex atrophies, in primary or secondary adrenal insufficiency the response to ACTH stimulation is suppressed. In the short ACTH stimulation test 0.25 mg(25 units) of cosyntropin, synthetic short ACTH)α^{1-24}-ACTH), which retains the biological activity of ACTH, is injected intravenously or intramuscularly and plasma cortisol is measured just before and at 30 and 60 minutes after injection. An increment of $\geq$

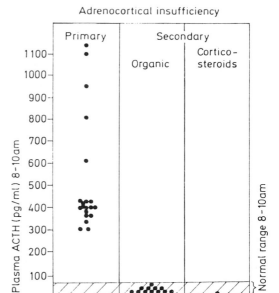

Figure 8.7. Plasma ACTH levels in normal subjects (hatched area) and patients with primary and secondary adrenal cortical insufficiency. (From Rees L.H., Holdaway I.M., Phenekos C., *et al.* ACTH secretion and clinical investigations.In: Some aspects of hypothalamic regulation of endocrine functions. Symposium, Vienna, June 3–6, 1973. Stuttgart, F Schattaur Verlag, 1974).

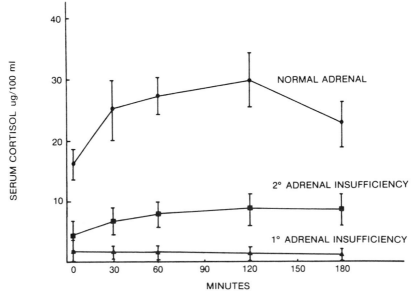

Figure 8.6. ACTH-stimulation test to confirm the diagnosis of adrenal insufficiency. Serum cortisol response to 0.25 mg of cosyntropin (synthetic ACTH$_{1-24}$) in normal subjects (n = 9), hypopituitarism (n = 8), and Addison's disease (n; eq 7). (From Speckart P.F., Nicoloff J.T., Bethune J.E. Screening for adrenocortical insufficiency with cosyntropin (synthetic ACTH). Arch. Intern. Med., *128*:761–XX, 1971.)

7μg/dl over basal levels or a peak value of ≥ 20 μg/dl is expected in normal subjects. In contrast, patients with ACTH deficiency or suppression have a definited, but blunted, response and patients with primary adrenal insufficiency generally have no response (Fig. 8.6.). When the diagnosi of adrenal insufficiency is confirmed, basal plasma ACTH measurements (Fig. 8.7.) and the CRH stimulation test (Fig. 8.8.) are used to establish the location and etiology of the disorder. In primary adrenal insufficiency, because di-

minished cortisol production provides reduced negative feedback of the pituitary corticotrophs, basal plasma ACTH levels are high and the ACTH response to CRH is exaggerated (Figs. 8.7 and 8.8) (303). On the other hand, with pituitary disease (secondary adrenal insufficiency) or after prolonged excess glucocorticoid exposure, basal plasma ACTH levels are low and do not respond, or respond minimally, to CRH infusion, whereas patients with hypothalamic disorders (tertiary adrenal insufficiency) have an

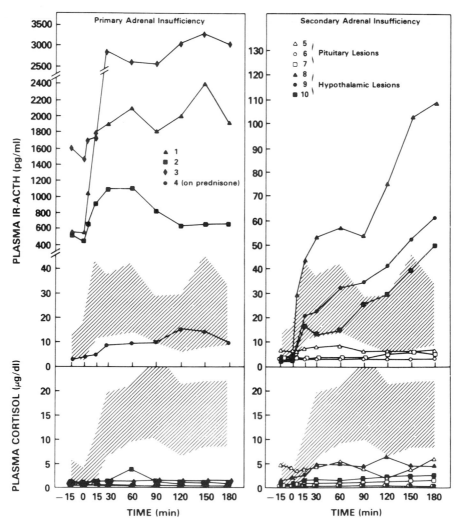

Figure 8.8. CRH-stimulation test in adrenal insufficiency. Plasma ACTH (top) and cortisol (bottom) responses to oCRH (1 μg/kg iv) in patients with primary (left) and secondary (right) adrenal insufficiency. (From Schulte H.M., Chrousos G.P., Avgerinos P.C., Oldfield E.H., Gold P.W., Cutler G.B. Jr., Loriaux D.L. 1984. The corticotropin-releasing factor stimulation test: an aid in the evaluation of patients with adrenal insufficiency. J. Clin. Endocrinol. Metab., 58:1064–1067.)

exaggerated and prolonged ACTH response to CRH (Figs. 8.7 and 8.8.).

By their enlarged size and occasional calcification, tuberculous adrenal glands can be distinguished by CT from the small, fibrotic glands associated with autoimmunity. Asymmetry and alterations of contour of the adrenal surface can occur with many benign disorders as well as with adrenal tumors and nodular adrenal disease. In such circumstances, needle aspiration under CT guidance is often diagnostic.

HYPERSECRETION OF CORTISOL

Etiology

The most common cause of Cushing's syndrome is iatrogenic by exogenous administration of glucocorticoids to patients with inflammatory disorders and other diseases. Endogenous hypercortisolism arises in three general circumstances (Fig. 8.9): 1) The pituitary may secrete an excess amount of ACTH, most commonly when it harbors an ACTH-secreting adenoma; 2) ectopic ACTH secretion may occur from tumors that arise from tissues other than the pituitary; and 3) there may be autonomous secretion of cortisol by a benign or malignant tumor of the adrenal cortex or due to bilateral nodular adrenal disease.

Cushing's syndrome is the eponym for the general clinical syndrome produced by chronic hypercortisolism. Hypercortisolism resulting from excess pituitary secretion of ACTH has the title of Cushing's disease.

About 70-80% of patients with endogenous hypercortisolism have a pituitary tumor, about 10-15% have an adrenal tumor, and about 10-15% harbor an extrapituitary tumor producing ACTH (Table 8.3.) (244, 250). Most children below the age of seven years with hypercortisolism have an adrenal carcinoma.

Primary Adrenal Disease (ACTH-Independent Cushing's Syndrome)

Cortisol-secreting tumors of the adrenal cortex produce cortisol autonomously and, by suppressing pituitary ACTH secretion, cause atrophy of the remaining normal adrenal tissue in the ipsilateral and contralateral glands. ACTH levels often fall below the limit of detection in modern radioimmunoassays (Fig. 8.10) (62, 261, 269). The diurnal variation of plasma cortisol is lost. Exogenous corticosteroid administration will not suppress cortisol production by adrenal tu-

TABLE 8.3.
Etiology of Cushing's Syndrome

ACTH-dependent	85%
Cushing's disease	80–85%
Ectopic ACTH-secreting tumor	15–20%
Ectopic CRH-secreting tumor	rare
ACTH-independent	15%
Adrenal adenoma	7%
Adrenocortical carcinoma	7%
Bilateral micronodular adrenocortical hyperplasia	rare
Bilateral macronodular adrenocortical hyperplasia	rare

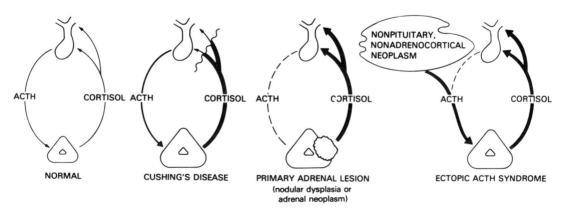

Figure 8.9. Pathophysiology of hypercortisolism. (From Loriaux D.L. and Cutler G.B. Jr. Diseases of the adrenal glands. In: *Clinical Endocrinology,* edited by Peter O. Kohler, M.D., pp. 167–238, John Wiley and Sons, Inc., 1986).

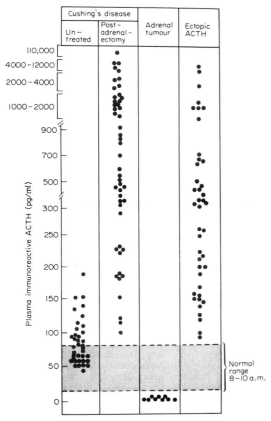

Figure 8.10. Plasma ACTH levels distinguish patients with ACTH-independent (primary adrenal disease) and ACTH-dependent forms of Cushing's syndrome. Plasma ACTH levels in 137 patients with Cushing's syndrome. (From Besser G.M., Edwards C.R.W. Cushing's syndrome. Clinics Endocrinol. Metab., *1*:451–490, 1972).

mors, nor will it affect plasma ACTH levels (which are already suppressed to low or undetectable levels by the endogenous cortisol excess). However, ACTH administration will increase plasma cortisol concentration in 5-15% of patients with adrenal carcinoma and perhaps a quarter of patients with an adrenal adenoma (176, 183, 270). This implies that some cortisol-secreting adrenal tumors can still respond to ACTH, despite autonomous cortisol secretion, whereas others cannot, perhaps due to loss of functional ACTH receptors (17).

Adrenal carinomas often attain a large size before producing sufficient steroid to cause clinically evident hypercortisolism. For this reason, as many as half of these patients have

no clinical endocrine disturbance when the adrenal carcinoma is diagnosed (17, 183, 193, 224), and the majority of tumors are palpable on abdominal exam at diagnosis. Many of these tumors have deficiency of one or more of the various enzymes involved in the pathways of steroid synthesis, particularly deficiency of 11-hydroxylation, which leads to increased secretion of 11–deoxycortisol (184), and deficiency of 21-hydroxylation, which results in diversion of steroid intermediates into androgen synthesis. In these patients, changes in secondary sex characteristics arise before clinical evidence of hypercortisolism appears (17, 100, 183, 192, 224, 362, 364). Some adrenal carcinomas also produce deoxycorticosterone, aldosterone, and other mineralocorticoids, and may do so primarily, without producing glucocorticoids (6, 265). Although the histology of adrenal carcinomas often indicates malignancy, their behavior is unpredictable and the only true indicators of clinical malignancy are local invasion of venous channels or direct extension of tumor through the adrenal capsule (349). Furthermore, histologically benign tumors may metastasize and histologically malignant tumors may remain quiescent and receive successful surgical cure (71, 193, 349).

Since adrenal adenomas produce steroids more efficiently than carcinomas, they are usually smaller at diagnosis (245) and they have less tendency than adrenal carcinomas to produce mineralocorticoids and androgens, because of the relative absence of specific enzyme defects. However, they, too, may cause virilism (100, 101, 301) associated with minimal excess cortisol production. The histology of adrenal adenomas is variable. Occasionally, there is such overlap in the histological appearance between adenoma and carcinoma that precise diagnosis demands consideration not only of the histological appearance but also of the clinical presentation and pattern of steroid secretion.

The diffuse primary (ACTH-independent) multinodular adrenal diseases, bilateral micronodular and macronodular adrenal hyperplasia, are also endogenous etiologies of Cushing's syndrome. These entities occur much less commonly than adrenal adenomas and carcinomas. In micronodular disease, nodules of adrenal cortical tissue several millimeters in diameter are found bilaterally (172, 211, 313). They function identically to adrenal adenomas, but are much smaller. Micronodular adrenal disease usually affects patients under the age of 20 years and may be familial (139). Bilateral ACTH-independent macronodular adrenal cortical hyperplasia, in which the adrenal cortex appears hyperplastic and contains macroscopic nodules, is very rare (5, 157, 172, 194, 319).

In patients with diffuse micronodular adrenal disease, cortisol secretion usually does not respond to ACTH stimulation. In the few patients who do respond to ACTH, it is unclear whether the response is from the nodules or the normal tissue between them. In patients with bilateral macronodular disease, cortisol secretion may increase in response to ACTH stimulation, but is not suppressed with high-dose dexamethasone.

Excess ACTH Secretion (ACTH-Dependent Cushing's Syndrome)

PITUITARY (Cushing's disease). In Cushing's disease, excess ACTH is usually produced by corticotroph tumors within the anterior lobe of the pituitary gland. In the large pathological series of pituitary tumors, Kovacs and his colleagues classified 4-10% of all tumors as ACTH adenomas by immunohistochemical staining (158, 159). However, 14.6% of the pituitary adenomas in the surgical specimens of the same group of pathologists were corticotrophic adenomas (141). Two–thirds were in patients with Cushing's syndrome and the remainder had been hormonally silent by clinical assessment (141). Surgical series contain an even greater fraction of clinically evident hormonally-active tumors, as they are more likely to be detected in life and to require removal (279).

About four-fifths of the patients with Cushing's syndrome who undergo transsphenoidal exploration of the pituitary after endocrinologic testing indicates Cushing's disease have a pituitary adenoma identified at surgery. Most (80-90%) of the tumors found at surgery are microadenomas (<10mm maximum diameter) (29, 48, 126, 195, 241, 264, 289). In 15-20% of patients in whom endocrine testing indicates Cushing's disease,

surgical exploration discloses no adenoma. In these patients, the ACTH-secreting lesion may be a tumor that is too small to be delineated from the surrounding normal pituitary tissue. Some ACTH-secreting tumors arise in ectopic rests of pituitary tissue located outside the sella, usually within the sphenoid sinus (28, 150).

Although it is rare, patients with hypercortisolism and non-adenomatous hyperplasia of ACTH-containing cells have been described (61, 69, 208, 368). It is now evident that some of these patients have ectopic secretion of CRH by a tumor. Others may have excess hypothalamic secretion of CRH or represent multifocal early development of a microadenoma. However, these entities must be exceptionally rare, as they have, combined, occurred with a frequency of less than 0.3% in over 350 patients with Cushing's disease who received pituitary surgery by one of the authors (Oldfield, unpublished data).

In patients with endocrine testing indicating Cushing's disease, an adenoma may not be identified at surgery despite careful exploration of the entire pituitary gland. In some of these patients, surgical success can be achieved by removing the median one-third of the anterior lobe (126), by removing most of the pituitary gland leaving a small amount attached to the stalk (248), or by excising the lateral 40 to 50% of the gland on the side corresponding to the side of highest ACTH concentration during petrosal sinus sampling (240). However, in many patients whose hypercortisolism resolves after such treatment, the excised specimen contains no identifiable adenoma or evidence of corticotroph hyperplasia and the etiology of hypercortisolism remains undefined.

Before it was evident that most patients with Cushing's syndrome had a pituitary adenoma, and prior to the availability of radioimmunoassays and the recent refinements in provocative endocrine testing, patients with Cushing's disease were treated with bilateral adrenalectomy (129). Ten to 20% of them later developed florid symptoms of pituitary hypersecretion of ACTH and growth of a pituitary tumor (Nelson's syndrome) (226). Negative feedback by cortisol and/or other unknown, substances secreted by the adrenal glands exert a restraining influence on tumor growth as well as on its ACTH secretion (219, 226, 269, 357). After adrenalectomy, pituitary ACTH secretion increases, plasma ACTH levels may reach 110,000 pg/ml or more, the ACTH response to CRH increases despite glucocorticoid replacement (Fig. 8.11.) (243), and hyperpigmentation occurs from crossreactivity of ACTH with the receptors of MSH in the melanocytes of the skin. Nelson's syndrome may be delayed for as long as 15 years after adrenalectomy. Although it occurs rarely, in Nelson's syndrome and with ACTH-secreting pituitary carcinomas the tumor can metastasize within the central nervous system and extracranially to the liver, bones, and lungs (44, 243, 267).

Mild hyperprolactinemia occasionally occurs with Cushing's disease (366). In most patients, it is probably due to the compression of portal blood flow within the pituitary stalk or is a result of an "isolated" segment of anterior pituitary gland, produced by the corticotroph adenoma, that no longer has access to prolactin-inhibiting factor (dopamine) from the hypothalamus. However, some tumors secrete prolactin and ACTH, as immunohistochemistry occasionally reveals staining of prolactin and ACTH within the same tumor (314). Although staining for multiple glycoprotein hormones is common in hormonally silent pituitary tumors, plurihormonal adenomas rarely contain ACTH (22, 89, 296) and coproduction of ACTH and other functional pituitary hormones is exceptional in Cushing's disease (124). Only the hormonally inactive α-subunit is coproduced with any frequency in the corticotropinomas (15), which is an observation that has uncertain clinical significance. In this sense, the corticotrophic adenomas form a more highly differentiated family of tumors than do their counterparts that produce growth hormone, prolactin, or the glycoprotein hormones (TSH, FSH, LH).

In an attempt to establish the biological basis of the various causes of Cushing's syndrome, ACTH secretion has been extensively analyzed. In Cushing's disease, ACTH levels are in the normal range or are only slightly elevated (Fig. 8.10.). In contrast, after adrenalectomy, patients with Cushing's disease

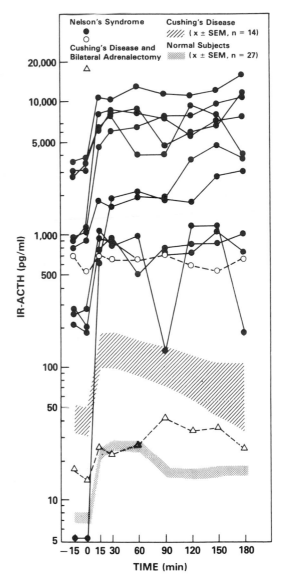

Figure 8.11. Basal plasma ACTH levels and the response to oCRH (1 μ/kg iv) in 11 patients with Nelson's syndrome (•) compared to 1 patient with Cushing's disease after bilateral adrenalectomy ($\triangle$), 27 normal subjects ($\square$; mean $\pm$ 1 SEM), and 14 patients with Cushing's disease (▨; mean $\pm$ 1 SEM). One patient with Nelson's syndrome received 0.5 mg of dexamethasone 2 h before the CRH-stimulation test. (From Oldfield E.H., Schulte H.M., Chrousos G.P., et al. Corticotropin-releasing hormone (CRH) stimulation in Nelson's syndrome: response of adrenocorticotropin secretion to pulse injection and continuous infusion of CRH. An aid in the evaluation of patients with Cushing's syndrome. J. Clin. Endocrinol. Metab., *62:*1020–1026, 1986).

and patients with Nelson's syndrome always have markedly elevated plasma ACTH levels; patients with ectopic secretion of ACTH usually have levels exceeding the normal range; and those with adrenal tumors have levels in the subnormal range (Fig. 8.10.) (18). Plasma ACTH levels are interpreted in conjunction with the levels of cortisol; if hypercortisolism is present, an ACTH level in the normal range represents an inappropriate elevation.

In Cushing's disease, although dampening of the normal diurnal variation of plasma ACTH and cortisol occurs, the diurnal rhythm usually is not eliminated altogether (Fig. 8. 12.). ACTH (55, 185, 272, 269, 352) and cortisol (23, 130, 310, 346, 351, 367) still show pulsatile secretion and episodic fluctuations about their mean values. When low doses of exogenous glucocorticoids are administered to patients with Cushing's disease, secretion of ACTH fails to suppress normally (55, 175, 272). Although corticotropin secretion is more resistant to the negative-feedback effects of dexamethasone than are the normal corticotrophs, ACTH secretion is suppressed when higher doses of dexamethasone are administered (Fig. 8.13.). Thus, in ACTH-secreting pituitary adenomas, the negative feedback effect of glucocorticoids is retained, but the threshold of the concentration required for suppression of ACTH secretion is set at a higher level than in normal corticotrophs.

The hypothalamus once was considered a potential site for the pathophysiology of Cushing's disease. The negative feedback effects of cortisol occur not only at the pitu-

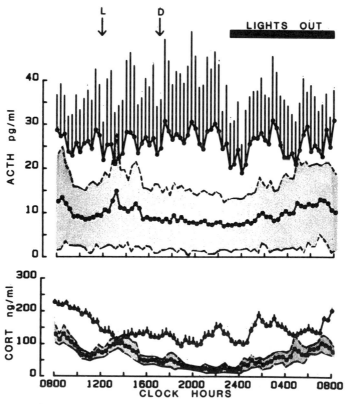

Figure 8.12. Diurnal rhythms of ACTH and cortisol in Cushing's disease. Plasma ACTH and cortisol levels in nine normal women (shaded area; ± 95% confidence limits) and in five women with Cushing's disease (mean ± SD). (From Liu J.H., Kazer R.R., Rasmussen D.D. Characterization of the twenty-four hour secretion patterns of adrenocorticotropin and cortisol in normal women and patients with Cushing's disease. J. Clin. Endocrinol. Metab., *64:*1027–1035, 1987).

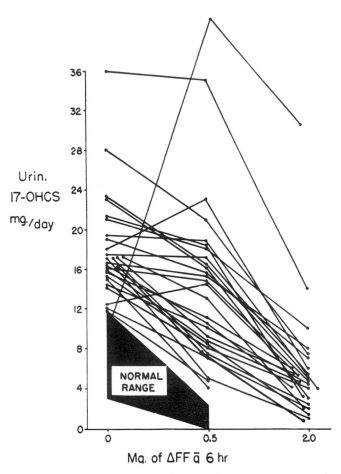

Figure 8.13. Standard six-day dexamethasone-suppression test (Liddle test) to detect patients with Cushing's syndrome. Normal subjects, but not patients with Cushing's syndrome, have suppression of 17-hydroxycorticosteroid (17-OHCS) excretion to less than 2.5 mg during the second day of low-dose (0.5 mg) dexamethasone administration. Urinary 17-OHCS in patients with Cushing's disease. Left: average basal levels; middle: values observed during the second day of suppression with 0.5 mg dexamethasone every 6 h; right: values observed during the second day of suppression with 2 mg dexamethasone every 6 h (From Liddle G.W., Island D., Meador C.K. Normal and abnormal regulation of corticotropin secretion in man. Recent Progr. Hormone Res., *18*:125–166, 1962).

itary gland but also at the hypothalamus. The failure of plasma ACTH levels to rise during stress (352) and the loss of circadian rhythmicity of ACTH and cortisol could also be attributed to either pituitary or hypothalamic abnormality. In Cushing's disease, most adenomas respond to CRH with an immediate ACTH response. The higher set-point of the threshold for negative feedback by cortisol (156, 258), the loss of circadian rhythms of cortisol and ACTH, the failure of stress to induce a cortisol response, and the ACTH response to CRH are, therefore, theoretically consistent with an abnormality in the pituitary or the hypothalamus. Although examination of the clonal composition of ACTH-secreting pituitary tumors in patients with Cushing's disease indicates that most patients have a tumor of monoclonal origin, some patients have polyclonal tumors, suggesting hormonal influence in a multicellular origin. The normal circadian rhythm of growth hormone secretion is also lost in Cushing's disease; but this defective regulation gradually disappears after removal of the pituitary adenoma (167, 300) and argues against a hypothalamic abnormality affecting both cortisol and growth hormone regulation. Furthermore, repeated measurements for CRH in the blood from the inferior petrosal sinuses, which drain the blood from the pituitary, have failed to reveal detectable CRH levels in patients with Cushing's disease (Oldfield *et al.,* unpublished). And neither has a role of excess hypothalamic secretion of an ACTH-releasing factor (i.e., CRH or vasopressin) been established for the rare patient with Cushing's disease and diffuse corticotroph hyperplasia. Although it has been difficult to confirm or refute a contributing role of the hypothalamus in all patients with Cushing's disease, almost all patients with Cushing's disease have a primary pituitary abnormality.

Cushing found pituitary adenomas in six of his eight autopsied patients and was the first person to suggest that there was a link between the intrasellar pituitary neoplasm and the hyperplasia of the adrenal cortex that all his patients had bilaterally (64). However, because of the small size of these tumors, they could usually not be demonstrated with contemporary diagnostic techniques; but, theories of the primary role of the adrenal gland soon developed. In the modern era, early evidence favoring a pituitary etiology for Cushing's disease came from a patient treated by Liddle (176). In this patient with Cushing's disease the hypercortisolism continued unabated, despite transsection of the pituitary stalk at surgery, resulting in complete hypothalamic-pituitary disconnection (confirmed by the absence of secretion of thyrotropin or gonadotropins postoperatively). At autopsy, a small pituitary adenoma was found.

Additional evidence favoring an intrinsic pituitary defect comes from the low incidence of postoperative recurrence of ACTH-secreting pituitary tumors and from the biochemical and clinical effects of selective adenomectomy. Patients cured by selective adenomectomy eventually return to a normal circadian cortisol rhythm and to normal feedback regulation of cortisol (16, 167, 289, 300), indicating that the ACTH-secreting pituitary adenoma caused the disease. Furthermore, preoperative stimulation of ACTH secretion with intravenous administration of CRH in Cushing's disease usually shows hyperresponsiveness, whereas after selective adenomectomy the ACTH response to CRH is flat. Recovery of normal pituitary responsiveness to CRH usually takes months after the removal of the tumor, but it occurs almost always (9, 10, 142, 223).

Nearly all patients successfully treated by pituitary surgery immediately develop hypocortisolism, which implies suppression of either the endogenous release of CRH from the hypothalamus, or inhibition of the ACTH response of the pituitary to CRH, or both (92). When insulin tolerance testing is performed (354) or when CRH is administered to such patients, subnormal or no pituitary secretion of ACTH occurs, despite coexisting secondary adrenal insufficiency (9, 10, 51). These observations indicate that the CRH-secreting neurons and the normal corticotrophs are suppressed by hypercortisolism in Cushing's disease, and that the origin of the disease is in the pituitary rather than in the hypothalamus. Finally, the results of anatomic studies of the vascularization of pituitary tumors also support the concept of an intrinsic pituitary defect: Two–thirds of microadenomas have an extraportal arterial supply and, thus, grow outside the part of the anterior lobe influenced by hypothalamic factors (111).

Thus, although a role for hypothalamic stimulation as an initiating factor in stimulating the transformation of a locus of hyperplasia into an adenoma cannot be excluded, it seems highly unlikely. When a tumor has formed, it secretes ACTH autonomously and elicits excess cortisol secretion from the adrenal cortex, which suppresses CRH release from the hypothalamus and ACTH release from the normal corticotrophs. Over several months after successful pituitary surgery, almost all patients recover normal function and regulation of the hypothalamic-pituitary–adrenal axis (10, 11, 300).

ECTOPIC ADRENOCORTICOTROPIN PRODUCTION. Since not all autopsied patients in Cushing's original series had demonstrable pituitary adenomas, Cushing may have included patients with occult ectopic ACTH-secreting tumors in his original description of Cushing's syndrome. The first identified extrapituitary tumor associated with Cushing's syndrome was an oat-cell carcinoma reported by Brown in 1928 (26). Not until the mid 1960s did investigators discover that the plasma and the tumors of these patients contained ACTH-like activity that was similar to that of pituitary ACTH (178, 272). In many patients, electrophoretic analysis of ACTH extracted from an ectopic tumor was identical to the ACTH from a normal human pituitary (334) and the amino acid composition was similar (188), suggesting that the same gene (the POMC gene, now known to be on chromosome 2 in humans) (252) codes for the ACTH in normal corticotrophs and in the extrapituitary tumors. However, in some patients with ectopic ACTH-secreting tumors, the tumor produces ACTH of a larger size than the 39 amino acid ACTH produced by the pituitary gland and by corticotroph adenomas (105). The question of whether the abnormal tumoral ACTH results from differences in splicing from the normal POMC gene, or whether the differences originate from abnormal genomic tumor DNA, is only now being answered.

Although patients with ectopic secretion of ACTH who have occult tumors often present with the typical features of Cushing's syndrome, others harbor malignant and rapidly progressive tumors and the primary symptoms are those of malignancy. ACTH is also occasionally detected in plasma in these patients, but in most instances, it produces no clinical manifestations because it is biologically inactive. "Big ACTH" and other byproducts of POMC may be the predominant moiety of these tumors (161). Many ectopic-ACTH secreting tumors also secrete other hormones, such as gastrin (191, 245), antidiuretic hormone (ADH) (58, 246, 273, 274), serotonin, and calcitonin (246) and thus cause Cushing's syndrome combined with Zollinger-Ellison syndrome or with the syndrome of inappropriate ADH secretion. Tumors in patients with multiple endocrine neoplasia type I may secrete gastrin and ACTH (170); however, a similar combined syndrome may also occur with the ACTH originating from a pituitary adenoma (299).

In most patients with rapidly progressing tumors, the site of the ectopic ACTH-secreting tumors is a malignancy that is obvious and is most commonly, a small cell lung carcinoma (Table 8.4.). In others, however, the origin of the ectopic ACTH production caus-

TABLE 8.4.
Ectopic ACTH-secreting Tumors

Common ectopic ACTH-secreting tumors[a]	
Oat cell carcinoma of the bronchus	50%
Endocrine tumors of the foregut	36%
Bronchial carcinoid	
Thymic carcinoid	
Pancreatic islet-cell carcinoma	
Medullary carcinoma of the thyroid	
Pheochromocytoma	4%
Ovarian tumors	2%
Sources of occult ectopic ACTH-secreting tumors[b, c]	
Bronchial carcinoids	53%
Other carcinoids (thymic, gut)	16%
Islet-cell carcinoma	12%
Medullary carcinoma of the thyroid	4%
Pheochromocytoma	5%
Adrenocarcinoma and miscellaneous carcinomas	9%

[a]Adapted from Loriaux D. L. and Cutler G. B., Jr. Diseases of the adrenal glands. In: *Clinical Endocrinology,* edited by Peter O. Kohler, M.D., pp. 167–238, John Wiley and Sons, Inc., 1986.
[b]Excluding small-cell lung carcinoma and patients with an unknown diagnosis.
[c]Reprinted with permission from Doppman J. L., Nieman L. K. and Miller D. L., *et al.* Ectopic adrenocorticotropic hormone syndrome: localization studies in 28 patients. Radiology, *172:*115–124, 1989.

ing Cushing's syndrome may not be obvious, even with complete clinical, laboratory, and radiologic evaluation, because of the small size of the tumor. In one-third of the reported cases of ectopic ACTH production by medullary thyroid carcinoma, the diagnosis was made only at autopsy (280). The most common tumors with occult ectopic ACTH production are bronchial carcinoids (76, 202). Other ectopic tumors that produce ACTH occultly include pancreatic islet cell tumors (54), ovarian carcinoids (298), medullary carcinoma of the thyroid (280, 315), thymic carcinoids, and parathyroid carcinoma (97). In addition, adrenal pheochromocytomas occasionally secrete ACTH (our reports). This possibility should be recognized because of the potential for misdiagnosis of an adrenal mass as an adrenal adenoma in a hypercortisolemic patient, and the possibility of the sudden onset of malignant hypertension and cardiac arrythmias during surgery on such patients (324). Another potential source of misdiagnosis that may lead to unnecessary thoractomy and thymic exploration, is misdiagnosis of the rebound thymic hyperplasia, which occurs after treatment of hypercortisolism, as a thymic tumor (77).

During administration of dexamethasone in high doses, 3% to 6% of patients with ectopic ACTH syndrome demonstrate suppression of cortisol production in a fashion identical to patients with Cushing's disease (179, 202, 241). These tumors only rarely respond to CRH (50, 51, 233, 234, 235, 241).

Clinical Presentation of Hypercortisolism

Nearly all organ systems are affected by hypercortisolism, but the effects are not similar in all patients (Table 8.5.). Clinical presentation is altered by age, susceptibility to obesity, the presence of diabetes mellitus, and, particularly, by gender. Cushing's syndrome occurs in women many times more frequently than in men. It is often more difficult to detect in men because the signs and symptoms tend to be less intense. Because many of the features of Cushing's syndrome (e.g., muscle weakness, hypertension, diabetes, and obesity) occur separately in patients without hypercortisolism, the early signs of Cushing's syndrome are often overlooked (161). The manifestations of Cushing's syndrome are usually progressive, but some ACTH-secreting tumors (pituitary adenomas and ectopic tumors) have alternating on and off intervals of ACTH secretion for several days, weeks, or months at a time, which produce periods of clinical exacerbation and quiescence (166, 311).

The obesity of Cushing's syndrome is "truncal," with increased fat deposition over the abdomen and the dorsal cervical area and decreased fat in the limbs. Muscle atrophy in the limbs and spinal osteoporosis, in combination with the increased fat, give the "buffalo hump." Patients with less advanced forms of the disease may have simple, generalized obesity instead of the typical redistribution (282). The "moon facies" that these patients acquire is caused by fat deposition in the cheeks and beneath the chin, which rounds out the face. Occasionally, hypertension is the presenting manifestation of Cushing's disease (282). Hypertension occurs because of increased mineralocorticoid activity (239) and is usually mild, but, occasionally, dangerously high pressures are reached (282). Abnormal glucose tolerance is common, but most patients do not have florid diabetes mellitus. The typical proximal muscle weakness of steroid etiology is often present and may be worsened by coexisting hypokalemia from the excess mineralocorticoid activity. Hirsutism, consisting of fine hair over the trunk, face, and arms in these patients must be distinguished from the virilization that suggests the presence of an adrenal carcinoma. Striae are common in Cushing's syndrome and are generally wide and purple. Menstrual irregularity in women and impotence in men (209) occur in at least half of patients with Cushing's syndrome. Mental changes, ranging from minor mood disturbances to severe psychosis, can influence affect and cognition (128, 274). There is a close correlation between the degree of hypercortisolism and the severity of psychiatric impairment (328). Osteoporosis, caused by inhibition of calcium absorption and bone matrix formation by cortisol (216), is sufficiently severe that 25% to 40% of patients have pathological vertebral or rib fractures (282). These patients may also develop renal calculi because of hypercalciuria associated with the calcium loss from bone. Glucocorticoid-induced impairment of the immune system may lead to susceptibility to opportunistic infection (114). Children with Cushing's syndrome generally show a combination of growth arrest and obesity (205, 330), and may also have hypertension and osteoporosis, although the latter complications seldom occur in the pediatric group.

The clinical presentation of hypercortisol-

TABLE 8.5.
Symptoms and Signs of Cushing's Syndrome

Fat distribution	Skin manifestations
centripetal obesity	purple stria
moon facies	plethora
"buffalo hump"	hirsutism
supraclavicular fat pads	acne
Musculoskeletal	bruising
osteoporis, fractures	pigmentation
proximal muscle	Metabolic/circulatory
weakness	hypertension
Pituitary dysfunction	glucose intolerance
menstrual disorder	hypokalemic alkalosis
decreased libido,	Mental Changes
Impotence	irritability
hypothyroidism	psychosis
dwarfism (children)	

ism is often atypical in patients with ectopic production of ACTH. Because the onset of hypercortisolism is often severe and of sudden onset, many of the most common features of the syndrome (obesity and striae) may not have sufficient time to develop (161, 178). Instead, hypokalemic alkalosis, diabetes mellitus, and hypertension are the dominant manifestations. Because of their tendency to have higher ACTH levels, pigmentation occurs much more frequently (178, 294) and cortisol production is higher in patients with the ectopic ACTH syndrome than in patients with Cushing's disease (62, 270, 360).

CLINICAL EVALUATION OF PATIENTS WITH HYPERCORTISOLISM

Correct interpretation of hormonal measurements in patients being evaluated for excess or insufficient cortisol production requires an understanding of the techniques used to make these measurements. Modern assessment of cortisol secretion has been described in recent reviews that, generally, present a consensus of the relative value of the many available tests (40, 187, 189, 247).

Endocrine Tests

Biochemical Measurements

Plasma Adrenocorticotropin Concentration (corticotropin, ACTH). Unfortunately, consistent and reliable radioimmunoassays of ACTH have been more difficult to develop than radioimmunoassays for most other peptide hormones. ACTH is unstable in plasma, with a half-life of 20 minutes (232), and must be protected from degradation by platelet-associated proteases if true values are to be obtained. Such protection is attained by cooling the specimen and by adding protease inhibitors to the sample. Repeated measurements are routinely made for determination of ACTH concentration.

If basal plasma ACTH concentration is elevated, the degree of elevation helps distinguish among the various causes of hypercortisolism (Fig. 8.10.). Very high levels (> 1000 pg/ml) imply ectopic ACTH secretion or Nelson's syndrome. Intermediate levels (> 300 pg/ml) occur in 60% of patients with

ectopic ACTH production, but in only 7% of patients with untreated ACTH-secreting pituitary adenomas, who usually have normal or slightly elevated plasma levels of ACTH. In ectopic ACTH syndrome, other products of POMC, including large forms of ACTH, β-MSH, corticotropin-like intermediate lobe peptide (CLIP), and γ-LPH, also are secreted excessively. The recent development of radioimmunoassays for β-LPH may provide a more stable alternative to ACTH measurement in patients with Cushing's syndrome and help to distinguish among the various etiologies of hypercortisolism (165).

Plasma Cortisol. The pulsatility of its secretion and the small fraction of cortisol in the biologically active, unbound, form limit the usefulness of random measurements of plasma cortisol. Cortisol is secreted episodically (356) and in a diurnal pattern (217, 249) such that plasma levels are highest in the early morning and lowest around midnight. Transcortin and albumin together bind 85-90% of available cortisol, permitting biologically active, free, cortisol to be held relatively constant, whereas the concentration of bound cortisol may vary widely (72). Plasma cortisol is measured by radioimmunoassay. The effects of medications and other drugs may alter the results, and cross-reactivity of the anticortisol antibody with other steroids can occur (285).

The diurnal variation of cortisol and ACTH levels tends to be blunted in hypercortisolism (108), although episodic secretion of ACTH (55, 269, 272, 359) and of cortisol (23, 130, 311, 346, 351, 367) still occurs in Cushing's disease (Fig. 8.12.). Very low plasma cortisol values in the late evening are counter to a diagnosis of Cushing's syndrome, whereas high evening values support the diagnosis. Consistently high-normal plasma cortisol levels in the morning and evening suggest Cushing's syndrome, the diagnosis of which requires confirmation by other tests, including multiple 24-hr collections for indirect analysis of 24-hr cortisol secretion.

Urinary Steroid Excretion. Changes in cortisol secretion are reflected in the urinary excretion of cortisol and in its breakdown products. Cortisol excretion into the urine depends on the concentration of the free, unbound, fraction of cortisol measured in the urine as urinary-free cortisol. Metabolites of cortisol, 17-OHCS, are also commonly measured. Liver disease affects degradation of cortisol and, with hepatic disorders, measurement of 17-OHCS is unreliable. Urinary measurements of 17-OHCS > 10 mg/24 h (> 7 mg/g creatinine excretion) or urinary-free cortisol > 100 μg/24 h indicates hypersecretion of cortisol (329).

Measurement of urinary 17-OHCS is by the Porter-Silber reaction (318), which involves the reaction of phenylhydrazine with the dihydroxyacetone moiety that is present in cortisol and in a number of its metabolites. Thus, urinary 17-hydroxysteroids include urinary-free cortisol and several additional chemical entities. Several confounding factors make this test valuable mainly as a screening test. First, although the 24-hr ex-

cretion of Porter-Silber chromagens (17-hydroxysteroids) correlates with the daily level of cortisol secretion, it measures only about one-third of the total cortisol secreted. Second, several medications artificially influence the values obtained. These include aspirin (which inhibits disconjugation of the steroid, a necessary preliminary step in the reaction), dilantin, and phenobarbital. The anticonvulsants decrease the efficiency of extraction and also are associated with falsely low results (31, 358). Because of the linear association of urinary 17-OHCS secretion with body mass, it is important to standardize the results of the 24-hr urinary 17-OHCS screening test to mg per gram of simultaneous urinary creatinine secretion (Fig. 8.14.).

Ideally, therefore, urinary-free cortisol should be measured. About 10-15% of plasma cortisol is not bound to transport

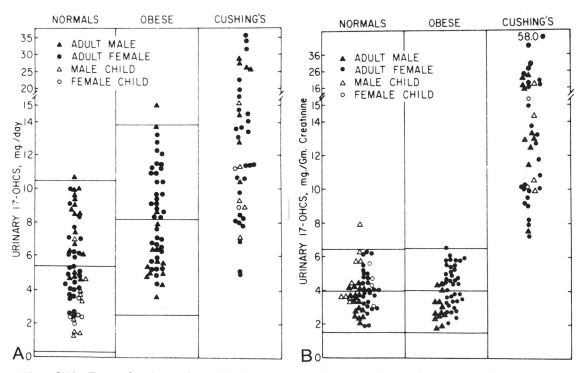

Figure 8.14. Twenty-four hour urinary 17-hydroxycorticosteroid (17-OHCS) excretion as a screening test for the presence of Cushing's syndrome. (**A**) Urinary 17-OHCS excretion expressed in milligrams per day in normal subjects, obese individuals, and patients with Cushing's syndrome. The overlap among the three groups is evident. (**B**) 17-OHCS excretion in the same subjects, but expressed in milligrams per gram of urinary creatinine. The overlap between patients with Cushing's syndrome and the non-Cushing's subjects has almost been eliminated by normalizing the 24-h 17-OHCS excretion per gram of simultaneous 24-h urinary creatinine excretion. (From Streeten D.H.P., Stevenson C.T., Dalakos T.G., *et al.* The diagnosis of hypercortisolism: biochemical criteria differentiating patients from lean and obese normal subjects and from females on oral contraceptives. J. Clin. Endocrinol. Metab., *29:*1191–1121, 1969).

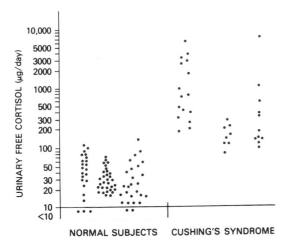

URINARY FREE CORTISOL (µg/day)

10,000
5000
3000
2000
1000
500
300
200
100
50
30
20
10
<10

NORMAL SUBJECTS   CUSHING'S SYNDROME

Figure 8.15. Twenty-four hour excretion of urine-free cortisol to screen patients for Cushing's syndrome. Comparison of 24-h excretion of urine-free cortisol value in normal subjects with that of patients with confirmed Cushing's syndrome. (From Loriaux D.L. and Cutler G.B. Jr. Diseases of the adrenal glands. In: *Clinical Endocrinology,* edited by Peter. O. Kohler, M.D., pp. 167–238, John Wiley and Sons, Inc., 1986).

proteins; it is filtered through the glomerular apparatus of the kidneys and about 2-4% is then excreted in the urine (285). The free cortisol thus produced can be extracted by organic solvents and measured by radioimmunoassay. Urinary-free cortisol measurement is the most reliable test to distinguish normal cortisol production from overproduction. It reflects the biologically active, unbound, component of plasma cortisol. It also shows an amplification effect, since, when saturation of cortisol-binding globulin occurs, even small increases in cortisol secretion produce large increases in urinary-free cortisol. Porter-Silber chromagens may be normal in patients with Cushing's syndrome, whereas the urinary-free cortisol is almost universally elevated (Fig. 8.15.) (83). However, misleading (high) results may occur in patients with depression or alcoholism and low results occur in renal failure, hypothyroidism, or with an incomplete urine collection.

Another group of steroids used to evaluate adrenal metabolism, but which is not useful for evaluating cortisol secretion, is that of the 17-ketosteroids. These are comprised of dehydroepiandrosterone and androstenedione and their byproducts, androsterone and etiocholanolone. Since dehydroepiandrosterone is principally produced by the adrenal glands (131) but androstenedione can also be produced by the gonads (157), 17-ketosteroid measurement reflects production of steroids by adrenal and gonadal tissue. The 17-ketosteroids are measured by the Zimmerman reaction (369), which depends on the presence of a ketone group in the 17 position of the sterol complex. This measurement is used as a screening test for adrenal tumors (342). Low values (<10 mg/24 h) suggest an adrenal adenoma; high values are associated with adrenal carcinoma in two–thirds, ectopic ACTH syndrome in one-sixth, and Cushing's disease in one-sixth of patients.

The 17-ketosteroids should not be confused with the 17-ketogenic steroids (which can be oxidized to the former), which are used principally to monitor therapy in patients with congenital adrenal hyperplasia.

Provocative Tests of the Hypothalamic-Pituitary-Adrenal Axis

The integrity of the hypothalamic-pituitary-adrenal axis requires adequate pituitary and adrenal reserve, both of which can be tested. Provocative testing is used to assess cortisol metabolism for two purposes. First, to establish whether true hypercortisolism is present, and second, if hypercortisolism is present, to determine the etiology of the cortisol excess. Since normal ACTH and cortisol secretion are episodic, with fluctuating values during the day, and are subject to influence by a variety of other factors, the provocative tests are particularly useful for identifying disease of the hypothalamic-pituitary-adrenal axis and have value in the differential diagnosis of hypercortisolism.

Dexamethasone-Suppression Tests. These tests examine the sensitivity of the pituitary and hypothalamus to negative feedback by glucocorticoids. The low-dose dexamethasone-suppression tests are used to confirm that the patient has Cushing's syndrome, whereas the high-dose tests are used to distinguish patients with the pituitary–dependent forms of Cushing's syndrome from those with ectopic ACTH syndrome and primary adrenal disease.

The overnight screening low–dose dexamethasone-suppression test is performed as a screening procedure to detect the presence of Cushing's syndrome. The patient takes 1 mg of dexamethasone at midnight and his plasma cortisol is measured eight hours later. If the hypothalamic–pituitary-adrenal axis is normal, the 8 AM plasma cortisol will be < 5 μg/dl; with Cushing's syndrome it will be > 10 μg/dl (Fig. 8.16.) (238). Values between 5 and 10 μg/dl indicate that retesting is necessary.

A low-dose suppression test and a high-dose suppression test are included as part of the six-day dexamethasone-suppression test, the standard (six-day) dexamethasone-suppression test, developed by Liddle *et al.* in 1960 (175). Basal measurements of 24-hr urinary 17-OHCS are obtained for two days (days one and two). The patient then takes 0.5 mg of dexamethasone by mouth every six hours for 48 hr (the low-dose phase, days three and four). The dexamethasone dose is then increased to 2 mg every six hours for the succeeding 48 hrs (the high-dose phase, days five and six). In normal subjects, the urinary

excretion of 17-OHCS falls to <2.5 mg/day during the second day of the low-dose phase of the test (day four) (175). The low-dose (days three and four) phase of this test is used to confirm the distinction between normal subjects and patients with Cushing's syndrome, who fail to suppress cortisol secretion during this phase of the test (Fig. 8.13.). The high-dose phase (days five and six) is used to separate patients with Cushing's disease from patients with ectopic ACTH syndrome and primary adrenal disease (Figures 8.13, 8.17, 8.18, and 8.20.). In Cushing's disease, urinary excretion of 17-OHCS does not fall during the low-dose phase, but drops to values that are <50% of the mean basal values during the second day of the high-dose phase (day six). On the other hand, with ectopic secretion of ACTH or primary adrenal disease, no suppression of 17-OHCS occurs during the second day of the high-dose phase (day six). The diagnostic accuracy of this test in the differential diagnosis of Cushing's syndrome is about 80% (83, 241).

Although the traditional measurement

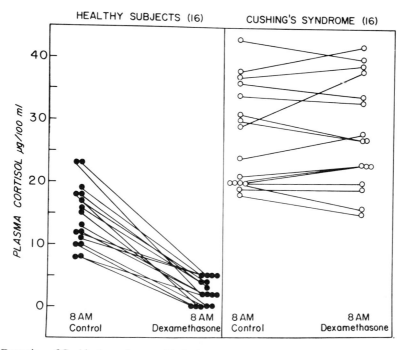

Figure 8.16.   Detection of Cushing's syndrome with the low-dose overnight dexamethasone-suppression test. Plasma cortisol levels at 8 AM on successive days before and after 1 mg dexamethasone given orally at 11:00 PM in healthy subjects and patients with Cushing's syndrome. (From Melby J.C.: Assessment of adrenocortical function. N. Eng. J. Med., *285*:735–739, 1971).

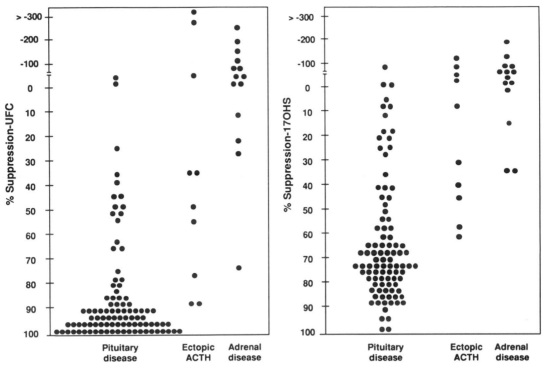

Figure 8.17. Comparison of suppression of urine-free cortisol (UFC) and urinary 17-hydroxycorticosteroid (17-OHCS) excretion during the standard six-day dexamethasone-suppression test in 118 patients with surgically confirmed causes of Cushing's syndrome. (From Flack M.R., Oldfield E.H., Cutler G.B. Jr., *et al.* Urine free cortisol in the high-dose dexamethasone suppression test for the differential diagnosis of the Cushing syndrome. Ann. Int. Med., *116*:211–217, 1992).

with this test is urinary 17-OHCS, many investigators used urine-free cortisol instead of 17-OHCS measurements when measurements of urine-free cortisol became available, but did so without altering the 50% ratio used to define a positive test. Flack *et al.* recently showed that the accuracy of use of urine-free cortisol is similar to that of 17-OHCS only if the degree of suppression used for diagnosing Cushing's disease is greater than the 50% traditionally used for 17-OHCS secretion (Fig. 8.17.) (93). The diagnostic performance of the test is significantly improved by measuring both urine-free cortisol and 17-OHCS and by requiring greater suppression of both steroids. When suppression of urine-free cortisol of > 90% and suppression of 17-OHCS of > 64% were combined as the criteria for a positive test, the percentage of correct predictions rose to 86%, higher

than the results obtained using either test alone (75%) or than the traditional criteria of 50% suppression with 17-OHCS (80%) (93).

The overnight high-dose dexamethasone-suppression test also distinguishes Cushing's disease from adrenal tumors and ectopic ACTH-secreting tumors by suppressing ACTH and cortisol production only in patients with Cushing's disease. Serum cortisol is obtained at 8 AM (basal value). That evening, 8 mg of dexamethasone is taken orally at 11 PM and serum cortisol is drawn at 8 AM the next morning. Suppression of plasma cortisol concentration the morning after dexamethasone to below 50% of the basal value indicates Cushing's disease (Fig. 8.18.). The sensitivity (89%), specificity (100% in the few patients that have been reported), and diagnostic accuracy (91%) compare favorably with the results of the Liddle

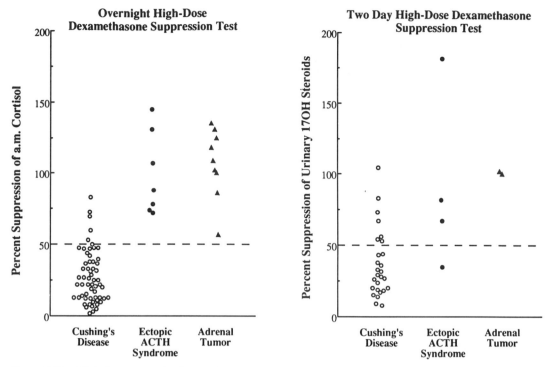

Figure 8.18. High-dose overnight dexamethasone-suppression test for the differential diagnosis of Cushing's syndrome. Comparison of the high-dose overnight dexamethasone-suppression test with the high-dose portion of the standard six-day dexamethasone-suppression test. (Graph created using data from Tyrrell J.B., Findling J.W., Aron D.C., Fitzgerald P.A., Forsham P.H. An overnight high-dose dexamethasone suppression test for rapid differential diagnosis of Cushing's syndrome. Ann. Int. Med., *104:*180–186, 1986.)

test (27, 40, 152, 343). It has not been established whether the ectopic ACTH-secreting tumors that have suppression of ACTH-secreting with high-dose dexamethasone (the bronchial carcinoids) during the Liddle test will suppress, with the same frequency, with 8 mg of dexamethasone overnight. The advantages of the overnight suppression are that it requires less time and cooperation from the patient and, since it can be performed easily on an outpatient basis, it is simple and cost-effective compared to the standard six-day test.

Interpretation. The results of the low-dose screening tests are occasionally misleading. For the overnight single-dose test, 12% to 30% of patients without suppression prove not to have Cushing's syndrome (false-positives), although the incidence of false-negative results, patients with suppression who do have Cushing's syndrome, is less than 3% (60). The false-negative results occur in patients with a slow rate of breakdown of dexa-

methasone (151), which leads to higher plasma dexamethasone levels than are usual, which, in turn, suppress cortisol secretion despite the presence of Cushing's syndrome. Patients who are receiving exogenous estrogens cannot be assessed reliably with the low-dose overnight test, as they have increased levels of cortisol-binding globulin and many false-positive results (238). False-positive results also occur in patients taking dilantin or phenobarbital (149, 215). Dilantin increase metabolism of dexamethasone and, therefore, the patient is not exposed to the usual degree of glucocorticoid suppression. In such patients, dexamethasone levels can be measured or a hydrocortisone suppression test may be used instead (213). Nonetheless, the low-dose overnight suppression test is quite useful because, if AM cortisol levels are suppressed, hypercortisolism can be assumed to be absent in at least 97% of patients.

The physical signs associated with obesity can suggest Cushing's syndrome (i.e., striae, amenorrhea, and hirsutism). Because of the association of urinary 17-OHCS secretion with body mass, as stated above, it is important to standardize the results of the 24-hr urinary 17-OHCS screening test to simulataneous creatinine secretion (Fig. 8.14.). Most obese patients have suppression of cortisol secretion during the low-dose dexamethasone tests. A few suppress only after a more prolonged low-dose dexamethasone administration (2 mg/day for four days).

Most patients in whom the dexamethasone suppression tests are misleading fall into one of the following four categories:

(a) Cushing's disease may be diagnosed falsely in the few patients with adrenal tumors (270) or ectopic ACTH secretion (179, 202, 241) who suppress cortisol secretion during high-dose dexamethasone administration. This occurs in as many as one-third to one-half of the patients with ectopic ACTH secretion by bronchial carcinoid tumors (40, 143, 202, 233, 241). Patients with ectopic ACTH syndrome who have episodic secretion of ACTH (periodic Cushing's syndrome) may also have misleading results if they are having an "off" period of their cyclic ACTH secretion during the test.

(b) As many as 20% of patients with Cushing's disease do not suppress during high-dose dexamethasone administration (35, 40, 119, 143, 233, 241). Since there is a spectrum of sensitivity of ACTH-secreting pituitary adenomas to dexamethasone suppression, the adenoma may be one that is relatively resistant. Some patients with Cushing's disease may show suppression of cortisol secretion only after longer dexamethasone administration, up to four days in some patients, or after higher doses of dexamethasone (16 to 100 mg/d). Patients with Cushing's disease also may have episodic secretion of ACTH, which may produce misleading negative results if their ACTH secretion is low during the basal collection interval (174). As stated previously, patients taking dilantin may also lack dexamethasone suppression during the high-dose tests.

(c) Some patients with Cushing's disease have normal suppression during the low-dose phase of the standard test (39). Some pituitary adenomas are at the sensitive end of the spectrum of pituitary sensitivity to dexa-

methasone. Episodic hormogenesis may provide an explanation in select patients (174), as can impaired dexamethasone catabolism, as described above (39, 155).

(d) Finally, failure of suppression may occur in the overnight low-dose dexamethasone screening test or during the low-dose phase of the standard six-day test in the absence of hypercortisolism and lead to a false diagnosis of Cushing's syndrome. Causes include treatment with dilantin (149), adrenal activation with psychiatric depression, alcoholism, stress, and low pituitary sensitivity to dexamethasone (53).

To reduce the risk of some of these errors, some experts recommend the routine collection of blood for dexamethasone assay when the dexamethasone suppression tests are performed (247). The measurement of dexamethasone eliminates the need for assumptions about its metabolism and the patient's sensitivity to it, and permits a more accurate interpretation of the tests (212).

It has recently been suggested that the accuracy of high-dose dexamethasone suppression may be improved by giving the drug as a continuous infusion (19). The initial results suggest a specificity of 90% and a sensitivity of 100% for Cushing's disease with this technique. Thus, the rate of misdiagnosis with this variant of the test may be lower than the 13% false-positive and 26% false-negative rates of the standard six-day suppression test described above (152).

Corticotrophin-Releasing Hormone Stimulation Test. This provocative test for examining the hypothalamic-pituitary-adrenal axis has only recently become available (51, 234, 134, 246). Synthetic ovine CRH (oCRH) is given intravenously (1 μg/kg) and then blood is drawn at frequent intervals over 90 min for measurement of plasma cortisol and ACTH. After oCRH in normal subjects, plasma ACTH should peak at 15-45 pg/ml and cortisol at 10-25 μg/dl in 15-30 min and 30-60 min, respectively (Fig. 8.19.) (50, 51, 68, 192, 225, 303). Although initially some endocrinologists suggested performing this test in the evening, when basal levels of ACTH and cortisol are lowest (109, 303), the incremental response is similar in the morning (312).

The oCRH test is most useful to distin-

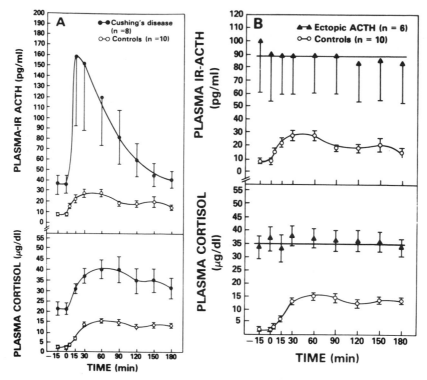

Figure 8.19. CRH-stimulation test for the differential diagnosis of Cushing's syndrome. Plasma ACTH (top) and cortisol (bottom) responses to oCRH in eight untreated patients with Cushing's disease (•), six patients with Cushing's syndrome due to ectopic ACTH secretion (▲), and 10 human controls (○). (From Chrousos G.P., Schulte H.M., Old-field E.H., Gold P.W., Cutler G.B. Jr., Loriaux D.L. The corticotropin-releasing factor stimulation test. An aid in the evaluation of patients with Cushing's syndrome. New Engl. J. Med., *310*:622–626, 1984).

guish between the differential diagnoses of Cushing's disease and ectopic ACTH syndrome (109). In Cushing's disease, plasma ACTH increases by at least 50% or cortisol rises ≥ 20% over basal levels in response to the oCRH bolus (Fig. 8.19.), whereas patients with ectopic ACTH syndrome and patients with adrenal tumors rarely respond to oCRH (Fig. 8.19.) (50, 51, 152, 109, 192, 221, 234, 235, 248, 256). Patients with psychiatric depression usually have a limited response, although the test fails to distinguish Cushing's disease from hypercortisolism associated with psychiatric depression in about 5% to 15% of patients (109) because ACTH-producing pituitary adenomas may have a response to CRH (119), which overlaps the responses that occur in patients with depression.

The criteria used for the definition of a positive test with the oCRH stimulation test

have recently been reexamined by Nieman *et al.,* who conclude that optimal results are achieved by analyzing the ACTH levels at − 5 and 0 min before and 15 and 30 min after oCRH (1 μ/kg body weight) administration. A response is defined as an increase of mean plasma ACTH levels of at least 35% at 15 and 30 min when compared to the mean basal values (− 5 and 0 min). The sensitivity of the oCRH test with this combination was 93% and the specificity was 100% (235).

When the CRH stimulation test is misleading, about 10% to 15% of the time (51, 109, 134, 222, 225, 233, 248, 256), it is usually as a false-negative result (no response to CRH) in a patient with Cushing's disease (Fig. 8.20.). Few patients with ectopic ACTH secretion have a false–positive result (50, 51, 134, 192, 222, 225, 233, 235, 248, 256, 306). The risk of an incorrect diagnosis of Cushing's disease with the oCRH test increases in patients with periodic hypercortisolism and in patients who have recently received pharmacological therapy, such as ketoconazole, metryapone (338), or mitotane, to reduce adrenal cortisol production. Since subjects with ectopic ACTH syndrome very rarely respond to oCRH, the diagnosis of Cushing's disease in patients who are hypercortisolemic during the test and who have a positive oCRH stimulation test is relatively secure (235).

Several groups have compared the relative efficacy of the CRH test and the high-dose dexamethasone suppression tests (Fig. 8.20.) to delineate Cushing's disease from other causes of Cushing's syndrome (93, 134, 233, 234, 235). Although the false-negative rate is 9% with the oCRH test and 11% with high-dose dexamethasone testing, patients with cctopic ACTH syndrome rarely respond to oCRH or suppress during high-dose dexamethasone administration. Either test used alone can be misleading, but all patients with

Cushing's disease have a true-positive result on one of these tests when the two are performed in the same individual (119, 143, 233).

Metyrapone Test. This, like the dexamethasone-suppression tests examines the integrity of the negative feedback system of the hypothalamic-pituitary-adrenal axis (177) and is a sensitive test for measuring the pituitary ACTH reserve. Metyrapone (2-methyl-1,2-*bis*-(3-pyridyl),-1-propanone) blocks the conversion of 11–deoxycortisol, which has minimal glucocorticoid activity, to cortisol (329). This decreases cortisol production, diminishes negative feedback by cortisol, and, thus, stimulates ACTH secretion. Urinary and/or plasma steroids are measured during the test (Fig. 8.21.). With an adequate ACTH reserve, the rise in ACTH causes increased production of 11–deoxycortisol, which cannot be converted to cortisol because of the metyrapone. Measurement of

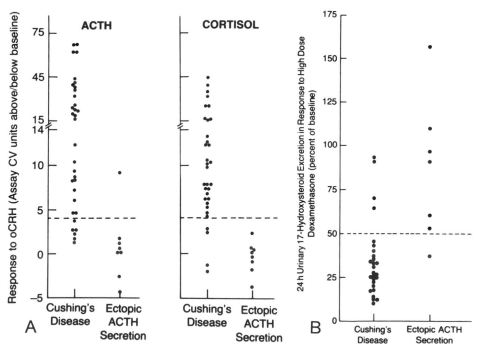

Figure 8.20. A. ACTH and cortisol responses to CRH in patients with Cushing's syndrome. Responses exceeding 4 coefficient of variation (CV) units above baseline values (dotted line) were considered positive. B. Twenty-four hour urinary 17-hydroxysteroid responses to high-dose dexamethasone in patients with Cushing's syndrome. Responses below 50% of the mean baseline level (dotted line) are considered positive. (From Nieman L.K., Chrousos G.P., Oldfield E.H., *et al.* The ovine corticotropin releasing hormone stimulation test and the dexamethasone suppression test in the differential diagnosis of Cushing's syndrome. Ann. Intern. Med., *105*:862–867, 1986).

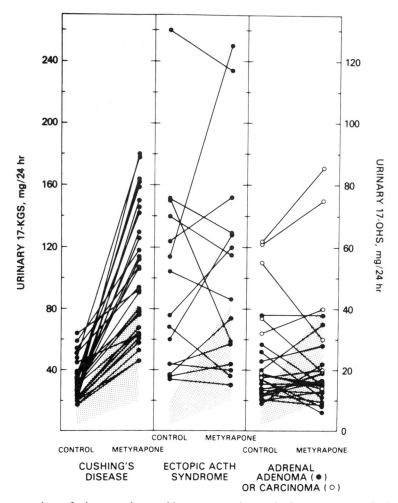

Figure 8.21. A comparison of urinary corticosteroid responses to the standard metyrapone test in Cushing's disease, the ectopic ACTH syndrome, and adrenal neoplasms; 750 mg of metyrapone was given by mouth every 4 h for six doses. The "metyrapone" value represents the highest value obtained during or on the day after the metyrapone was given. The responses shown represent 17-hydroxysteroid excretion in some patients and 17-ketogenic steroid excretion in others. (From Loriaux D.L. and Cutler G.B. Jr. Diseases of the adrenal glands. In: *Clinical Endocrinology,* edited by Peter O. Kohler, M.D., pp. 167–238, John Wiley and Sons, Inc., 1986, with permission.)

urinary 17-OHCS secretion rises because 11–deoxycortisol is as much a chromogen as is cortisol.

The test is performed by obtaining a 24-hr urine collection for 17-OHCS and then giving the patient 750 mg of metyrapone by mouth every 4 hr for 24 hr (329). Urinary 17-OHCS is measured on the day of metyrapone ingestion and on the following day. After metyrapone in normal individuals, urinary 17-OHCS increases by two to three times, compared to basal excretion, particularly on the day after metyrapone administration.

Plasma levels of 11–deoxycortisol, which normally are very low, should rise to 10-30 μg/dl when measured 4 hrs after the last dose of metyrapone (213). Because this test relies on the measurement of Porter-Silber chromogens, estrogen, phenytoin, and thyroid abnormalities may affect the results (149, 214). A single-dose version of this test has also been described, but is less commonly used (326).

Patients with adrenal insufficiency should not undergo metyrapone testing, as it does not differentiate between pituitary and adrenal disorders in patients with hypocortisolism, and because the test may induce an Addisonian crisis in these patients. The test is used to establish the differential diagnosis of Cushing's syndrome (Fig. 8.21.). In Cushing's disease, a normal or supranormal rise in urinary 17-hydroxysteroids occurs after metyrapone administration. Such rises do not occur in patients with ectopic ACTH secretion. Thus, a flat response (or decrease) after metyrapone administration helps to exclude a diagnosis of Cushing's disease.

Anatomic Imaging

Adrenal Gland

CT scanning allows noninvasive study of the adrenal glands and is a great improvement over older procedures, such as presacral pneumography (323) and adrenal venography (218), used to assess adrenal anatomy. It is now possible to diagnose virtually 100% of adrenal tumors with CT or MRI (Fig. 8.22.) (80, 321). If multiple thin slices are obtained, nodules as small as 3-5 mm can be de-

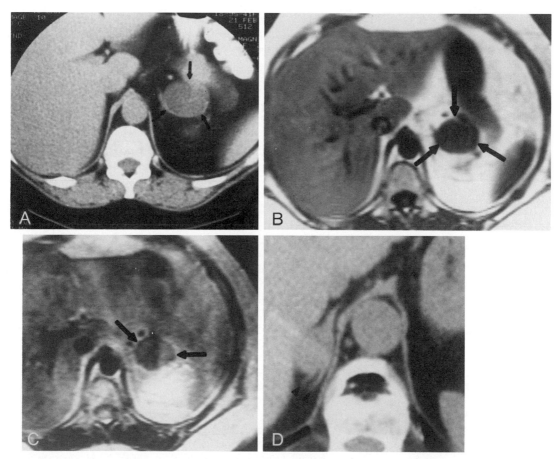

Figure 8.22. **A-C.** CT scan (A) and MRI (B and C) of an adenoma in the left adrenal gland of a patient with Cushing's syndrome. On the T1-weighted image (B) the adenoma is well visualized and has less signal intensity (darker) than the liver. Note on the T2-weighted image (C) the adenoma (arrows) retains its low signal intensity, similar to the liver. Malignant adrenal cortical tumors and metastases generally have increased signal intensity on T2-weighted images. **D.** CT scan of adenoma in right adrenal gland in patient with ACTH-independent Cushing's syndrome. Note the normal medial and lateral limbs (arrowheads) of the adrenal gland, evidence of lack of ACTH stimulation. (From Doppmann J.L., Miller D.L., Dwyer A.J., *et al.* Macronodular adrenal hyperplasia in Cushing disease. Radiology, *166:*347–352, 1988, with permission. Images are courtesy of John Doppmann.)

tected. Because of the safety and ease of establishing such diagnoses, adrenal CT is used early in the evaluation of patients with Cushing's syndrome (75, 78, 80, 316).

However, interpretation of adrenal imaging requires experience. Bilateral adrenal enlargement on CT scanning suggests hypersecretion of ACTH. In some patients, it can be difficult to distinguish adrenal hyperplasia from normal adrenal tissue by CT, but the presence of two normally shaped crescentic glands of normal size favors the latter possibility. In hypercortisolism, demonstration by CT or magnetic resonance imaging (MRI) of a unilateral adrenal mass, combined with very low levels of plasma ACTH, confirms the presence of an adrenal tumor (40, 75, 78, 79, 80). Diffuse nodular hyperplasia of the adrenal cortex can be incorrectly diagnosed in ACTH-dependent Cushing's syndrome if a unilateral dominant nodule exists on a background of diffuse hyperplasia. Furthermore, with diffuse primary micronodular disease and minimal change in the adrenal contour, the diagnosis can be overlooked. The distinction of adenoma from carcinoma is imperfect with CT and MRI, although MRI often distinguishes the malignant tumors (78, 106, 145, 275). Nonetheless, adrenal masses > 5 cm in diameter are much more likely to be malignant than smaller tumors. Adrenal hyperplasia or neoplasia can also arise in ectopic adrenal rests, but these are generally in the vicinity of the adrenal glands and can be detected by CT as well (45).

Abdominal ultrasound is also useful in some patients, although it does not have the accuracy of CT scanning (290). Because of its low sensitivity, excretory urography is no longer routinely used to assess suspected adrenal tumors. In the few patients in whom the provocative tests suggest adrenal tumors, but which CT and MRI do not reveal, adrenal arteriography or venography, with measurement of venous cortisol levels may be of value (82).

Scintigraphic studies with ^{131}I-labeled cholesterol derivatives are also helpful in localizing primary adrenal lesions. Such investigations have a threshold of detection of lesions that are at least 2 cm in maximum diameter. They are used to identify ectopic adrenal tissue, distinguish bilateral nodular hyperplasia from an adrenal adenoma (which suppresses the contralateral gland) (90), and localize remnants of adrenal tissue left behind after adrenalectomy in patients with persistent postoperative hypercortisolism. For these specific purposes, it has a higher yield than CT. This procedure can also be used to distinguish adrenal cortical carcinomas, in which hormone production and cholesterol utilization is relatively inefficient, from adrenal adenomas.

Masses within one or both adrenal glands are seen on abdominal CT in 1% to 10% of patients without signs or symptoms of endocrine disease. Most of these patients have normal pituitary–adrenal function and the incidental lesions are nonfunctioning. However, they merit assessment with serial CT or MRI or with scintigraphy. Needle biopsy may be warranted in certain instances (1, 57).

Pituitary

Skull x-rays, polytomography, and CT scanning have been superseded by MRI for pituitary imaging. Contrast-enhanced CT scans of the sella using recent-generation machines show the tumor directly or indirectly in only about 60% of patients with Cushing's disease (195, 198, 262, 293). The smaller the adenoma, the less likely it is to be detected with CT or MRI—and lesions less than 5 mm in diameter are often not detected with either technique. On contrast–enhanced CT scans, microadenomas generally have a density that is lower than that of the normal gland. When an adenoma is isodense with the pituitary gland, indirect signs, including such anatomic details as stalk deviation, unilateral superior convex shape of the superior surface of the gland, and sloping of the sella floor, have been used to suggest the side of the tumor. However, the indirect signs that have been used to indicate the presence of an adenoma with CT and MRI occur frequently in normal subjects. Those who have examined this issue in detail believe that such variations as stalk deviation and sloping of the sellar floor are minimally useful for determining the presence or location of pituitary microadenomas (201, 254, 336). Because ACTH-secreting adenomas are the smallest of the functioning pituitary tumors (mean diameter $\leq$ 5mm) (195), in Cushing's disease, the adenomas are less frequently detected than those that secrete prolactin or growth hormone (198–200).

MRI is more sensitive for detecting anatomical distortion than CT and also gives valuable information about water content and vascular flow that is useful to detect small tumors, define their extent, and plan their removal. Unenhanced MRI is better than enhanced CT for determining the extrasellar extent of the tumor, but it is no more effective than CT for the evaluation of intrasellar disease (229). On unenhanced MRI, pituitary tumors are indicated by a focal area of hypointense signal compared to the pituitary on short TR/TE (T_1-weighted) images. On long TR/TE (T_2-weighted) images, the adenoma pattern is variable with a mix of iso-, hypo-, and hyperintense signal (164). For this reason, T_2-weighted images are used only if a suspected adenoma is not seen on the standard, T_1-weighted, images.

Improvements in field strength and the introduction of gadolinium as a contrast agent have greatly improved the diagnostic sensitivity and accuracy of sellar MRI and have made it the investigation of choice in patients suspected of having pituitary adenomas (74, 228, 254). Infusion of gadolinium immediately enhances normal pituitary tissue. Because the relatively avascular microadenoma will not be enhanced for two to three minutes, for optimal detection of small pituitary tumors with MRI, scanning should be performed within 2 to 3 min of gadolinium injection (Fig. 8.23.). With proper scanning protocols, the sensitivity of MRI in Cushing's disease has been reported to reach 70-80%, and similar levels of specificity are obtained (75, 82, 254). Even with gadolinium, however, the sensitivity for determining cavernous sinus invasion by tumor is poor (254, 309). Furthermore, adenomas detected by CT or MRI may not be the source of the excess ACTH. Areas of low density within the sella may represent a cyst or artifact rather than a tumor, and about 12-27% of normal pituitary glands at autopsy contain incidental adenomas (30, 47, 253). With recent improvements in imaging, more such inciden-

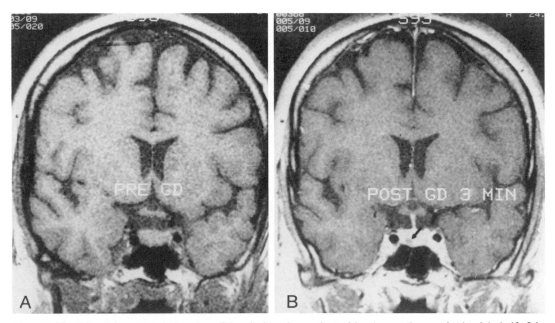

Figure 8.23. Magnetic resonance imaging of the pituitary in a patient with a 4-mm adenoma in the right half of the anterior lobe. These images were acquired before (**A**) and immediately after (**B**) infusion of gadolinium-DTPA (T1-weighted MRI, TR 500, TE 20). (From Doppman J.L., Frank J.A., Dwyer A.J., *et al.* Gadolinium DTPA enhanced imaging of ACTH-secreting microadenomas of the pituitary gland. Correlation of MR appearance with surgical findings. J. Comput. Assist. Tomogr., *12*:728–735, 1988).

tal adenomas will be detected. Thus, radiographic testing cannot be used in isolation, but must be interpreted with the results of the endocrine tests.

Anatomic Localization of Hormonal Secretion

Bilateral Simultaneous Inferior Petrosal Sinus Sampling

The most recent addition to the tests to localize ACTH secretion in Cushing's syndrome is simultaneous bilateral inferior petrosal sinus sampling (171, 196, 206, 240, 241, 322, 333). This test has the potential of providing two functions. It has been demonstrated to have utility for the differential diagnosis of Cushing's disease and ectopic ACTH syndrome and is being investigated to determine its role in the preoperative localization of pituitary microadenomas.

Differential Diagnosis of Cushing's Syndrome. The small, but significant, rate of false-positive and false-negative results

with the dexamethasone-suppression test, and the incidence of false-negative results with the CRH-stimulation test indicate that a test with higher diagnostic accuracy would be desirable. The short plasma half-life of ACTH in the peripheral blood permits an ACTH concentration gradient to be maintained between the pituitary venous drainage and the peripheral blood when ACTH is being secreted from the pituitary. Bilateral simultaneous inferior petrosal sinus (IPS) sampling successfully distinguishes patients with Cushing's disease from those with ectopic ACTH secretion with greater accuracy than any of the other tests (92, 240, 241, 302, 333).

Venous catheterization of both inferior petrosal sinuses is accomplished through a percutaneous bilateral femoral vein approach (Fig. 8.24.). After systemic heparinization both femoral veins are catheterized. Then, blood is slowly withdrawn simultaneously from both catheters and a peripheral vein for ACTH measurement. After two sets of basal

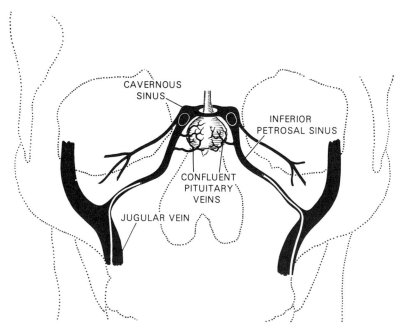

Figure 8.24. Anatomy and catheter placement in bilateral simultaneous blood sampling of the inferior petrosal sinuses. Confluent pituitary veins empty laterally into the cavernous sinuses, which drain into the inferior petrosal sinuses. (From Oldfield E.H., Chrousos G.P., Schulte H.M., *et al.* Preoperative lateralization of ACTH-secreting microadenomas by bilateral and simultaneous inferior petrosal sinus sampling. New Engl. J. Med., *312:*100–103, 1985, with permission.)

samples are obtained, CRH 1 μg/kg, is infused into a peripheral vein over one minute and samples are obtained simultaneously from both inferior petrosal sinuses and a peripheral vein at 2-3 and 5 min after injecting the CRH. Retrograde venograms, separately through each IPS catheter, are performed at the conclusion of blood sampling to document filling of the ipsilateral cavernous sinus from each catheter. The entire procedure usually requires 25-60 min.

The ACTH values are expressed as a ratio equal to the greater concentration of ACTH in the right or left IPS sample, divided by the simultaneous concentration in the peripheral blood (ACTH IPS:P). Representative data sets for patients with Cushing's disease and ectopic ACTH secretion are shown in Table 8.6.

In the typical patient with Cushing's disease, the ACTH level from one of the IPSs is greater than two-fold higher than the concurrent ACTH level in the peripheral blood in the basal samples (Fig. 8.25, Table 8.6). In contrast, patients with ectopic ACTH secretion, as in the patient with an ACTH-secreting bronchial carcinoid shown in Table 8.5, have suppression of ACTH secretion from the normal corticotrophs and therefore have no ACTH concentration gradient from the central to the peripheral samples.

In the largest series of patients in whom this procedure has been performed, 96% of 212 patients with Cushing's disease had a ratio of IPS ACTH levels to the simultaneous peripheral ACTH levels of > 2.0 in at least one of the two basal sets, whereas all 20 patients with ectopic ACTH secretion had a maximum ACTH IPS:P ratio of < 2.0 (Fig. 8.25).

CRH Stimulation during Bilateral Simultaneous Inferior Petrosal Sinus Sampling. With the peripheral CRH-stimulation test, diagnostic errors are almost all false-negative results in patients with Cushing's disease when no cortisol or ACTH response to CRH is detected in the peripheral blood. Very few patients with the ectopic ACTH syndrome have elevation of peripheral ACTH or cortisol concentrations. Because most misleading results with the peripheral CRH-stimulation test in Cushing's syndrome occur in patients

TABLE 8.6.
Representative Patients with Bilateral Simultaneous Inferior Petrosal Sinus (IPS) Sampling[a]

	A. Cushing's Disease						B. Ectopic ACTH Syndrome					
	ACTH (pg/ml)			Greater IPS:P[c] Ratio	Lesser IPS:P Ratio	ACTH gradient Between IPSs		ACTH (pg/ml)			Greater IPS:P Ratio	Lesser IPS:P Ratio
Time	R[b] IPS	L[c] IPS	Peripheral				Time	R IPS	L IPS	Peripheral		
Basal 1	81	24	23	3.5	1.0	3.4 to R	Basal 1	54	50	35	1.5	1.4
Basal 2	76	28	21	3.6	1.3	2.7 to R	Basal 2	59	57	45	1.3	1.3
			CRH,[d] 1 ug/kg IV							CRH, 1 μg/kg IV		
2–3 min	5,790	100	35	165.4	2.9	57.9 to R	2–3 min	57	56	49	1.2	1.2
5 min	3,680	122	77	30.2	1.6	30.2 to R	5 min	64	58	51	1.3	1.1
10 min	3,170	143	115	27.6	4.2	22.2 to R	10 min	59	53	42	1.4	1.3

Maximum basal IPS:P ACTH ratio, 3.6
Peak IPS:P ACTH ratio, 165.4
Maximum IPS:P ACTH ratio from side with lesser ratio, 4.2
Peak IPS ACTH concentration, 5790 pg/ml
Peak ACTH gradient between the IPSs:basal, 3.4 to R; after CRH, 57.9 to R.

Maximum basal IPS:P ACTH ratio, 1.5
Peak IPS:P ACTH ratio, 1.5
Maximum IPS:P ratio from side with lesser ratio, 1.4
Peak IPS ACTH concentration, 64 pg/ml

[a]Results typical of those for patients with Cushing's disease(A) and ectopic ACTH secretion(B). A. In many patients with Cushing's disease, the ACTH concentration from one IPS is higher than the concurrent ACTH level in the peripheral blood, but the ACTH level in the other IPS is not significantly different from that in peripheral blood. After CRH, the ACTH concentration from one IPS promptly increases and the response is greatest in the early samples after CRH. Simultaneous ACTH levels in the IPSs are higher on the same side as a 3 mm microadenoma found at transsphenoidal surgery. B. In patients with ectopic ACTH syndrome, the ACTH concentrations from both IPSs are less than 1.7-fold greater than those in the peripheral blood, both before and after CRH injection.
[b]R, right; [c]
L, left.[c]IPS:P, ratio of ACTH concentration in IPS to simultaneous ACTH concentration in peripheral blood (P).
[d]CRH, corticotropin-releasing hormone.

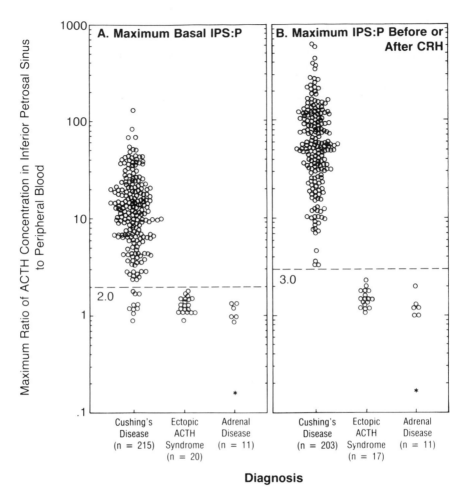

Figure 8.25.   Bilateral inferior petrosal vein sampling in the differential diagnosis of Cushing's syndrome. Maximum ratio of ACTH concentration from one of the inferior petrosal sinuses to the simultaneous peripheral venous ACTH concentration in patients with Cushing's syndrome **(A)** in basal samples and **(B)** in basal and CRH-stimulated samples. **A.** During basal sampling, the maximum IPS:P ACTH ratio was ≥ 2.0 in 205 of 215 patients with confirmed Cushing's disease, but was < 2.0 in all patients with ectopic ACTH syndrome or primary adrenal disease. **B.** All patients with Cushing's disease who received CRH had maximum IPS:P ACTH ratios of ≥ 3.0, whereas all patients with ectopic ACTH syndrome had IPS:P ratios of < 3.0. The asterisks represent five patients with primary adrenal disease in whom ACTH was undetectable in the peripheral blood before and after CRH administration. (From Oldfield E.H., Doppman J.L., Nieman L.K., *et al.* Bilateral inferior petrosal sinus sampling with and without corticotropin-releasing hormone for the differential diagnosis of Cushing's syndrome. N. Eng. J. Med., *325*:897–905, 1991).

with Cushing's disease who have false-negative results, a more sensitive method of detecting an ACTH response, such as selective catheterization of the venous drainage of the pituitary, should reduce the number of false-negative results with CRH stimulation. The administration of CRH during bilateral IPS sampling has been reported to increase the diagnostic accuracy of the test to 100% by eliciting an ACTH response in the few patients with Cushing's disease who did not have a diagnostic IPS:P gradient in the basal samples. In the NIH series, the patients who received CRH had a peak ACTH IPS:P of $>$ 3.0 in all 200 patients with Cushing's disease, whereas ACTH IPS:P was < 3.0 in all 17 patients with ectopic ACTH syndrome (Fig. 8.25.).

The absolute concentrations of ACTH in the inferior petrosal sinuses is also helpful in interpreting the IPS:P ratios. In Cushing's disease, the IPS:P ratios increase as IPS ACTH concentration increases. In contrast, in ectopic ACTH syndrome, the ACTH IPS:P ratios remain close to one regardless of the IPS ACTH concentration. Thus, the higher the IPS ACTH concentration, the greater is the separation between the ACTH IPS:P ratios of patients with Cushing's disease and patients with ectopic ACTH syndrome. Hence, even without CRH administration, the diagnostic accuracy of IPS sampling attains 100% when the basal IPS ACTH level is > 125 pg/ml (Fig. 8.26.).

For IPS sampling results to be reliable, the patient has to be hypercortisolemic at the time of the procedure and for the preceding three to four weeks. This is true both for the basal samples and for the CRH-stimulated samples, as the response of the normal corticotrophs to CRH must be suppressed. Suppression of ACTH secretion from the normal corticotrophs by the hypercortisolism present in the ectopic ACTH syndrome is responsible for the absence of a central-to-peripheral ACTH gradient. Thus, in patients who have received adrenalectomy or medical therapy—such as metyrapone, ketoconazole, or mitotane, to normalize cortisol production—in patients with intermittent Cushing's syndrome, in patients with ectopic CRH secretion, or in patients with pseudo-Cushing's syndrome—in whom hypercortisolism is caused by excess CRH secretion—

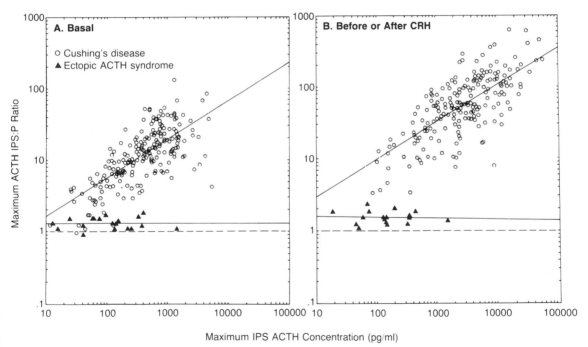

Figure 8.26. Bilateral inferior petrosal vein sampling in the differential diagnosis of Cushing's syndrome. Correlation of IPS:P ACTH ratios in relation to maximum petrosal vein ACTH levels in patients with Cushing's syndrome. **A.** The maximum basal ACTH IPS:P ratios correlated positively with the highest basal IPS ACTH level in patients with Cushing's disease, but not in those with ectopic ACTH secretion. All 171 patients with a maximum basal IPS ACTH level of > 125 pg/ml had IPS:P ACTH ratios of at least 2.9. **B.** In patients with Cushing's syndrome who received CRH, there was a linear relation between the peak ACTH concentration in the inferior petrosal sinuses and the maximum IPS:P ratio that was reached during sampling in Cushing's disease, but there was no such relation in the patients with ectopic ACTH syndrome. All 187 patients with Cushing's disease who had IPS ACTH levels ≥ 440 pg/ml had IPS:P ACTH ratios of ≥ 7.4, whereas none of the patients with ectopic ACTH syndrome had a maximum IPS:P ACTH ratio of > 2.3. (From Oldfield E.H., Doppman J.L., Nieman L.K., *et al.* Bilateral inferior petrosal sinus sampling with and without corticotropin-releasing hormone for the differential diagnosis of Cushing's syndrome. N. Eng. J. Med., *325*:897–905, 1991).

IPS sampling may show a central-to-peripheral gradient that could be misinterpreted as indicating a pituitary adenoma (241). Similar findings would likely occur in normal subjects if IPS sampling were performed.

Bilateral simultaneous IPS sampling is highly effective in distinguishing hypercortisolemic patients who have Cushing's disease from hypercortisolemic patients who have ectopic ACTH syndrome. However, it cannot be relied upon in any circumstance in which the normal corticotroph cells would be expected to be active, such as ectopic CRH syndrome or after medical or surgical normalization of cortisol levels.

Lateralization of Pituitary Microadenomas. The lateral origin of most microadenomas in Cushing's disease (196, 241) and the laterality of the venous drainage from the cavernous sinus (240) suggest the possibility of lateralization of microadenomas with venous sampling. In addition to its diagnostic utility, the results of bilateral IPS sampling can be used for predicting lateralization of pituitary microadenomas preoperatively. Although lateralization (defined as an ACTH gradient ≥ 1.4 between the IPSs) is not always correct (it is about 70% correct with microadenomas found at surgery), if no adenoma can be identified intraoperatively, excision of the half of the anterior lobe on the side with the higher ACTH level can be expected to provide remission of hypercortisolism in most patients (240, 241).

DIAGNOSTIC APPROACH FOR EVALUATION OF PATIENTS SUSPECTED TO HAVE CUSHING'S SYNDROME

The evaluation of the patient with hypercortisolism follows a logical sequence (Table 8.7) that, if applied correctly, usually separates patients who are appropriate for neurosurgical treatment from those needing other forms of therapy. Before initiating the evaluation however, patients who present with the symptoms of Cushing's syndrome should be questioned closely to exclude ingestion of exogenous glucocorticoids as the etiology. They should also be asked about the use of topical steroids, which may occasionally be absorbed in sufficient quantities to

TABLE 8.7.
Diagnostic Approach to Patients Suspected of Having Cushing's Syndrome

I. Establish presence of Cushing's syndrome
  A. Establish presence of hypercortisolism
    1. Plasma cortisol at 6–8 AM and 11 PM–1 AM
    2. 24-hour urine-free cortisol
    3. 24-hour urine 17-hydroxycorticosteroids/gm of urinary creatinine
  B. Establish resistance to dexamethasone suppression
    1. Overnight low-dose (1 mg) dexamethasone-suppression test
II. Differential diagnosis of Cushing's syndrome
  A. Plasma ACTH to distinguish ACTH-independent from ACTH-dependent forms of Cushing's syndrome
  B. If plasma ACTH levels indicate ACTH-independent Cushing's syndrome → adrenal disease
  1. Adrenal CT or MRI
  C. If plasma ACTH levels indicate ACTH-dependent Cushing's syndrome
    1. CRH stimulation test
    2. High-dose dexamethasone-suppression test
      a. Overnight high-dose (8 mg)
      b. Standard six-day low-dose, high-dose test (Liddle test)
    3. Anatomic confirmation of diagnosis
      1. If endocrine tests indicate Cushing's disease → pituitary MRI
      2. If endocrine tests indicate ectopic ACTH secretion → MRI of chest and abdomen
    4. Bilateral petrosal vein sampling for ACTH (with and without CRH stimulation) **if**:
      a) results of CRH test and dexamethasone-suppression test are discordant, **or**
      b) radiographic imaging is negative, **or**
      c) radiographic imaging results differ from results of CRH and dexamethasone-suppression test.

cause their symptoms and signs of hypercortisolism.

Establish the Presence of Hypercortisolism

If the history does not indicate iatrogenic or fictitious sources of Cushing's syndrome, the level of cortisol excretion must be evaluated to provide laboratory evidence for increased secretion of cortisol and, thus, to confirm or refute any clinical suggestions of a Cushing's syndrome. For this, 24-hr urine collections for urinary-free cortisol, 17-OHCS, and creatinine, and a low-dose overnight dexamethasone-suppression test are performed. Most patients without hypercortisolism will be excluded by these tests. However, about 10% of those with abnormal results in the outpatient screening tests prove not to have Cushing's syndrome with more detailed evaluation. Because psychiatric depression (42) and alcoholism (156, 169) are occasionally associated with excess cortisol production, false-positive results indicating Cushing's syndrome may occur in these patients.

Patients with Cushing's syndrome and intermittent hypercortisolism may have normal screening tests if they are studied during an interval in which hypersecretion of cortisol is not occurring. Intermittent Cushing's syndrome occurs with adrenal adenomas (115), ectopic production of ACTH (46), and ACTH-secreting pituitary adenomas (7, 25). When the clinical findings suggest Cushing's syndrome but the laboratory findings do not, the possibility of intermittent hypersecretion must be considered and the urinary-free cortisol should be repeatedly measured over longer periods of time.

If the clinical signs are equivocal and the laboratory findings are inconclusive, an immediate diagnosis may not be possible. These patients should be followed and re-evaluated after three to six months. In patients with only mild abnormalities in the screening tests and borderline clinical evidence of Cushing's syndrome, the possibility of pseudo-Cushing's syndrome and adrenal cortical activation by alcoholism or depression should be considered. Such patients may be separated from those with true Cushing's syndrome by the finding of physical evidence of Cushing's syndrome on the physical examination, which rarely occurs with depression, or by abnormal liver function tests, which occur universally in patients with pseudo-Cushing's syndrome associated with alcoholism (247), or by performing an insulin-tolerance test, which is almost always abnormal with Cushing's syndrome.

Establish Differential Diagnosis of Cushing's Syndrome

Patients with excess cortisol secretion in the outpatient testing should be hospitalized for further, detailed evaluation. This testing is done to confirm the presence of hypercortisolism and to determine its etiology. The insulin-tolerance test is performed if it is deemed necessary for the reasons cited above. Collection of urine over a 24-hr period for the measurement of urinary-free cortisol, 17-hydroxysteroids, and creatinine confirms hypercortisolism. Plasma cortisol and ACTH are measured with 6–8 AM and 11 PM–1 AM collections. These blood and urine measurements are performed on at least two successive days. While these data are collected, the sella turcica and adrenal glands are scanned with CT and/or MRI to provide anatomic evidence of the presence of a lesion. One each of the low-dose and high-dose dexamethasone-suppression tests are performed. If the plasma ACTH levels are low, there is no suppression of urinary 17-OHCS with high-dose dexamethasone suppression, and adrenal imaging reveals an adrenal tumor the diagnosis is established. With careful planning, preliminary inpatient evaluation can be completed in a week. At this point, most patients with adrenal tumors, and patients with an obvious source of ACTH-dependent hypercortisolism will have had the diagnosis of Cushing's syndrome confirmed and the etiology established.

Adrenal tumors present few diagnostic difficulties. When excess cortisol is produced by an adrenal tumor, plasma ACTH levels are usually undetectable or very low. The complete autonomy of cortisol secretion by the tumor results in failure of suppression during high-dose dexamethasone testing. Furthermore, the neoplasm is usually obvious with adrenal CT. Nonetheless, the subtleties of interpretation of CT and MRI of the adrenal must not be overlooked. Exceptions to these expectations occur with diffuse primary micronodular adrenal disease, in which adrenal CT is normal; adrenal neoplasms, which suppress with dexamethasone and which are rare; and ACTH-secreting pheochromocytomas, which resemble adrenal adenomas on dexamethasone suppression testing and radiological imaging, but which secrete ACTH rather than cortisol and, thus, cause hypertrophy, rather than atrophy, of the opposite adrenal cortex.

If the hypercortisolism is ACTH-dependent, it is important to identify the source of the excess ACTH before undertaking therapy. Most patients with Cushing's disease have normal (or slightly elevated) plasma ACTH levels, fail to suppress with low-dose dexamethasone-suppression tests, but suppress with the high-dose dexamethasone-suppression tests. Bilateral adrenal enlargement may be present on CT scans, and a gadolinium-enhanced MRI scan shows a pituitary lesion in more than half of the patients. A CRH-stimulation test can be used instead of the high-dose dexamethasone-suppression test. An ACTH response occurs in 95% of patients with Cushing's disease. In patients with negative pituitary MRI, patients with conflicting results of the CRH tests and the high–dose dexamethasone-suppression tests, and patients in whom the results of the endocrine tests and the imaging tests are in conflict, bilateral simultaneous sampling from the inferior petrosal veins with central and peripheral measurement of ACTH can confirm the presence of a pituitary microadenoma if radiological studies are unrevealing. Although there is some overlap in the biochemical profile of patients with pituitary and extrapituitary hypersecretion of ACTH, CRH-stimulation testing and petrosal sinus sampling will generally obviate the need to pursue the possibility of an ectopic tumor mimicking Cushing's disease.

In patients with ectopic secretion of ACTH, the radiological appearance of the adrenal glands is similar to that seen in Cushing's disease, imaging of the pituitary shows no tumor, and plasma ACTH levels have a wider range than in Cushing's disease, tending to be higher (often more than 300 pg/ml), although many patients have normal values. If patients with bronchial carcinoids are excluded, a high-dose dexamethasone-suppression test fails to suppress cortisol secretion in the great majority of patients. On the other hand, about one-third to one-half of bronchial carcinoids will suppress in the same manner as patients with an ACTH-secreting pituitary tumor. When the diagnosis of ectopic ACTH secretion is suspected, a CT of the chest and abdomen, and, if negative, an MRI, should be obtained to look for a neoplasm (76), and urinary catecholamines should be measured to screen for pheochromocytoma. If the MRI and CT are negative, selective arteriography, portal venous sampling, and scintigraphy reveal the site of a tumor so infrequently that they are not useful (76). On clinical grounds alone, patients with ectopic ACTH secretion can be identified in many instances by the systemic effects of the tumor and by the presence of a hypokalemic alkalosis, which is uncommon in Cushing's disease.

Metyrapone testing is useful when other inpatient investigations fail to clearly distinguish between ectopic and pituitary sources of ACTH hypersecretion. When urinary 17-OHCS do not respond, or decrease, after metyrapone, the patient is almost certain not to have Cushing's disease. Patients with a supranormal response are almost sure *not* to have an adrenal tumor. Although patients with ACTH-secreting pituitary adenomas usually have a response that is equal to, or slightly greater than, the response of normal subjects, similar responses occasionally occur with the ectopic ACTH syndrome. The metyrapone test is useful only as a supplementary test and can only be interpreted in conjunction with the results of the other dynamic tests.

The results of endocrine testing in the rare patient with Cushing's syndrome due to an ectopic CRH-secreting tumor indicate Cushing's disease. In fact, this diagnosis is often made only after pituitary surgery indicates diffuse corticotroph hyperplasia. Measurement of elevated plasma CRH levels in a patient with an extrapituitary tumor, but endocrine testing that indicates Cushing's disease, should provide the correct diagnosis in these patients (36).

It is critical to establish the presence of Cushing's syndrome before proceeding with the differential diagnostic portion of the endocrine evaluation described above. Since, in normal subjects, ACTH secretion from the pituitary is suppressed by dexamethasone, responds to CRH and metyrapone, and the concentration of ACTH is greater in the inferior petrosal sinuses than in peripheral blood, the results of these endocrine tests will suggest, erroneously, Cushing's disease, which could potentially result in pituitary surgery in a normal subject.

Summary. Complete evaluation of patients suspected of having hypercortisolism can be time-consuming and complex. If, however, a few simple questions are addressed in logical sequence, in most patients the diagnosis can be elucidated in a straightforward manner. Are the symptoms those of cortisol excess? If so, iatrogenic causes are excluded and the cortisol excess is biochemically quantified, initially by outpatient studies. If hypercortisolism is present, static and dynamic tests of hormonal function are performed on an inpatient basis to classify the problem as either pituitary hypersecretion of ACTH, ectopic hypersecretion of ACTH, or adrenal hypersecretion of cortisol. Imaging with CT or MRI, if positive, confirms the location of the lesion, although normal form does not exclude abnormal function in the hypothalamic-pituitary-adrenal axis. Only with biochemical and/or anatomic evidence of the site of the lesion should surgery be performed. Successful management of patients with hypercortisolism requires cooperation between endocrinologist, radiologist, and surgeon if curative treatment is to be achieved with consistency.

REFERENCES

1. Abecassis M., McLoughlin M., Langer B., and Kudlow J.E. Serendipitous adrenal masses: prevalence, significance, and management. Am. J. Surg., *149:*783–788, 1985.
2. Addison T. On the Constitutional and Local Effects of Disease of the Supra-renal Capsules, edited by Samuel Highley, London, 1855.
3. Allen J.P., Allen C.F. Role of the amygdaloid complexes in the stress-induced release of ACTH in the rat. Neuroendocrinology, *15:*220–230, 1974.
4. Andreis P.G., Neri G., Belloni A.S., Mazzocchi G., Kasprzak A., Nussdorfer G.G. Interleukin-1β enhances corticosterone secretion by acting directly on the rat adrenal gland. Endocrinology, *129:*53–57, 1991.
5. Aron D.C., Findling J.W., Fitzgerald P.A., *et al.* Pituitary ACTH dependency of nodular adrenal hyperplasia in Cushing's syndrome. Report of two cases and review of the literature. Am. J. Med., *71:*302–306, 1981.
6. Arteaga E., Biglieri E.G., Kater C.E., Lopez J.M., Schambelan M. Aldosterone-producing adrenocortical carcinoma. Preoperative recognition and courses in three cases. Ann. Int. Med., *101:*316–321, 1984.
7. Atkinson A.B., Chestnutt A., Crothers E., *et al.* Cyclical Cushing's disease. Two distinct rhythms in a patient with a basophil adenoma. J. Clin. Endocrinol. Metab., *60:*328–332, 1985.
8. Autelitano D.J., Lundblad J.R., Blum M., Roberts J.L. Hormonal regulation of POMC gene expression. Ann. Rev. Physiol., *51:*715–726, 1989.
9. Avgerinos P.C., Chrousos G.P., Nieman L.K., Oldfield E.H., Loriaux D.L., Cutler G.B. Jr. The corticotropin-releasing hormone test in the postoperative evaluation of patients with Cushing's syndrome. J. Clin. Endocrinol. Metab., *65:*906–913, 1987.
10. Avgerinos P.C., Nieman L.K., Oldfield E.H., *et al.* The effect of pulsatile human corticotropin-releasing hormone administration on the adrenal insufficiency that follows cure of Cushing's disease. J. Clin. Endocrinol. Metab., *68:*912–916, 1989.
11. Baker B.L. Functional cytology of the hypophysial pars distalis and pars intermedia. In: *Handbook of Physiology,* Section 7, Endocrinology. Vol IV. The Pituitary Gland and its Neuroendocrine Control, part 1, edited by R.O. Greep and E.B. Atwood, pp. 45–80, Washington, D.C., American Physiological Society, 1974.
12. Bateman A., Singh A., Kral T., Solomon S. The immune-hypothalamic-pituitary-adrenal axis. Endocr. Rev., *10:*92–112, 1989.
13. Baxter J.D. Glucocorticoid hormone action. Pharmacol. Ther., *2:*605–659, 1976.
14. Baxter J.D., Forsham P.H. Tissue effects of glucocorticoids. Am. J. Med., *53:*573–589, 1972.
15. Berg K.K., Scheithauer B.W., Felix I., *et al.* Pituitary adenomas that produce adrenocorticotropic hormone and α-subunit: Clinicopathological, immunohistochemical, ultrastructural, and immunoelectron microscopic studies in nine cases. Neurosurgery, *26:*397–403, 1990.
16. Berlinger F.G., Ruder H.L., Wilber J.F. Cushing's syndrome associated with galactorrhea, amenorrhea, and hypothyroidism. A primary hypothalamic disorder. J. Clin. Endocrinol. Metab., *45:*1205–1210, 1977.
17. Bertagna C., Orth D.N. Clinical and laboratory findings and results of therapy in 58 patients with adrenocortical tumors admitted to a single medical center (1951 to 1978). Am. J. Med., *71:*855–875, 1981.
18. Besser G.M., Edwards C.R.W. Cushing's syndrome. Clinics Endocrinol. Metab., *1:*451–490, 1972.
19. Biemond P., deJong F.H., Lamberts S.W.J. Continuous dexamethasone infusion for seven hours in patients with the Cushing's syndrome. Ann. Int. Med., *112:*738–742, 1990.
20. Bilezikjian L.M., Vale W. Glucocorticoids inhibit corticotropin-releasing factor-induced production of cyclic adenosine 3′,5′-monophosphate in cultured anterior pituitary cells. Endocrinology, *113:*657–662, 1983.
21. Birnberg N.C., Lissitzky J.C., Hinman M., Herbert. Glucocorticoids regulate proopiomelanocortin gene expression *in vivo* at the levels of transcription and secretion. Proc. Nat. Acad. Sci., *80:*6982–6986, 1983.
22. Black P.Mc.L., Hsu D.W., Klibanski A., *et al.* Hormone production in clinically nonfunctioning pituitary adenomas. J. Neurosurg., *66:*244–250, 1987.

23. Boyar R.M., Witkin A., Carruth A., Ramsey J. Circadian cortisol secretory rhythms in Cushing's disease. J. Clin. Endocrinol. Metab., *48:*760–765, 1979.

24. Brown J.D., Doe R.P. Pituitary pigmentary hormones. Relationship of melanocyte-stimulating hormone to lipotropic hormone. J.A.M.A., *240:*1273–1278, 1978.

25. Brown R.D., van Loon G.R., Orth D.N., Liddle G.W. Cushing's disease with periodic hormonogenesis. One explanation for paradoxical response to dexamethasone. J. Clin. Endocrinol. Metab., *36:*445–451, 1973.

26. Brown W.H. A case of pluriglandular syndrome. Diabetes in bearded women. Lancet, *2:*1022–1023, 1928.

27. Bruno O.D., Rossi M.A., Conteras L.N., *et al.* Nocturnal high dose dexamethasone suppression test in the aetiological diagnosis of Cushing's syndrome. Acta Endocrinol. (Copenh.), *109:*158–162, 1985.

28. Burch W.M., Kramer R.S., Kenan P.D., Hammond C.B. Cushing's disease caused by an ectopic pituitary adenoma within the sphenoid sinus. New Engl. J. Med., *312:*587–588, 1985.

29. Burke C.W., Adams C.B., Esiri M.M., Morris C., Bevan J.S. Transsphenoidal surgery for Cushing's disease: does what is removed determine the endocrine outcome? Clin. Endocrinol. (Oxf.), *33:*525–537, 1990.

30. Burrow G.N., Wortzman G., Rewcastle N.B., Holgate R.C., Kovacs K. Microadenomas of the pituitary and abnormal sellar tomograms in an unselected autopsy series. New Engl. J. Med., *304:*156–158, 1981.

31. Burstein S., Klaiber E.L. Phenobarbital-induced increase in 6-hydroxycortisol excretion. Clue to its significance in human urine. J. Clin. Endocrinol. Metab., *25:*293–296, 1965.

32. Cahill G.F. Jr. Action of adrenal corticol steroids on carbohydrate metabolism. In: *The Human Adrenal Cortex.* edited by N.P. Christy, pp. 205–239, New York, Harper and Row, 1971.

33. Calogero A., Kamilaris T.C., Gomez M.T., *et al.* The muscarinic cholinergic agonist arecoline stimulates the rat hypothalamic-pituitary-adrenal axis through a centrally-mediated corticotropin-releasing hormone-dependent mechanism. Endocrinology, *125:*2445–2553, 1990.

34. Campbell E.A., Altaher A.R.H., Scraggs P.R., Gilham B., Jones M.T. Effect of GABA transaminase inhibitors on the hypothalamo-pituitary-adrenal axis in the rat. Neuroendocrine. Perspectives, *5:*303–307, 1986.

35. Carey R.M. Suppression of ACTH by cortisol in dexamethasone-nonsuppressible Cushing's disease. New Engl. J. Med., *302:*275–279, 1980.

36. Carey R.M., Varma S.K., Drake C.R. Jr., *et al.* Ectopic secretion of corticotropin-releasing factor as a cause of Cushing's syndrome. A clinical, morphological and biochemical study. New Engl. J. Med., *311:*13–20, 1984.

37. Carlson D.E., Dornhorst A., Gann D.S. Organization of the lateral hypothalamus for control of adrenocorticotropin release in the cat. Endocrinology, *107:*961–969, 1980.

38. Carnes M., Lent S.J., Goodman B., Mueller C., Saydoff J., Erisman S. Effects of immunoneutralization of corticotropin-releasing hormone on ultradian rhythms of plasma adrenocorticotropin. Endocrinology, *126:*1904–1913, 1990.

39. Caro J.F., Meikle A.W., Check J.H., Cohen S.N. "Normal suppression" to dexamethasone in Cushing's disease. An expression of decreased metabolic clearance for dexamethasone. J. Clin. Endocrinol. Metab., *47:*667–670, 1978.

40. Carpenter P.C. Cushing's syndrome. An update of diagnosis and management. Mayo Clin. Proc., *61:*49–58, 1986.

41. Carroll B.J. The dexamethasone suppression test for melancholia. Br. J. Psychiatry, *140:*292–304, 1982.

42. Carroll B.J., Curtis G.C., Mendels J. Neuroendocrine regulation in depression. I. Limbic system-adrenocortical dysfunction. Arch. Gen. Psych., *33:*1039–1044, 1976.

43. Carroll B.J., Feinberg M., Greden J.R., *et al.* A specific laboratory test for the diagnosis of melancholia. Standardization, validation, and clinical utility. Arch. Gen. Psych., *38:*15–22, 1981.

44. Casson I.F., Walker B.A., Hipkin L.J., Davis J.C., Buxton P.H., Jeffreys R.V. An intrasellar pituitary tumor producing metastases in liver, bone and lymph glands and demonstration of ACTH in the metastatic deposits. Acta Endocrinol. (Copenh.), *111:*300–304, 1986.

45. Chaffee W.R., Moses A.M., Lloyd D.W., Rogers L.S. Cushing's syndrome with accessory adrenocortical tissue. J.A.M.A., *186:*799–801, 1963.

46. Chajek T., Romanoff H. Cushing syndrome with cyclic edema and periodic secretion of corticosteroids. Arch. Int. Med., *136:*441–443, 1976.

47. Chambers E.F., Turski P.A., LaMasters D., Newton T.H. Regions of low density in the contrast-enhanced pituitary gland. Normal and pathological processes. Radiology, *144:*109–113, 1982.

48. Chandler W.F., Schteingart D.E., Lloyd R.V., McKeever P.E., Ibarra-Perez G. Surgical treatment of Cushing's disease. J. Neurosurg., *66:*204–212, 1987.

49. Chernow B., Alexander R., Smallridge R., *et al.* Hormonal responses to graded surgical stress. Arch. Int. Med., *147:*1273–1278, 1987.

50. Chrousos G.P., Schuermeyer T.H., Doppman J.L., Oldfield E.H., Schulte H.M., Gold P.W., Loriaux D.L. Clinical applications of corticotropin-releasing factor. Ann. Intern. Med., *102:*344–358, 1985.

51. Chrousos G.P., Schulte H.M., Oldfield E.H., Gold P.W., Cutler G.B. Jr., Loriaux D.L. The corticotropin-releasing factor stimulation test. An aid in the evaluation of patients with Cushing's syndrome. New Engl. J. Med., *310:*622–626, 1984.

52. Chrousos G.P., Schulte H.M., Oldfield E.H., Loriaux D.L., Cutler G.B. Jr., Gold P.W. Corticotropin-releasing factor: basic and clinical studies. Psychopharm. Bull., *19:*416–421, 1983.

53. Chrousos G.P., Vingerhoeds A., Brandon D., *et al.*

Primary cortisol resistance in man. A glucocorticoid receptor-mediated disease. J. Clin. Invest., 69:1261–1269, 1982.

54. Clark E.S., Carney J.A. Pancreatic islet cell tumor associated with Cushing's syndrome. Am. J. Surg. Pathol., 8:917–924, 1984.
55. Cook D.M., Kendall J.W., Allen J.P., Lagerquist L.G. Nyctohemeral variation and suppressibility of plasma ACTH in various stages of Cushing's disease. Clin. Endocrinol. (Oxf.), 5:303–312, 1976.
56. Cooper C.E., Nelson D.H. ACTH levels in plasma in preoperative and surgically stressed patients. J. Clin. Invest., 41:1599–1605, 1962.
57. Copeland P.M. The incidentally discovered adrenal mass. Ann. Int. Med., 98:940–945, 1983.
58. Coscia M., Brown R.D., Miller M., et al. Ectopic production of antidiuretic hormone (ADH), adrenocorticotropic hormone (ACTH) and beta-melanocyte stimulating hormone (β-MSH) by an oat cell carcinoma of the lung. Am. J. Med., 62:303–307, 1977.
59. Crispell K.R., Parson W., Hamlin J., Hollifield G. Addison's disease associated with histoplasmosis. Report of four cases and review of the literature. Am. J. Med., 20:23–29, 1956.
60. Cronin C., Igoe D., Duffy M.J., Cunningham S.K., McKenna T.J. The overnight dexamethasone test is a worthwhile procedure. Clin. Endocrinol. (Oxf.), 33:27–33, 1990.
61. Croughs R.J.M., Kopperschaar H.P.F., van't Verlaat J.W., McNicol A.M. Bromocriptine-responsive Cushing's disease associated with anterior pituitary corticotroph hyperplasia or normal pituitary gland. J. Clin. Endocrinol. Metab., 68:495–498, 1989.
62. Croughs R.J.M., Tops C.F., DeJong F.H. Radioimmunoassay of plasma adrenocorticotrophin in Cushing's syndrome. J. Endocrinol., 59:439–449, 1973.
63. Cushing H. The Pituitary Body and its Disorders. Philadelphia, J.B. Lippincott Co., 1912.
64. Cushing H. The basophil adenomas of the pituitary body and their clinical manifestations (pituitary basophilism). Bull. Johns Hopkins Hosp., 50:137–195, 1932.
65. Cushman P. Jr. Hypothalamic-pituitary-adrenal function in thyroid disorders. Effects of methopyrapone infusion on plasma corticosteroids. Metabolism, 17:263–270, 1968.
66. Danowski T.S., Bonessi J.V., Sabek G., Sutton R.D., Webster M.W. Jr., Sarver M.E. Probabilities of pituitary-adrenal responsiveness after steroid therapy. Ann. Int. Med., 61:11–26, 1964.
67. Dave J.R., Eiden L.E., Eskay R.L. Corticotropin-releasing factor binding to peripheral tissue and activation of the adenylate cyclase-adenosine 3',5'-monophosphate system. Endocrinology, 116:2152–2159, 1985.
68. DeBold C.R., DeCherney G.S., Jackson R.V., et al. Effect of synthetic ovine corticotropin-releasing factor: prolonged duration of action and biphasic response of plasma adrenocorticotropin and cortisol. J. Clin. Endocrinol. Metab., 57:294–298, 1983.
69. DeBold C.R., Sheldon W.R., DeCherney G.S., et al. Arginine vasopressin potentiates adrenocorticotropin release induced by ovine corticotropin-releasing factor. J. Clin. Invest., 73:533–538, 1984.
70. Didolkar M.S., Bescher R.A., Elias E.G., Moore R.H. Natural history of adrenal cortical carcinoma. A clinicopathologic study of 42 patients. Cancer, 47:2153–2161, 1981.
71. Dobrakovová M., Kvetnansky R., Torda T., Murgas K. Changes of plasma and adrenal catecholamines and corticosterone in stressed rats with septal lesions. Physiol. Behav., 29:41–45, 1982.
72. Doe R.P., Zinneman H.H., Flink E.B., Ulstrom R.A. Significance of the concentration of nonprotein bound plasma cortisol in normal subjects, Cushing's syndrome, pregnancy and during estrogen therapy. J. Clin. Endocrinol. Metab., 20:1484–1492, 1960.
73. Donald R.A. Plasma immunoreactive corticotrophin and cortisol response to insulin hypoglycemia in normal subjects and patients with pituitary disease. J. Clin. Endocrinol. Metab., 32:225–231, 1971.
74. Doppman J.L., Frank J.A., Dwyer A.J., et al. Gadolinium DTPA enhanced imaging of ACTH-secreting microadenomas of the pituitary gland. Correlation of MR appearance with surgical findings. J. Comput. Assist. Tomogr., 12:728–735, 1988.
75. Doppman J.L., Miller D.L., Dwyer A.J., et al. Macronodular adrenal hyperplasia in Cushing disease. Radiology, 166:347–352, 1988.
76. Doppman J.L., Nieman L.K., Miller D.L., et al. Ectopic adrenocorticotropic hormone syndrome: localization studies in 28 patients. Radiology, 172:115–124, 1989.
77. Doppman J.L., Oldfield E.H., Chrousos G.P., Cutler G.B. Jr., Loriaux D.L. Rebound thymic hyperplasia after treatment of Cushing's syndrome. A.J.R., 147:1145–1147, 1986.
78. Doppman J.L., Reinig J.W., Dwyer A.J., et al. Differentiation of adrenal masses by magnetic resonance imaging. Surgery, 102:1018–1026, 1987.
79. Doppman J.L., Travis W.D., Nieman L., et al. Cushing's syndrome due to pigmented nodular adrenocortical disease: findings at CT and MR imaging. Radiology, 172:415–424, 1989.
80. Dunnick N.R., Schaner E.G., Doppman J.L., Strott C.A., Gill J.R. Jr., Javadpour N. Computed tomography in adrenal tumors. AJR, 132:43–46, 1979.
81. Dunnick N.R., Doppman J.L., Gill J.R. Jr., Strott C.A., Keiser H.R., Brennan M.F. Localization of functional adrenal tumors by computed tomography and venous sampling. Radiology, 142:429–433, 1982.
82. Dwyer A.J., Frank J.A., Doppman J.L., et al. Pituitary adenomas in patients with Cushing's disease: initial experience with Gd-DTPA-enhanced MR imaging. Radiology, 163:421–426, 1987.
83. Eddy R.L., Jones A.L., Gilliland P.F., Ibarra J.D. Jr., Thompson J.Q., McMurry J.F. Jr. Cushing's syndrome: a prospective study of diagnostic methods. Am. J. Med., 55:621–630, 1973.

84. Ellis M.J., Schmidli R.S., Donald R.A., Livesey J.H., Espiner E.A. Plasma corticotrophin-releasing factor and vasopressin responses to hypoglycaemia in normal man. Clin. Endocrinol. (Oxf.), *32:*93–100, 1990.

85. Estep H.L., Island D.P., Ney R.L., Liddle G.W. Pituitary-adrenal dynamics during surgical stress. J. Clin. Endocrinol. Metab., *23:*419–425, 1963.

86. Estour B., Pugeat M., Land F., *et al.* Rapid escape of cortisol from suppression in response to i.v. dexamethasone in anorexia nervosa. Clin. Endocrinol. (Oxf.), *33:*45–52, 1990.

87. Fehm H.L., Klein E., Holl R., Voight K.H. Evidence for extrapituitary mechanisms mediating the morning peak of plasma cortisol in man. J. Clin. Endocrinol. Metab., *58:*410–414, 1984.

88. Feldman S. Neural pathways mediating adrenocortical responses. Fed. Proc., *44:*169–175, 1985.

89. Felix I., Asa S.L., Kovacs K., Horvath E. Changes in hormone production of a recurrent silent corticotroph adenoma of the pituitary: A histologic, immunohistochemical, ultrastructural, and tissue culture study. Hum. Pathol., *22:*719–721, 1991.

90. Fig L.M., Gross M.D., Shapiro B., *et al.* Adrenal localization in the adrenocorticotropic hormone-independent Cushing's syndrome. Ann. Int. Med., *109:*547–553, 1988.

91. Findling J.W., Kehoe M.E., Shaker J.L., Raff. Routine inferior petrosal sinus sampling in the differential diagnosis of adrenocorticotropin (ACTH)-dependent Cushing's syndrome: early recognition of the occult ectopic ACTH syndrome. J. Clin. Endocrinol. Metab., *73:*408–413, 1991.

92. Fitzgerald P.A., Aron D.C., Findling J.W., *et al.* Cushing's disease: transient secondary adrenal insufficiency after selective removal of pituitary microadenomas; evidence for a pituitary origin. J. Clin. Endocrinol. Metab., *54:*413–422, 1982.

93. Flack M.R., Oldfield E.H., Cutler G.B. Jr., *et al.* Urine free cortisol in the high-dose dexamethasone suppression test for the differential diagnosis of the Cushing's syndrome. Ann. Int. Med., *116:*211–217, 1992.

94. Forbus W.D., Bestebreurtje A.M. Coccidiomycosis. A study of 95 cases of the disseminated type with special reference to the pathogenesis of the disease. Military Surg., *99:*653–719, 1946.

95. Fortier C., Selye H. Adrenocorticotrophic effect of stress after severance of the hypothalamo-hypophyseal pathways. Am. J. Physiol., *159:*433–439, 1949.

96. Franks R.C. Diurnal variation of plasma 17-hydroxycorticosteroids in children. J. Clin. Endocrinol. Metab., *27:*75–78, 1967.

97. Friedman M., Marshall-Jones P., Ross E.J. Cushing's syndrome. Adrenocortical hyperactivity secondary to neoplasm arising outside the pituitary-adrenal system. Q. J. Med., *35:*193–214, 1966.

98. Fuller R.W. Serotonin receptors and neuroendocrine responses. Neuropsychopharmacology, *3:*495–502, 1990.

99. Fuxe K., Wikstrol A.C., Okret S., *et al.* Mapping of glucocorticoid receptor immunoreactive neurons in the rat tel- and diencephalon using a monoclonal antibody against rat liver glucocorticoid receptor. Endocrinology, *117:*1803–1812, 1985.

100. Gabrilove J.L., Seman A.T., Sabet R., Mitty H.A., Nicolis G.L. Virilizing adrenal adenoma with studies on the steroid content of the adrenal venous effluent and review of the literature. Endocr. Rev., *2:*462–470, 1981.

101. Gabrilove J.L., Sharma D.C., Wotiz H.H., Dorfman R.I. Feminizing adrenocortical tumors in the male. A review of 52 cases including a case report. Medicine (Baltimore), *44:*37–79, 1965.

102. Gallagher T.F., Hellman L., Finkelstein J., *et al.* Hyperthyroidism and cortisol secretion in man. J. Clin. Endocrinol. Metab., *34:*919–927, 1972.

103. Gallagher T.F., Yoshida K., Roffwarg H.D., Fukushima D.K., Weitzman E.D., Hellman L. ACTH and cortisol secretory patterns in man. J. Clin. Endocrinol. Metab., *36:*1058–1073, 1973.

104. Gann D.S., Bereiter D.A., Carlson D.E., Thrivikamen D.V. Neural interaction in control of adrenocorticotropin. Fed. Proc., *44:*161–168, 1985.

105. Gerwicz G., Yalow R.S. Ectopic ACTH production in carcinoma of the lung. J. Clin. Invest., *53:*1022–1032, 1974.

106. Glazer G.M., Woolsey E.J., Borrello J., *et al.* Adrenal tissue characterization using MR imaging. Radiology, *158:*73–79, 1986.

107. Glasgow B.J., Steinsapir K.D., Anders K., Layfield L.J. Adrenal pathology in the acquired immunodeficiency syndrome. Am. J. Clin. Pathol., *84:*594–597, 1985.

108. Glass A.R., Zavadil A.P. III, Halberg F., Cornelissen G., Schaaf M. Circadian rhythm of serum cortisol in Cushing's disease. J. Clin. Endocrinol. Metab., *59:*161–165, 1984.

109. Gold P.W., Loriaux L.D., Roy A., *et al.* Responses to corticotropin-releasing hormone in the hypercortisolism of depression and Cushing's disease. Pathophysiologic and diagnostic implications. New Engl. J. Med., *314:*1329–1335, 1986.

110. Goodwin R.A. Jr., Shapiro J.L., Thurman G.H., Thurman S.S., Des Prez R.M. Disseminated histoplasmosis: Clinical and pathological correlations. Medicine (Baltimore), *59:*1–33, 1980.

111. Gorczyca W., Hardy J. Microadenomas of the human pituitary and their vascularization. Neurosurgery, *22:*1–6, 1988.

112. Gordon D., Semple C.G., Beastall G.H., Thomson J.A. A study of hypothalamic-pituitary-adrenal axis suppression following curative surgery for Cushing's syndrome due to adrenal adenoma. Acta Endocrinol. (Copenh.), *114:*166–170, 1987.

113. Graber A.L., Ney R.L., Nicholson W.E., Island D.P., Liddle G.W. Natural history of pituitary-adrenal recovery following long-term suppression with corticosteroids. J. Clin. Endocrinol. Metab., *25:*11–16, 1965.

114. Graham B.S., Tucker W.S. Jr. Opportunistic infections in endogenous Cushing's syndrome. Ann. Int. Med. *101:*334–338, 1984.

115. Green J.R.B., van't Hoff W. Cushing's syndrome with fluctuation due to adrenal adenoma. J. Clin. Endocrinol. Metab., *41:*235–240, 1975.

116. Greene L.W., Cole W., Greene J.B., *et al.* Adrenal

insufficiency as a complication of the acquired immunodeficiency syndrome. Ann. Int. Med., *101:*497–499, 1984.

117. Greenwood F.C., Landon J., Stamp T.C.B. The plasma sugar, free fatty acid, cortisol and growth hormone response to insulin. I. In control subjects. J. Clin. Invest., *45:*429–436, 1966.

118. Greep R.O., Atwood E.B., Blaschko H., Sayers G., Smith A.D., eds. Handbook of Physiology. Section 7. Endocrinology. Vol VI. Adrenal Gland. Washington, D.C., American Physiological Society, 135–270, 1975.

119. Grossman A.B., Howlett T.A., Perry L., *et al.* CRF in the differential diagnosis of Cushing's syndrome: a comparison with the dexamethasone suppression test. Clin. Endocrinol. (Oxf.), *19:*167–178, 1988.

120. Guillemin R., Rosenberg B. Humoral hypothalamic control of anterior pituitary: a study with combined tissue cultures. Endocrinology, *57:*599–607, 1955.

121. Gustafsson J-Å., Carlstedt-Duke J., Poellinger L., *et al.* Biochemistry, molecular biology, and physiology of the glucocorticoid receptor. Endocr. Rev., *8:*185–234, 1987.

122. Gwosdow A.R., Kumar M.S.A., Bode N.H. Interleukin 1 stimulation of the hypothalamic-pituitary-adrenal axis. Am. J. Physiol., *258:*E65–E70, 1990.

123. Haas D.A., Sturtridge W.C., George S.R. Differential alpha-1 and alpha-2 adrenergic effects on hypothalamic corticotropin-releasing factor and plasma adrenocorticotropin. Neuroscience, *38:*693–701, 1990.

124. Hale A.C., Coates P.J., Doniach I., *et al.* A bromocriptine-responsive corticotroph adenoma secreting α-MSH in a patient with Cushing's disease. Clin. Endocrinol. (Oxf.), *28:*215–233, 1988.

125. Halmi N.S., Moriarty G.C. The cells of origin of ACTH in man. Ann. N.Y. Acad. Sci., *297:*167–181, 1977.

126. Hardy J. Cushing's disease: 50 years later. Can. J. Neurol. Sci., *4:*375–380, 1982.

127. Harris M.J., Baker R.T., McRoberts J.W., Mohler J.L. The adrenal response to trauma, operation and cosyntropin stimulation. Surg. Gynecol. Obstet., *170:*513–516, 1990.

128. Haskett R. Diagnostic categorization of psychiatric disturbance in Cushing's syndrome. Am. J. Psychiatry, *142:*911–916, 1985.

129. Heinbecker P. The pathogenesis of Cushing's disease. Medicine (Baltimore), *23:*225–247, 1944.

130. Hellman L., Weitzman E.D., Roffwarg H., Fukushima D.K., Yoshida K., Gallagher T.F. Cortisol is secreted episodically in Cushing's syndrome. J. Clin. Endocrinol. Metab., *30:*686–689, 1970.

131. Hemsell D.L., Edman C.D., Marks J.F., Siiteri P.K., MacDonald P.C. Massive extraglandular aromatization of plasma androstenedione resulting in feminization of a prepubertal boy. J. Clin. Invest., *60:*455–464, 1977.

132. Herman J.P., Schäfer M.K.-H., Young E.A., *et al.* Evidence for hippocampal regulation of neuroendocrine neurons of the hypothalamo-pituitary-ad-

renocortical axis. J. Neurosci., *9:*3072–3082, 1989.

133. Herman J.P., Wiegand S.J., Watson S.J. Regulation of basal corticotropin-releasing hormone and arginine vasopressin messenger ribonucleic expression in the paraventricular nucleus: Effects of selective hypothalamic deafferentation. Endocrinology, *127:*2408–2417, 1990.

134. Hermus A.R., Pieters G.F., Pesman G.J., Smals A.G., Benraad T.J., Kloppenborg P.W. The corticotropin-releasing hormone test versus the high dose dexamethasone test in the differential diagnosis of Cushing's syndrome. Lancet, *2:*540–544, 1986.

135. Hermus A.R., Pieters G.F.F.M., Smals A.G.H., Benraad T.J., Kloppenborg P.W.C. Plasma adrenocorticotropin, cortisol, and aldosterone responses to corticotropin-releasing factor: modulatory effect of basal cortisol levels. J. Clin. Endocrinol. Metab., *58:*187–191, 1984.

136. Higuchi T., Takahashi Y., Takahashi K., Niimi Y., Miyasita A. Twenty-four-hour secretory patterns of growth hormone, prolactin, and cortisol in narcolepsy. J. Clin. Endocrinol. Metab., *49:*197–204, 1979.

137. Hillman D.A., Giroud C.J.P. Plasma cortisone and cortisol levels at birth and during the neonatal period. J. Clin. Endocrinol. Metab., *25:*243–248, 1965.

138. Hilton C.W., Harrington P.T., Prasad C., Svec F. Adrenal insufficiency in the acquired immunodeficiency syndrome. South Med. J., *81:*1493–1495, 1988.

139. Hodge B.O., Froesch T.A. Familial Cushing's syndrome. Micronodular adrenocortical dysplasia. Arch. Int. Med., *148:*1133–1136, 1988.

140. Horrocks P.M., Jones A.F., Ratcliffe W.A., *et al.* Patterns of ACTH pulsatility over twenty-four hours in normal males and females. Clin. Endocrinol. (Oxf.), *32:*127–134, 1990.

141. Horvath E., Kovacs K., Killinger D.W., Smyth H.S., Platts M.Z., Singer W. Silent corticotropic adenomas of the human pituitary gland. A histologic, immunocytologic, and ultrastructural study. Am. J. Pathol., *98:*617–638, 1980.

142. Hotta M.N., Shibasaki T., Suda T., Ling N., Shizume K. The use of the corticotropin-releasing hormone test to monitor the recovery of patients with Cushing's disease or Cushing's syndrome due to an adrenal adenoma after adenectomy. Endocrinol. Jpn., *32:*113–125, 1985.

143. Howlett T.A., Drury P.L., Perry L., Doniach I., Rees L.H., Besser G.M. Diagnosis and management of ACTH-dependent Cushing's syndrome: comparison of the features in ectopic and pituitary ACTH production. Clin. Endocrinol. (Oxf.), *24:*699–713, 1986.

144. Huminer D., Garty M., Lapidot M., Leiba S., Borohov H., Rosenfeld J.B. Lymphoma presenting with adrenal insufficiency. Adrenal enlargement on computed tomographic scanning as a clue to the diagnosis. Am. J. Med., *84:*169–172, 1988.

145. Hussain S., Belldegrun A., Seltzer S.E., Richie J.P., Gittes R.F., Adams H.L. Differentiation of malig-

nant from benign adrenal masses: Predictive indices on computed tomography. A.J.R., *144*:61–65, 1985.

146. Iranmadesh A., Lizarralde G., Johnson M.L., Veldhuis J.D. Dynamics of 24-hour endogenous cortisol secretion and clearance in primary hypothyroidism assessed before and after partial thyroid hormone replacement. J. Clin. Endocrinol. Metab., *70*:155–161, 1990.

147. Irvine W.J., Stewart A.G., Scarth L. A clinical and immunological study of adrenocortical insufficiency (Addison's disease). Clin. Exp. Immunol., *2*:31–70, 1967.

148. Jones M.T., Gillham B. Factors involved in the regulation of adrenocorticotropic hormone/β-lipotropic hormone. Physiol. Rev., *68*:743–818, 1988.

149. Jubiz W., Levinson R.A., Meikle A.W., West C.D., Tyler F.H. Absorption and conjugation of metyrapone during diphenylhydantoin therapy: mechanism of the abnormal response to oral metyrapone. Endocrinology, *86*:328–331, 1970.

150. Kammer H., George R. Cushing's disease in a patient with an ectopic pituitary adenoma. J.A.M.A., *246*:2722–2724, 1981.

151. Kapcala L.P., Hamilton S.M., Meikle A.W. Cushing's disease with "normal suppression" due to decreased dexamethasone clearance. Arch. Int. Med., *144*:636–637, 1984.

152. Kaye T.B., Crapo L. The Cushing's syndrome: An update on diagnostic tests. Ann. Int. Med., *112*:434–444, 1990.

153. Kehlet H., Binder C. Adrenocortical function and clinical course during and after surgery in unsupplemented glucocorticoid-treated patients. Br. J. Anaesth., *45*:1043–1048, 1973.

154. Keller-Wood M.E., Dallman M.F. Corticosteroid inhibition of ACTH secretion. Endocr. Rev., *5*:1–14, 1984.

155. King L.W., Post K.D., Yust J.Y., Reichlin S. Suppression of cortisol secretion by low-dose dexamethasone testing in Cushing's disease. Case report. J. Neurosurg., *58*:129–132, 1983.

156. Kirkman S., Nelson D.H. Alcohol-induced pseudo-Cushing's disease: A study of prevalence with review of the literature. Metabolism, *37*:390–394, 1988.

157. Kirschner M.A., Powell R.D. Jr., Lipsett M.B. Cushing's syndrome. Nodular cortical hyperplasia of adrenal glands with clinical and pathological features suggesting adrenocortical tumor. J. Clin. Endocrinol. Metab., *24*:947–955, 1964.

158. Kovacs K. Light and electron microscopic pathology of pituitary tumors: immunohistochemistry. In: *Tumors of the Pituitary Gland,* edited by P.M. Black, N.T. Zervas, E.C. Ridgway, and J.B. Martin, pp. 365–376, New York, Raven Press, 1984.

159. Kovacs K., Horvath E. Tumors of the Pituitary Gland. Washington, D.C., Armed Forces Institute of Pathology, 70–178, 1986.

160. Krieger D.T. Pathophysiology of central nervous system regulation of anterior pituitary function. In: *Biology of Brain Dysfunction,* edited by G.E. Gaull, pp. 351–407, New York, Plenum Press, 1973.

161. Krieger D.T. Physiopathology of Cushing's disease. Endocr. Rev., *4*:22–43, 1983.

162. Krieger D.T., Allen W., Rizzo F., Krieger H.P. Characterization of the normal temporal pattern of plasma corticosteroid levels. J. Clin. Endocrinol. Metab., *32*:266–284, 1971.

163. Krieger D.T., Glick S., Silverberg A., Krieger H.P. A comparative study of endocrine tests in hypothalamic disease. Circadian periodicity of plasma 11-OHCS levels, plasma 11-OHCS and growth hormone response to insulin hypoglycemia and metyrapone responsiveness. J. Clin. Endocrinol. Metab., *28*:1589–1597, 1968.

164. Kucharczyk W., Davis D.O., Kelly W.M., Sze G., Norman D., Newton. Pituitary adenomas: High-resolution MR imaging at 1.5T. Radiology, *161*:761–765, 1986.

165. Kuhn J.M., Proeschel M.F., Seurin D.F., Bertagna X.Y., Luton J.P., Girard F.L. Comparative assessment of ACTH and lipotropin plasma levels in the diagnosis and follow-up of patients with Cushing's syndrome: A study of 210 cases. Am. J. Med., *86*:678–684, 1989.

166. LaCivita K.A., McDonald S., Jacobson J. Cyclic Cushing's disease in association with a pituitary stone. South Med. J., *82*:1174–1176, 1989.

167. Lagerquist L.G., Meikle A.W., West C.D., Tyler F.H. Cushing's disease with cure by resection of pituitary adenoma. Evidence against a primary hypothalamic defect. Am. J. Med., *57*:826–830, 1974.

168. Lamberts S.W.J., Klign J.G.M., de Jong F.H., *et al.* Hormone secretion in alcohol-induced pseudo-Cushing's syndrome. Differential diagnosis with Cushing's disease. J. Am. Med. Assoc., *242*:1640–1643, 1979.

169. Lamberts S.W., Stefanko S.Z., de Lange S.A., *et al.* Failure of clinical remission after transsphenoidal removal of a microadenoma in a patient with Cushing's disease: multiple hyperplastic and adenomatous cell nests in surrounding pituitary tissue. J. Clin. Endocrinol. Metab., *50*:793–795, 1980.

170. Lamers C.B., Stadil F., van Tongeren J.H. Prevalence of endocrine abnormalities in patients with the Zollinger-Ellison syndrome and in their families. Am. J. Med., *64*:607–612, 1978.

171. Landolt A.M., Valavanis A., Girard J., Eberle A.N. Corticotropin-releasing factor-test used with bilateral simultaneous inferior petrosal sinus blood sampling for the diagnosis of pituitary-dependent Cushing's disease. Clin. Endocrinol. (Oxf.), *25*:687–696, 1986.

172. Larsen J.L., Cathey W.J., Odell W.D. Primary adrenocortical nodular dysplasia, a distinct subtype of Cushing's syndrome. Case report and review of the literature. Am. J. Med., *80*:976–984, 1986.

173. Lesch K.-P., Söhnle K., Poten B., Schoellnhammer G., Rupprecht R., Schulte H.M. Corticotropin and cortisol secretion after central 5-hydroxytryptamine-1A (5-HT$_{1A}$) receptor activation: Effects of 5-HT receptor and β-adrenoceptor antagonists. J. Clin. Endocrinol. Metab., *70*:670–674, 1990.

174. Liberman B., Wajchenberg B.L., Tambascia M.A.,

Mesquita C.H. Periodic remission in Cushing's disease with paradoxical dexamethasone response. An expression of periodic hormonogenesis. J. Clin. Endocrinol. Metab., *43*:913–918, 1976.

175. Liddle G.W. Tests of pituitary-adrenal suppressibility in the diagnosis of Cushing's syndrome. J. Clin. Endocrinol. Metab., *20*:1539–1560, 1960.

176. Liddle G.W. Pathogenesis of glucocorticoid disorders. Am. J. Med., *53*:638–648, 1972.

177. Liddle G.W., Estep H.L., Kendall T.W., Williams W.C. Jr., Townes A.W. Clinical application of a new test of pituitary reserve. J. Clin. Endocrinol. Metab., *19*:875–894, 1959.

178. Liddle G.W., Givens J.R., Nicholson W.E., Island D.P. The ectopic ACTH syndrome. Cancer Res., *25*:1057–1061, 1965.

179. Liddle G.W., Nicholson W.E., Island D.P., *et al.* Clinical and laboratory studies of ectopic humoral syndromes. Recent Prog. Horm. Res., *25*:283–305, 1969.

180. Linkowski P., Mendlewicz J., Kerkhofs M., *et al.* 24-hour profiles of adrenocorticotropin, cortisol, and growth hormone in major depressive illness: Effect of antidepressant treatment. J. Clin. Endocrinol. Metab., *65*:141–152, 1987.

181. Linkowski P., Mendlewicz J., Leclerq R., *et al.* The 24-hour profile of adrenocorticotropin and cortisol in major depressive illness. J. Clin. Endocrinol. Metab., *61*:429–438, 1985.

182. Linton E.A., Lowry P.J. Corticotrophin releasing factor in man and its measurement: A review. Clin. Endocrinol. (Oxf.), *31*:225–249, 1989.

183. Lipsett M.B., Hertz R., Ross G.T. Clinical and pathophysiologic aspects of adrenocortical carcinoma. Am. J. Med., *35*:374–383, 1963.

184. Lipsett M.B., Wilson H. Adrenocortical cancer. Steroid biosynthesis and metabolism evaluated by urinary metabolites. J. Clin. Endocrinol. Metab., *22*:906–915, 1962.

185. Liu J.H., Kazer R.R., Rasmussen D.D. Characterization of the twenty-four hour secretion patterns of adrenocorticotropin and cortisol in normal women and patients with Cushing's disease. J. Clin. Endocrinol. Metab., *64*:1027–1035, 1987.

186. Loriaux D.L. The polyendocrine deficiency syndromes. New Engl. J. Med., *312*:1568–1569, 1985.

187. Loriaux D.L., and Cutler G.B. Jr. Diseases of the adrenal glands. In: *Clinical Endocrinology,* edited by O. Peter and M.D. Kohler, pp. 167–238, John Wiley and Sons, Inc., 1986.

188. Lowry P.J., Rees L.H., Tomlin S., Gillies G., Landon J. Chemical characterization of ectopic ACTH purified from a malignant thymic carcinoid tumor. J. Clin. Endocrinol. Metab., *43*:831–835, 1976.

189. Luciano M., Oldfield E.H. The diagnosis of Cushing's disease. In: *Contemporary Diagnosis and Management of Pituitary Adenomas,* edited by P. Cooper, pp. 101–123, American Association of Neurological Surgeons, 1991.

190. Lumpkin M.D. The regulation of ACTH secretion by IL-1. Science, *238*:452–454, 1987.

191. Lyons D.F., Eisen B.R., Clark M.R., Pysher T.J., Welsh J.D., Kem D.C. Concurrent Cushing's and Zollinger-Ellison syndromes in a patient with islet cell carcinoma. Case report and review of the literature. Am. J. Med., *76*:729–733, 1984.

192. Lytras N., Grossman A., Perry L., *et al.* Corticotropin releasing factor: responses in normal subjects and patients with disorders of the hypothalamus and pituitary. Clin. Endocrinol. (Oxf.), *20*:71–84, 1984.

193. Macfarlane D.A. Cancer of the adrenal cortex. The natural history, prognosis and treatment in a study of fifty-five cases. Ann. R. Coll. Surg. Engl., *23*:155–186, 1958.

194. Malchoff C.D., Rosa J., DeBold C.R., *et al.* Adrenocorticotropin-independent bilateral macronodular adrenal hyperplasia: An unusual cause of Cushing's syndrome. J. Clin. Endocrinol. Metab., *68*:855–860, 1989.

195. Mampalam T.J., Tyrrell J.B., Wilson C.B. Transsphenoidal microsurgery for Cushing's disease. A report of 216 cases. Ann. Int. Med., *109*:487–493, 1988.

196. Manni A., Latshaw R.F., Page R., Santen R.J. Simultaneous bilateral venous sampling for adrenocorticotropin in pituitary-dependent Cushing's disease: evidence for lateralization of pituitary venous drainage. J. Clin. Endocrinol. Metab., *57*:1070–1073, 1983.

197. Maran J.W., Carlson D.E., Grizzle W.E., Ward D.G., Gann D.S. Organization of the medial hypothalamus for control of adrenocorticotropin in the cat. Endocrinology, *103*:957–970, 1979.

198. Marcovitz S., Wee R., Chan J., Hardy J. The diagnostic accuracy of preoperative CT scanning in the evaluation of pituitary ACTH-secreting adenomas. AJNR, *8*:641–644, 1987.

199. Marcovitz S., Wee R., Chan J., Hardy J. Diagnostic accuracy of preoperative CT scanning of pituitary prolactinomas. AJNR, *9*:13–17, 1988.

200. Marcovitz S., Wee R., Chan J., Hardy J. Diagnostic accuracy of preoperative CT scanning of pituitary somatotroph adenomas. AJNR, *9*:19–22, 1988.

201. Mark L., Pech P., Daniels D., Charles C., Williams A., Haughton V. The pituitary fossa: A correlative anatomic and MR study. Radiology, *153*:453–457, 1984.

202. Mason A.M.S., Ratcliffe J.G., Buckle R.M., Mason A.S. ACTH secretion by bronchial carcinoid tumours. Clin. Endocrinol. (Oxf.), *1*:3–25, 1972.

203. Matheson G.K., Branch B.J., Taylor A.N. Effects of amygdaloid stimulation on pituitary-adrenal activity in conscious cats. Brain Res., *32*:151–167, 1971.

204. Mattingly D., Tyler C. Plasma 11-hydroxycorticoid levels in surgical stress. Proc. R. Soc. Med., *58*:1010–1012, 1965.

205. McArthur R.G., Cloutier M.D., Hayles A.B., Sprague R.G. Cushing's disease in children. Findings in 13 cases. Mayo Clin. Proc., *47*:318–326, 1972.

206. McCance D.R., McIlrath E., McNeill A., *et al.* Bilateral inferior petrosal sinus sampling as a routine procedure in ACTH-dependent Cushing's syndrome. Clin. Endocrinol. (Oxf.), *30*:157–160, 1989.

207. McIntosh T.K., Lothrop D.A., Lee A., Jackson

B.T., Nasbeth D., Egdahl R.E. Circadian rhythm of cortisol is altered in postsurgical patients. J. Clin. Endocrinol. Metab., *53:*117–122, 1981.

208. McKeever P.E., Koppelman M.C., Metcalf D., *et al.* Refractory Cushing's disease caused by multinodular ACTH-cell hyperplasia. J. Neuropathol. Exp. Neurol., *41:*490–499, 1982.

209. McKenna T.J., Lorber D., LaCroix A., Rabin D. Testicular activity in Cushing's disease. Acta Endocrinol. (Copenh.), *91:*501–501, 1979.

210. McMahon M., Gerich J., Rizza R. Effects of glucocorticoids on carbohydrate metabolism. Diabetes Metab. Rev., *4:*17–30, 1988.

211. Meador C.K., Bowdoin B., Owen W.C. Jr., Farmer T.A. Jr. Primary adrenocortical nodular dysplasia: a rare cause of Cushing's syndrome. J. Clin. Endocrinol. Metab., *27:*1255–1263, 1967.

212. Meikle A.W. Dexamethasone suppression tests: Usefulness of simultaneous measurement of plasma cortisol and dexamethasone. Clin. Endocrinol. (Copenh.), *16:*401–408, 1982.

213. Meikle A.W., Jubiz W., Hutchings M.P., West C.D., Tyler F.H. A simplified metyrapone test with determination of plasma 11-deoxycortisol (metyrapone test with plasma S). J. Clin. Endocrinol. Metab., *29:*985–987, 1969.

214. Meikle A.W., Jubiz W., Matsukura S., Harada G., West C.D., Tyler, F.H. Effect of estrogen on the metabolism of metyrapone and release of ACTH. J. Clin. Endocrinol. Metab., *30:*259–263, 1970.

215. Meikle A.W., Stanchfield J.B., West C.D., Tyler F.H. Hydrocortisone suppression test for Cushing's syndrome. Therapy with anticonvulsants. Arch. Int. Med., *134:*1068–1071, 1974.

216. Meunier P.J., Dempster D.W., Edouard C., Chapuy M.C., Arlot M., Charhon S. Bone histomorphometry in corticosteroid-induced osteoporosis and Cushing's syndrome. Adv. Exp. Med. Biol., *171:*191–200, 1984.

217. Migeon C.J., Tyler F.H., Mahoney T.P., *et al.* The diurnal variation of plasma levels and urinary excretion of 17-hydroxycorticosteroids in normal subjects, night workers and blind subjects. J. Clin. Endocrinol. Metab., *16:*622–633, 1956.

218. Mitty H.A., Nicolis G.L., Gabrilove J.L. Adrenal venography: clinical-roentgenographic correlation in 80 patients. AJR, *119:*564–575, 1973.

219. Moore T.J., Dluhy R.G., Williams G.H., Cain J.P. Nelson's syndrome: frequency, prognosis and effect of prior pituitary irradiation. Ann. Int. Med., *85:*731–734, 1976.

220. Moser H.W., Moser A.E., Singh I., O'Neill B.P. Adrenoleukodystrophy: survey of 303 cases: biochemistry, diagnosis, and therapy. Ann. Neurol., *16:*628–641, 1984.

221. Müller O.A., Stalla G.K., Werder K. Corticotropin-releasing factor: a new tool for the differential diagnosis of Cushing's syndrome. J. Clin. Endocrinol. Metab., *57:*227–229, 1983.

222. Müller O.A., Hartwimmer J., Hauer A., *et al.* Corticotropin-releasing factor (CRF): stimulation in normal controls and in patients with Cushing's syndrome. Psychoneuroendocrinology, *11:*49–60, 1986.

223. Müller O.A., Stalla G.K., Hartwimmer J., Schopol J., von Werder K. Corticotropin releasing factor (CRF): diagnostic implications. Acta Neurochir. (Wein), *75:*49–59, 1985.

224. Nader S., Hickey R.C., Sellin R.V., Samaan N.A. Adrenal cortical carcinoma. A study of 77 cases. Cancer, *52:*707–711, 1983.

225. Nakahara M., Shibasaki T., Shizume K., *et al.* Corticotropin-releasing factor test in normal subjects and patients with hypothalamic-pituitary-adrenal disorders. J. Clin. Endocrinol. Metab., *57:*963–968, 1983.

226. Nelson D.H., Meakin J.W., Thorn G.W. ACTH-producing tumors following adrenalectomy for Cushing's syndrome. Ann. Int. Med., *52:*560–569, 1960.

227. Nerup J. Addison's disease—serological studies. Acta Endocrinol. (Copenh.), *76:*142–158, 1974.

228. Newton D.R., Dillon W.P., Norman D., Newton T.H., Wilson C.B. Gd-DTPA-enhanced MR imaging of pituitary adenomas. AJNR, *10:*949–954, 1989.

229. Nichols D.A., Laws E.R. Jr., Houser O.W., Abboud C.A. Comparison of magnetic resonance imaging and computed tomography in the preoperative evaluation of pituitary adenomas. Neurosurgery, *22:*380–385, 1988.

230. Nichols T., Nugent C.A., Tyler F.H. Diurnal variation in suppression of adrenal function by glucocorticoids. J. Clin. Endocrinol. Metab., *25:*343–349, 1965.

231. Nicholson W.E., DeCherney G.S., Jackson R.V., *et al.* Plasma distribution, disappearance half-time, metabolic clearance rate, and degradation of synthetic corticotropin-releasing factor in man. J. Clin. Endocrinol. Metab., *57:*1263–1269, 1983.

232. Nicholson W.E., Liddle R.A., Puett D., Liddle G.W. Adrenocorticotropic hormone biotransformation, clearance, and catabolism. Endocrinology, *103:*1344–1351, 1978.

233. Nieman L.K., Chrousos G.P., Oldfield E.H., Avgerinos P.C., Cutler G.B. Jr., Loriaux D.L. The ovine corticotropin-releasing hormone stimulation test and the dexamethasone suppression test in the differential diagnosis of Cushing's syndrome. Ann. Int. Med., *105:*862–867, 1986.

234. Nieman L.K., Cutler G.B., Oldfield E.H., Loriaux D.L., Chrouson G.P. The ovine corticotropin-releasing hormone (CRH) stimulation test is superior to the human CRH stimulation test for the diagnosis of Cushing's disease. J. Clin. Endocrinol. Metab., *69:*165–176, 1989.

235. Nieman L.K., Oldfield E.H., Wesley R., Loriaux D.L., Cutler G.B. Jr. The morning oCRH test: A practical tool for the differential diagnosis Cushing's syndrome. Clin. Res., *38:*475A, 1990.

236. Nolten W.E., Lindheimer M.D., Rueckert P.A., Oparil S., Ehrlich E.N. Diurnal patterns and regulation of cortisol secretion in pregnancy. J. Clin. Endocrinol. Metab., *51:*466–472, 1980.

237. Nosadini R., Del Prato S., Tiengo A., *et al.* Insulin resistance in Cushing's syndrome. J. Clin. Endocrinol. Metab., *57:*529–536, 1983.

238. Nugent C.A., Nichols T., Tyler F.H. Diagnosis of

Cushing's syndrome. Single dose dexamethasone suppression test. Arch. Int. Med., *116:*172–176, 1965.

239. Oddie C.J., Coghlan J.P., Scoggins B.A. Plasma deoxycorticosterone levels in man with simultaneous measurement of aldosterone, corticosterone, cortisol and 11-deoxycortisol. J. Clin. Endocrinol. Metab., *34:*1039–1054, 1972.

240. Oldfield E.H., Chrousos G.P., Schulte H.M., *et al.* Preoperative lateralization of ACTH-secreting microadenomas by bilateral and simultaneous inferior petrosal sinus sampling. New Engl. J. Med., *312:*100–103, 1985.

241. Oldfield E.H., Doppman J.L., Nieman L.K., *et al.* Bilateral inferior petrosal sinus sampling with and without corticotropin-releasing hormone for the differential diagnosis of Cushing's syndrome. N. Eng. J. Med., *325:*897–905, 1991.

242. Oldfield E.H., Girton M.E., Doppman. Absence of intercavernous venous mixing: evidence supporting lateralization of pituitary microadenomas by venous sampling. J. Clin. Endocrinol. Metab., *61:*644–647, 1985.

243. Oldfield E.H., Schulte H.M., Chrousos G.P., Cutler G.P. Jr., Loriaux D.L. Corticotropin releasing factor stimulates ACTH secretion in Nelson's syndrome. J. Clin. Endocrinol. Metab., *62:*1020–1026, 1986.

244. O'Neal L.W. Pathologic anatomy in Cushing's syndrome. Ann. Surg., *160:*860–869, 1964.

245. O'Neal L.W., Kipnis D.M., Luse S.A., Lacy P.E., Jarett L. Secretion of various endocrine substances by ACTH-secreting tumors—gastrin, melanotropin, norepinephrine, serotonin, parathormone, vasopressin, glucagon. Cancer, *21:*1219–1232, 1968.

246. Orth D.N., DeBold C.R., DeCherney G.S., *et al.* Pituitary microadenoma causing Cushing's disease is responsive to corticotropin-releasing factor. J. Clin. Endocrinol. Metab., *55:*1017–1019, 1982.

247. Orth D.N., Kovacs W.J., DeBold C.R. The adrenal cortex. In: *Textbook of Endocrinology,* edited by J.D. Wilson and D.W. Foster, pp. 489–620, Philadelphia, PA, W.B. Saunders Co., 1992.

248. Orth D.N., DeBold C.R., DeCherney G.S., *et al.* Clinical studies with synthetic ovine corticotropin-releasing factor. Fed. Proc., *44:*197–202, 1985.

249. Orth D.N., Island D.P., Liddle G.W. Experimental alteration of circadian rhythm in plasma cortisol (17-OHCS) concentration in man. J. Clin. Endocrinol. Metab., *27:*549–555, 1967.

250. Orth D.N., Liddle G.W. Results of treatment in 108 patients with Cushing's syndrome. New Engl. J. Med., *285:*243–247, 1971.

251. Ovadia H., Abramsky O., Barak V., Conforti N., Saphier D., Weidenfeld J. Effect of interleukin-1 on adrenocortical activity in intact and hypothalamic deafferented male rats. Exp. Brain Res., *76:*246–249, 1989.

252. Owerbach D., Rutter W.J., Roberts J.L., *et al.* The proopiocortin gene is located on chromosome 2 in humans. Somat. Cell. Mol. Genet., *7:*359–369, 1981.

253. Parent A.D., Bebin J., Smith R.R. Incidental pituitary microadenomas. J. Neurosurg., *54:*228–231, 1981.

254. Peck W.W., Dillon W.P., Norman D., Newton T.H., Wilson C.B. High-resolution MR imaging of microadenomas at 1.5T: experience with Cushing's disease. AJNR, *9:*1085–1091, 1988.

255. Peterson R.E. The influence of the thyroid on adrenal cortical function. J. Clin. Invest., *37:*736–743, 1958.

256. Pieters G.F.F.M., Hermus A.R.M.M., Smals A.G.H., Bartelink A.K.M., Benraad T.J., Kloppenborg P.W.C. Responsiveness of the hypophyseal-adrenocortical axis to corticotropin-releasing factor in pituitary dependent Cushing's disease. J. Clin. Endocrinol. Metab., *57:*513–516, 1983.

257. Pieters G.F.F.M., Hermus A.R.M.M., Smals A.G.H., Kloppenborg P.W.C. Paradoxical responsiveness of growth hormone to corticotropin-releasing factor in acromegaly. J. Clin. Endocrinol. Metab., *58:*560–562, 1984.

258. Plotsky P.M. Hypophyseotropic regulation of adenohypophyseal adrenocorticotropin secretion. Fed. Proc., *44:*207–213, 1984.

259. Plotsky P.M., Otto S., Sutton S. Neurotransmitter modulation of corticotropin-releasing factor secretion into the hypophysial-portal circulation. Life Sci., *41:*1311–1317, 1987.

260. Plotsky P.M., Sawchenko P.E. Hypophysial-portal plasma levels, median eminence content, and immunohistochemical staining of corticotropin-releasing factor, arginine vasopressin, and oxytocin after pharmacological adrenalectomy. Endocrinology, *120:*1361–1369, 1987.

261. Plotz C.M., Knowlton A.L., Ragan C. The natural history of Cushing's syndrome. Am. J. Med., *13:*597–614, 1952.

262. Pojunas K.W., Daniels D.L., Williams A.L., Thorsen M.K., Haughton V.M. Pituitary and adrenal CT of Cushing's syndrome. AJR, *146:*1235–1238, 1986.

263. Pon L.A., Orme-Johnson N.R. Protein synthesis requirement for acute ACTH stimulation of adrenal corticosteroidogenesis. Endocr. Res., *10:*585–590, 1985.

264. Post K.E., Habas J.-E. Comparison of long term results between prolactin secreting adenomas and ACTH secreting adenomas. Can. J. Neurol. Sci., *17:*74–77, 1990.

265. Powell-Jackson J.D., Calin A., Fraser R., *et al.* Excess deoxycorticosterone secretion from adrenocortical carcinoma. BMJ, *2:*32–33, 1974.

266. Pulakhandam U., Dincsoy H.D. Cytomegaloviral adrenalitis and adrenal insufficiency in AIDS. Am. J. Clin. Pathol., *93:*651–656, 1990.

267. Queiroz L., Facure N.O., Facure J.J., Modesto N.P., de Faria J.L. Pituitary carcinoma with liver metastases and Cushing's syndrome. Report of a case. Arch. Pathol. Lab. Med., *99:*32–35, 1975.

268. Ramachandran J. Corticotropin receptors, cyclic AMP and steroidogenesis. Endocr. Res., *10:*347–363, 1985.

269. Raux M.C., Binoux M., Luton J.P., Gourmelen M., Girard F. Studies of ACTH secretion control

in 116 cases of Cushing's syndrome. J. Clin. Endocrinol. Metab., *40:*186–197, 1975.

270. Rayfield E.J., Rose L.I., Cain J.P., Dluhy R.G., Williams G.H. ACTH-responsive, dexamethasone-suppressible adrenocortical carcinoma. New Engl. J. Med., *284:*591–592, 1971.

271. Reader S.C., Daly J.R., Alaghband-Zadeh J., Robertson W.R. Negative feedback effects on ACTH secretion by cortisol in Cushing's disease. Clin. Endocrinol. (Oxf.), *18:*43–49, 1983.

272. Rees L.H., Bloomfield G.A., Rees G.M., Corrin B., Franks L.M., Ratcliffe J.G. Multiple hormones in a bronchial tumor. J. Clin. Endocrinol. Metab., *38:*1090–1097, 1974.

273. Rees L.H., Ratcliffe J.G. Ectopic hormone production by non-endocrine tumors. Clin. Endocrinol. (Oxf.), *3:*263–299, 1974.

274. Regenstein Q.R., Rose L.I., Williams G. Psychopathology in Cushing's syndrome. Arch. Int. Med., *130:*114–117, 1972.

275. Reinig J.W., Doppman J.L., Dwyer A.J., Johnson A.R., Knop R.H. Adrenal masses differentiated by MR. Radiology, *158:*81–84, 1986.

276. Reincke M., Allolio B., Saeger W., Kaulen D., Winkelmann W. A pituitary adenoma secreting high molecular weight adrenocorticotropin without evidence of Cushing's disease. J. Clin. Endocrinol. Metab., *65:*1296–1300, 1987.

277. Reynolds J.W., Colle E., Ulstrom R.A. Adrenocortical steroid metabolism in newborn infants. V. Physiologic disposition of endogenous cortisol loads in the early neonatal period. J. Clin. Endocrinol. Metab., *22:*245–254, 1962.

278. Rivier C., Vale W. Effects of corticotropin-releasing factor, neurohypophyseal peptides, and catecholamines on pituitary function. Fed. Proc., *44:*189–195, 1985.

279. Robert F., Pelletier G., Hardy J. Pituitary adenomas in Cushing's disease. Arch. Pathol. Lab. Med., *102:*448–455, 1978.

280. Rosenberg E.M., Hahn T.J., Orth D.N., Deftos L.J., Tanaka K. ACTH-secreting medullary carcinoma of the thyroid presenting as severe idiopathic osteoporosis and senile purpura: report of a case and review of the literature. J. Clin. Endocrinol. Metab., *47:*255–262, 1978.

281. Rosman P.M., Farag A., Benn R., Ttio J., Mishik A., Wallace E.Z. Modulation of pituitary-adrenocortical function: Decreased secretory episodes and blunted circadian rhythmicity in patients with alcoholic liver disease. J. Clin. Endocrinol. Metab., *55:*709–717, 1981.

282. Ross E.J., Marshall-Jones P., Friedman M. Cushing's syndrome: diagnostic criteria. Q. J. Med., *35:*149–192, 1966.

283. Roth J., Grunfeld C. Mechanism of action of peptide hormones and catecholamines. In: *Williams' Textbook of Endocrinology,* 7th ed., edited by J.D. Wilson and D.W. Foster, pp. 76–122, Philadelphia, W.B. Saunders, 1985.

284. Rousseau G.G. Structure and regulation of the glucocorticoid hormone receptor. Mol. Cell Endocrinol., *38:*1–11, 1984.

285. Ruder H.J., Guy R.L., Lipsett M.B. A radioimmunoassay for cortisol in plasma and urine. J. Clin. Endocrinol. Metab., *35:*219–224, 1972.

286. Rupprecht R., Lesch K.-P., Müller U, Beck G., Beckmann H., Schulte H.M. Blunted adrenocorticotropin but normal β-endorphin release after human corticotropin-releasing hormone administration in depression. J. Clin. Endocrinol. Metab., *69:*600–603, 1989.

287. Sacks J., Sazbon L., Lunenfeld B., Najenson T. Hypothalamic-pituitary function in patients with prolonged coma. J. Clin. Endocrinol. Metab., *56:*635–638, 1983.

288. Saffran M., Schally A.V. Release of corticotropin by anterior pituitary tissue in vitro. Biochem. Cell Biol., *33:*408–415, 1955.

289. Salassa R.M., Laws E.R. Jr., Carpenter P.C., Northcutt R.C. Transsphenoidal removal of pituitary microadenoma in Cushing's disease. Mayo Clin. Proc., *53:*24–28, 1978.

290. Sample W.F. Adrenal ultrasonography. Radiology, *127:*461–466, 1978.

291. Sandberg A.A., Slaunwhite W.R. Physical state of adrenal cortical hormones in plasma. In: *The Human Adrenal Cortex,* edited by N.P. Christy, pp. 69–86, New York, Harper and Row, 1971.

292. Sapolsky R., Rivier C., Yamamoto G., Plotsky P., Vale W. Interleukin-1 stimulates the secretion of hypothalamic corticotropin-releasing factor. Science, *238:*522–524, 1987.

293. Saris S.C., Patronas N.J., Doppman J.L., *et al.* Cushing's syndrome: pituitary CT scanning. Radiology, *162:*775–777, 1986.

294. Sawin C.T., Abe K., Orth D.N. Hyperpigmentation due solely to increased plasma beta-melanotropin. Arch. Int. Med., *125:*708–710, 1970.

295. Schaumberg H., Powers J.M., Raine C.S, Suzuki K., Richardson E.P. Jr. Adrenoleukodystrophy. A clinical and pathological study of 17 cases. Arch. Neurol., *32:*577–591, 1975.

296. Scheithauer B.W., Horvath E., Kovacs K., Laws E.R. Jr., Randall R.V., Ryan N. Plurihormonal pituitary adenomas. Sem. Diag. Pathol., *3:*69–82, 1986.

297. Schlaghecke R., Kornely E., Santen R.T., Riddreskamp P. The effect of long-term glucocorticoid therapy on pituitary-adrenal responses to exogenous corticotropin-releasing hormone. N. Eng. J. Med., *326:*226–230, 1992.

298. Schlaghecke R., Krenzpaintner G., Bürrig K.F., Juli E., Kley H.K. Cushing's syndrome due to ACTH-production of an ovarian carcinoid. Klin. Wochenschr., *67:*640–644, 1989.

299. Schmid J.R., Labhart A., Rossier P.H. Relationship of multiple endocrine adenomas to the syndrome of ulcerogenic islet cell adenomas (Zollinger-Ellison). Am. J. Med., *31:*343–353, 1961.

300. Schnall A.M., Brodkey J.S., Kaufman B., Pearson O.H. Pituitary function after removal of pituitary microadenomas in Cushing's disease. J. Clin. Endocrinol. Metab., *47:*410–417, 1978.

301. Schteingart D.E., Woodbury M., Tsao H.S., McKenzie A.K. Virilizing syndrome associated

with an adrenal cortical adenoma secreting predominantly testosterone. Am. J. Med., *67:*140–146, 1979.

302. Schulte H.M., Allolia B., Gunther R.W., *et al.* Selective bilateral and simultaneous catheterization of the inferior petrosal sinus: CRF stimulates prolactin secretion from ACTH-producing microadenomas in Cushing's disease. Clinical Endocrinol. (Oxf.), *28:*289–295, 1988.

303. Schulte H.M., Chrousos G.P., Avgerinos P.C., Oldfield E.H., Gold P.W., Cutler G.B. Jr., Loriaux D.L. The corticotropin-releasing factor stimulation test: an aid in the evaluation of patients with adrenal insufficiency. J. Clin. Endocrinol. Metab., *58:*1064–1067, 1984.

304. Schulte H.M., Chrousos G.P., Booth J.D., *et al.* Corticotropin-releasing factor: pharmacokinetics in man. J. Clin. Endocrinol. Metab., *58:*192–196, 1984.

305. Schulte H.M., Chrousos G.P., Oldfield E.H., Gold P.W., Cutler G.B. Jr., Loriaux D.L. The effects of corticotropin-releasing factor on the pituitary function of stalk-sectioned cynomolgus macaques: dose response of cortisol secretion. J. Clin. Endocrinol. Metab., *55:*810–812, 1982.

306. Schulte H.M., Chrousos G.P., Oldfield E.H., Gold P.W., Cutler G.B. Jr., Loriaux D.L. Ovine corticotropin-releasing factor administration in normal men; pituitary and adrenal responses in the morning and evening. Horm. Res., *21:*69–74, 1985.

307. Schulte H.M., Oldfield E.H., Allolio E.H., Katz D.A., Berkman R., Ali I.U. Clonal composition of pituitary adenomas in patients with Cushing's disease. J. Clin. Endocrinol. Metab., *73:*1302–1308, 1991.

308. Scott E.M., McGarrigle H.H.G., Lachelin G.C.L. The increase in plasma and saliva cortisol levels in pregnancy is not due to the increase in corticosteroid-binding globulin levels. J. Clin. Endocrinol. Metab., *71:*639–644, 1990.

309. Scotti G., Yu C.-Y., Dillon W.P., *et al.* MR imaging of cavernous sinus involvement by pituitary adenomas. A.J.N.R., *9:*657–664, 1988.

310. Sederberg-Olsen P., Binder C., Kehlet H., Neville A.M., Nielsen L.M. Episodic variation in plasma corticosteroids in subjects with Cushing's syndrome of differing etiology. J. Clin. Endocrinol. Metab., *36:*906–910, 1973.

311. Shapiro M.S., Shenkman L. Variable hormonogenesis in Cushing's syndrome. Q. J. Med., *79:*351–363, 1991.

312. Sheeler L.R., Myers J.M., Eversman J.J., Taylor H.C. Adrenal insufficiency secondary to carcinoma metastatic to the adrenal gland. Cancer, *52:*1312–1316, 1983.

313. Shenoy B.V., Carpenter B.C., Carney J.A. Bilateral primary pigmented nodular adrenocortical disease. Rare cause of the Cushing syndrome. Am. J. Surg. Pathol., *8:*335–344, 1984.

314. Sherry S.H., Guay A.T., Lee A.K., *et al.* Concurrent production of adrenocorticotropin and prolactin from two distinct cell lines in a single pituitary adenoma: A detailed immunohistochemical analysis. J. Clin. Endocrinol. Metab., *55:*947–955, 1982.

315. Shimatsu A., Kato Y., Tanaka I., Nakai Y., Fukunaga M., Imura H. Plasma calcitonin and ACTH responses to lysine vasopressin, calcium and pentagastrin in a patient with medullary thyroid carcinoma associated with Cushing's syndrome. Clin. Endocrinol. (Oxf.), *18:*119–125, 1983.

316. Shirkhoda A. Current diagnostic approach to adrenal abnormalities. J. Comput. Assist. Tomogr., *8:*277–285, 1985.

317. Silber R.H., Porter C.C. The determination of 17,21-dihydroxy-20-ketosteroids in urine and plasma. J. Biol. Chem., *210:*923–932, 1954.

318. Sippel W.G., Dörr H.G., Bidlingmaier F., Knorr D. Plasma levels of aldosterone, corticosterone, 11-deoxycorticosterone, progesterone, 17-hydroxyprogesterone, cortisol, and cortisone during infancy and childhood. Pediatric Res., *14:*39–46, 1980.

319. Smals A.G.H., Pieters G.F.F.M., van Haelst U.J.G., Kloppenborg P.W.C. Macronodular adrenocortical hyperplasia in long-standing Cushing's disease. J. Clin. Endocrinol. Metab., *58:*25–31, 1984.

320. Smith A.I., Funder J.W. Proopiomelanocortin processing in the pituitary, central nervous system, and peripheral tissues. Endocr. Rev., *9:*159–179, 1988.

321. Snell M.E., Lawrence R., Sutton D., Sever P.S., Peart W.S. Advances in the techniques of localization of adrenal tumors and their influence on the surgical approach to the tumor. Br. J. Urol., *55:*617–621, 1983.

322. Snow R.B., Patterson R.H., Horwith M., Saint Louis L., Fraser R.A.R. Usefulness of preoperative inferior petrosal vein sampling in Cushing's disease. Surg. Neurol., *29:*17–21, 1988.

323. Soffer L.J., Iannaccone A., Gabrilove J.L. Cushing's syndrome. A study of fifty patients. Am. J. Med., *30:*129–146, 1961.

324. Spark R.F., Connolly P.B., Gluckin D.S., White R., Sacks B., Landsberg L. ACTH secretion from a functioning pheochromocytoma. New Engl. J. Med., *301:*416–418, 1979.

325. Spiegel R.J., Vigersky R.A., Oliff A.I., Echelberger C.K., Bruton J., Poplack D.G. Adrenal suppression after short term corticosteroid therapy. Lancet, *1:*630–633, 1979.

326. Spiger M., Jubiz W., Meikle W., West C.D., Tyler F.H. Single-dose metyrapone test. Review of a four-year experience. Arch. Int. Med., *135:*698–700, 1975.

327. Stacpoole P.W., Interlandi J.W., Nicholson W.E., Rabin D. Isolated ACTH deficiency: a heterogeneous disorder. Critical review and report of four new cases. Medicine (Baltimore), *61:*13–24, 1982.

328. Starkman M.N., Schteingart D.E., Schork M.A. Depressed mood and other psychiatric manifestations of Cushing's syndrome. Relationship to hormone levels. Psychosom. Med., *43:*3–18, 1981.

329. Streeten D.H.P., Anderson G.H. Jr., Dalakos

T.G., *et al.* Normal and abnormal function of the hypothalamic-pituitary-adrenocortical system in man. Endocr. Rev., *5:*371–394, 1984.

330. Styne D.M., Grumbach M.M., Kaplan S.L., Wilson C.B., Conte F.A. Treatment of Cushing's disease in childhood and adolescence by transsphenoidal microadenomectomy. New Engl. J. Med., *310:*889–893, 1984.

331. Szafarczyk A., Alonso G., Ixart G., Malaval F., Nouguier-Soule J., Assenmacher I. Serotoninergic system and circadian rhythms of ACTH and corticosterone in rats. Am. J. Physiol., *239:*E482–E489, 1980.

332. Szafarczyk A., Malaval F., Laurent A., Gibauld R., Assenmacher I. Further evidence for a central stimulatory action of catecholamines on adrenocorticotropin release in the rat. Endocrinology, *121:*883–892, 1987.

333. Tabarin A., Greselle J.F., San-Galli F., *et al.* Usefulness of the corticotropin-releasing hormone test during bilateral inferior petrosal sinus sampling for the diagnosis of Cushing's disease. J. Clin. Endocrinol. Metab., *73:*53–59, 1991.

334. Tanaka N., Abe K., Miyakawa S., Ohnami S., Tanaka M., Takeachi T. Analysis of human pituitary and tumor adrenocorticotropin using isoelectric focusing. J. Clin. Endocrinol. Metab., *48:*559–565, 1979.

335. Taylor T., Dluhy R.G., Williams G.H. Beta-endorphin suppresses adrenocorticotropin and cortisol levels in normal human subjects. J. Clin. Endocrinol. Metab., *57:*592–596, 1983.

336. Teasdale E., Teasdale G., Mohsen F., MacPherson P. High-resolution computed tomography in pituitary microadenoma: is seeing believing? Clin. Radiol., *37:*227–232, 1986.

337. Tomori N., Suda T., Nakagami Y., *et al.* Adrenergic modulation of adrenocorticotropin responses to insulin-induced hypoglycemia and corticotropin-releasing hormone. J. Clin. Endocrinol. Metab., *68:*87–93, 1989.

338. Totani Y., Niinomi M., Takatsuki K., Oiso Y., Tomita A. Effect of metyrapone pretreatment on adrenocorticotropin secretion induced by corticotropin-releasing hormone in normal subjects and patients with Cushing's disease. J. Clin. Endocrinol. Metab., *70:*798–803, 1990.

339. Tsagarakis S., Gillies G., Rees L.H., Besser M., Grossman A. Interleukin-1 directly stimulates the release of corticotrophin releasing factor from rat hypothalamus. Neuroendocrinology, *49:*98–101, 1989.

340. Tsukada T., Nakai Y., Koh T., Tsuji S., Imura H. Plasma adrenocorticotropin and cortisol responses to intravenous injection of corticotropin-releasing factor in the morning and evening. J. Clin. Endocrinol. Metab., *57:*869–871, 1983.

341. Tuomisto J., Männistö P. Neurotransmitter regulation of pituitary hormones. Pharmacol. Rev., *37:*249–332, 1985.

342. Tyler F.H., West C.D. Laboratory evaluation of disorders of the adrenal cortex. Am. J. Med., *53:*664–672, 1972.

343. Tyrrell J.B., Findling J.W., Aron D.C., Fitzgerald P.A., Forsham P.H. An overnight high-dose dexamethasone suppression test for rapid differential diagnosis of Cushing's syndrome. Ann. Int. Med., *104:*180–186, 1986.

344. Vale W., Spiess J., Rivier C., Rivier J. Characterization of a 41-residue ovine hypothalamic peptide that stimulates secretion of corticotropin and β-endorphin. Science, *213:*1394–1397, 1981.

345. Van Cauter E.W., Golstein J., Vanhaelst L., Leclerq R. Effects of oral contraceptive therapy on the circadian patterns of cortisol and thyrotropin (TSH). Eur. J. Clin. Invest., *5:*115–121, 1975.

346. Van Cauter E.W., Refetoff S. Evidence for two subtypes of Cushing's disease based on the analysis of episodic cortisol secretion. New Engl. J. Med., *312:*1343–1344, 1985.

347. Van Cauter E.W., Virasoro E., Leclerq R., Copinschi G. Seasonal, circadian and episodic variations of human immunoreactive β-MSH, ACTH and cortisol. Int. J. Pept. Prot. Res., *17:*3–13, 1981.

348. Vance M.L., Thorner M.O. Fasting alters pulsatile and rhythmic cortisol release in normal man. J. Clin. Endocrinol. Metab., *68:*1013–1018, 1989.

349. Van Slooten H., Schaberg A., Smeenk D., Moolenaar A.J. Morphological characteristics of benign and malignant adrenocortical tumors. Cancer, *55:*766–773, 1985.

350. Veldhuis J.D., Iranmanesh A., Johnson M.L., Lizarralde G., Amplitude, but not frequency, modulation of adrenocorticotropin secretory bursts gives rise to the nyctohemeral rhythm of the corticotropic axis in man. J. Clin. Endocrinol. Metab., *71:*452–463, 1990.

351. Vetter H., Strass R., Bayer J.M., Beckerhoff R., Armbruster H., Vetter W. Short-term fluctuations in plasma cortisol in Cushing's syndrome. Clin. Endocrinol. (Oxf.), *6:*1–4, 1977.

352. Von Werder K., Smilo R.P., Hane S., Forsham P.H. Pituitary response to stress in Cushing's disease. Acta Endocrinol. (Copenh.), *67:*127–140, 1971.

353. Walker B.F., Gunthel C.J., Bryan J.A., Watts N.B., Clark R.V. Disseminated cryptooccosis in an apparently normal host presenting as primary adrenal insufficiency: Diagnosis by fine needle aspiration. Am. J. Med., *86:*715–717, 1989.

354. Watanabe T., Tanaka K., Kumagae M., *et al.* Hormonal response to insulin-induced hypoglycemia in man. J. Clin. Endocrinol. Metab., *65:*1187–1191, 1987.

355. Weiner H., Katz J.L. The hypothalamic-pituitary-adrenal axis in anorexia nervosa: a reassessment. In: *Anorexia Nervosa: Recent Developments in Research,* edited by P.L. Darby, P.E. Garfinkel, D.M. Garner, and D.V. Coscina, pp. 249–270, New York, Alan R. Liss Inc., 1983.

356. Weitzman E.D., Fukushima D., Nogeire C., Roffwarg H., Gallagher T.F., Hellman L. Twenty-four hour pattern of the episodic secretion of cortisol in normal subjects. J. Clin. Endocrinol. Metab., *33:*14–22, 1971.

357. Welbourn R.B., Montgomery D.A.D., Kennedy T.L. The natural history of treated Cushing's syndrome. Br. J. Surg., *58:*1–16, 1971.

358. Werk E.E., MacGee T., Sholiton L.J. Effect of diphenylhydantoin on cortisol metabolism in man. J. Clin. Invest., *43:*1824–1835, 1964.

359. West C.D., Dolman L.I. Plasma ACTH radioimmunoassays in the diagnosis of pituitary-adrenal dysfunction. Ann. N.Y. Acad. Sci., *297:*205–217, 1977.

360. Whitnall M.H., Smyth D., Gainer H. Vasopressin coexists in half of the corticotropin-releasing factor axons present in the external zone of the median eminence in normal rats. Neuroendocrinology, *45:*420–424, 1988.

361. Whitworth J.A., Stewart P.M., Burt D., Atherden S.M., Edwards C.R.W. The kidney is the major site of cortisone production in man. Clin. Endocrinol. (Oxf.), *31:*355–361, 1989.

362. Wilkins L. A feminizing adrenal tumor causing gynecomastia in a boy of five years contrasted with a virilizing tumor in a five year old girl. Classification of seventy cases of adrenal tumor in children according to their hormonal manifestations and a review of eleven cases of feminizing adrenal tumor in adults. J. Clin. Endocrinol. Metab., *8:*111–132, 1948.

363. Wilkinson C.W., Shinsako J., Dallman M.F. Daily rhythms in adrenal responsiveness to adrenocorticotropin are determined primarily by the time of feeding in the rat. Endocrinology, *104:*350–359, 1979.

364. Wohltmann H., Mathur R.S., Williamson H.O. Sexual precocity in a female infant due to a feminizing adrenal carcinoma. J. Clin. Endocrinol. Metab., *50:*186–189, 1980.

365. Wynn P.C., Harwood J.P., Catt K.J., Aguilera G. Regulation of corticotropin-releasing factor (CRF) receptors in the rat pituitary gland: Effects of adrenalectomy on CRF receptors and corticotroph responses. Endocrinology, *116:*1653–1659, 1985.

366. Yamaji T., Ishibashi M., Teramoto A., Fukushima T. Hyperprolactinemia in Cushing's disease and Nelson's syndrome. J. Clin. Endocrinol. Metab., *58:*790–795, 1984.

367. Yoshida K., Satowa H., Sato A., *et al.* Plasma cortisol profiles in Cushing's syndrome. Acta Endocrinol. (Copenh.), *91:*319–328, 1979.

368. Young W.F. Jr., Scheithauer B.W., Gharib H., Laws E.R. Jr., Carpenter P.C. Cushing's syndrome due to primary multinodular corticotrope hyperplasia. Mayo Clin. Proc., *63:*256–262, 1988.

369. Zimmerman W. Eine Farbreaktion der Sexualhormone und ihre Anwendung zur Quantitativen Colorimetrischen Bestimmung. Hoppe-Seylers Zeitschr. Physiol. Chem., *233:*257–264, 1935.

CHAPTER 9

Specific Hormones: Regulation, Disorders, and Clinical Evaluation—Thyroid

STEVEN A. SMITH, M.D.

INTRODUCTION

Thyroid hormone is regulated by the hypothalamic-pituitary-thyroid axis. This neuroendocrine axis is controlled primarily by thyroid hormone itself in a classical negative-feedback endocrine system (49). Recent advances in the understanding of the molecular action of thyroid hormone and the clinical use of newer, more specific and sensitive assays for thyrotropin (TSH) have provided a greater understanding of the disorders of thyroid hormone and facilitated their clinical evaluation.

This review will update what is known about central nervous system control of thyroid hormone production and secretion in light of disorders of regulation and discuss the clinical assessment of these disorders. The emphasis will be on disorders of thyrotropin-releasing hormone (TRH) and TSH secretion, including central hyperthyroidism and hypothyroidism.

REGULATION: HYPOTHALAMIC-PITUITARY-THYROID HORMONAL AXIS

The production and secretion of "normal" quantities of thyroid hormone depend on the secretion of "appropriate" amounts of TRH from the hypothalamus, pituitary thyrotrophs that respond to TRH with the appropriate secretion of TSH, and a thyroid gland that is normally responsive to TSH stimulation (110).

TRH

TRH, the first hypothalamic releasing factor to be isolated (11, 71), serves as the highest specific neuroendocrine level of control for thyroid hormone production and secretion, whereas other neurologic and hormonal input (dopamine, somatostatin, and cortisol) inhibit TRH secretion (110). TRH is synthesized in the paraventricular nucleus of the hypothalamus and is released into the portal capillary plexus; it then travels to the anterior pituitary. The main function of hypothalamic TRH is to stimulate TSH release. Direct effects of TRH on the control of cycling secretory granules, alterations in membrane structure, and second messages (protein kinase [A and C], calcium fluxes, and prostaglandins) have been postulated as the mechanism(s) by which TRH stimulates TSH release from the pituitary thyrotroph (9, 32, 70).

TRH is a ubiquitous neurotransmitter found not only in the hypothalamus, but also in other neuronal and non-neuronal tissue. Assays for circulating TRH have not been reliable (54, 63, 67, 73) and because circulating TRH is almost exclusively from nonhypothalamic sources, it has had limited clinical utility in the assessment of the hypothalamic-pituitary-thyroid axis (67). However, because small increases in "free" thyroid hormone concentrations decrease the thyrotroph's sensitivity to TRH (see section on Thyroid Hormone and the Thyroid Hormone Receptor) (86), the use of synthetic TRH as a stimulus for TSH secretion via the TRH-stimulation test (200 to 500 μg TRH given intravenously and followed by TSH measurements every 30 min, usually for 90 min) has become a standard for assessing disorders of thyroid hormone excess (45).

TSH

TSH was first identified by Crew and Wiesner (19). It is a glycoprotein made of two subunits (α and β) (75). The α subunit is common to other glycoprotein hormones—luteinizing hormone (LH), follicle-stimulating hormone(FSH), and human chorionic gonadotropin (hCG)—and is synthesized separately and in excess of the β subunit. The hypothalamus provides a tonic stimulus for TSH release via TRH (32), whereas other hypothalamic peptides (dopamine, somatostatin), neuropeptides (neurotensin, serotonin, norepinephrine, cholecystokinin), and steroid hormones (estrogens, cortisol) directly or indirectly affect release of TSH (70).

The biological effects of TSH are dependent on the appropriate association of the α and β subunit and the binding of TSH to its receptor (specifically determined by the β subunit). The TSH receptor contains two subunits (A and B) linked by a disulfide bridge. The TSH receptor A subunit forms the binding site for TSH on the outside surface of the thyroid cell membrane, and the B subunit penetrates the cell membrane and, through its cytoplasmic domain, interacts with the regulatory subunits of adenylate cyclase (101). Glycosylation of both the α and β subunit, along with primary sequence specificity, influences binding of TSH to its receptor and hormone action (75, 107). This glycosylation is also under hormonal control by TRH and thyroid hormone (117).

TSH secretion leads to thyroid gland enlargement and increased formation and secretion of tetraiodothyronine (thyroxine) (T_4) and, to a lesser extent, triiodothyronine (T_3). The effect of TSH on the growth of thyroid follicular cells (both direct and permissive for other growth-promoting agents) operates independently of its effect on thyroid hormone production (106, 120).

Thyroid Hormone and the Thyroid Hormone Receptor

T_4 is the major hormone secreted by the thyroid gland, whereas T_3 (which is principally formed in target tissue from outer ring [5'] deiodinase of circulating T_4) is the metabolically active hormone (95). Although thyroid hormone has activity at the cell membrane (96) and mitochondria (23), its primary action in tissue involves T_3 binding to specific nuclear receptors. Thyroid hormones control development, growth, and metabolic rate.

The discovery that the product of a cellular oncogene (c-*erb* A) binds T_3 with the affinity and specificity characteristic of the T_3 receptor (91, 115) suggested that the thyroid hormone receptor should have a structure and a function similar to it and the homologous superfamily of intracellular steroid hormone and retinoic acid receptors. Molecular cloning techniques have found two distinct nuclear thyroid hormone receptors (α and β) with additional subtypes (61). The tissue patterns of expression of each form of the thyroid hormone receptor and unique thyroid hormone response elements determine the biological effects of thyroid hormone by increasing or decreasing the rates of transcription of target genes. For example, thyroid hormone has a profound effect on brain development, including neuron cytostructure and neurotransmitter synthesis, binding, and degradation in a tissue-specific manner (38). This appears to involve the expression of an alternatively spliced, tissue-specific transcript from the thyroid receptor α gene (c-*erb* Aα2) which does not bind T_3 (61, 69).

Thyroid hormone is also the most important regulator of its own secretion, primarily by inhibiting the transcription of the α and β subunit genes of TSH at the pituitary. Thyroid hormone appears also to inhibit the transcription, translation, and secretion of TRH in the hypothalamus (52, 97, 122), although this may have little clinical importance in so much as wide variations in serum levels of T_4 and TSH appear to have little effect on hypothalamic TRH content (2, 15). Thyroid receptor binding to target genes is mediated by two highly conserved "zinc finger" structures formed by the tetrahedral coordination of zinc with four cysteine residues (26). Heterodimer and homodimer formation of the T_3 receptor (in particular with the retinoic acid receptor) in a leucine zipperlike motif appears to be necessary for some of its effect on transcriptional activity (30, 39).

It has been reported that several disorders of thyroid hormone resistance are a result of single gene deletions of the thyroid hormone receptor (see section on Hypothyroidism—Generalized Thyroid Hormone Resistance). Based on the clinical observations of individuals with selective (pituitary) and generalized thyroid hormone resistance, it has become apparent that the primary control of thyroid hormone is not based on its peripheral metabolic effects but on a tissue-specific effect of "free" hormone. Individuals have been reported with severe pituitary and peripheral thyroid hormone resistance who are clinically hypothyroid (55, 62, 80), partial pituitary and peripheral thyroid hormone resistance who are euthyroid (48, 77, 80, 108), and selective resistance at the level of the pituitary who are hyperthyroid (14, 24, 25, 27, 35, 102, 116).

DISORDERS AND CLINICAL EVALUATION

Hyperthyroidism

Hyperthyroidism or thyrotoxicosis is a hypermetabolic state that is secondary to the peripheral tissue effects of thyroid hormone excess. Tachycardia, heat intolerance, weight loss, diarrhea, tremor, polyuria, and emotional lability define the clinical syndrome, although it can occasionally be subtle and elderly patients can present with apathy or primary cardiac problems.

In the most common conditions causing hyperthyroidism (Graves' disease, toxic multinodular goiter, and toxic adenoma), serum TSH is suppressed and not measurable after the administration of TRH. In central hyperthyroidism, the level of basal or TRH-stimulated TSH is inappropriately normal or elevated in the presence of an elevated thyroid hormone level. This has been referred to as "inappropriate" secretion of TSH (116). More sensitive measurements of TSH by

chemoluminescence or immunoradiometric sandwich assays (which can measure normal and low levels of TSH) have facilitated the recognition of central hyperthyroidism.

Central hyperthyroidism must be distinguished from other causes of hyperthyroxinemia that are not associated with goiter or the clinical syndrome of thyrotoxicosis (euthyroid hyperthyroxinemia). The most frequently occurring of these disorders are thyroxine-binding abnormalities (acquired and congenital), transient hyperthyroxinemia of acute medical or psychiatric illness, and generalized thyroid hormone resistance. Because the symptoms of hyperthyroidism are not unique to thyrotoxicosis, the clinical diagnosis can often be difficult to make. Commercially available assays of "free thyroxine" levels are not reliable in confirming the diagnosis of thyrotoxicosis, unless performed by equilibrium dialysis. Sex-hormone-binding globulin, angiotensin-converting enzyme, and ferritin are hepatic proteins whose levels are increased by thyroid hormone, and their measurements, along with basal metabolic rate, deep tendon reflex relaxation time, and cardiac systolic time intervals have been used to help distinguish hyperthyroidism from euthyroid hyperthyroxinemia (7, 105).

Inappropriate Secretion of TSH

Clinical syndromes of inappropriate TSH secretion and hyperthyroidism have been divided into those that are associated with pituitary TSH-secreting adenomas and nontumor selective (pituitary) thyroid hormone resistance.

TSH-Secreting Pituitary Adenomas.— Since the first reported case in 1970 (42), almost 100 additional cases of TSH-secreting adenomas have been reported in the world literature, and estimates suggest that these cases account for less than 1% of all pituitary tumors (3, 87). The clinical presentation is usually that of hyperthyroidism in individuals with a symmetrical goiter who, often, are treated as if they have Graves' disease or autoimmune thyroid disease (with antithyroid drugs, radioactive iodine, or thyroid operation) before the true diagnosis is made (99, 116). However, patients can be euthyroid

(37, 57, 87, 93) or hypothyroid without a history of hyperthyroidism (21, 29, 112).

The time to diagnosis after the onset of symptoms has ranged from two to nine years (3, 68). The age at presentation has been reported to range from 17 to 84 years, with an almost equal sex distribution (3). Most individuals present with macroadenomas (although microadenomas have been reported), sellar erosion, and extrasellar extension (3, 27, 68). Headaches, facial pain, visual-field abnormalities, loss of vision, and cranial nerve palsies (in particular the sixth cranial nerve) are commonly associated with these large aggressive tumors (68).

TSH levels have been reported to range from 1.5 to 565 mIU/L (3, 27, 34, 99), with one series reporting a TSH value (mean ± standard deviation) of 12.7 ± 14 mIU/L (3). TSH has been shown to "up-regulate" the TSH receptor in the thyroid at these levels reported for TSH-secreting adenomas; this might explain the clinical observation of hyperthyroidism as opposed to euthyroidism or hypothyroidism that might result from "down-regulation" of the TSH receptor after prolonged exposure to TSH (20, 50, 104). Individuals with TSH-producing pituitary tumors may secrete disproportionate amounts of α subunit (58), and a molar ratio (α subunit-to-TSH) greater than 1 has been one of the better discriminating factors for TSH-secreting adenomas (3). TSH-secreting adenomas have generally not been found to have TRH receptors (98), and TRH does not usually stimulate TSH secretion in individuals with such adenomas (27, 99). However, individuals with proven TSH-secreting adenomas have been reported to have TSH and α subunit increases of as high as 100% above the baseline after TRH stimulation (3, 27, 34, 99). Thus, the presence of a TSH response to TRH cannot be used to exclude the diagnosis of a TSH-secreting adenoma.

TSH-secreting adenomas can cosecrete other hormones besides TSH and its α subunit. Growth hormone (with clinical acromegaly being the most frequent syndrome), prolactin, and the gonadotropins are the most commonly cosecreted hormones. Prolactin elevations are frequently less than 100 pg/mL and not always diagnostic of cosecretion, but they raise the possibility of a hypothalamic or "stalk" effect. Immunostaining the TSH-secreting adenomas often demonstrates the presence of growth hormone, prolactin, and FSH or LH within tumor cells. Paradoxical responses of TSH secretion to gonadotropin-releasing hormone (GnRH) and growth hormone releasing hormone (GHRH) can also be seen (3, 60). The significance of the colocalization of various other neuroendocrine peptides (including substance P, neuropeptide-Y, neuromedin-B, galanin, and met-enkephalin) to the thyrotroph and TSH-secreting adenomas is not understood (84, 85). These peptides have short half-lives and are not clinically measurable, suggesting a possible paracrine or autocrine function. It is uncertain whether this colocalization is an expression of neoplastic transformation or of peptides found in a common progenitor cell.

Localization should be by high-resolution computed tomography with contrast material or by gadolinium-enhanced magnetic resonance imaging of the sella. Macroadenomas and microadenomas are usually visible by these techniques, whereas preoperative lateralization of microadenomas has been detected with petrosal sinus sampling and simultaneous TRH testing (31).

The growth of TSH-secreting adenomas is poorly understood. Thyrotroph hyperplasia and possibly progression to adenoma formation are known to occur in the setting of primary hypothyroidism because of the loss of thyroxine's negative feedback on the pituitary and hypothalamus (68, 94). TSH-secreting adenomas (microadenomas and macroadenomas) appear more aggressive than non-TSH-secreting pituitary tumors (68). Therapy directed to the hyperthyroidism only, without considering the possible secondary growth effects that this treatment may have on these adenomas, could potentiate their aggressiveness. For this reason, neurosurgery is the treatment of choice for TSH-secreting pituitary adenomas. Surgical cure rates (defined as a resolution of hyperthyroidism; normalization of TSH, α subunit, or other cosecreted hormones; and lack of recurrence noted at follow-up radiographic examination) have been as high as

50%, with a mean follow-up period after surgery of 54 months and relapses occurring as late as 5 years after surgery (3, 27, 68). Surgical approaches have required both transsphenoidal and transcranial approaches (68). Successful resection is more likely to occur when the size of the tumor is less than 2 cm (68).

Although radiotherapy has been advocated after subtotal resection of TSH-secreting tumors (27, 68), limited numbers of patients make it difficult to determine if it has a significant effect on the growth and secretion of these tumors (68). Somatostatin has shown the most promise for the presurgical treatment of hyperthyroidism and as an adjunctive medical therapy for surgically unresected tissue (5, 17, 40, 66, 98, 118). Although reports have suggested improvement in visual fields with somatostatin (68), it has caused measurable regression in tumor size infrequently (4, 98). The long-term administration of dopaminergic drugs (i.e., bromocriptine) has had limited success and generally, at best, has been associated with modest clinical improvement and reduction in TSH and thyroid hormone levels (27).

Selective (Pituitary) Thyroid Hormone Resistance

Central hyperthyroidism secondary to selective (pituitary) thyroid hormone resistance (non-neoplastic central hyperthyroidism) was first reported by Gershengorn and Weintraub (33) and, since that time, has been described in approximately 30 individuals (27). The typical presentation of a patient with this syndrome is a symmetrical goiter with hyperthyroidism. Symptoms of hyperthyroidism are typically mild, possibly due to a degree of coexisting peripheral resistance (14, 27). The male-to-female ratio was reported as 2:1 and the age range was from 3 months to 80 years (27, 74).

No structural abnormalities have been noted in the hypothalamus or pituitary of individuals with selective (pituitary) thyroid hormone resistance, except for two individuals with an "empty sella" (27, 47). Selective (pituitary) thyroid hormone resistance has also been described in isolated cases with pregnancy (76, 103), autoimmune thyroid

disease (with hypothyroidism and hyperthyroidism) (47, 76), multinodular goiter (111), hypergonadotrophic hypogonadism (92), and cystinosis (8).

TSH levels have ranged from 1 to 180 mIU/L (25% within the normal range) and α subunit:TSH molar ratios have been reported to be less than 1 (14, 27). TSH response to TRH stimulation is normal or exaggerated in selective (pituitary) thyroid hormone resistance (14, 27, 83, 116).

Lowering thyroid hormone levels with antithyroid drugs, radioactive iodine, or thyroid surgery may control the symptoms of hyperthyroidism but it has frequently led to increases in TSH levels (27). These forms of treatment alone are not recommended because of the concern that this could induce thyrotroph hyperplasia and adenoma formation. T_3, which has no effect on the secretion of TSH from TSH-secreting adenomas, has been used diagnostically and therapeutically to lower TSH levels in individuals with pituitary thyroid hormone resistance (53, 83), but, because of its metabolic effects, an increase in the symptoms of hyperthyroidism often occurs (59). Although dopamine agonists and antagonists have acutely decreased and increased TSH, respectively (6, 27, 64), the long-term success of bromocriptine has not been consistent (33, 89, 92). Somatostatin has had variable success in lowering TSH levels in selective (pituitary) thyroid hormone resistance (5, 14, 121). Pharmacologic doses of glucocorticoids have been required to suppress TSH secretion and, in general, have not been used because of the subsequent undesirable side effects (33, 59, 102). TRIAC (3,5,3'-triiodothyroacetic acid), a metabolite of T_3, and D-thyroxine have been shown to inhibit TSH release and, at the same time, lack the peripheral metabolic effects of thyroid hormone (10, 22, 43, 59, 80, 89). It may be that these drugs, along with primary management of the hyperthyroidism, will be the treatment of choice for selective (pituitary) thyroid hormone resistance.

The precise genetic abnormality in selective (pituitary) thyroid hormone resistance has yet to be determined, despite the clinical observation of a familial pattern in some patients (83). Multiple genetic abnormalities have been postulated (109), including mutations in the pituitary-specific, β thyroid hormone receptor (β2 isoform). Two cases have been attributed to hypersecretion of hypothalamic TRH (18, 25).

Hypothyrodism

The diagnosis of central hypothyroidism requires a high index of suspicion. Thyroid hormone deficiency causes mental retardation in infants, growth delay in children, and the clinical syndrome of myxedema in adults. Symptoms of thyroid deficiency (cold intolerance, constipation, increased sleep demand, and lethargy) are common for both primary and secondary forms of hypothyroidism and can be very protean. In primary hypothyroidism, low T_3 and T_4 levels are accompanied by increased TSH levels, whereas a low or normal TSH measurement should make one suspect a central form of hypothyroidism. TSH levels are normal or slightly elevated in hypothyroidism associated with generalized thyroid hormone resistance.

TRH/TSH Deficiency

Hypothyroidism from TRH or TSH deficiency often results from destructive hypothalamic or pituitary processes (neoplastic, infectious, granulomatous, vascular, traumatic, autoimmune, and radiation necrosis) (27). Lesions involving the hypothalamus and pituitary and presenting with TRH and/or TSH deficiency are usually not subtle and are often associated with partial or total pituitary insufficiency. There appears to be a teleologic hierarchy of hormonal loss starting with the gonadotropins and then followed by TSH and corticotropin. The clinical presentation may also be dominated by hormonal hypersecretion (prolactin from prolactinomas, most commonly) or visual field loss. Neurologic symptoms (mental status changes, somnolence, and seizures) can occur but are not common unless there is an acute infarction or bleeding (apoplexy) (27).

The diagnosis of central hypothyroidism is often supported by an appropriate structural evaluation. Magnetic resonance imaging is much better than computed tomography in the assessment of the hypothalamus and is equally sensitive in the detection of micro-adenomas of the pituitary if sufficiently thin cuts are made. A standard magnetic resonance image or computed tomography of the brain is not sufficient and may miss even large abnormalities if careful attention is not given to the hypothalamus and pituitary region.

Under normal conditions, it has been reported (56) that there is a log-linear relationship between TSH and T_4. Although a certain percentage of the normal population can have low T_4 levels, a value less than 3 μg/dL is almost invariably associated with hypothyroidism (56). An elevated TSH value (the standard in securing the diagnosis of primary hypothyroidism) is not helpful in diagnosing central hypothyroidism, although levels of TSH reaching up to 10 mIU/L (27) and often lacking biological activity (28, 51) have been reported. TRH-stimulation testing has been reported to be potentially helpful in making the diagnosis of pituitary or hypothalamic hypothyroidism, but the decreased TSH responsiveness seen in the aging population (particularly elderly men) and the delayed peak often seen in euthyroid individuals has limited its clinical usefulness, thus it cannot be routinely recommended. An accompanying mild-to-moderate increase in serum prolactin values (less than 150 ng/mL) (secondary to the loss of the tonic inhibition by dopamine) or accompanying diabetes insipidus should lead one to consider hypothalamic dysfunction.

Generalized Thyroid Hormone Resistance

More than 200 patients with combined pituitary and peripheral thyroid hormone resistance (generalized thyroid hormone resistance) have been reported since it was first described in 1967 (80, 88). Although patients with generalized thyroid hormone resistance present with hyperthyroxinemia and a goiter, they are symptomatically euthyroid or have subtle findings of hypothyroidism (goiter, cognitive impairment, deaf mutism, retarded growth, and delayed skeletal maturation) (48, 80). Most often, individuals have already received inappropriate treatment for their hyperthyroxinemia prior to the recognition of their thyroid hormone resistance and have become clinically hypothyroid.

Autosomal dominant (36, 48, 62, 100) and

autosomal recessive (78) inheritance patterns have been described with this syndrome. Three affected families have been found to have single nucleic acid base mutations resulting in single amino acid substitutions in the hormone-binding domain of the β form of the T_3 receptor (88, 108, 109). The location of point mutations in these three families suggested abnormalities in their receptor dimerization, receptor affinity for thyroid hormone, or decreased receptor interaction with other transactivation factors (108). Other kindreds with generalized thyroid hormone resistance have been suspected of having prereceptor and postreceptor defects (13, 23, 123). The diversity of symptoms and presentations among families with generalized thyroid hormone resistance suggests that thyroid hormone resistance results from heterogeneous genetic abnormalities. It has been suggested, but not generally accepted, that the degree of thyroid hormone resistance may improve over time (65, 80). Individuals with generalized hormone resistance have been reported in families with selective (pituitary) thyroid hormone resistance (74).

Patients with generalized resistance to thyroid hormone have high serum free and total T_4 and T_3 levels, with normal or elevated TSH levels that respond to TRH stimulation and T_3 suppression. Basal TSH levels in one series were 4.1 ± 3.5 mIU/L (mean $\pm$ standard deviation) (100), with values reported to be as high as 350 mIU/L (81). Most individuals have elevated values for 24-hour radioactive iodine uptake (30% to 60%) (100).

In most cases, the individual with generalized thyroid hormone resistance does not require treatment because of adequate compensation by an already increased endogenous thyroid hormone level. Treatment designed to decrease thyroid hormone secretion is likely to be harmful and has been associated with iatrogenic growth failure, thyroid gland enlargement, and symptomatic hypothyroidism (81). Treatment with thyroid hormone replacement (particularly in infants and children) may be appropriate to avoid neuropsychologic sequelae that may result from subtle hypothyroidism, but it is not generally agreed that there is a relationship between mental dysfunction and thyroid hormone resistance (65, 81, 100, 119). It has been recognized clinically that athyrotic children are resistant to the negative feedback of T_4 and T_3 treatment and the lowering of TSH, without demonstrating peripheral resistance (12, 82). Because of this, in infancy, doses of thyroid hormone sufficient to suppress TSH may cause craniosynostosis and other peripheral manifestations of thyroid hormone excess. Clinical judgment and close monitoring of the dose of thyroid hormone given to children are essential. If an adult with generalized resistance to thyroid hormone has been treated with thyroid ablation (^{131}I or operation), large doses of thyroid hormone replacement are often needed to normalize serum TSH and TSH responses to TRH, and it is thought that these would be the best criteria for adequate thyroid hormone replacement (46).

Nonthyroidal Illness

The control of the peripheral metabolic effects of thyroid hormone and the neuroendocrine axis also appears to be important in an adaptive survival response to nonthyroidal illness by a transient expression of hypothyroidism (110).

Reduced extrathyroidal T_3 production resulting from (5') deiodinase inhibition occurs in almost all illnesses, and an accompanying reduced T_4 production from the thyroid is seen in the seriously ill (110). Reduced serum T_4 levels usually can be attributed to a decreased production of thyroid hormone binding proteins or to an inhibitor of binding of thyroid hormone (16, 110), whereas "free" thyroid hormone levels remain normal. In many seriously ill patients, however, low levels of "free" thyroxine and T_3, with decreased basal and TRH-stimulated TSH levels, have been reported (113, 114). Increases in T_4 and T_3 levels have correlated with the return of TSH secretion and clinical recovery (41, 110).

It is likely that alterations in one or more of the hypothalamic factors (glucocorticoids, dopamine, somatostatin) that regulate TSH secretion account for the normal or low levels of TSH seen despite the low thyroid hormone levels (T_3 and T_4) common to nonthyroidal illness. For example, cortisol secretion rates have been shown to influence the circadian rhythm of TSH physiologically as well as in stress and depression (1).

Because of the possible adaptive effect of diminished TSH secretion and subsequent decreased T_4 production, thyroid hormone replacement in the euthyroid sick syndrome is thought to be contraindicated. Although an increased TSH level can be seen in the recovery phase of nonthyroidal illness, its increase in an acutely ill patient is an indication for hormonal replacement. Significantly, low T_4 levels in the seriously ill intensive care patient are not reliable in predicting hypothyroidism, but they can be used as a marker of increased mortality (113).

SUMMARY

Thyroid hormone is controlled primarily by a neuroendocrine axis that is regulated in a classical negative-feedback manner. The introduction of sensitive and specific assays for TSH has greatly simplified the clinical assessment of primary hyperthyroidism and hypothyroidism to a point where a single measurement of TSH has been reported to be the best screening test for thyroid hormone dysfunction (44). The clinical recognition and assessment of central (secondary) forms of hyperthyroidism (TSH-secreting adenoma and selective [pituitary] thyroid hormone resistance) and hypothyroidism (TRH and/or TSH deficiency, generalized thyroid hormone resistance, and nonthyroidal illness) also have been facilitated by these more sensitive measures of TSH. Continued advances in our understanding of the molecular mechanisms of thyroid hormone action, along with an increasing ability to recognize syndromes of secondary thyroid hormone dysfunction, reinforce the important relationship between molecular and cellular biology and clinical practice.

REFERENCES

1. Aygerinos P.C., Tsekes G.A., Tzanela M., Vasilatou E., Nicolou C., Tzavara I., and Thalassinos N.C. Evidence for coordinated diurnal variations of ACTH and TSH in patients with Addison's disease. 73rd Annual Meeting. The Endocrine Society. June 1991; Abstract #761: Washington, D.C.
2. Bassiri R.M., and Utiger R.D. Thyrotropin-releasing hormone in the hypothalamus of the rat. Endocrinology, *94:*188–197, 1974.
3. Beckers A., Abs R., Mahler C., Vandalem J.-L., Pirens G., Hennen G., and Stevenaert A. Thyrotropin-secreting pituitary adenomas: report of seven cases. J. Clin. Endocrinol. Metab., *72:*477–483, 1991.
4. Beckers A., Hennen G., Reznik M., Thibaut A., and Stevenaert A. Les adénomes hypophysaires à TSH. Rev. Med. Liege, *43:*396–402, 1988.
5. Beck-Peccoz P., Mariotti S., Guillausseau P.J., Medri G., Piscitelli G., Bertoli A., Barbarino A., Rondena M., Chanson P., Pinchera A., and Faglia G. Treatment of hyperthyroidism due to inappropriate secretion of thyrotropin with the somatostatin analog SMS 201–995. J. Clin. Endocrinol. Metab., *68:*208–214, 1989.
6. Beck-Peccoz P., Piscitelli G., Cattaneo M.G., and Faglia G. Successful treatment of hyperthyroidism due to nonneoplastic pituitary TSH hypersecretion with 3,5,3'-triiodothyroacetic acid (TRIAC). J. Endocrinol. Invest., *6:*217–223, 1983.
7. Beck-Peccoz P., Roncoroni R., Mariotti S., Medri G., Marcocci C., Brabant G., Forloni F., Pinchera A., and Faglia G. Sex hormone-binding globulin measurement in patients with inappropriate secretion of thyrotropin (IST): evidence against selective pituitary thyroid hormone resistance in nonneoplastic IST. J. Clin. Endocrinol. Metab., *71:*19–25, 1990.
8. Bercu B.B., Orloff S., and Schulman J.D. Pituitary resistance to thyroid hormone in cystinosis. J. Clin. Endocrinol. Metab., *51:*1262–1268, 1980.
9. Brenner-Gati L., and Gershengorn M.C. Effects of thyrotropin-releasing hormone on phosphoinositides and cytoplasmic free calcium in thyrotropic pituitary cells. Endocrinology, *118:*163–169, 1986.
10. Burger A.G., Engler D., Sakoloff C., and Staeheli V. The effects of tetraiodothyroacetic and triiodothyroacetic acids on thyroid function in euthyroid and hyperthyroid subjects. Acta Endocrinol. (Copenh.), *92:*455–467, 1979.
11. Burgus R., Dunn T.F., Desiderio D., Ward D.N., Vale W., and Guillemin R. Characterization of ovine hypothalamic hypophysiotropic TSH-releasing factor. Nature, *226:*321–325, 1970.
12. Cavaliere H., Medeiros-Neto G.A., Rosner W., and Kourides I.A. Persistent pituitary resistance to thyroid hormone in congenital versus later-onset hypothyroidism. J. Endocrinol. Invest., *8:*527–532, 1985.
13. Chait A., Kanter R., Green W., and Kenny M. Defective thyroid hormone action in fibroblasts cultured from subjects with the syndrome of resistance to thyroid hormones. J. Clin. Endocrinol. Metab., *54:*767–772, 1982.
14. Chan A.W., MacFarlane I.A., van Heyningen C., and Foy P.M. Clinical hyperthyroidism due to non-neoplastic inappropriate thyrotrophin secretion. Postgrad. Med. J., *66:*743–746, 1990.
15. Ching M.C.-H., and Utiger R.D. Hypothalamic portal blood immunoreactive TRH in the rat: lack of effect of hypothyroidism and thyroid hormone treatment. J. Endocrinol. Invest., *6:*347–352, 1983.
16. Chopra I.J., Hershman J.M., Pardridge W.M., and

Nicoloff J.T. Thyroid function in nonthyroidal illnesses. Ann. Intern. Med., *98:*946–957, 1983.

17. Comi R.J., Gesundheit N., Murray L., Gorden P., and Weintraub B.D. Response of thyrotropin-secreting pituitary adenomas to a long-acting somatostatin analogue. N. Engl. J. Med., *317:*12–17, 1987.

18. Connell J.M.C., McCruden D.C., Davis D.L., and Alexander W.D. Bromocriptine for inappropriate thyrotropin secretion (letter to the editor). Ann. Intern. Med., *96:*251–252, 1982.

19. Crew F.A.E., and Wiesner B.P. On the existence of a fourth hormone, thyreotropic in nature, of the anterior pituitary. BMJ, *1:*777–778, 1930.

20. Davies T.F. Positive regulation of the guinea pig thyrotropin receptor. Endocrinology, *117:*201–207, 1985.

21. Dickstein G., and Barzilai D. Hypothyroidism secondary to biologically inactive thyroid-stimulating hormone secretion by a pituitary chromophobe adenoma: recovery after removal of the tumor. Arch. Intern. Med., *142:*1544–1545, 1982.

22. Dorey F., Strauch G., and Gayno J.P. Thyrotoxicosis due to pituitary resistance to thyroid hormones. Successful control with D thyroxine: a study in three patients. Clin. Endocrinol. (Oxf.), *32:*221–228, 1990.

23. Eil C., Fein H.G., Smith T.J., Furlanetto R.W., Bourgeois M., Stelling M.W., and Weintraub B.D. Nuclear binding of [^{125}I]triiodothyronine in dispersed cultured skin fibroblasts from patients with resistance to thyroid hormone. J. Clin. Endocrinol. Metab., *55:*502–510, 1982.

24. Emerson C.H. Central hypothyroidism and hyperthyroidism. Med. Clin. North Am., *69:*1019–1034, 1985 Sept.

25. Emerson C.H., and Utiger R.D. Hyperthyroidism and excessive thyrotrophin secretion. N. Engl. J. Med., *287:*328–333, 1972.

26. Evans R.M., Hollenberg S.M. Zinc fingers: gilt by association. Cell, *52:*1–3, 1988.

27. Faglia G., Beck-Peccoz P., Piscitelli G., and Medri G. Inappropriate secretion of thyrotropin by the pituitary. Horm. Res., *26:*79–99, 1987.

28. Faglia G., Bitensky L., Pinchera A., Ferrari C., Paracchi A., Beck-Peccoz P., Ambrosi B., and Spada A. Thyrotropin secretion in patients with central hypothyroidism: evidence for reduced biological activity of immunoreactive thyrotropin. J. Clin. Endocrinol. Metab., 48:989–998, 1979.

29. Fatourechi V., Gharib H., Scheithauer B.W., Meybody N.A., and Gharib M. Pituitary thyrotropic adenoma associated with congenital hypothyroidism: report of two cases. Am. J. Med., *76:*725–728, 1984.

30. Forman B.M., Yang C.-r., Au M., Casanova J., Ghysdael J., and Samuels H.H. A domain containing leucine-zipper-like motifs mediate novel *in vivo* interactions between the thyroid hormone and retinoic acid receptors. Mol. Endocrinol., *3:*1610–1626, 1989.

31. Frank S.J., Gesundheit N., Doppman J.L., Miller D.L., Merriam G.R., Oldfield E.H., and Weintraub B.D. Preoperative lateralization of pituitary

microadenomas by petrosal sinus sampling: utility in two patients with non-ACTH-secreting tumors. Am. J. Med., *87:*679–682, 1989.

32. Gershengorn M.C. Thyrotropin releasing hormone: a review of the mechanisms of acute stimulation of pituitary hormone release. Mol. Cell. Biochem., *45:*163–179, 1982.

33. Gershengorn M.C., and Weintraub B.D. Thyrotropin-induced hyperthyroidism caused by selective pituitary resistance to thyroid hormone: a new syndrome of "inappropriate secretion of TSH." J. Clin. Invest., *56:*633–642, 1975.

34. Gesundheit N., Petrick P.A., Nissim M., Dahlberg P.A., Doppman J.L., Emerson C.H., Braverman L.E., Oldfield E.H., and Weintraub B.D. Thyrotropin-secreting pituitary adenomas: clinical and biochemical heterogeneity: case reports and follow-up of nine patients. Ann. Intern. Med., *111:*827–835, 1989.

35. Gharib H., Carpenter P.C., Scheithauer B.W., and Service F.J. The spectrum of inappropriate pituitary thyrotropin secretion associated with hyperthyroidism. Mayo Clin. Proc., *57:*556–563, 1982.

36. Gharib H., and Klee G.G. Familial euthyroid hyperthyroxinemia secondary to pituitary and peripheral resistance to thyroid hormones. Mayo Clin. Proc., *60:*9–15, 1985.

37. Girod C., Trouillas J., and Claustrat B. The human thyrotropic adenoma: pathologic diagnosis in five cases and critical review of the literature. Semin. Diagn. Pathol., *3:*58–68, 1986.

38. Glass C.K., and Holloway J.M. Regulation of gene expression by the thyroid hormone receptor. Biochim. Biophys. Acta, *1032:*157–176, 1990.

39. Glass C.K., Lipkin S.M., Devary O.V., and Rosenfeld M.G. Positive and negative regulation of gene transcription by a retinoic acid-thyroid hormone receptor heterodimer. Cell, *59:*697–708, 1989.

40. Guillausseau P.J., Chanson P., Timsit J., Warnet A., Lajeunie E., Duet M., and Lubetski J. Visual improvement with SMS 201–995 in a patient with a thyrotropin-secreting pituitary adenoma (letter to the editor). N. Engl. J. Med., *317:*53–54, 1987.

41. Hamblin P.S., Dyer S.A., Mohr V.S., Le Grand B.A., Lim C.-F., Tuxen D.V., Topliss D.J., and Stockigt J.R. Relationship between thyrotropin and thyroxine changes during recovery from severe hypothyroxinemia of critical illness. J. Clin. Endocrinol. Metab., *62:*717–722, 1986.

42. Hamilton C.R. Jr., Adams L.C., and Maloof F. Hyperthyroidism due to thyrotropin-producing pituitary chromophobe adenoma. N. Engl. J. Med., *283:*1077–1080, 1970.

43. Hamon P., Bovier-Lapierre M., Robert M., Peynaud D., Pugeat M., and Orgiazzi J. Hyperthyroidism due to selective pituitary resistance to thyroid hormones in a 15-month-old boy: efficacy of D-thyroxine therapy. J. Clin. Endocrinol. Metab., *67:*1089–1093, 1988.

44. Hay I.D., and Klee G.G. Thyroid dysfunction. Endocrinol. Metab. Clin. North Am., *17:*473–509, 1988.

45. Hershman J.M. Clinical application of thyrotro-

pin-releasing hormone. N. Engl. J. Med., *290:*886–890, 1974.

46. Hoffman D.P., Surks M.I., Oppenheimer J.H., and Weitzman E.D. Response to thyrotropin releasing hormone: an objective criterion for the adequacy of thyrotropin suppression therapy. J. Clin. Endocrinol. Metab., *44:*892–901, 1977.

47. Hoffman W.H., England B.G., Gomez L.M., Rosculet G., and Gala R.R. Empty sella associated with inappropriate TSH secretion. Neuropediatrics, *18:*37–39, 1987.

48. Hopwood N.J., Sauder S.E., Shapiro B., and Sisson J.C. Familial partial peripheral and pituitary resistance to thyroid hormone: a frequently missed diagnosis? Pediatrics, *78:*1114–1122, 1986.

49. Hoskins R.G. The thyroid-pituitary apparatus as a servo (feed-back) mechanism (editorial). J. Clin. Endocrinol., *9:*1429–1431, 1949.

50. Huber G.K., Concepcion E.S., Graves P.N., and Davies T.F. Positive regulation of human thyrotropin receptor mRNA by thyrotropin. J. Clin. Endocrinol. Metab., *72:*1394–1396, 1991.

51. Illig R., Krawczynska H., Torresani T., and Prader A. Elevated plasma TSH and hypothyroidism in children with hypothalamic hypopituitarism. J. Clin. Endocrinol. Metab., *41:*722–728, 1975.

52. Iriuchijima T., Rogers D., and Wilber J.F. L-triiodothyronine (L-T_3) can inhibit thyrotropin-releasing hormone (TRH) secretion from rat hypothalami in vitro [Abstract]. Clin. Res., *32:*865A, 1984.

53. Isales C.M., Tamborlane W., Gertner J.M., Genel M., Insogna K.L. Effect of short-term somatostatin and long-term triiodothyronine administration in a child with nontumorous inappropriate thyrotropin secretion. J. Pediatr., *112:*51–55, 1988.

54. Iversen E. Thyrotropin-releasing hormone cannot be detected in plasma from normal subjects. J. Clin. Endocrinol. Metab., *63:*516–519, 1986.

55. Kaplan M.M., Swartz S.L., and Larsen P.R. Partial peripheral resistance to thyroid hormone. Am. J. Med., *70:*1115–1121, 1981.

56. Klee G.G., and Hay I.D. Sensitive thyrotropin assays: analytic and clinical performance criteria. Mayo Clin. Proc., *63:*1123–1132, 1988.

57. Koide Y., Kugai N., Kimura S., Fujita T., Kameya T., Azukizawa M., Ogata E., Tomono Y., and Yamashita K. A case of pituitary adenoma with possible simultaneous secretion of thyrotropin and follicle-stimulating hormone. J. Clin. Endocrinol. Metab., *54:*397–403, 1982.

58. Kourides I.A., Ridgway E.C., Weintraub B.D., Bigos S.T., Gershengorn M.C., and Maloof F. Thyrotropin-induced hyperthyroidism: use of alpha and beta subunit levels to identify patients with pituitary tumors. J. Clin. Endocrinol. Metab., *45:*534–543, 1977.

59. Kunitake J.M., Hartman N., Henson L.C., Lieberman J., Williams D.E., Wong M., and Hershman J.M. 3,5,3'-Triiodothyroacetic acid therapy for thyroid hormone resistance. J. Clin. Endocrinol. Metab., *69:*461–466, 1989.

60. Kuzuya N., Inoue K., Ishibashi M., Murayama Y., Koide Y., Ito K., Yamaji T., and Yamashita K.

Endocrine and immunohistochemical studies on thyrotropin (TSH)-secreting pituitary adenomas: responses of TSH, α-subunit, and growth hormone to hypothalamic releasing hormones and their distribution in adenoma cells. J. Clin. Endocrinol. Metab., *71:*1103–1111, 1990.

61. Lazar M.A., Chin W.W. Nuclear thyroid hormone receptors. J. Clin. Invest., *86:*1777–1782, 1990.

62. Linde R., Alexander N., Island D.P., and Rabin D. Familial insensitivity of the pituitary and periphery to thyroid hormone: a case report in two generations and a review of the literature. Metabolism, *31:*510–513, 1982.

63. Lombardi G., Lupoli G., Scopacasa F., Panza R., and Minozzi M. Plasma immunoreactive thyrotropin releasing hormone (TRH) values in normal newborns. J. Endocrinol. Invest., *1:*69–72, 1978.

64. Magee B., Sheridan B., Scanlon M.F., and Atkinson A.B. Inappropriate thyrotrophin secretion, increased dopaminergic tone and preservation of the diurnal rhythm in serum TSH. Clin. Endocrinol. (Oxf.), *24:*209–215, 1986.

65. Magner J.A., Petrick P., Menezes-Ferreira M.M., Stelling M., and Weintraub B.D. Familial generalized resistance to thyroid hormones: report of three kindreds and correlation of patterns of affected tissues with the binding of [^{125}I] triiodothyronine to fibroblast nuclei. J. Endocrinol. Invest., *9:*459–470, 1986.

66. Malarkey W.B., Kovacs K., and O'Dorisio T.M. Response of a GH- and TSH-secreting pituitary adenoma to a somatostatin analogue (SMS 201-995): evidence that GH and TSH coexist in the same cell and secretory granules. Neuroendocrinology, *49:*267–274, 1989.

67. Mallik T.K., Wilber J.F., and Pegues J. Measurements of thyrotropin-releasing hormone-like material in human peripheral blood by affinity chromatography and radioimmunoassay. J. Clin. Endocrinol. Metab., *54:*1194–1198, 1982.

68. McCutcheon I.E., Weintraub B.D., and Oldfield E.H. Surgical treatment of thyrotropin-secreting pituitary adenomas. J. Neurosurg., *73:*674–683, 1990.

69. Mitsuhashi T., and Nikodem V.M. Regulation of expression of the alternative mRNAs of the rat α-thyroid hormone receptor gene. J. Biol. Chem., *264:*8900–8904, 1989.

70. Morley J.E. Neuroendocrine control of thyrotropin secretion. Endocr. Rev., *2:*396–436, 1981.

71. Nair R.M.G., Barrett J.F., Bowers C.Y., and Schally A.V. Structure of porcine thyrotropin releasing hormone. Biochemistry, *9:*1103–1106, 1970.

72. Nelson B.D. Thyroid hormone regulation of mitochondrial function. Comments on the mechanism of signal transduction. Biochim. Biophys. Acta, *1018:*275–277, 1990.

73. Oliver C., Charvet J.P., Codaccioni J.-L., and Vague J. Radioimmunoassay of thyrotropin-releasing hormone (TRH) in human plasma and urine. J. Clin. Endocrinol. Metab., *39:*406–409, 1974.

74. Pagliara A.S., Caplan R.H., Gundersen C.B.,

Wickus G.G., and Elston A.C.V. III. Peripheral resistance to thyroid hormone in a family: heterogeneity of clinical presentation. J. Pediatr., *103*:228–232, 1983.

75. Pierce J.G., and Parsons T.F. Glycoprotein hormones: structure and function. Annu. Rev. Biochem., *50*:465–495, 1981.

76. Pillay N.L., Jialal I., Governder P.A., Green-Thompson R.W., and Joubert S.M. Graves' disease and selective resistance of pituitary thyrotroph to thyroid hormone: a case report. S. Afr. Med. J., *70*:360–361, 1986.

77. Refetoff S. Syndromes of thyroid hormone resistance. Am. J. Physiol., *243*:E88–E98, 1982.

78. Refetoff S., DeGroot L.J., and Barsano C.P. Defective thyroid hormone feedback regulation in the syndrome of peripheral resistance to thyroid hormone. J. Clin. Endocrinol. Metab., *51*:41–45, 1980.

79. Refetoff S., DeGroot L.J., Benard B., and DeWind L.T. Studies of a sibship with apparent hereditary resistance to the intracellular action of thyroid hormone. Metabolism, *21*:723–756, 1972.

80. Refetoff S., DeWind L.T., and DeGroot L.J. Familial syndrome combining deaf-mutism, stippled epiphyses, goiter and abnormally high PBI: possible target organ refractoriness to thyroid hormone. J. Clin. Endocrinol. Metab., *27*:279–294, 1967.

81. Refetoff S., Salazar A., Smith T.J., and Scherberg N.H. The consequences of inappropriate treatment because of failure to recognize the syndrome of pituitary and peripheral tissue resistance to thyroid hormone. Metabolism, *32*:822–834, 1983.

82. Rettig K.R., Sargeant D.T., and Kemp S.F. Resistance to the effects of thyroid hormone in children. South. Med. J., *80*:1316–1318, 1987.

83. Rösler A., Litvin Y., Hage C., Gross J., and Cerasi E. Familial hyperthyroidism due to inappropriate thyrotropin secretion successfully treated with triiodothyronine. J. Clin. Endocrinol. Metab., *54*:76–82, 1982.

84. Roth K.A., and Krause J.E. Substance-P is present in a subset of thyrotrophs in the human pituitary. J. Clin. Endocrinol. Metab., *71*:1089–1095, 1990.

85. Roth K.A., Lorenz R.G., McKeel D.W., Leykam J., Barchas J.D., and Tyler A.N. Methionine-enkephalin and thyrotropin-stimulating hormone are intimately related in the human anterior pituitary. J. Clin. Endocrinol. Metab., *66*:804–810, 1988.

86. Saberi M., and Utiger R.D. Augmentation of thyrotropin responses to thyrotropin-releasing hormone following small decreases in serum thyroid hormone concentrations. J. Clin. Endocrinol. Metab., *40*:435–441, 1975.

87. Saeger W., and Lüdecke D.K. Pituitary adenomas with hyperfunction of TSH. Frequency, histological classification, immunocytochemistry and ultrastructure. Virchows Arch. [A]., *394*:255–267, 1982.

88. Sakurai A., Takeda K., Ain K., Ceccarelli P., Nakai A., Seino S., Bell G.I., Refetoff S., and DeGroot L.J. Generalized resistance to thyroid hormone associated with a mutation in the ligand-binding domain of the human thyroid hormone receptor β. Proc. Natl. Acad. Sci. USA, *86*:8977–8981, 1989.

89. Salmela P.I., Wide L., Juustila H., and Ruokonen A. Effects of thyroid hormones (T_4,T_3), bromocriptine and TRIAC on inappropriate TSH hypersecretion. Clin. Endocrinol. (Oxf.), *28*:497–507, 1988.

90. Samuels M.H., Wood W.M., Gordon D.F., Kleinschmidt-DeMasters B.K., Lillehei K., and Ridgway E.C. Clinical and molecular studies of a thyrotropin-secreting pituitary adenoma. J. Clin. Endocrinol. Metab., *68*:1211–1215, 1989.

91. Sap J., Muñoz A., Damm K., Goldberg Y., Ghysdael J., Leutz A., Beug H., Vennström B. The c-erb-*A* protein is a high-affinity receptor for thyroid hormone. Nature, *324*:635–640, 1986.

92. Sato M., Otokida K., and Kato M. A case of hyperthyroidism caused by the syndrome of inappropriate secretion of thyroid stimulating hormone: association of primary hypergonadotropic hypogonadism. Jpn. J. Med., *28*:223–227, 1989.

93. Scanlon M.F., Howells S., Peters J.R., Williams E.D., Richards S., Hall R., and Thomas J.P. Hyperprolactinaemia, amenorrhoea and galactorrhoea due to a pituitary thyrotroph adenoma. Clin. Endocrinol. (Oxf.), *23*:35–42, 1985.

94. Scheithauer B.W., Kovacs K., Randall R.V., and Ryan N. Pituitary gland in hypothyroidism: histologic and immunocytologic study. Arch. Pathol. Lab. Med., *109*:499–504, 1985.

95. Schimmel M., and Utiger R.D. Thyroidal and peripheral production of thyroid hormones: review of recent findings and their clinical implications. Ann. Intern. Med., *87*:760–768, 1977.

96. Segal J., Schwartz H., and Gordon A. The effect of triiodothyronine on 2-deoxy-D-[1-^{3}H] glucose uptake in cultured chick embryo heart cells. Endocrinology, *101*:143–149, 1977.

97. Segerson T.P., Kauer J., Wolfe H.C., Mobtaker H., Wu P., Jackson I.M.D., and Lechan R.M. Thyroid hormone regulates TRH biosynthesis in the paraventricular nucleus of the rat hypothalamus. Science, *238*:78–80, 1987.

98. Shaker J.L., Brickner R.C., Sirus S.R., and Cerletty J.M. Octreotide acetate-induced size reduction of a large thyrotropin (TSH)-secreting pituitary tumor with correction of hyperthyroidism and hypopituitarism. 73rd Annual Meeting [Abstract # 1138]. The Endocrine Society. Washington, D.C. June 1991.

99. Smallridge R.C. Thyrotropin-secreting pituitary tumors. Endocrinol. Metab. Clin. North Am., *16*:765–792, 1987 Sept.

100. Smallridge R.C., Parker R.A., Wiggs E.A., Rajagopal K.R., and Fein H.G. Thyroid hormone resistance in a large kindred: physiologic, biochemical, pharmacologic, and neuropsychologic studies. Am. J. Med., *86*:289–296, 1989.

101. Smith B.R., and Furmaniak J. Structural analysis of the TSH receptor. Horm. Metab. Res. Suppl., *23*:28–32, 1990.

102. Spanheimer R.G., Bar R.S., and Hayford J.C. Hyperthyroidism caused by inappropriate thyrotro-

pin hypersecretion: studies in patients with selective pituitary resistance to thyroid hormone. Arch. Intern. Med., *142:*1283–1286, 1982.

103. Spitz I.M., Sheinfeld M., Glasser B., and Hirsch H.J. Hyperthyroidism due to inappropriate TSH secretion with associated hyperprolactinaemia—a case report and review of the literature. Postgrad. Med. J., *60:*328–335, 1984.

104. Takasu N., Charrier B., Mauchamp J., and Lissitzky S. Positive and negative regulation by thyrotropin of thyroid cyclic AMP response to thyrotropin in porcine thyroid cells. FEBS Lett., *84:*191–194, 1977.

105. Terzolo M., Orlandi F., Bassetti M., Medri G., Paccotti P., Cortelazzi D., Angeli A., and Beck-Peccoz P. Hyperthyroidism due to a pituitary adenoma composed of two different cell types, one secreting α-subunit alone and another cosecreting α-subunit and thyrotropin. J. Clin. Endocrinol. Metab., *72:*415–421, 1991.

106. Teuscher J., Peter H.-J., Gerber H., Berchtold R., and Studer H. Pathogenesis of nodular goiter and its implications for surgical management. Surgery, *103:*87–93, 1988.

107. Thotakura N.R., Desai R.K., and Szkudlinski M.W. The role of carbohydrate chains of TSH alpha and beta subunits in hormone activity. 73rd Annual Meeting [Abstract #824]. The Endocrine Society. Washington, D.C., June 1991.

108. Usala S.J., Menke J.B., Watson T.L., Bérard J., Bradley W.E.C., Bale A.E., Lash R.W., and Weintraub B.D. A new point mutation in the 3,5,3'-triiodothyronine-binding domain of the c-*erb*Aβ thyroid hormone receptor is tightly linked to generalized thyroid hormone resistance. J. Clin. Endocrinol. Metab., *72:*32–38, 1991.

109. Usala S.J., Tennyson G.E., Bale A.E., Lash R.W., Gesundheit N., Wondisford F.E., Accilli D., Hauser P., and Weintraub B.D. A base mutation of the C-erbAβ thyroid hormone receptor in a kindred with generalized thyroid hormone resistance: molecular heterogeneity in two other kindreds. J. Clin. Invest., *85:*93–100, 1990.

110. Utiger R.D. Thyrotropin-releasing hormone and thyrotropin secretion. J. Lab. Clin. Med., *109:*327–335, 1987.

111. Vesely D.L. Selective pituitary resistance to thyroid hormone after treatment of a toxic multinodular goiter. South. Med. J., *81:*1173–1176, 1988.

112. Wajchenberg B.L., Tsanaclis A.M.C., and Marino R. Jr. TSH-containing pituitary adenoma associated with primary hypothyroidism manifested by amenorrhoea and galactorrhoea. Acta Endocrinol. (Copenh.), *106:*61–66, 1984.

113. Wartofsky L., and Burman K.D. Alterations in thyroid function in patients with systemic illness: the "euthyroid sick syndrome." Endocr. Rev., *3:*164–217, 1982.

114. Wehmann R.E., Gregerman R.I., Burns W.H., Saral R., and Santos G.W. Suppression of thyrotropin in the low-thyroxine state of severe nonthyroidal illness. N. Engl. J. Med., *312:*546–552, 1985.

115. Weinberger C., Thompson C.C., Ong E.S., Lebo R., Gruol D.J., and Evans R.M. The c-erb-*A* gene encodes a thyroid hormone receptor. Nature, *324:*641–646, 1986.

116. Weintraub B.D., Gershengorn M.C., Kourides I.A., and Fein H. Inappropriate secretion of thyroid-stimulating hormone. Ann. Intern. Med., *95:*339–351, 1981.

117. Weintraub B.D., Stannard B.S., Magner J.A., Ronin C., Taylor T., Joshi L., Constant R.B., Menezes-Ferreira M.M., Petrick P., and Gesundheit N. Glycosylation and posttranslational processing of thyroid-stimulating hormone: clinical implications. Recent Prog. Horm. Res., *41:*577–606, 1985.

118. Wémeau J.L., Dewailly D., Leroy R., D'Herbomez M., Mazzuca M., Decoulx M., and Jaquet P. Long term treatment with the somatostatin analog SMS 201–995 in a patient with a thyrotropin- and growth hormone-secreting pituitary adenoma. J. Clin. Endocrinol. Metab., *66:*636–639, 1988.

119. Weiss R.E., Balzano S., Scherberg N.H., and Refetoff S. Neonatal detection of generalized resistance to thyroid hormone. JAMA, *264:*2245–2250, 1990.

120. Wilders-Truschnig M.M., Drexhage H.A., Leb G., Ober O., Brezinschek H.P., Dohr G., Lanzer G., and Krejs G.J. Chromatographically purified immunoglobulin G of endemic and sporadic goiter patients stimulates FRTL5 cell growth in a mitotic arrest assay. J. Clin. Endocrinol. Metab., *70:*444–452, 1990.

121. Williams G., Kraenzlin M., Sandler L., Burrin J., Law A., Bloom S., and Joplin G.F. Hyperthyroidism due to non-tumoural inappropriate TSH secretion: effect of a long-acting somatostatin analogue (SMS 201–995). Acta Endocrinol. (Copenh.), *113:*42–46, 1986.

122. Wondisford F.E., Farr E.A., Radovick S., Steinfelder H.J., Moates J.M., McClaskey J.H., and Weintraub B.D. Thyroid hormone inhibition of human thyrotropin β-subunit gene expression is mediated by a cis-acting element located in the first exon. J. Biol. Chem., *264:*14601–14604, 1989.

123. Wortsman J., Premachandra B.N., Williams K., Burman K.D., Hay I.D., and Davis P.J. Familial resistance to thyroid hormone associated with decreased transport across the plasma membrane. Ann. Intern. Med., *98:*904–909, 1983.

CHAPTER 10

Gonadotrophs: Regulation, Disorders and Clinical Evaluation

Mary H. Samuels, M.D.

REGULATION

The Hypothalamic-Pituitary-Gonadal (HPG) Axis

The gonadotropins, luteinizing hormone (LH) and follicle-stimulating hormone (FSH), are glycoproteins synthesized by the gonadotrophs of the anterior pituitary. Along with thyroid-stimulating hormone (TSH) and the placental glycoprotein, human chorionic gonadotropin (hCG), they are each composed of an α and a β subunit (14). The α subunit is common to all four glycoproteins, whereas the unique β subunits confer biological specificity to each hormone. Although uncombined subunits are secreted by the pituitary in normal and disease states, only the intact hormones are bioactive.

LH and FSH are regulated by the hypothalamic-pituitary-gonadal (HPG) axis (46). The major hypothalamic hormone that controls gonadotropin production is gonadotropin releasing hormone (GnRH), a decapeptide that is synthesized in the hypothalamus, travels down the median eminence via portal blood vessels, and stimulates LH and FSH synthesis and secretion. LH and FSH, in turn, travel through the systemic circulation and stimulate gonadal steroid (testosterone, estradiol, and progesterone) and peptide (the inhibins and activins) production, as well as gametogenesis. The gonadal hormones exert negative feedback on the pituitary and hypothalamus to decrease GnRH and gonadotropin levels. The sex steroids suppress LH to a greater extent than FSH, whereas the inhibins appear to preferentially suppress FSH levels. In addition to tonic negative feedback at the time of ovulation there is also positive feedback of estradiol to the pituitary, which initiates the LH surge and causes ovulation.

Pulsatile Release of Gonadotropins

The gonadotropins are secreted by the pituitary gland in a series of discrete pulses over 24 hrs. In normal men, this pulsatile pattern is relatively constant over time, with an average LH pulse interval of 90 to 120 min (65). In contrast, the gonadotropin pulse pattern in women changes during the menstrual cycle (11, 34, 68). The early follicular phase is characterized by LH pulses of moderate amplitude and an interpulse interval of 90 min. During the mid-follicular phase, LH pulse amplitude decreases, whereas frequency increases to approximately every 60 min, probably due to increasing estrogen production by the dominant follicle. During the late follicular phase, LH pulse frequency and amplitude both increase, resulting in the mid-cycle LH surge and ovulation. Finally, the luteal phase is characterized by infrequent LH pulses of high amplitude, probably due to progesterone production by the corpus luteum. FSH pulses are preferentially secreted during the early follicular phase, leading to follicle recruitment. During the mid-follicular phase, FSH pulses are selectively inhibited, and plasma FSH levels fall and remain low until the next follicular phase. Figure 10.1 illustrates representative 24-hr pul-

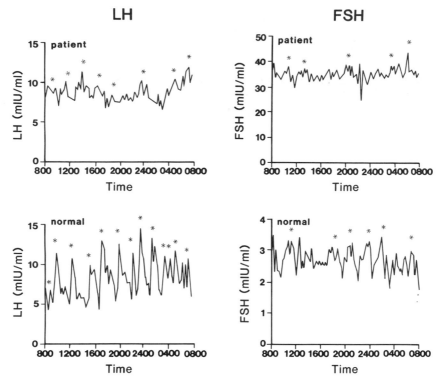

Figure 10.1   24-hr serum LH and FSH levels in the patient described in the case history (upper), compared to those in a normal male (lower). Blood samples were taken every 15 min over 24 hr, and LH and FSH levess were measured by immunoradiometric assays. Note the different y-axis scale for FSH in the patient. Significant hormone pulses were located by an objective pulse algorithm and are indicated by asterisks.

satile LH and FSH secretion in a normal individual.

Pulsatile LH and FSH secretion is due to the pulsatile release of GnRH from the hypothalamus, which, in turn, arises from the intermittent stimulation of GnRH neurons (34, 65). The relative predominance of LH or FSH secretion during the menstrual cycle seems to depend upon the frequency of GnRH pulses and circulating gonadal hormone levels, but may also be due to other, undefined factors (16, 17, 34). Recent evidence has shown that sex steroids are secreted from the gonad in pulses that are temporally linked to, and probably arise from, LH pulses (49, 68). The gonadal steroids, in turn, exert negative feedback on gonadotropin pulses by decreasing gonadotropin pulse amplitude and, in some cases, pulse frequency (43, 65). GnRH pulses also appear to regulate normal gonadotropin subunit synthesis, since maximal stimulation of LH gene

expression occurs over a narrow range of GnRH pulse patterns (17).

The pulsatile mode of GnRH secretion is essential to maintain gonadotropin pulses. In GnRH-deficient patients, pulses of GnRH at the correct frequency restore LH and FSH secretion, while continuous GnRH infusions suppress gonadotropin release (34, 62). Hypogonadism can result from disordered pulse patterns, even when basal hormone levels are normal (34, 53, 63, 65). In addition, recent data show that gonadotropin bioactivity, as well as immunoactivity, changes with GnRH pulse frequency and is altered in many hypothalamic-pituitary diseases that cause abnormal GnRH pulses (10).

Other Regulators of Gonadotroph Function

In addition to the HPG feedback loop, other central and peripheral factors affect gonadotropin production. For example, prolactin inhibits GnRH release and causes hypogonadism with altered gonadotropin pulses (56). During lactation, this postpones ovulation and subsequent pregnancy. However, in states of pathologic hyperprolactinemia, this leads to oligomenorrhea in women and impotence in men.

Exogenous opiates decrease gonadotropin release and may contribute to hypogonadism in habitual users of these drugs. In addition, endogenous opioids probably inhibit GnRH under normal conditions, since administration of opioid antagonists leads to increased gonadotropin pulses and increased bioactivity in healthy subjects. Therefore, increased endogenous opioids may contribute to hypogonadism, which is seen in conditions such as chronic illness or stress (9, 54, 65, 76).

Similarly, some studies have suggested that glucocorticoids suppress the HPG axis (32, 33, 38, 39, 69). If true, this may contribute to the high incidence of gonadal dysfunction seen in Cushing's syndrome (32, 38) and in patients receiving chronic glucocorticoid therapy (33). Physiologic activation of the hypothalamic-pituitary-adrenal axis due to severe stress or illness may result in similar reductions in gonadotroph function. Whether this is due to direct effects of cortisol or to suppression of the gonadal axis by corticotropin releasing hormone (CRH), adrenocorticotropin (ACTH), or other central mediators of stress, is unclear (5, 71).

Other central mediators of gonadotropin release are dopamine and somatostatin, which decrease LH levels and have minor effects on FSH levels (18, 22, 35, 52). Administration of dopamine antagonists increases LH levels (2, 56), suggesting that endogenous dopamine tone affects gonadotroph function in healthy subjects. The potential role of increased endogenous dopamine or somatostatin levels in the hypogonadism associated with certain diseases is unclear. (6)

DISORDERS

Hypogonadism

Clinical manifestations of hypogonadism depend on the sex and age of the patient. In prepubertal children, hypogonadism causes no symptoms, whereas in adolescents, it leads to delayed or absent pubertal development. In adult women, hypogonadism classically causes amenorrhea (arbitrarily defined as lack of menses for six months) but can also present as oligomenorrhea, anovulatory cycles, short luteal phase, or infertility. Other symptoms in women include loss of libido, vaginal dryness, and hot flashes. Physical examination may reveal breast atrophy and atrophic vaginitis. In men, hypogonadism causes loss of libido, erectile dysfunction, and infertility. Physical examination can reveal loss of lean body mass and muscle strength, gynecomastia, decreased beard growth, and testicular atrophy. Laboratory tests may show a mild anemia due to lack of the usual stimulation of erythropoiesis by testosterone.

The above findings occur in any patient with hypogonadism, whether it is central (pituitary or hypothalamic) or primary (gonadal) in origin. Further clues to possible central causes of hypogonadism include headaches, visual changes, galactorrhea, or dysfunction of other pituitary hormones. In addition, in women with hypogonadism, a careful history should be taken to check for possible "stress," exercise, or weight changes that could have caused the central hypogonadism. On the other hand, clues to possible peripheral causes of hypogonadism include a history of mumps, gonadal trauma, chemotherapy, or autoimmune diseases.

Primary hypogonadism occurs when the testis or ovary ceases functioning, such that sex hormones and sperm or ova are no longer produced. This interrupts the normal negative feedback to the pituitary and hypothalamus, and FSH and LH levels rise. FSH levels usually rise to a much greater extent (possibly due to loss of inhibin feedback) and, therefore, provide the most sensitive laboratory indicator of primary hypogonadism. If a patient with primary hypogonadism is studied over a 24-hr period, FSH and LH pulse frequency and amplitude are increased, confirming the loss of negative feedback by gonadal hormones (65). Thus, in a hypogonadal subject, a low testosterone or estradiol level and an elevated FSH level are virtually diagnostic of primary hypogonadism, except for the rare patient with a gonadotropin-secreting tumor (see below). In addition, when evaluating a woman with oligomenorrhea, care must be taken not to obtain gonadotropin levels near the tim of possible ovulation, since the ovulatory surge may cause gonadotropin levels to reach those seen in primary hypogonadism (11).

The causes of primary hypogonadism are diverse (Table 10.1). The most common cause in women is menopause, which occurs at an average age of approximately 51 years. Premature menopause is defined as primary hypogonadism before the age of 40 years and is due to genetic factors (for example, Turner's syndrome), or to autoimmune, viral, radiation, or drug-induced damage to the ovary. Similar diseases affect the testes; for example, men with Kleinfelter's syndrome (XXY) present with primary gonadal failure, decreased virilization, and gynecomastia. There also appears to be an age-related decline in testicular function in men, but the origins and clinical consequences of this entity are currently being debated (69).

Central hypogonadism occurs when the pituitary does not produce gonadotropins in sufficient amounts or in the normal pulsatile patterns. This leads to insufficient stimulation of the gonad, which, in turn, decreases gonadal hormone and germ cell production. Because normal gonadotropin pulses are essential for gonadal function, central hypogonadism is often seen with "normal" basal levels of LH and FSH. If these patients are studied over 24 hrs, however, abnormal pulse patterns are usually seen (53, 63). Therefore, a diagnosis of central hypogonadism is made when sex steroid levels are decreased and when basal gonadotropin levels are either decreased or normal. Central hypogonadism occurs in approximately 5% of adult women but is much less common in men. Causes can be divided into diseases that affect the pituitary and those that affect the hypothalamus (Table 10.1).

The most common pituitary disease associated with loss of gonadotroph function is a pituitary adenoma. These benign tumors, when large enough, compress or destroy normal gonadotrophs or interfere with normal hypothalamic input of GnRH by compressing the pituitary stalk. In addition, pituitary adenomas of any size that cause hyperprolactinemia may present with hypogonadism. Other pituitary mass lesions that lead to hypogonadism include meningiomas, craniopharyngiomas, dysgerminomas, Rathke's cleft cysts, metastatic tumors, and abscesses. Clues to the presence of a pituitary mass include headaches, visual changes, or extraocular movement disorders, since cranial nerves II, III, IV, or VI can be compressed by masses growing superiorly or laterally out of the sella. However, the absence of such symptoms in a patient with central hypogonadism does not exclude the diagnosis of a mass lesion, since gonadotroph function is often disrupted before the tumor reaches the optic chiasm or cavernous sinus. Therefore, unless there is an obvious reason for a patient's central hypogonadism (see discussion below on hypothalamic amenorrhea), a radiologic procedure should be performed to rule out a mass lesion.

Other diseases of the pituitary that cause hypogonadism include trauma or infarction. Head injury may lead to pituitary, pituitary stalk, or hypothalamic contusion and temporary or permanent hypogonadism (74), while pituitary infarction may follow obstet-

TABLE 10.1.
Causes of Hypogonadism

A. Primary hypogonadism
   Menopause (natural or surgical)
   Genetic (Turner's, Kleinfelter's)
   Autoimmune
   Viral (especially mumps)
   Radiation
   Chemotherapeutic agents (especially
     cyclophosphamide, busulfan)
B. Central hypogonadism
   Pituitary diseases
     Pituitary adenomas
     Other pituitary masses
     Trauma, infarction
     Lymphocytic hypophysitis
     Empty sella
   Hypothalamic diseases
     Hypothalamic tumors
     Infiltrative diseases
     Radiation
     Genetic (Kallman's syndrome)
     Hyperprolactinemia
     "Hypothalamic amenorrhea" (weight loss,
      exercise, stress)
   Systemic diseases
     Serious acute illness
     Chronic illnesses
     Adrenal disorders
     Thyroid disorders

rical catastrophes (Sheehan's syndrome), anticoagulant use, or bleeding into preexisting, sometimes undiagnosed, adenomas (pituitary apoplexy) (13, 67). Some cases of central hypogonadism may be autoimmune in nature, since antibodies to pituitary cells have been found in the serum of patients with lymphocytic hypophysitis or empty sella syndrome (3, 27). When no obvious cause for loss of gonadotroph function is apparent, the disease is termed "idiopathic" central hypogonadism.

Any hypothalamic process that disrupts normal production or secretion of GnRH can cause hypothalamic hypogonadism. These processes include infiltrative diseases such as hemochromatosis, sarcoidosis, tuberculosis, and Wegener's granulomatosis, as well as hypothalamic tumors that include gliomas, meningiomas, craniopharyngiomas, or metastases (21, 57). In addition, radiation therapy of the pituitary/hypothalamic region often leads to the gradual development of central hypogonadism, thought to be due primarily to hypothalamic damage (29).

Many conditions not associated with infiltrative or mass lesions can also suppress GnRH production. Kallman's syndrome, or idiopathic hypogonadotropic hypogonadism, is a congenital disease characterized by a lack of GnRH neuronal development and therefore a lack of GnRH pulses. Affected individuals fail to undergo normal pubertal development but can be successfully treated with pulsatile GnRH administration. This disease often is accompanied by anosmia and, occasionally, by other developmental defects of the central nervous system (cleft lip and palate, cranial nerve defects, and color blindness) (53, 63).

Another broad category of hypothalamic hypogonadism, seen in women, is often termed "hypothalamic amenorrhea." This common condition accounts for approximately 60% of all cases of secondary amenorrhea and is associated with fasting, weight loss, anorexia nervosa, bulimia, exercise, or stressful conditions. There have been several excellent studies demonstrating that this disorder is due to defects in pulsatile GnRH secretion (45, 53). The spectrum of defects ranges from complete lack of GnRH pulses

to disorders of pulse amplitude or frequency alone. The specific neuroendocrine modulators of this defect are unknown, but postulated causes include increased endogenous opiates or activation of the hypothalamic-pituitary-adrenal axis. The condition remits when weight is regained, exercise is decreased, or the stressful condition is alleviated. Interestingly, men may also develop hypothalamic hypogonadism under stress or with intensive exercise, although this entity is less well understood.

Finally, as discussed above, elevated prolactin levels suppress GnRH pulses and, in effect, lead to hypothalamic hypogonadism (65). Although galactorrhea often accompanies hyperprolactinemia, its absence does not rule out the diagnosis. Since hyperprolactinemia is common, especially in young women (where it accounts for approximately 30% of all cases of secondary amenorrhea) (57), a serum prolactin level should be obtained in anyone with central hypogonadism.

It is obvious then that the HPG axis is exquisitely sensitive to suppression by external factors. Thus, many patients with acute or chronic diseases manifest temporary or permanent central hypogonadism (Table 10.1). In fact, in patients with serious acute illnesses, gonadotropins and gonadal hormone levels begin to fall within hours of the onset of illness (72, 75). Similarly, a large proportion of patients with chronic diseases, such as diabetes mellitus, chronic obstructive pulmonary disease, inflammatory bowel disease, inflammatory arthritis, or chronic renal failure, have hypogonadism (41, 65). Endocrine disorders often associated with hypogonadism include over- or underactivity of the thyroid and adrenal glands. While hypogonadism in these conditions is often multifactorial, derangement of hypothalamic GnRH output may play a role in many cases (23, 32, 38, 70, 76).

Overproduction of Gonadotropins

Gonadotropin-Producing Pituitary Tumors

Case Report. A 54-year-old man presented with a long history of intense bifrontal headaches, decreasing vision, and loss of libido. He had been previously healthy and had fathered two children. Physical examination revealed a well-developed, well-virilized man with a dense bitemporal hemianopsia. There was no physical evidence of acromegaly or Cushing's syndrome. Laboratory examination revealed a serum FSH level of 63 IU/L (normal 1-14), LH of 11 IU/L (normal 2-12), α subunit of 2.2 ng/mL (normal 0.5-2.1), testosterone of 863 ng/dL (normal 300-1000), and prolactin of 48 ng/mL (normal 1-10). Thyroid and adrenal function were normal, and there was no evidence of diabetes insipidus. Computerized tomography (CT) showed a huge tumor filling an enlarged sella, with extensive superior extension beyond the hypothalamus into frontal and temporal lobes (Fig. 10.2). The patient underwent transsphenoidal debulking of the tumor, followed by radiation therapy. Immunocytochemistry of tumor tissue was diffusely and intensely positive for LH-β, FSH-β, and α subunit and was negative for all other pituitary hormones. Northern blot analysis of tumor mRNA was positive for the same hormones. Six months following surgery and radiation therapy, the patient's serum gonadotropin, α subunit, and testosterone levels were below normal, although there was a significant amount of residual tumor by CT. The patient was started on bromocriptine and has remained stable for two years.

Until recently, gonadotropin-producing tumors were thought to be rare. However, as more sensitive techniques of tumor classification have been developed, it has become clear that most previously classified "nonfunctioning" pituitary tumors are in fact gonadotropin-producing (60). These tumors usually present as macroadenomas in middle-aged or elderly patients, although they have been reported in subjects of all ages. In most series, men with gonadotropin tumors outnumber women. Whether gonadotropin adenomas really occur more frequently in men or are merely more difficult to diagnose in postmenopausal women is unclear. Since the tumors often grow to be quite large before detection, the most common presenting complaints include headaches and visual field defects. In fact, many of these patients are initially evaluated by ophthalmologists for decreasing vision. Loss of normal pituitary function due to pituitary or stalk com-

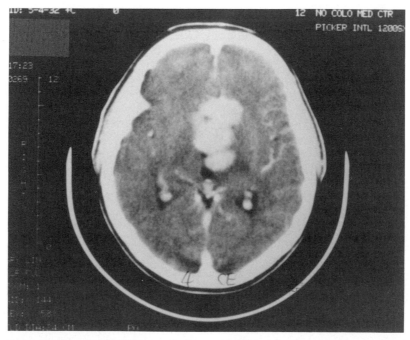

Figure 10.2   Contrast-enhanced axial CT scan showing tumor filling enlarged sella with extension into frontal and temporal lobes.

pression is also common, and many patients have central hypothyroidism and/or hypoadrenalism on presentation. In addition, although the tumors produce gonadotropins, almost all of these patients have symptoms of hypogonadism. This may be due to secretion of gonadotropins of altered structure and with decreased bioactivity (60, 61). Diabetes insipidus is less common, but can be seen in patients with very large tumors that involve the hypothalamus.

Many tumors previously classified as nonfunctioning adenomas actually produce gonadotropins (60); this misclassification arose for a number of reasons. In contrast to tumors producing other hormones, such as growth hormone, there is no typical clinical syndrome associated with gonadotropin tumors. In addition, serum gonadotropin levels can be normal, although closer scrutiny reveals that they are often higher than expected in a patient with a large pituitary adenoma (for example, LH levels in the case history). These normal serum levels may occur because the tumor secretes hormones with altered glycosylation or uncombined subunits (61), neither of which may be measured by conventional gonadotropin assays, or because hormone secretion is relatively inefficient compared to synthesis. Finally, when these tumors present in postmenopausal women, elevated serum gonadotropin levels often overlap those seen in the normal menopausal state. In this case, divergence of gonadotropin levels, such as elevated FSH and low LH levels, may provide a clue to the diagnosis.

Given these diagnostic hazards, it is not surprising that an accurate preoperative diagnosis of gonadotropin-producing tumors is difficult. However, the true nature of these tumors becomes apparent when tumor tissue is subjected to pathologic analysis (as in the case history) (60). Immunocytochemistry and immuno-electron microscopy using antibodies to LH and FSH show that tumor cell granules contain gonadotropins, and RNA analysis reveals the presence of LH-β, FSH-β, and/or α subunit mRNA species (20). In addition, when these tumors (as well as many tumors with no immunocytochemical staining) are placed in cell culture, they secrete LH, FSH, and/or α subunit into the me-

dium, confirming that they are indeed gonadotropin-producing (4, 28, 60, 77).

When the diagnostic techniques described above are applied to large series of macroadenomas, it becomes apparent that gonadotropin tumors probably represent a significant minority of all such tumors and the majority of clinically "nonfunctioning" adenomas. Recognition of this frequency is important for patient management (60). Serum concentrations of LH, FSH, and α-subunit can be used to aid in distinguishing pituitary adenomas from nonpituitary sellar lesions, such as craniopharyngiomas, which may affect treatment decisions. In addition, serum gonadotropin levels can be used to measure treatment efficacy. Finally, new therapeutic modalities directed specifically toward gonadotroph cells are currently under investigation.

When patients with gonadotropin tumors are studied over time, the gonadotropins appear to be secreted in pulses, as they are in normal individuals (Fig 10.1) (50). Pulse frequency is relatively preserved, although pulse amplitude and contours vary widely. This raises some interesting questions regarding possible hypothalamic contributions to the development of pituitary adenomas. The clinical relevance here is that serum gonadotropin levels may vary in untreated patients and that moderate decreases in levels may not signify improvement.

FSH-Producing Tumors. Although gonadotropin-producing tumors may secrete any combination of FSH and/or LH, those secreting FSH alone are the most common (60). In these patients, serum FSH levels are usually elevated, although they may be within the normal range. LH levels are normal or low, testosterone or estradiol levels are almost always low, and α subunit levels are normal or elevated. Although not routinely measured, serum concentrations of FSH-β subunit are also often elevated.

LH-Producing Tumors. Pituitary adenomas that produce only LH are rare (60). In these cases, serum LH levels are usually elevated, FSH levels are normal or low, and α subunit levels are usually elevated. Because the LH secreted from these tumors is bioactive, some of these patients have high testosterone or estradiol levels, which can be a clue to the nature of the tumor. However, for unclear reasons and despite the elevated sex hormone levels, many of these patients have symptoms of hypogonadism.

FSH- and LH-Producing Tumors. In tumors that produce both gonadotropins (as in the case history), serum FSH levels are usually elevated, LH levels are normal to elevated, and α subunit levels are usually normal or slightly elevated (60). Sex hormone levels are normal or elevated, depending on the amount of bioactive LH produced.

α**-Subunit-Producing Tumors.** A significant number of pituitary tumors secrete excess amounts of free α subunit (19, 48). Since α subunit is not bioactive, there are no symptoms directly related to the hormone, and most patients present with symptoms related to the tumor mass. In addition, some α subunit tumors also produce growth hormone, ACTH, or prolactin and present with symptoms of overproduction of those hormones. Other α subunit tumors also produce intact gonadotropins, but some produce only α subunit. In fact, when sensitive monoclonal assays for α subunit are used, over 20% of patients with clinically nonfunctioning tumors have elevated serum α subunit levels (42). When placed in cell culture, these tumors often produce intact FSH as well as free α subunit. Therefore, many α subunit tumors probably derive from gonadotroph cells (60). Despite its lack of clinical effects, α subunit can provide a valuable tumor marker in patients with macroadenomas.

Polycystic Ovarian Disease

Polycystic ovarian disease (Stein-Leventhal syndrome) is a common disorder in reproductive-aged women. Classically, it presents with menstrual irregularities starting at puberty, infertility, obesity, hirsutism, and multiple ovarian cysts. However, milder forms may present with only irregular menstrual periods or infertility. Laboratory examination usually reveals normal or elevated estradiol levels, mildly elevated androgen levels, normal to increased LH levels, and normal to decreased FSH levels (LH to FSH ratio usually > 3). Up to one-third of affected women also have mild elevations in prolactin. Pelvic ultrasound may show multiple small ovarian cysts. Interestingly, many of these patients have insulin resistance and acanthosis nigricans (37).

The etiology of polycystic ovarian disease is unclear. Some authors have postulated an ovarian or adrenal abnormality, with overproduction of androgens (31, 37). Others believe that the defect arises from the hypothalamus, with a rapid GnRH pulse generator causing a predominance of LH over FSH secretion (73). Whatever the underlying cause, affected women tend to have high-normal or mildly elevated LH levels. However, there is no diagnostic confusion between this syndrome and LH-producing tumors, since the clinical presentation is quite different.

EVALUATION

History and Physical Examination

In a patient with a suspected gonadal disorder, a careful history should include information about present and past sexual and reproductive function. Female patients should be asked about menstrual patterns, previous pregnancies, decreased libido, acne, hirsutism, vaginal dryness, and hot flashes (thought to be relatively specific for primary gonadal failure). Male patients should be asked about decreased libido, difficulties in achieving or maintaining erections or emissions, semen volume, and beard growth. All patients should be questioned regarding headaches, changes in vision, and the presence of galactorrhea. Further information that is often helpful includes a history of change in weight, exercise, stress, medication or illicit drug use, or symptoms of systemic disease. For example, oligoamenorrhea is often a presenting symptom in young women with hyperthyroidism.

On physical examination, women with hypogonadism may have breast atrophy and dry vaginal mucosa. Men may have decreased muscle strength, decreased beard growth, and small, soft testes. Other important clues on examination include expressible galactorrhea (more common in women with hyperprolactinemia, but also seen in men), visual field defects, ophthalmoplegia, changes in hair distribution (hirsutism in women, decreased sexual hair in men), acne in women (a sign of androgen excess), or signs of systemic illness.

Initial Laboratory Examination

Normal menstrual cycles in a woman rule out any pathology of the HPG axis, and no further evaluation is needed. In a woman with oligoamenorrhea, initial laboratory evaluation includes serum prolactin level, thyroid function tests, and a pregnancy test. If they are normal, further evaluation may proceed along one of two pathways: 1) The patient receives a short course of progesterone and is monitored for withdrawal bleeding following discontinuation of the medication. A positive test indicates that the patient produces sufficient estrogen to cause the uterine lining to develop, while a negative test indicates severe estrogen deficiency or an anatomic defect. If the test is negative, serum FSH and LH should be measured. 2) Alternatively, serum estradiol, FSH, and LH levels may be measured at baseline (immediately following a menstrual cycle if the patient has oligomenorrhea). Elevated gonadotropin levels (especially FSH) almost always indicate primary gonadal failure, except for the rare gonadotropin tumor. Young patients with primary gonadal failure should have a karyotype performed to exclude gonadal dysgenesis. Normal or low serum gonadotropin levels indicate a central defect. Optional studies in women with gonadal disorders include serum androgen levels (in women with hirsutism, acne, and/or suspected polycystic ovaries) and pelvic ultrasound (in women with suspected polycystic ovarian disease).

Most young women with central hypogonadism have hypothalamic amenorrhea without structural defects of the HPG axis. Therefore, it may be difficult to decide whether to perform expensive imaging studies of the hypothalamus and pituitary in these patients. The author reserves imaging studies for women with hyperprolactinemia, headaches, or other neurologic symptoms, or no history of obvious causes of hypothalamic amenorrhea (intensive exercise, weight loss, etc.). However, this decision must be individualized.

Initial laboratory evaluation in men with complaints of hypogonadism or impotence includes serum testosterone and prolactin as well as thyroid function tests. If testosterone is low, serum FSH and LH levels should be measured. As in women, elevated serum gonadotropins almost always signify primary gonadal failure (except for gonadotropin tumors), while normal or low levels suggest a central defect. Men with central hypogonadism and/or hyperprolactinemia usually have structural lesions and an imaging study should be performed in all such patients.

In any patient with a pituitary macroadenoma, serum FSH, LH, and α subunit levels should be measured. Abnormalities in these hormone levels can alert the physician to the presence of a secretory adenoma. While the treatment of such tumors is currently the same as that for nonsecreting tumors, abnormal hormone levels provide valuable tumor markers when assessing treatment efficacy. In addition, medical treatment of gonadotropin tumors, currently experimental, may eventually offer another therapeutic option for these patients.

Dynamic Tests of Serum Gonadotropins

GnRH tests have been used in attempts to localize central hypogonadism to the pituitary or hypothalamus. In these tests, serum LH and FSH levels are measured for one to two hours following injection of synthetic GnRH. In theory, patients with pituitary disorders should not respond to GnRH, whereas patients with hypothalamic or pituitary stalk disorders should have normal or exaggerated responses. Unfortunately, in practice, there is overlap between patient groups, and the GnRH test has little utility in localizing sites of central hypogonadism (40).

GnRH tests have also been used in attempts to characterize gonadotropin tumors. In theory, such tumors should produce LH and/or FSH in an autonomous fashion, and serum gonadotropin levels should not respond to administered GnRH. However, responses are quite variable in patients with proven gonadotropin tumors, and the GnRH test has not proven to be useful in these patients (28).

TRH, or thyrotropin-releasing hormone, is the hypothalamic factor responsible for normal TSH secretion from the pituitary gland. In normal subjects, FSH and LH do not increase following TRH injection. In contrast, some patients with gonadotropin tumors show paradoxic increases in intact gonadotropin or β subunit levels during TRH tests, even when baseline serum gonadotropin levels are normal. Therefore, TRH testing can be used to further characterize suspected gonadotropin tumors and to follow such patients after surgery or radiation therapy (60).

As discussed above, gonadotropin pulses have been measured in many cases of primary and central hypogonadism, as well as in patients with gonadotropin tumors. While such studies provide insights into the dynamic control of gonadotropin pulses in disease states, they are primarily research tools and are not indicated for clinical management of patients with gonadal disorders.

Radiologic Studies

In the past, imaging of the pituitary and hypothalamus involved imprecise studies, such as skull films, or invasive studies, such as pneumoencephalography and angiography. These studies have largely been replaced by CT and magnetic resonance imaging (MRI), and one of these modalities should be used in patients with central hypogonadism or suspected gonadotropin tumors. Since tumors or infiltrative processes may be missed by conventional CT or MRI views, the radiologist should be alerted to the diagnosis of pituitary disease and should perform coronal CT or MRI with special cuts.

TREATMENT

The treatment of patients with gonadal disorders involves three separate issues: the replacement of sex steroids, the restoration of fertility, and the treatment of gonadotropin tumors when they are present.

Hormone Therapy

Hypogonadal men and women not only have distressing symptoms due to sex steroid deficiency, but, over the long term, are at risk for significant osteoporosis (12, 44, 57). In addition, hypogonadal women lose the protective effects of estrogens against cardiovascular disease (36). Therefore, unless there is a contraindication, patients of both sexes should be treated with sex steroids.

Currently, hypogonadal men are best treated with intramuscular injections of long-acting testosterone preparations, given every two or three weeks. Although this regimen leads to nonphysiologic variability in serum testosterone levels, it is well tolerated and clinically satisfactory for most men. Oral androgens have fallen into disfavor due to variable absorption and hepatic toxicity. While not yet available, trials of transdermal testosterone preparations have been promising and may eventually offer a more physiologic treatment for these patients (1, 15).

Young hypogonadal women may be treated with low-dose oral contraceptives, whereas older women are usually given conjugated estrogens and progestins in lower doses. An alternative treatment for older women is the recently developed transdermal estrogen patch.

The restoration of fertility is more difficult than the treatment of sex steroid deficiency in hypogonadal individuals. With rare exceptions, patients with primary hypogonadism cannot be treated, since the gonad no longer produces germ cells. Women with mild defects in gonadotropin production may respond to clomiphene, an estrogen agonist/antagonist that increases LH pulse frequency and initiates folliculogenesis if sufficient endogenous estrogen is present. Women with hypothalamic amenorrhea can be encouraged to gain weight, decrease exercise in intensity, or otherwise reverse the abnormality that caused the amenorrhea. Fertility has been induced in patients with hypothalamic defects (for example, Kallman's syndrome and hypothalamic amenorrhea) by long-term subcutaneous administration of pulsatile GnRH via a portable pump, but this requires a highly motivated patient and a medical team experienced in such treatment (7, 53). Patients with either hypothalamic or pituitary defects can also be given injections of exogenous gonadotropins (human menopausal gonadotropins, hCG); these hormones should be administered by a physician with adequate training and laboratory support, since they carry a risk of multiple gestations.

Treatment of Gonadotropin-Producing Pituitary Tumors

Optimal treatment of gonadotropin tumors requires the combined approach of specialists in neurosurgery, radiation therapy, and neuroendocrinology. Unless there is a contraindication to surgery, the initial management of such tumors usually involves transsphenoidal surgery. As in other types of pituitary adenomas, surgical success rates depend on the size and location of the tumor and on the experience of the surgeon. Even very large tumors can be significantly debulked via the transsphenoidal approach, and craniotomy is therefore rarely indicated, at least as the initial procedure (60).

Following transsphenoidal surgery, any patient with signs of residual tumor by laboratory or radiologic tests may be considered for radiation therapy. In addition, many experts believe that the surgical cure rate for macroadenomas is low and that the risk of recurrence is high. Therefore, even patients with gross total resection of gonadotropin macroadenomas may be considered for postoperative radiation therapy (47). The morbidity of radiation therapy, when performed by experienced therapists, is low. The most common long-term side effect involves gradual loss of normal pituitary function, which can be treated with hormone replacement therapy. Loss of normal gonadotropin function is of greater concern in young patients who desire fertility, and, after discussing the risks, they may wish to delay or forego radiation therapy. However, this concern rarely arises, since most patients are older, and many younger patients have already lost normal gonadotroph function from effects of the tumor or surgery. Nevertheless, with improvements in non-invasive imaging, a period of observation for direct signs of tumor growth may be considered before instituting radiation therapy.

There is currently no standard medical therapy for gonadotropin-producing pituitary adenomas. However, there are case reports of decreases in serum hormone levels, improvement in visual fields, and/or tumor shrinkage with dopamine or dopamine agonists (26, 30, 60). In these reports, most of the patients had received prior radiation therapy and reduction of tumor size was quite variable (0% to 50%). Therefore, bromocriptine may be tried in a patient with residual tumor following surgery and radiation therapy, especially with continued visual compromise. However, primary therapy with bromocriptine or other dopamine agonists should not be utilized unless other therapies are refused, unavailable, or contraindicated.

Recently, long–acting GnRH analogs have been developed to treat many conditions. These drugs initially act as GnRH agonists but eventually cause decreases in gonadotropin secretion and bioactivity, leading to hypogonadism.

As such, they have been used to treat prostatic cancer, endometriosis, precocious puberty, and other sex-steroid dependent diseases (7). Patients with gonadotropin tumors have been given these GnRH agonists in attempts to reduce tumorous hormone secretion and tumor size. Despite occasional reports of efficacy (79), such studies have produced disappointing results, especially in patients with α-subunit tumors (24, 25, 55, 60). In fact, most patients have had sustained elevations in gonadotropin and/or α-subunit levels when given GnRH agonists, and these drugs may be deleterious (24, 25, 55).

More promising have been the recently developed pure GnRH antagonists, which do not have initial agonist effects. Preliminary studies suggest that these new drugs may be effective as adjuvant therapy in patients with gonadotropin tumors (8). Whether these drugs will be successful as primary therapy in patients with gonadotropin tumors, as bromocriptine has been in patients with prolactinomas, remains to be seen.

REFERENCES

1. Ahmed S.R., Boucher A.E., Manni A., *et al.* Transdermal testosterone therapy in the treatment of male hypogonadism. J. Clin. Endocrinol. Metab., 66:546–551, 1988.
2. Andersen A.N., Hagen C., Lange P., *et al.* Dopaminergic regulation of gonadotropin levels and pulsatility in normal women. Fertil. Steril., 47:391–397, 1987.
3. Asa S.L., Bilbao J.M., Kovacs K., *et al.* Lymphocytic hypophysitis of pregnancy resulting in hypopituitarism: a distinct clinicopathologic entity. Ann. Intern. Med., 95:166–171, 1981.

4. Asa S.L., Gerrie B.M., Singer W., *et al.* Gonadotropin secretion *in vitro* by human pituitary null cell adenomas and oncocytomas. J. Clin. Endocrinol. Metab., *62*:1011–1019, 1986.

5. Barabarino A., De Marinis L., Tofani., *et al.* Corticotropin-releasing hormone inhibition of gonadotropin release and the effect of opioid blockade. J. Clin. Endocrinol. Metab., *68*:523–528, 1986.

6. Besga S.L., Loucks A.B., Rossmanith W.G., Kettel C.M., Laughlin G.A., Yen S.S.C. Acceleration of luternizing hormone pulse frequency in functional hypothalamic amenorrhea by dopaminergic blockade. J. Clin. Endocrinol. Metab., *72*:151–6, 1991.

7. Cutler G.B. Jr., Hoffman A.R., Swerdloff R.S., *et al.* Therapeutic applications of luteinizing-hormone-releasing hormone and its analogs. Ann. Intern. Med., *102*:643–657, 1985.

8. Daneshdoost L., Pavlou S.N., Molitch M.E., *et al.* Inhibition of follicle-stimulating hormone secretion from gonadotroph adenomas by repetitive administration of a gonadotropin-releasing hormone antagonist. J. Clin. Endocrinol. Metab., *71*:92–97, 1990.

9. Delitala G., Giusti M., Mazzocchi G., *et al.* Participation of endogenous opiates in regulation of the hypothalamic-pituitary-testicular axis in normal men. J. Clin. Endocrinol. Metab., *57*:1277–1281, 1983.

10. Fabbri A., Jannini E.A., Ulisse S., *et al.* Low serum bioactive luteinizing hormone in nonorganic male impotence: Possible relationship with altered gonadotropin-releasing hormone pulsatility. J. Clin. Endocrinol. Metab., *67*:867–875, 1988.

11. Filicori M., Santoro N., Merriam G.R., *et al.* Characterization of the physiological pattern of episodic gonadotropin secretion throughout the human menstrual cycle. J. Clin. Endocrinol. Metab., *62*:1136–1144, 1986.

12. Finkelstein J.S., Klibanski A., Neer R.M., *et al.* Osteoporosis in men with idiopathic hypogonadotropic hypogonadism. Ann. Intern. Med., *106*:354–361, 1987.

13. Fleckman A.M., Schubart U.K., Danziger A., *et al.* Empty sella of normal size in Sheehan's syndrome. Am. J. Med., *75*:585–591, 1983.

14. Gharib S.D., Wierman M.E., Shupnik M.A., *et al.* Molecular biology of the pituitaly gonadotropins. Endocr. Rev., *11*:177–199, 1990

15. Ghusn H.F. and Cunningham G.R. Evaluation and treatment of androgen deficiency in males. The Endocrinologist *1*:399–408, 1991.

16. Gross K.M., Matsumo A.M., and Bremner W.J. Differential control of luteinizing hormone and follicle-stimulating hormone secretion by luteinizing hormone-releasing hormone pulse frequency in man. J. Clin. Endocrinol. Metab., *64*:675–680, 1987.

17. Haisenleder D.J., Katt J.A., Ortolano G.A., *et al.* Influence of gonadotropin-releasing hormone pulse amplitude, frequency, and treatment duration on the regulation of luteinizing hormone (LH) subunit messenger ribonucleic acids and LH secretion. Mol. Endocrinol., *2*:338–343, 1988.

18. Huseman C.A., Kugler J.A., and Schneider I.G. Mechanism of dopaminergic suppression of gonadotropin secretion in men. J. Clin. Endocrinol. Metab., *51*:209–214, 1980.

19. Ishibashi M., Yamaji T., Takaku F., *et al.* Secretion of glycoprotein hormone α-subunit by pituitary tumors. J. Clin. Endocrinol. Metab., *64*:1187–1193, 1987.

20. Jameson J.L., Kilbanski A., Black P.McL., *et al.* Glycoprotein hormone genes are expressed in clinically nonfunctioning pituitary adenomas. J. Clin. Invest., *80*:1472–1478, 1987.

21. Jenkins J.S., Gilbert C.J., and Ang V. Hypothalamic-pituitary function in patients with craniopharyngiomas. J. Clin. Endocrinol. Metab., *43*:394–399, 1974.

22. Kaptein E.M., Kletzky O.A., Spencer C.A., *et al.* Effects of prolonged dopamine infusion on anterior pituitary function in normal males. J. Clin. Endocrinol. Metab., *51*:488–491, 1980.

23. Kidd G.S., Glass A.R., and Vigersky R.A. The hypothalamic-pituitary-testicular axis in thyrotoxicosis. J. Clin. Endocrinol. Metab., *48*:798–802, 1979.

24. Klibanski A., Deutsch P.J., Jameson J.L., *et al.* Luteinizing hormone-secreting pituitary tumor: biosynthetic characterization and clinical studies. J. Clin. Endocrinol. Metab., *64*:536–542, 1987.

25. Klibanski A., Jameson J.L., Biller B.M.K., *et al.* Gonadotropin and δ-subunit responses to chronic gonadotropin-releasing hormone analog administration in patients with glycoprotein hormone-secreting pituitary tumors. J. Clin. Endocrinol. Metab., *68*:81–86, 1989.

26. Klibanski A., Shupnik M.A., Bikkal H.A., *et al.* Dopaminergic regulation of α-subunit secretion and messenger ribonucleic acid levels in δ-secreting pituitary tumors. J. Clin. Endocrinol. Metab., *66*:96–102, 1988.

27. Komatsu M., Kondo T., Yamauchi K., *et al.* Antipituitary antibodies in patients with the primary empty sella syndrome. J. Clin. Endocrinol. Metab., *67*:633–638, 1988.

28. Kwekkeboom D.J., de Jong F.H., and Lamberts S.W.J. Gonadotropin release by clinically nonfunctioning and gonadotroph pituitary adenomas *in vivo* and *in vitro:* relation to sex and effects of thyrotropin-releasing hormone, gonadotropin-releasing hormone, and bromocriptine. J. Clin. Endocrinol. Metab., *68*:1128–1135, 1989.

29. Lam K.S.L., Tse V.K.C., Wang C., *et al.* Early effects of cranial irradiation on hypothalamic pituitary function. J. Clin. Endocrinol. Metab., *64*:418–424, 1987.

30. Lamberts S.W.J., Verleun T., Osterom R., *et al.* The effects of bromocriptine, thyrotropin-releasing hormone, and gonadotropin-releasing hormone on hormone secretion by gonadotropin-secreting pituitary adenomas *in vivo* and *in vitro.* J. Clin. Endocrinol. Metab., *64*:524–530, 1987.

31. Loughlin T., Cunningham S., Moore A., *et al.* Adrenal abnormalities in polycystic ovary syndrome. J. Clin. Endocrinol. Metab., *62*:142–147, 1986.

32. Luton J.P., Thieblot P., Valcke J.C., *et al.* Reversible gonadotropin deficiency in male Cushing's disease. J. Clin. Endocrinol. Metab., *45*:488–495, 1977.

33. MacAdams M.R., White R.H., and Chipps B.E. Reduction of serum testosterone levels during chronic glucocorticoid therapy. Ann. Intern. Med., *104:*648–651, 1986.

34. Marshall J.C., and Kelch R.P. Gonadotropin-releasing hormone: role of pulsatile secretion in the regulation of reproduction. N. Engl. J. Med., *315:*1459–1468, 1986.

35. Matsubara M., Tango M., and Nakagawa K. Effects of dopaminergic agonists on plasma luteinizing hormone-releasing hormone (LRH) and gonadotropins in man. Horm. Metab. Res., *19:*31–34, 1987.

36. Matthews K.A., Meilahn E., Kuller L.H., et al. Menopause and risk factors for coronary heart disease. N. Engl. J. Med., *321:*641–646, 1989.

37. McKenna T.J. Pathogenesis and treatment of polycystic ovary syndrome. N. Engl. J. Med., *318:*558–562, 1988.

38. McKenna T.J., Lorber D., Lacroix A., et al. Testicular activity in Cushing's disease. Acta. Endocrinol. (Copenh) *91:*501–510, 1979.

39. Melis G.B., Mais V., Gambacciani M., et al. Dexamethasone reduces the postcastration gonadotropin rise in women. J. Clin. Endocrinol. Metab., *65:*237–241, 1987.

40. Mortimer C.H., Besser G.M., McNeilly A.S., et al. Luteinizing hormone and follicle stimulating hormone-releasing hormone test in patients with hypothalamic-pituitary-gonadal dysfunction. B. M. J., *4:*73–77, 1973.

41. O'Hare J.A., Eichold B.H. II., and Vignati L. Hypogonadotropic secondary amenorrhea in diabetes: effects of central opiate blockade and improved metabolic control. Am. J. Med., *83:*1080–1084, 1987.

42. Oppenheim D.S., Kana A.R., Sangha J.S., et al. Prevalence of α-subunit hypersecretion in patients with pituitary tumors: Clinically nonfunctioning and somatotroph adenomas. J. Clin. Endocrinol. Metab., *70:*859–864, 1990.

43. Plant T.M. Gonadal regulation of hypothalamic gonadotropin-releasing hormone release in primates. Endocr. Rev., *7:*75–88, 1986.

44. Raisz L.G. Local and systemic factors in the pathogenesis of osteoporosis. N. Engl. J. Med. 818–828, 1988.

45. Reame N.E., Sauder S.E., Case G.D., et al. Pulsatile gonadotropin secretion in women with hypothalamic amenorrhea: evidence that reduced frequency of gonadotropin-releasing hormone secretion is the mechanism of persistent anovulation. J. Clin. Endocrinol. Metab., *61:*851–858, 1985.

46. Reichlin S. Neuroendocrine control of thyrotropin and gonadotropin secretion. In: *Secretory Tumors of the Pituitary Gland* (progress in Endocrine Research and Therapy, Vol 1), edited by P. McL. Black, N.T. Zervas, E.C. Ridgway, and J.B. Martin, pp. 309–325, New York, Raven Press, 1984.

47. Ridgway E.C. Glycoprotein hormone production by pituitary tumors. In: *Secretory Tumors of the Pituitary Gland* (Progress in Endocrine Research and Therapy, Vol 1), edited by P. McL. Black, N.T. Zervas, E.C. Ridgway, and J.B. Martin, pp. 343–363, New York, Raven Press, 1984.

48. Ridway E.C. Klibanski A., Landenson P.W., et al. Pure alpha-secreting pituitary adenomas. N. Engl. J. Med., *304:*1254–1259, 1981.

49. Rossmanith W.G., Laughlin G.A., Mortola J.F., et al. Pulsatile cosecretion of estradiol and progesterone by the midluteal phase corpus luteum: Temporal link to luteinizing hormone pulses. J. Clin. Endocrinol. Metab., *70:*990–995, 1990.

50. Samuels M.H., Henry P., Kleinschmidt-Demasters B.K., Lillehei K., and Ridgway E.C. Pulsatile glycoprotein hormone secretion in glycoprotein-producing pituitary tumors. J. Clin. Endocrinol. Metab., *73:*1281–8, 1991.

51. Samuels M.H., Lillehei K., Kleinschmidt-Demasters B.K., et al. Patterns of pulsatile pituitary glycoprotein secretion in central hypothyroidism and hypogonadism. J. Clin. Endocrinol. Metab., *70:*391–395, 1990.

52. Samuels M.H., Henry P., and Ridgway E.C. Effects of dopamine and somatostatin on pulsatile pituitary glycoprotein secretion. J. Clin. Endocrinol. Metab., *74:*217–22, 1992.

53. Santoro N, Filicori M., and Crowley W.F. Jr. Hypogonadotropic disorders in men and women: diagnosis and therapy with pulsatile gonadotropin-releasing hormone. Endocr. Rev., *7:*11–23, 1986.

54. Sapolsky R.M., and Krey L.C. Stress-induced suppression of luteinizing hormone concentrations in wild baboons: role of opiates. J. Clin. Endocrinol. Metab., *66:*722–726, 1988.

55. Sassolas G., Lejeune H., Trouillas J., et al. Gonadotropin-releasing hormone agonists are unsuccessful in reducing tumoral gonadotropin secretion in two patients with gonadotropin-secreting pituitary adenomas. J. Clin. Endocrinol. Metab., *67:*180–185, 1988.

56. Sauder S.E., Frager M., Case G.D., et al. Abnormal patterns of pulsatile luteinizing hormone secretion in women with hyperprolactinemia and amenorrhea: responses to bromocriptine. J. Clin. Endocrinol. Metab., *59:*941–948, 1984.

57. Scharla S.H., Minne H.W., Waibel-Treber S., et al. Bone mass reduction after estrogen deprivation by long-acting gonadotropin-releasing hormone agonists and its relation to pretreatment serum concentrations of 1,25-dihydroxyvitamin D₃. J. Clin. Endocrinol. Metab., *70:*1055–1061, 1990.

58. Schlechte J., Sherman B., Halmi N., et al. Prolactin-secreting pituitary tumors in amenorrheic women: A comprehensive study. Endocr. Rev., *1*(3):295–308, 1980.

59. Seki K., and Nagata I. Effects of a dopamine antagonist (metoclopramide) on the release of LH, FSH, TSH, and Prl in normal women throughout the menstrual cycle. Acta. Endocrinol. (Copenh) *2:*211–216, 1990.

60. Snyder P.J. Gonadotroph cell adenomas of the pituitary. Endocr. Rev., *6:*552–563, 1985.

61. Snyder P.J., Bashey H.M., Kim S.U., et al. Secretion of uncombined subunits of luteinizing hormone by gonadotroph cell adenomas. J. Clin. Endocrinol. Metab., *59:*1169–1175, 1984.

62. Southworth M.B., Matsumoto .M., Gross K.M., Soules M.R., and Bremner W.J. The importance of

signal pattern in the transmission of endocrine information: pituitary gonadotropin responses to continuous and pulsatile gonadotropin-releasing hormone. J. Clin. Endocrinol. Metab., *72:*1286–89, 1991.

63. Spratt D.I., Carr D.B., Merriam G.R., *et al.* The spectrum of abnormal patterns of gonadotropin-releasing hormone secretion in men with idiopathic hypogonadotropic hypogonadism: clinical and laboratory correlations. J. Clin. Endocrinol. Metab., *64:*283–291, 1987.

64. Tsitouras P.D. Effects of age on testicular function. Endocrinol. Metab. Clin. North. Am., *16:*1045–1059, 1987.

65. Urban R.J., Evans W.S., Rogol A.D., *et al.* Contemporary aspects of discrete peak-detection algorithms. I. The paradigm of the luteinizing hormone pulse signal in men. Endocr. Rev., *9:*3–37, 1988.

66. Veldhuis J.D., Beitins I.Z., Johnson M.L., *et al.* Biologically active luteinizing hormone is secreted in episodic pulsations that vary in relation to stage of the menstrual cycle. J. Clin. Endocrinol. Metab., *58:*1050–1058, 1984.

67. Veldhuis J.D., and Hammond J.M. Endocrine function after spontaneous infarction of the human pituitary: report, review, and reappraisal. Endocr. Rev., *1:*100–107, 1980.

68. Veldhuis J.D., King J.C., Urban R.J., *et al.* Operating characteristics of the male hypothalamo-pituitary-gonadal axis: pulsatile release of testosterone and follicle-stimulating hormone and their temporal coupling with luteinizing hormone. J. Clin. Endocrinol. Metab., *65:*929–941, 1987.

69. Veldhuis J.D., Lizarralde G., Iranmanesh A. Divergent effects of short term glucocorticoid excess on the gonadotropic and somatotropic axes in normal men. J. Clin. Endocrinol. Metab., *74:*96–102, 1992.

70. Vierhapper H, Waldhausl W, and Nowotny P. Gonadotrophin-secretion in adrenocortical insufficiency: impact of glucocorticoid substitution. Acta Endocrinol. (Copenh) *101:*580–585, 1982.

71. Vierhapper H., Waldhausl W., and Nowotny P. Suppression of luteinizing hormone induced by adrenocorticotrophin in healthy women. J. Endocrinol., *91:*399–403, 1981.

72. Vogel A.V., Peake G.T., and Rada R.T. Pituitary-testicular axis dysfunction in burned men. J. Clin. Endocrinol. Metab., *60:*658–665, 1985.

73. Waldstreicher J., Santoro N.F., Hall J.E., *et al.* Hyperfunction of the hypothalamic-pituitary axis in women with polycystic ovarian disease: indirect evidence for partial gonadotroph desensitization. J. Clin. Endocrinol. Metab., *66:*165–172, 1988.

74. Winternitz W.W. and Dzur J.A. Pituitary failure secondary to head trauma. Case Report. J. Neurosurg., *44:*504–5, 1976.

75. Woolf P.D., Hamill R.W., McDonald J.V., *et al.* Transient hypogonadotropic hypogonadism caused by critical illness. J. Clin. Endocrinol. Metab., *60:*444–450, 1985.

76. Wortsman J., Rosner W., and Dufau M.L. Abnormal testicular function in men with primary hypothyroidism. Am. J. Med., *82:*207–212, 1987.

77. Yamada S., Asa S.L., Kovacs K., *et al.* Analysis of hormone secretion by clinically nonfunctioning human pituitary adenomas using the reverse hemolytic plaque assay. J. Clin. Endocrinol. Metab. 73–80, 1989.

78. Yen S.S.C., Quigley M.E., Reid R.L., *et al.* Neuroendocrinology of opioid peptides and their role in the control of gonadotropin and prolactin secretion. Am. J. Obstet. Gynecol., *152:*485–493, 1985.

79. Zarate A., Fonseca M.E., Mason M., *et al.* Gonadotropin-secreting pituitary adenoma with concomitant hypersecretion of testosterone and elevated sperm count. Treatment with LRH agonist. Acta Endocrinol. (Copenh) *113:*29–34, 1986.

Chapter 11

Antidiuretic Hormone

PAUL B. NELSON, M.D.

NORMAL PHYSIOLOGY

Antidiuretic hormone, or vasopressin, is synthesized as a prohormone, which includes the hormone, a neurophysin, and a glycopeptide. (13, 14) The entire prohormone is packaged into neurosecretory granules. These are enzymatically converted to the mature, approximately 1 kilodalton (kd) hormone, the 10 kd neurophysin, and 12 kd glycopeptide. The prohormones are synthesized in the magnocellular neurons in the paired supraoptic and paraventricular nuclei of the hypothalamus. Neurosecretory granules are transported down axons that extend to the posterior pituitary; here the hormones are stored. (Fig. 11.1)

Neurosynapses regulating hormonal release are on the cell bodies in the hypothalamus. With secretion of vasopressin, there is simultaneous secretion of the neurophysin and the glycopeptide. Neurophysin and glycopeptide are carriers or markers for antidiuretic hormone but have no known biological function.

The osmotic regulation of antidiuretic hormone secretion is highly sensitive. (8, 11, 12, 13, 14) Osmotic receptors are located in the anterior aspect of the hypothalamus. The normal range of plasma osmolality is between 285 and 295 mosm/kg water. An increase of as little as 1% in plasma osmolality will stimulate the osmotic receptors to release antidiuretic hormone. Extracellular sodium is the major ion to which these receptors respond.

The volume regulation of antidiuretic hormone secretion is less sensitive. (8, 11, 12, 13, 14) Receptors are located in the chest, with pressure receptors in the aorta and carotid sinus and volume receptors in the left atrium. The information is passed by the vagal and glossopharyngeal nerves to the brain stem and, probably, through multisynaptic pathways that eventually go to the magnocellular neurons, where they have a predominantly inhibitory action. A 10- to 15% reduction in blood pressure is needed to stimulate release of vasopressin. Other nonosmotic stimuli, such as nausea and intestinal traction, may also release vasopressin.

Once secreted into the bloodstream, antidiuretic hormone is carried to the kidney where it causes water retention. The hormone binds to antidiuretic receptors of the renal collecting ducts to stimulate cyclic adenosine monophosphate. The renal tubule cells are extremely sensitive to small changes in plasma vasopressin. Free water is absorbed from the distal convoluted tubules and collecting ducts. Without antidiuretic hormone function, 20 to 30 liters of urine would be lost daily.

Vasopressin and neurophysin have been found outside the usual hypothalamic hypophyseal tract. (8) In addition, the magnacellular neurons have been shown to project to the median eminence and near to the organum vasculosum of the lamina terminales. Therefore, vasopressin may be secreted directly into the third ventricle. The function of vasopressin in this area of the brain is poorly understood.

HYPONATREMIA

Hyponatremia indicates an excess of water relative to sodium and other solutes in the extracellular fluid. (17) Approximately 20% of patients become hyponatremic during their hospital course. Sodium is the most osmotically-active substance in the plasma. The following formula indicates the importance of

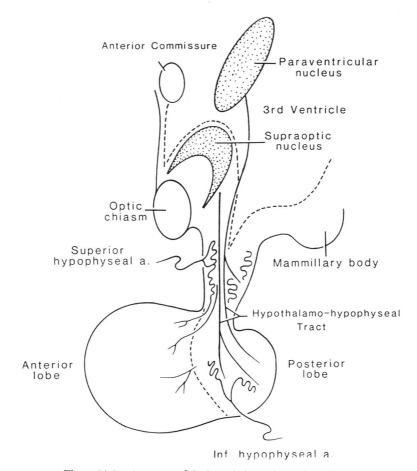

Figure 11.1.   Anatomy of the hypothalamo–hypophyseal tract.

plasma sodium in determining the plasma osmolality:

Posm (mosm/kg H_2O) = 2 × Na^+ (mmol/L)+ glucose (mmol/L).

There are two exceptions in which hyponatremia will not reflect plasma osmolality. These are cases associated with 1) marked elevations of lipids or proteins or 2) high concentrations of glucose. The syndrome of inappropriate secretion of antidiuretic hormone (SIADH) is by far the most common cause of hyponatremia.

The Syndrome of Inappropriate Secretion of Antidiuretic Hormone (SIADH)

In 1957, Schwartz *et al.* described a syndrome of renal sodium loss with hyponatremia that was thought to represent SIADH. This report was based on the study of two patients with bronchogenic carcinoma who

were thought to have antidiuretic-hormone-producing tumors. Since then, it has generally been accepted that patients with intracranial disorders who exhibit hyponatremia and excessive loss of sodium from the urine suffer from SIADH. Before this syndrome was defined, investigators felt that patients with intracranial disorders who developed hyponatremia and the inability to prevent the loss of sodium in their urine had cerebral salt wasting. It was felt that the abnormality was due either to an adrenal corticotropic hormone (ACTH) deficiency or to direct influence from the central nervous system on the renal absorption of salt. True cerebral salt wasting (without SIADH) is still a legitimate diagnosis; these patients are more likely to have a contracted intravascular volume.

SIADH is defined as a continued secretion of antidiuretic hormone despite a low serum osmolality. (8, 11, 12, 13, 14, 17) The diagnosis of SIADH assumes that there is a normal state of hydration; that there is normal renal, thyroid, and adrenal function; and that the patient is not taking diuretics. In all cases the patients are hyponatremic, with less than complete suppression of plasma vasopressin and a urine osmolality that is not maximally dilute. In general, the urine osmolality must be inappropriate for the plasma osmolality (i.e., > 100 mosm/kg H2O). Serum sodium is less than 135 mmol/L, urine sodium is generally greater than 25 mmol/L, and the serum osmolality is less than 280 mosm/kg.

Possible causes of the natriuresis seen in SIADH include an increased glomerular filtration rate with increased filter load of sodium, a decreased aldosterone secretion, and a decreased reabsorption of sodium in the proximal tubule secondary to a "third factor." Despite the need for high urinary sodium in making the diagnosis of SIADH, a low urinary sodium may develop with prolongation of the syndrome if sodium intake is low.

Both elevated antidiuretic hormone levels and water intake are necessary for hyponatremia to develop. Increased urinary sodium and water retention are not reflections of increased levels of antidiuretic hormone alone. In the absence of fluid intake, high levels of antidiuretic hormone may be present, but hyponatremia will not develop. If the levels of antidiuretic hormone are extremely high, even normal amounts of water intake may cause water retention and hyponatremia.

An oral water load test is usually not done to confirm the diagnosis of SIADH because of the concerns of exacerbating the hyponatremia and its symptoms. If a normal individual is given an oral load of 20 ml/kg of water, he will excrete 80% of the water by the fifth hour and the urine osmolality should be less than 100 mosm/kg.

There are both non-central nervous system and central nervous system causes of SIADH. The most common non-central nervous system cause of SIADH is autonomous secretion of antidiuretic hormone by malignant tumors. This is seen primarily with small cell-type bronchogenic carcinomas of the lung, although the syndrome may be as-sociated with cancers of the pancreas, duodenum, thymus, and with lymphoma. Abdominal surgery has been associated with elevation of antidiuretic hormone, which usually lasts three to four days. Hyponatremia is common in general surgery patients during their early postoperative period. Tuberculosis, chronic obstructive pulmonary disease, and positive end expiratory pressure breathing have also been associated with SIADH. Numerous drugs have been associated with SIADH, including phenothiazines, tricyclic antidepressants, the prostaglandin inhibitors, chlorpropamide, carbamazepine, and nicotine. On the other hand, dilantin and ethanol inhibit the release of antidiuretic hormone. Lithium and demeclocycline have been shown to inhibit the action of antidiuretic hormone in the kidney.

A number of central nervous system disorders are associated with SIADH. In fact, almost all intracranial disorders have been associated with hyponatremia and SIADH. One possible cause of this frequent association is that the magnacellular neurons appear to be under inhibitory regulatory influences, from brain stem cardiovascular regulatory centers. Therefore, any diffuse central nervous system disorder can potentially disrupt this chronic inhibition, causing antidiuretic hormone hypersecretion and SIADH.

The clinical manifestations of hyponatremia associated with SIADH generally depend upon how rapidly the hyponatremia develops and upon how low the serum sodium level drops. If the onset is slow, the symptoms may be vague and nonspecific. Confusion, stupor, coma, and seizures have been described. Increased focal neurologic deficits may be seen in patients who already have underlying central nervous system damage. Generally, symptoms do not develop in a normal individual until the sodium falls below 125 mmol/L. The mean plasma sodium of patients who develop seizures is generally reported to be between 110 and 115 mmol/L. The clinical manifestations probably represent brain edema caused by the osmotic water shifts into the brain due to the decreased plasma osmolality.

Treatment of SIADH most commonly involves water restriction. In general, unless the patient is extremely symptomatic with coma and seizures, correction of the hypo-natremia should not be too rapid. In the last 10 to 15 years, a number of patients have been reported to develop a rare demyelinating disorder of central pontine myelinolysis with quadriparesis and bulbar palsies after rapid correction of plasma sodium. Although this is not common, it is generally accepted that rapid correction of hyponatremia may cause brain demyelination in some patients. If it is necessary to correct the sodium rapidly because of coma, impaired consciousness, and seizures, it should probably not be corrected any faster than .5-2 mmol liter/hr; 3% hypertonic saline is generally used if rapid correction is needed. The following formula may be used to approximate the amount of sodium required: Total body water X desired correction rate = mmol/h Na^+. The body water is generally felt to be .6 of the body weight. The desired correction rate is generally .5 to 2 mmol liter/hr, and 3% saline contains .513 mmol/ml.

While the patient is receiving hypertonic saline, electrolytes should be checked at least every two hours. If the patient improves clinically and/or the sodium reaches a level of approximately 120 mmol/liter, the hypertonic saline should be stopped and the usual treatment of water restriction should be implemented. Occasionally, patients may be given a combination of furosemide and hypertonic saline. The patients are given furosemide 1 mg/kg body weight intravenously. Urinary losses of sodium and potassium are measured and replaced with 3% saline over an eight-hour period.

The most common treatment involves restricting water to 600 to 800 ml per day. Normal saline is usually used if intravenous fluids are necessary. Generally, the serum sodium will gradually increase over a two-to-three day period. Refractory chronic SIADH, which is sometimes seen in patients with head injuries, may benefit from demeclocycline (60–1200 mg/day). This tetracycline derivative causes a nephrogenic form of diabetes insipidus. It generally takes several days for demeclocycline to have an effect. Because of the drug's potential nephrotoxicity, renal function should be monitored regularly. Alcohol and phenytoin are known to inhibit antidiuretic hormone reduction, but,

therapeutically, they generally have been ineffectual.

DIABETES INSIPIDUS
Hyposecretion of vasopressin)

Diabetes insipidus is the excretion of dilute urine. (4, 12, 13, 14, 18) Once an osmotic diuresis is excluded, hypotonic polyuria may be caused by the absence of vasopressin (hypothalamic or central diabetes insipidus), lack of renal response to vasopressin (nephrogenic diabetes insipidus), or excessive ingestion of water (primary polydipsia).

Most patients with central diabetes insipidus who are awake and alert have a normal thirst mechanism and are able to drink sufficient water to maintain a relatively normal state of metabolic balance. Treatment in these patients is generally to prevent polyuria and nocturia and to allow the patient to sleep and carry on with normal daily activities. In the patient who has a decreased state of consciousness, however, large volumes of urine may produce severe dehydration and cardiovascular collapse in just a few hours.

Eighty-five percent of the secretory capacity of antidiuretic hormone must be impaired for central diabetes insipidus to occur. Damage to the posterior lobe of the pituitary of the lower stalk seldom causes permanent diabetes insipidus. However, upper pituitary stalk and basal hypothalamic damage are more likely to give a permanent disorder. The patient presents with polyuria, nocturia, polydipsia, and thirst. Urine output may vary from 3 to 5 liters per day, depending on the severity of the syndrome.

Although the diagnosis is usually obvious, one may confirm the diagnosis and the severity of the antidiuretic hormone deficit by performing a water deprivation test. This is usually done in the clinical laboratory but should not be done if the patient cannot tolerate the dehydration. The patient is deprived of water for six to eight hours or until the urine osmolality reaches a plateau. The patient is not allowed to lose more than 3% of body weight. A normal response is a decrease in the urine volume with associated increase in the urine osmolality. Normal individuals will concentrate urine to about 600 to 800 mosm/kg within eight to 10 hours of water restriction. If the patient fails to decrease the urine output and concentrate urine maximally, exogenous antidiuretic hormone is given. The normal response to vasopressin is a decrease in the urine volume or an increase in the urine osmolality to at least 300 to 350 mosm/kg.

After pituitary stalk section, a triphasic response may be seen. Polyuria and polydipsia with elevated serum sodium may be present for four to five days. The second phase of antidiuresis, with decreased urinary output and lower serum sodium, may be seen for the next four to five days. This is eventually followed by permanent diabetes insipidus.

Treatment of partial diabetes insipidus may be controlled by the patient's regulation of his intake and by the administration of agents that enhance antidiuretic hormone, such as chlorpropamide, hydrochlorothiazide, and clofibrate. If the patient is on parenteral fluids, the previous hour's urine output may be replaced with IV fluids. Generally, hypotonic fluids are used for fluid replacement.

When the urine output exceeds 300 ml/h, is associated with specific gravities less than 1.003 and elevated serum sodium, and it has become difficult to keep up with fluid losses either orally or with parenteral fluids, vasopressin or a vasopressin analog may be given.

L-Arginine vasopressin (AVP) is the natural human vasopressin. Aqueous vasopressin is a buffered solution of AVP that can be given parenterally. It is usually given subcutaneously. Its onset of action lies within one to two hours and its effects last four to eight hours. Intravenous bolus administration should not be given because of an even shorter duration of action and because of the potential significant pressor effects. Aqueous pitressin is generally provided in 1 ml vials at a concentration of 20 units/ml.

Pitressin tannate in oil is a crude extract of the posterior pituitary that contains AVP in a suspension of peanut oil. It generally comes in vials of 5 u/ml. Because this is a suspension, sedimentation of the active portion occurs during storage. The vial should be warmed and shaken. A single dose of five to 10 units provides 24 to 72 hrs of antidiuresis. The delayed absorption is due to the oily suspension.

Desmopressin (1-Deamine-8-D-arginine vasopressin—DDAVP) is a synthetic analog of L-Arginine vasopressin. It has a longer action than L-Arginine vasopressin and has less pressor activity. It is available for use intranasally, subcutaneously, or intravenously. The intranasal preparation is a buffered aqueous solution containing 100 mg/ml. Fifty to 200 μl can be loaded into a soft plastic tube and administered by inhaling into the nose. The onset of action is rapid and the duration of effect is from six to 24 hrs. Desmopressin is also available in 2 ml vials of 4 μg/ml for parenteral injection. When administered parenterally, 10% to 20% of the agent produces an effect similar to that produced when administered intranasally.

Oral agents may be used in patients with partial diabetes insipidus. Chloropropamide (Diabinese) was found to decrease free water excretion in patients with diabetes insipidus. It enhances the effect of vasopressin on the renal tubule. The usual dose is 100 to 500 mg orally per day. One must be cautious of the development of hypoglycemia. Carbamazepine (Tegretol) has been shown to cause release of antidiuretic hormone in patients with partial diabetes insipidus. The usual dose is 200 to 600 mg/day. Blood counts should be followed with long-term use of carbamazepine.

In acute postsurgical diabetes insipidus, treatment begins with parenteral administration of desmopressin at a dose of 1 to 4 μg subcutaneously or intramuscularly. The patient should experience a return of polyuria before subsequent doses are administered. The postoperative diabetes insipidus may be transient, and the second antidiuretic phase of triphasic diabetes insipidus must be anticipated.

Once it is established that the patient will have chronic diabetes insipidus, a maintenance therapy should be set up. Intranasal desmopressin is the best drug to use for chronic diabetes insipidus. The patient should be trained in the proper administration of intranasal DDAVP. Initially, test doses of 50, 100, and 200 μl of the drug are given, and after each of the test doses, a record of the action and duration of the drug may be made. Generally, the effects of the drug last 12 hrs. After three test doses, the optimal dosage and time of the day to administer the drug should become apparent. The protocol has to be individualized for each patient. Occasionally, patients can be controlled with a single dose per day, but, usually, two doses are required.

OTHER APPLICATIONS OF ANTIDIURETIC HORMONE AND DDAVP

Gastrointestinal Hemorrhage

Intravenous vasopressin is used to control human upper gastrointentinal hemorrhage. (5, 15) It is a potent vasoconstrictor and greatly reduces mesenteric blood flow. Its primary application has been in the control of variceal hemorrhage. Vasopressin will temporarily reduce portal pressure and slow or stop the variceal hemorrhage. This may give the physician time to start more definitive therapy, since this is only a temporary effect. Intravenous vasopressin appears to be as effective as intra-arterial administration and is associated with fewer complications. Its use in controlling nonvariceal hemorrhages is less clear. Intra-arterial administration may decrease bleeding in hemorrhagic gastritis; however, treatment of bleeding from peptic ulcers has not produced good results. Gastrointestinal side effects of vasopressin include abdominal pain and diarrhea. Cardiovascular complications include hypertension, cardiac arrhythmias, and congestive heart failure.

The drug is prepared by mixing 40 units of aqueous pitressin in 250 ml of 5% dextrose in water. The administration rate is .2–.4 μg/minute, and treatment may be maintained for 24 hr after bleeding is controlled.

Hemostasis

In concentrations 10 times higher than those used for antidiuretic applications, DDAVP raises circulatory levels of Factor VIII and of von Willebrand's factor. (9) Vasopressin may be used in the treatment of patients with mild-to-moderate hemophelia A and von Willebrand's disease. The recommended intravenous dose of desmopressin for these disorders is 0.3 μg/kg of body weight. Patients with severe deficiencies do not respond to this therapy.

Desmopressin can also reduce blood loss and transfusion requirements for individuals who have no hematological disorders and are undergoing cardiopulmonary bypass surgery. DDAVP shortens bleeding time in patients with uremia and liver cirrhosis, and may also be useful in patients with excessive operative bleeding related to previous aspirin ingestion.

Memory

Animal studies have shown that vasopressin may enhance both the consolidation and retrieval of memory. (7) The memory-enhancing effects in adult humans have been less consistent. (2, 3, 7, 10) Additional studies will need to be done to determine whether or not antidiuretic hormone should be used in patients with memory disorders.

Enuresis

Desmopressin has been used in the management of nocturnal enuresis in children because it reduces the volume of urine produced during the night. (1, 6, 16) Several double-blind studies have shown that it will decrease nocturnal enuresis without serious side effects. In general, 20 to 40 μg was given intranasally at bedtime depending on the child's age and body weight. Theoretically, the pathogenesis of nocturnal enuresis may be the inability of enuretic patients to experience a nocturnal increase in the secretion of endogenous vasopressin. The drug may be useful in the treatment of older children with enuresis.

REFERENCES

1. Abramowicz, M. (ed) Desmopressin for nocturnal enuresis. Med. Lett. Drugs. Ther., *32(816)*:38–39, Apr. 20, 1990.
2. Brambilla, F., Bondiolotti G.P., Maggioni M., *et al.* Vasopressin (DDAVP) therapy in chronic schizophrenia; effects on negative symptoms and memory. Neuropsychobiology, *20(3)*:113–119, 1989.
3. Dons R.E., House J.F., Hood D., *et al.* Assessment of desmopressin-enhanced cognitive function in a neurosurgical patient. Milit. Med., *154(2)*:83–85, 1989.
4. Harris A.S. Clinical experience with desmopressin: efficacy and safety in central diabetes insipidus and other conditions. J. Pediatr., *114(4Pt2)*:711–718, 1989.
5. Jacoby A.G., Wiegman M.V. Cardiovascular complications of intravenous vasopressin therapy. Focus. Crit. Care., *17(1)*:63–66, 1990.

6. Klauber G.T. Clinical efficacy and safety of desmopressin in the treatment of nocturnal enuresis. J. Pedeatr., *114(4Pt2):*719–722, 1989.

7. Legros J.J., Timsit-Berthier M. Vasopressin and vasopressin analogues for treatment of memory disorders in clinical practice. Prog. Neuropsychopharmacol. Biol. Psychiatry, *12(Suppl S):*71–86, 1988.

8. Lester M.C., Nelson P.B. Neurological aspects of vasopressin release and the syndrome of inappropriate secretion of antidiuretic hormone. Neurosurgery., *8(6):*735–7740, 1981.

9. Mannucci,P.M. Desmopressin: A nontransfusional hemostatic agent. Annu. Rev. Med., *41:*55–64, 1990.

10. Mattes J.A., Pettinati H.M., Nilsen S.M., *et al.* Vasopressin for ECT-induced memory impairment: a placebo-controlled comparison. Phychopharmacol. bull. *25(1):*80–84, 1989.

11. Nelson P.B. Etiology, recognition, and current management of the syndrome of inappropriate secretion of antidiuretic hormone. Cont. Neurosurg., *2(14):*1–6, 1980.

12. Nelson P.B. Fluid and clcctrolyte physiology, pathophysiology, and management. In: *Neurosur-gical. Critical. Care. Volume 1, Concepts in Neurosurgery.* Edited by F.P. Wirth and R.A. Ratcheson, pp. 69–80, Baltimore, Williams and Wilkins, 1987.

13. Robinson A.G. Disorders of the posterior pituitary. In: *Textbook of Internal Medicine.,* edited by W.N. Kelley, pp. 2172–2177, Philadelphia, J.B. Lippincott Co., 1989.

14. Robinson A.G. Regulation and pathophysiology of posterior pituitary function. In: *Clinical Neruoendocrinology.,* edited by R. Collu and G.M. Brown, pp. 65–90, Boston, Blackwell Scientific, 1988.

15. Stump D.L., Hardin T.C. The use of vasopressin in the treatment of upper gastrointestinal hemorrhage. Drugs., *39(1):*38–53, 1990.

16. Sukhai R.N., Mol J., Harris A.S. Combined therapy of enuresis alarm and desmopressin in the treatment of nocturnal enuresis. Eur. J. Pediatr., *148(5):*465–467, 1989.

17. Verbalis J.G. Hyponatraemia. Baillier's Clin. Endocrinol. Metab., *3(2):*499–530, 1989.

18. Verbalis J.G., Robinson A.G. Hypothalamic disease. In: *Currrent Therapy in Endocrinology and Metabolism.,* edited by C.W. Bardin, pp. 1–6, New York, Population Council, 1987.

CHAPTER 12

Neuro-Ophthalmic Manifestations of Endocrine Disease

DENNIS C. MATZKIN, M.D., RONALD M. BURDE, M.D.

INTRODUCTION

Patients with endocrine disease may have visual symptoms related to a primary hypothalamic-pituitary axis space occupying lesion. Alternatively, they may be afflicted with ocular disease as part of a peripheral endocrinopathy. The eye findings associated with thyroid disease are legion. The association of cataract and glaucoma with Cushing's syndrome is well recognized. This chapter, however, will confine itself to providing the reader with insights into the afferent and efferent visual system and manifestations of sellar and parasellar mass lesions. We will not discuss Graves orbitopathy or other remote endocrine ophthalmopathies.

The close anatomical relationship between the optic chiasm, the pituitary gland, the hypothalamus, and the cavernous sinus, renders the afferent and efferent visual system vulnerable to expanding tumors of the pituitary gland, craniopharyngiomas, and ectopic dysgerminomas. Signs and symptoms depend on the direction of growth and degree of compression or distortion of surrounding structures. Other lesions in this area, such as aneurysms, basal tumors—such as chordomas, meningiomas, and a variety of cysts may also cause such symptoms.

The effect of such lesions can be categorized as follows:

a) Loss of visual acuity or visual field (afferent system).
b) Onset of diplopia with or without pupillary abnormalities (cranial nerves III, IV, VI).
c) Facial pain syndromes (cranial nerve V).
d) Ptosis and miosis (Horner's syndrome).
e) Headache, field loss, or transient obscurations of vision due to obstruction of cerebrospinal fluid outflow, which produces papilledema.
f) Abnormalities of endocrine function, with syndromes of excess or deficiency.
g) Any combination of the above.

Traditional ophthalmic teaching emphasizes the importance of early visual symptoms in the diagnosis of parasellar tumors. This emphasis has been based upon the early reports of Chamlin et al. in 1955 (9), and Hollenhorst and Young (33). The latter series consisted of 1,000 cases seen at the Mayo Clinic between 1940 and 1964. In these reports, approximately 70% of patients had visual disturbance. However, in recent years, refined diagnostic techniques, such as neuroimaging and radioimmune assays for the various pituitary and hypothalamic hormones, have enabled the diagnosis of secretory pituitary adenomas to be made while such tumors remain within the sella, i.e., before symptoms related to the visual system would be expected. A tumor has to extend 10–12 mm above the diaphragma sellae in order for it to cause chiasmal compression. The decline of visual manifestations associated with sellar tumors can be substantiated by looking at the series of patients reported by Wray (85) and Anderson et al. (2). Wray examined 100 patients with pituitary tumors between 1974 and 1978 and could demonstrate visual field defects in 31%. Anderson published a series of 200 such cases in 1983, only 9% had visual field defects, 2% had optic atrophy, and 1% had diplopia.

The identification of prolactin as a distinct entity, and the elucidation of the physiology of its release and secretion through the use of highly sensitive radioimmunoassay techniques, has drastically changed the diagnostic and therapeutic approach to prolactin-secreting pituitary tumors. It is now known that prolactin hypersecretion produces both the amenorrhea-galactorrhea syndrome in women, and impotence, infertility, and occasionally galactorrhea in men. Since these adenomas represent a large proportion of all pituitary tumors, most of them can now be identified before they became large enough to cause sella enlargement and be seen on plain skull X-rays, or produce visual field defects or diplopia. The hyperprolactinemia state can be reversed and the size of the adenoma reduced with the use of drugs like the ergot derivative bromocriptine. These drugs mimic the action of prolactin inhibitory factor, a substance released by the hypothalamus into the pituitary portal circulation. Such drugs can be used to treat prolactinomas medically for an indefinite period, providing an alternative, as well as an adjunct, to surgery (i.e., shrink a tumor that has expanded extrasellarly back into the pituitary fossa). Modern transsphenoidal microsurgery has so reduced the morbidity and increased the success rate of neurosurgical intervention in cases of pituitary tumors, that the endocrinologist can refer his patients confident that he is offering a viable alternative to long-term medical therapy.

Many small (3-4mm) tumors are detected nowadays as incidental findings. Nonsecreting tumors can simply be followed radiologically and the patients can be monitored for endocrine dysfunction. Patients with secretory tumors can be treated either pharmacologically or surgically, and they can be followed serologically as well as with neuroimaging. Thus, today, far fewer patients with biologically active tumors should present with visual dysfunction.

The ophthalmologist's role in the diagnosis of sellar tumors would therefore appear to be changing, especially in the case of secretory pituitary tumors. Nevertheless, a detailed neuro-ophthalmic exam, including perimetry, remains an essential part of the clinical evaluation. The visual field examination suggests the extent of compression if any, and, in certain instances, the location of the tumor. Serial examinations are used to follow the effect of the compressive process in response to treatment. It is often the level of visual function that determines the nature and timing of the medical or surgical intervention.

REGIONAL NEUROANATOMY

Optic Chiasm

The optic chiasm, a midline structure formed by the junction and partial crossing over (decussation) of the intracranial portions of the optic nerves, is 10-20mm wide, 4-13mm long, and 3-5mm thick. Its posterior extension bilaterally constitutes the optic tracts and forms the anterior wall of the third ventricle. Despite the surrounding basilar cisterns containing cerebrospinal fluid, the chiasm is close to many critical structures. It has a variable relationship to the underlying pituitary gland and stalk, which accounts for the confusing array of visual field loss that can be seen with pituitary tumors. In most cases, the chiasm lies directly over the sella, but in 12-17% of patients it is anterior to the sella (prefixed), and in 4-5%, it is relatively posterior (postfixed) (6). Since the average distance between the chiasm and the diaphragma sellae (which forms a roof over the pituitary gland) is 8-13mm, pituitary masses must have significant suprasellar extension before producing visual signs and symptoms. Thus visual fields play little role in following patients with microadenomas.

The optic nerves ascend at an angle of 45° as they leave the optic canal and enter the cranium approaching the chiasm. Therefore, the anterior portion of the chiasm is measurably closer to the structures underlying the diaphragma sellae and is usually the first structure to become involved by an expanding mass. Within the chiasm, fibers from the nasal half of the retina, comprising 53% of the approximately 1 million axons in each optic nerve, decussate. The most anterior of these fibers subserve the inferior nasal retina and carry information from the superotemporal visual fields. These fibers loop forward into the opposite optic nerve medially, making up the so-called "Willebrand's knee." The practical significance of this neuroanatomy is that a compressive lesion affecting "Willebrand's knee" produces an ipsilateral central scotoma, with a contralateral supertemporal field defect (see case 2). This exquisitely localizes the lesion to the junction between the optic nerve and chiasm. Macular fibers predominate (25% of axons come from the central five degrees of the retina) and cross throughout the chiasm, although they are more prominent centrally and posteriorly (35, 36, 37).

Cavernous Sinus

The cavernous sinus, with its contents, is separated from the pituitary fossa by the soft tissue of the dura. In the medial aspect of the sinus lies the internal carotid artery surrounded by postganglionic sympathetic fibers. Closely applied to the artery laterally and anteriorly within the sinus is the abducens nerve. The postganglionic sympathetic fibers join the sixth nerve for a short distance before joining the nasociliary branch of V_1. In the lateral wall of the anterior part of the sinus, superiorly to inferiorly, are found the oculomotor nerve, the trochlear nerve, and the ophthalmic division of the trigeminal nerve. The maxillary branch of the fifth cranial nerve is also present posteriorly in the lateral wall of the cavernous sinus.

The pituitary gland is surrounded anteriorly, posteriorly, and inferiorly by bone. Expansion due to tumor formation will take the path of least resistance, which occurs most frequently in a superior direction and, more rarely, laterally into the cavernous sinus. Therefore, the afferent and efferent visual systems should be carefully examined in all patients suspected of harboring a pituitary or parasellar tumor.

CLINICAL FEATURES OF THE CHIASMAL SYNDROME

Visual Loss

Progressive Visual Loss

Visual symptoms due to parasellar disease may be unilateral or bilateral and result from loss of central acuity or visual field. In the majority of patients, it is insidious in onset and slowly progressive. Fluctuation of vision may occur, in particular with craniopharyngioma of both the solid and cystic varieties. Frequently, there may be only vague complaints of visual difficulty, such as decreased depth perception, inability to focus, or missing part of the sentence while reading. Occasional repeated mishaps while walking or driving may lead the patient to seek an ophthalmic evaluation. Bitemporal hemianopia is a frequent accompanying ailment in these patients. The observation of the pattern of the letters that patients miss while reading the Snellen chart at a distance is a clue to the presence of a neurological visual field defect. The patient with a bitemporal defect will tend to miss the right half of the chart while reading with his right eye, and the left half while reading with his left eye.

As long as central acuity is spared in one eye, patients may not be aware of any visual deficit. In such instances, it is only when the good eye is closed incidentally that the visual loss is discovered by the patient. One must differentiate between sudden visual loss and the sudden discovery of visual loss. Obtaining an accurate history in such instances may be difficult. In a study comprising 149 patients with visual loss due to parasellar tumors, nearly 25% had undiagnosed visual complaints varying between two and 10 years in duration (70).

The reason for the delay in the diagnosis of a compressive optic neuropathy is multifactorial. Low clinical suspicion of "minor visual ailments" by physicians or optometrists and patient reluctance to pursue "minimal" visual difficulty with a second opinion, are among the causes. In an interesting review of 100 cases of proven pituitary tumor by Lyle and Clover in 1961 (47), the initial visual diagnosis in the medical records of 14 out of 30 cases was "refractive error;" other diagnoses included tobacco amblyopia, optic neuritis, glaucoma, "hemorrhage behind the eye," migraine, and optic atrophy. Two patients were simply reassured. In a similar study (83), visual complaints were misinterpreted in 26 out of 45 patients. One patient allegedly had been given prescriptions for eight pairs of glasses over the year during which he experienced progressive visual loss. This particular patient had good central acuity and normal optic discs, but a profound bitemporal hemianopia on visual field testing. Admittedly, these cases were reported prior to the availability of modern neuroimaging and before automated visual tests were widely available. Nevertheless, it is important to have a high index of suspicion when a patient presents with minor visual complaints. In any patient presenting with a visual disturbance that is not explained during a routine examination, a visual field test is mandatory.

Bilateral progressive loss of vision, with central and centrocecal scotomata is usually due to demyelinating disease, toxins, nutritional disorders, or is hereditary. However, if there is no clue to such an etiology, the existence of a parasellar tumor must be considered in the differential diagnosis. Bilateral central and centrocecal scotomata due to suprasellar mass lesions are atypical but well documented in the literature (27). Prompt referral to a neuro-ophthalmologist will rapidly determine the extent of a visual defect. In close consultation with a neuroradiologist, neuroimaging of a specific anatomical region can then be performed.

Acute Visual Loss

There are patients in which the first evidence of tumor is rapid visual loss (51, 59) (i.e., pituitary apoplexy or expansion of a craniopharyngiomal cyst). When visual loss is unilateral and isolated, a misdiagnosis of retrobulbar neuritis may be made. Vision may improve somewhat over the first few weeks following the ictus, which typifies optic neuritis even more. In these cases, the correct diagnosis of a compressive lesion may be missed for weeks or even months, until symptoms of visual loss or a visual field defect is noted in the other eye.

Acute visual loss sometimes occurs in patients who are already known to have a pituitary tumor. A sudden infarction or hemorrhage into the tumor may cause a rapid expansion, producing a compressive neuropathy. This is termed "pituitary apoplexy," and has been reported in association with trauma (34), radiotherapy (56), angiography, anticoagulant therapy, estrogen therapy, bromocriptine therapy, and craniopharyn-

gioma (40, 44). The classical symptoms include rapid and usually bilateral visual loss, diplopia, severe headache, confusion, and even coma if the diagnosis is delayed. Apoplexy may also be subacute, presenting as progressive visual loss; or silent, without any symptoms or signs (71). The visual prognosis in pituitary apoplexy is generally excellent.

Examination of the patient with either acute or progressive visual loss reveals a variable acuity, ranging from 20/20, to near or complete blindness. Visual function is usually affected differently in each eye. The ability to discriminate colors grossly, especially in the red and green axis, is particularly sensitive to optic nerve dysfunction. Comparing the appreciation of color, one eye against the other, as well as across the vertical midline, is helpful in identifying optic nerve versus chiasm or retrochiasmal disease. Such testing may be done with Ishihara color plates or with the red top of a mydriatic bottle. This method has been found to be a useful adjunctive screening test for compressive optic neuropathies.

Positive Visual Phenomenon

Visual hallucinations were first reported as occurring in patients with pituitary adenomas in 1940 (81). Numerous reports since then have further characterized the nature of the photopsias. They may be formed, consisting of recognizable shapes, or unformed, and they may include visual sensations, such as sparks, flashes, or colored lights (15, 54, 64). Other patients may experience photophobia, which is the subjective sensation of visual discomfort in bright light, and an awareness of improved visual function in dim light. The history should be aimed at elucidating this occurrence.

In a study comprising 45 consecutive patients with positive visual phenomenon, nine patients had compressive optic neuropathy. Two experienced photopsias and seven suffered from photophobia (64). More recently, three patients were described as having visual hallucinations as their presenting symptom of pituitary adenoma (54). One patient reported only simple unformed hallucinations, whereas the other two patients experienced complex formed visual hallucinations.

Visual Field Defects

Visual field defects due to neuroendocrine disorders are the result, in most part, of a compressive neuropathy involving the optic nerve, optic chiasm, or optic tract, depending on the anatomical relationship between the chiasm and the pituitary gland. Accurate plotting of the visual field enables clinical localization of the lesion and helps direct subsequent neuroimaging studies. It also permits meaningful follow-up of tumor progression and of its response to treatment.

While the visual acuity is a test of the patient's central vision, perimetry is a test of the patient's paracentral and peripheral visual function. Accurate recording depends to a large extent on the ability of the patient to cooperate with the examiner as well as on his subjective response to test stimuli. In young children and mentally retarded or semicomatose individuals, accurate quantitative assessment of the visual field may be impossible. Unconventional methods utilizing confrontation techniques, such as finger counting or mimicking, may be tried to obtain a sense of the visual field loss.

In order to familiarize the reader with neuro-ophthalmic jargon related to visual field testing, a brief description of the various tests used clinically will be discussed (Table 12.1). It is important to remember that during the examination each eye is tested separately, with fixation of the eye maintained centrally. Often, the most difficult part of the test is to prevent the patient's eyes from wandering.

Manual Perimetry

Confrontation Field. The simplest and most rapid way of assessing whether a field defect is present is by the confrontation method. With the patient having one eye closed, the examiner simply asks the patient to maintain eye contact with him and acknowledge whether he is able to see peripheral objects or count fingers presented in the four quadrants. In asphasic adults and in children over the age of two, finger mimicking, as in the game "Simon Says," is a useful technique. The patient may be asked to compare two objects for clarity or color, i.e., two hands, or red-topped mydriatic bottle tops across the vertical meridian in the nasal and temporal fields. This test will rapidly detect a bitemporal, homonymous, or quadrantic field defect.

Confrontation techniques in the uncooperative patient make use of saccadic reflexes to assess whether an image falling on the peripheral retina has been seen. An object of interest i.e., a doll or brightly colored ball, is presented in the peripheral field. If the patient simply looks toward this object, one can assume that the field in that particular quadrant is intact. Similarly, a threatening motion can be made by looking for a blink reflex. A time-tested technique is for the physician to use his or her own face as a target, with the nose as a point of fixation. One then enquires whether the eyes, ears, mouth, and chin are visible. If the patient reports missing portions of the face, a visual field defect is suggested that can be definitively explored with more refined techniques.

Confrontation field techniques are used to obtain an initial sense, in the office or at the bedside, of the visual field. Once a qualitative appreciation of the defect has been obtained, a decision can be made as to which type of formal field test should be used for more accurate recording. Manual perimetry has the advantage of tailoring the test to the patient's physical and visual capabilities. For exam-

TABLE 12.1.
Types of Visual Field Tests

i) Manual	Confrontation		
	Kinetic-	Tangent screen	
		Goldmann perimeter	
	Static	Amsler grid	
ii) Automated	Static-	Humphrey }	Threshold
			versus
	Octopus }	suprathreshold
		}	strategies

ple, an elderly patient with poor vision and short endurance would be far better suited to a manual kinetic field performed on the Goldmann perimeter than to an automated threshold test that may take an hour to perform.

Kinetic Perimetry. Kinetic perimetry is usually performed with the manual technique and involves moving a target from the far periphery towards fixation. The point at which a patient first sees the target in his peripheral visual field is recorded. The visual field is tested in a number of different meridians. The size and configuration of the field depend on the object's size, color, and speed. The ability of the patient to react promptly to the recognition of the stimulus and to maintain fixation centrally is crucial to accurate testing. "Spot checks" can be performed with static techniques in order to check the accuracy of the responses. Close cooperation between the examiner and the patient determines the reliability and reproducibility of the visual field.

Kinetic and static perimetry measure different retinal functions. Kinetic fields test movement and directional sensitivity, which are two aspects of retinal ganglion cell physiology. Static fields test the ability to detect a given light intensity against background illumination, which is another function of ganglion cells. The size of a kinetic visual field is always larger than the static field, and the different tests are performed to complement each other if necessary.

The Goldmann perimeter is the most widely used kinetic perimeter. It consists of a hemispheric bowl one-third of a meter in diameter. A chin rest on the concave side enables the patient to sit comfortably, maintaining fixation on a central spot within the concavity of the bowl. The examiner is able to ensure fixation of the patient by observing him from the opposite side through a telescope. A standard recording chart is fixed to the convex side and a controlling arm with a pointer is moved across the chart. The arm is connected to a light that projects from behind the patient into the concavity of the bowl. The position of the pointer on the chart corresponds to the specific point in the patient's visual field that is being tested. The

TABLE 12.2.
Goldmann Perimetry Target Parameters

Spot Size (mm)		Light Intensity of Target (Log unit of neutral density filter)			
0	1/16	1	1.5	a	0.4
I	1/4	2	1.0	b	0.3
II	1	3	0.5	c	0.2
III	4	4	0	d	0.1
IV	16			e	0
V	64				

projected target consists of a light that can be varied in size, intensity, and color. Large bright targets, designated as V_4e by convention (Table 12.2), test peripheral field, whereas small dim targets (I_2e) are used to explore the central and paracentral fields.

An isopter connects various points in the visual field to which the patient responds when tested with an object of specified size and luminance intensity. Various points in the field may be checked with static techniques across the midline in a more formal fashion.

Another commonly used manual kinetic field technique is a "Tangent" or "Bjerrum" Screen. The patient is placed at one or two meters in front of a black screen and maintains fixation on the center spot; one eye is tested at a time. A wand is then moved from the periphery towards the point of fixation along different meridians (usually eight). Various target sizes attached to the end of the wand are used to plot different isopters. Again, points in the visual field may be checked with static techniques. The resultant field is plotted on the screen with black pins and then transferred to a chart for permanent record.

The tangent screen is inexpensive and enables rapid and accurate plotting of the field. The patient is placed at either one or two meters from the screen, as compared to field tests performed on a bowl perimeter conducted at a distance of one-third of a meter. The resultant field defect is therefore much larger and easier to detect. This is especially useful with small central and paracentral defects. In addition, there is close observation and interaction between the examiner and the patient, who can sit in a wheelchair if necessary. Recording of a field defect in a sick patient who is unable to sit within the confines of a Goldmann, Humphrey, or Octopus perimeter is possible utilizing the tangent screen.

Static Amsler Grid Test. The Amsler test consists of a sheet of paper printed with a grid pattern and held by the patient one-third of a meter away. With one eye closed, the patient fixates on a central point on the grid and observes whether the entire grid is visible without shifting his gaze. The patient is also asked whether the lines of the grid are straight or appear distorted. The other eye is then tested in a similar fashion. A cooperative patient can easily map out his own field defect with this simple test. The Amsler Grid is a screening test for a central or paracentral scotoma that extends to within 20° of fixation if held at arms length. The field defect may be due to an optic neuropathy or a retinal maculopathy, and other tests (i.e., afferent pupillary defect, fundoscopy) may be necessary in order to differentiate the two conditions. Distortion of the grid (metamorphopsia) implies a maculopathy, whereas a central or paracentral scotoma may be due to either a maculopathy or an optic neuropathy.

The Amsler grid is printed in dark ink and is readily visible by a patient who has normal central as well as paracentral vision. This test is therefore considered a suprathreshold test, as compared to a threshold test, where a target is increased in intensity until it becomes visible.

Automated Perimetry

Currently, most static fields are obtained utilizing automated threshold parameters. The Humphrey and the Octopus machines are the most popular. In static perimetry, targets of different illumination intensity and size are projected into a concave bowl similar to the Goldmann perimeter. The points that a patient either sees or misses are recorded by a computer and the resultant field is plotted. The computer is able to compensate for the slow response time of a given patient and, therefore, the rate of response should not adversely affect the field as compared to kinetic perimetry. Computerized perimetry frequently rechecks various points and therefore assesses the consistency of responses. It

is able to keep track of the number of times a patient registers seeing a target that was not projected, i.e., false-positives, and, similarly, it is able to compute the incidence of false-negatives by checking previously recognized targets. Furthermore, age-matched statistics are available to compare the response of a patient to the average for his age. Therefore, in a reliable patient, an extremely accurate assessment of threshold visual field is possible. This permits accurate serial studies for monitoring a patient's progression of disease or response to therapy. A certain amount of clinical acumen is needed for the clinician to determine which visual field test is most suited to a particular patient. Often, both automated and manual field tests are required in order to make a definitive diagnosis. A substandard field test gives little basis for comparative analysis.

When interpreting a visual field test, it must be remembered that it is recorded from the patient's perspective. Therefore, when analyzing the result, the patient's left visual field is on the left, and his right field on the right. Both blind spots, which represent the optic discs void of photoreceptors, should be plotted, and they will be located temporal to fixation in both eyes. The inability to plot the blind spot adequately sheds doubt on the validity of the visual field test.

Field Defects in Parasellar Tumors (cases 1-7) Four patterns of field defects are typically seen in association with parasellar tumors. Both the size of the tumor and the direction of spread will determine the nature of the field loss. In patients with craniopharyngiomas, the nature of the visual field defect may change with time as fluid within the tumor resorbs and reaccumulates (41).

Bitemporal Hemianopia (case 1)

Bitemporal hemianopia (Fig. 12.1) is the most common visual field defect seen in patients with pituitary or parasellar tumors (50%), in contrast to craniopharyngioma, in which bitemporal hemianopia is less common (27%) (41). Because macular fibers predominate in the chiasm, the bitemporal hemianopia is frequently accompanied by a variable central or paracentral scotoma. Asymmetry of field loss is almost the rule, and it is rare to see a pure bitemporal hemi-anopia with no loss of central acuity in at least one eye. Bitemporal hemianopias may be complete (Fig. 12.1) or incomplete (see Fig. 12.16), symmetrical or asymmetrical. The hemianopia may be so subtle that it can be more easily detected when explored with a small red target. Bitemporal central hemi-anopic scotomas are typical of posterior chiasmal interference and may be missed if the central field is not tested with suitable thresh-old strategies.

Theoretically, when the chiasm is com-pressed from below, the decussating fibers originating from the inferior and nasal retina are affected first. The expected visual field loss begins in the superior temporal quad-rants. As the tumor continues to grow, the upper nasal fibers become involved and the superior field defect extends into the inferior temporal quadrants. Thus, the visual field defect progresses in an anticlockwise direc-tion in the left eye, and in a clockwise direc-tion in the right eye. An important feature is that the field defect obeys the vertical merid-ian. In practice, because most patients have variable loss of vision in one eye, true sym-metry of visual field loss in both eyes is not often seen. Most visual field defects are, in fact, variations on a theme of bitemporal or homonymous hemianopias. Pseudo-bitem-poral hemianopias may be caused by anom-alous optic discs, retinal pathology, or even excessive eyelid skin folds.

Central Scotoma

If the chiasm is significantly retroplaced, or if the mass projects in an anterior direc-tion, a pure prechiasmal compressive optic neuropathy with a central scotoma will re-sult. The visual field in the contralateral eye will be full. More rarely, however, bilateral optic nerves will be affected, causing bilateral central or cecocentral scotomata (27).

Junctional Scotoma (case 2)

A central scotoma in one eye, with a con-tralateral superior temporal field defect, is due to a compressive neuropathy involving Willebrand's knee (see Fig. 12.3). This field defect exquisitely localizes the lesion to the anatomical junction of the posterior optic nerve and the anterior chiasm (see II Re-gional Anatomy).

Homonymous Hemianopia (cases 3, 4, 5)

Where there is a prefixed chiasm or a pos-terior expanding tumor, the mass will com-press both the posterior angle of the chiasm and the optic tract on one side, causing an in-congruous homonymous hemianopia (See Fig. 12.6). The affected ipsilateral temporal fibers and the contralateral nasal fibers form-ing the optic tract will cause a contralateral field defect, i.e., a left-sided lesion will pro-duce a right-sided homonymous field defect. Lesions producing this type of defect are usu-ally large and involve the ipsilateral optic nerve, lateral chiasm, and tract, causing both asymmetric visual and visual field loss (See Figs. 12.6, 12.12, 12.13).

Eye Movement Disorders

Neurogenic/Paralytic Strabismus

Double vision is usually binocular and oc-curs when there is misalignment of the visual axis of both eyes. Causes include restrictive myopathies, i.e., Graves orbitopathy or trauma; neuromuscular junction conduc-tion defects, as in myasthenia gravis; or com-pressive neuropathies of the cranial nerves innervating the ocular muscles.

Parasellar tumors invading the cavernous sinus will produce pressure effects on the III, IV, and VI cranial nerves, as well as the first and second divisions of the V cranial nerve. Cases of pure motility disturbances without detectable visual field defects as the only pre-senting sign of a pituitary tumor are rare. Re-ports have varied considerably in the stated frequency of paralysis of ocular muscles. In 1910, de Lapersonne and Cantonnet re-ported ocular motility complications in 27% of patients with pituitary tumors (16). Since then, other investigators have published sim-ilar results with ocular motility difficulty oc-curring in 8% to 25% of patients (78, 82). In-terestingly, Davidoff, in 1926, found no ocular motility disturbance in his series of 100 patients (14). Most commonly affected is the third cranial nerve, either partially or to-tally and with or without pupillary involvement (case 2). There have been instances where the sixth nerve has been affected isolatedly, but it is usually associated with a third nerve paresis. When the fourth nerve is affected it is always accompanied by a third, fifth, or sixth nerve palsy. Corneal sensation should always be tested in these patients, as there may be involvement of the first division of the trigeminal nerve (29, 31, 34).

Although pituitary tumors are uncommon in adolescents, cranial neuropathies are more likely to be seen. In a review of 115 patients with pituitary adenomas, only four were adolescent, but all had invasive tumors with ocular motility palsies and three had trigeminal involvement (52).

Comitant Strabismus

Strabismus may occur in association with a sellar mass that has no cavernous sinus extension and compression of the nerves innervating ocular muscles. Where there is profound unilateral loss of vision involving both central and peripheral vision, the non-seeing eye will have no stimulus to keep it aligned with its fellow. Under such circumstances, a nonparalytic strabismus, usually a divergent squint, will result. The deviation measures the same in all directions of gaze, and is termed a comitant strabismus. By contrast, in a paralytic strabismus, the deviation will be worse in the field of action of the paretic muscle. Comitant strabismus has been reported to occur in up to 30% of children with craniopharyngioma (41), but may occur in anyone with a blind eye.

Non-Paretic Diplopia/Hemi-Field Slide Phenomenon

Occasionally, patients with profound bitemporal hemianopias will complain of double vision without an apparent motility abnormality. Elkington (19), described 98 of 260 patients with pituitary tumors who complained of double vision. Only 14 had a definite ocular motor palsy. It is presumed that patients with bitemporal field loss are unable to hold the two nasal visual fields in juxtaposition. This may lead to slippage in both the vertical and horizontal planes, and is termed the hemifield slide phenomenon (42).

Other

Other eye movement disorders are rarely seen in association with parasellar tumors. See-saw nystagmus, where one eye rises and intorts while the other falls and extorts, may be evident in children with gliomas involving the chiasm.

Headache

Headache has been found to be a constant finding in a large series of patients with parasellar tumors (19, 33). The headache is usually frontal in location and attributed to the stretching of the diaphragma sella. Chronic headache may be undiagnosed for months or years. It is imperative for all physicians to be aware of the headache associated with visual and endocrine abnormalities and initiate the appropriate investigations or referral.

Pupil Abnormalities

Afferent Pupillary Defect

In any affliction of the optic nerve (including compression) where the III cranial nerve and ciliary ganglion are spared, the pupils will be equal in size, although there will be a difference in pupil reactivity. The hallmark of optic nerve dysfunction is an afferent pupillary defect. Clinically, this can be most easily demonstrated using the swinging flashlight test. This test will objectively detect asymmetrical conduction along the anterior afferent visual pathway. Assuming there is no retinal pathology, if a light is shined into one eye there will normally be constriction of both pupils. If the light is then shifted to the other eye a similar response should be obtained. However, if dilatation of both pupils is observed while alternately swinging the flashlight, the stimulated eye that allows the pupillary dilatation probably has a relative conduction defect compared to the other. In the absence of retinal pathology, this test is extremely sensitive for unilateral optic nerve disease. Because there is a relatively greater decussation, i.e., crossed versus uncrossed retinal fibers (53% vs 47%), a profound homonymous field defect due to a tract lesion may give rise to a contralateral afferent pupillary defect (case 3). This finding will rarely be seen with homonymous defects from a pituitary adenoma.

Anisocoria

Anisocoria refers to a difference in pupil size between the two eyes. In the context of this chapter, it can occur with dysfunction of either the parasympathetic or sympathetic innervation of the pupil.

Pupillary constriction is controlled by parasympathetic nerves that course from the midbrain via cranial nerve III to the nerve's inferior division and then to the ciliary ganglion. A compressive lesion of the chiasm causing a third nerve palsy will typically cause the pupil on the involved side to be larger than the contralateral pupil (case 2).

Pupillary dilatation on the other hand, is mediated by the sympathetic nervous system. The third order neurons are intimately adherent to the internal carotid artery as it winds through the cavernous sinus, joins the sixth nerve for a short distance, and then joins the first division of the fifth nerve to enter the orbit. A space-occupying lesion compressing the carotid artery, sixth nerve, or sympathetics will theoretically cause a third-order neuronal Horner's syndrome, manifesting as miosis, ptosis, and failure to dilate with hydroxyamphetamine (1%). There are instances where minimal mydriasis is present in association with a III nerve palsy. In such a case, the sympathetic nerves within the cavernous sinus may also be compromised, resulting in a combined Horner's-third-nerve palsy picture.

Fundus Findings

Optic Atrophy

Optic atrophy occurs in approximately 50% of patients with chiasmal compression (9, 83). It is found only where there has been longstanding compression (33). If there has been a compressive neuropathy, such that the fibers subserving either the nasal or temporal field are damaged, so-called "bow-tie" or "winged" atrophy of the disc may be apparent.

The diagnosis of optic atrophy however, is notoriously subjective. When compression of the anterior visual system has advanced to the stage of optic atrophy there will be drop-

out of the retinal nerve fiber layer. Careful examination of the retinal nerve fiber layer has been found to be a more accurate way of documenting the extent of the neuronal damage than trying to assess the severity of the optic atrophy by the pallor of the disc. The reason for this is as follows: Normally, the nerve-fiber bundles are most prominent immediately around the optic disk, where the contrast is greatest. As they enter the optic disc, fibers are not readily discernible because of poor contrast. The optic atrophy or the loss of axons can be more accurately evaluated by the appearance of nerve-fiber layers in the peripapillary region then by the appearance of the optic disk alone. The technique of examining the retinal nerve-fiber layer with a so-called red-free light, (green light on the ophthalmoscope), has become popular and has been found to correlate well with the final visual outcome of patients with compressive optic neuropathy (38, 45, 46). Photographing the nerve-fiber layer in black and white with a red-free filter, has enabled very accurate recording of the degree of nerve-fiber dropout and, perhaps, has more relevance to optic nerve dysfunction than assessing disc pallor alone.

Before this technique was popularized, the prognostic significance of optic atrophy was not certain. Surprisingly, even in cases with distinct pallor, visual improvement has been documented (83). Conversely, the absence of optic atrophy does not in itself necessarily imply a good visual prognosis.

Papilledema

Papilledema is described as the swelling and elevation of the optic nerve head, with obscuration of the physiological cup and blurring of the disc margins. It is caused by increased intracranial pressure transmitted along the subdural space and producing obstruction of venous return and of axoplasmic flow along the nerve. It may be associated with transient loss of vision lasting a few seconds (transient obscurations), but it is not associated with prolonged visual loss until longstanding papilledema has caused ischemic damage to the nerve. Optic atrophy, in this instance, occurs as a result of gliosis, without defervescence of the disc elevation.

Papilledema secondary to pituitary tumors is extremely rare and is associated with florid extrasellar extension or anomalous venous connections between the sella and the orbit. A pituitary tumor might induce papilledema by extending above the sella and applying direct pressure on the optic nerves or by interrupting the cerebrospinal fluid (CSF) circulation and, thereby, increasing CSF pressure. In any event, the incidence of papilledema with pituitary tumor is between 0.3–8% (49). However, 4% of patients with craniopharyngioma may have raised intracranial pressure as manifested by swollen discs (41).

Incidentaloma—The Asymptomatic Patient

Autopsy studies have revealed that the incidence of asymptomatic pituitary adenomas in the general population is between 2-27% (8, 50). The term "incidentaloma," was coined by Reinecke *et al.* (57) to describe small pituitary tumors diagnosed incidentally on magnetic resonance imaging or computerized tomographic scanning. These authors had recommended initially that, if no growth was documented of an asymptomatic microadenoma after one year, no further surveillance would be necessary. However, a subsequent report (23) documented unexpected late tumor growth that caused chiasmal compression due to the lack of close follow-up. Whereas annual neuroimaging studies are expensive and therefore relatively contraindicated, clinical observation with sequential recording of visual acuity and perimetry is recommended on a yearly basis for both asymptomatic patients without prior treatment and for those who have had therapy.

THE CHIASMAL SYNDROME IN PREGNANCY

The chiasmal syndrome in pregnancy may result from a number of different circumstances involving pituitary gland function. Visual disturbances during pregnancy may also be related to other ocular as well as nonocular causes (69), but will not be discussed in the confines of this chapter.

Pregnancy increases the size of the normal pituitary gland without chiasmal compro-

mise (20, 67). This hypertrophic gland is vulnerable to hemorrhagic infarction in situations of obstetrically induced hypotension and is known as Sheehans's Syndrome. The hypopituitarism that follows may be associated with visual symptoms, not unlike pituitary apoplexy, due to a chiasmal syndrome. Sight-threatening loss of vision during pregnancy may be caused by the rapid growth of a preexisting asymptomatic pituitary adenoma, recurrence of a previously treated secreting adenoma—such as a prolactinoma—or, more rarely, a meningioma (case 7).

Pituitary Adenoma

In women who have asymptomatic pituitary tumors, visual complications during pregnancy may develop. In a review of 91 pregnancies in women with previously untreated microadenomas, only 5.5% developed symptoms related to enlargement. These symptoms consist of headache, visual disturbance, and diabetes insipidus (24), and usually develop late in pregnancy.

Infertile women who have prolactin-secreting adenomas may become pregnant with medical treatment. These patients have been found to be at slight risk for developing symptomatic pituitary enlargement during their pregnancy especially if bromocriptine is withdrawn (5, 21). Fortunately however, although sometimes poorly tolerated, this drug appears to be safe for both the mother and the fetus in all trimesters of pregnancy (74).

Women undergoing treatment to induce ovulation should be informed of the possibility that they may have a pituitary tumor (13). Most authors recommend an initial evaluation of serum prolactin levels prior to inducing ovulation as well as neuroimaging studies to exclude the presence of a tumor. If a microadenoma is detected, some authors recommend watching the patient for an additional few months to make sure that there is no evidence of growth. Induction of ovulation may then be attempted. During the course of a pregnancy in a woman with a known pituitary adenoma, monthly ophthalmic assessment of visual acuity and fields is recommended. If deterioration is detected, the various treatment options, including observation, should be evaluated by the medical team, which should consist of an endocrinologist, an obstetrician, an ophthalmologist, a radiologist, and a neurosurgeon.

Meningioma (Case 7)

There are many reports of patients presenting with a meningioma during pregnancy (7, 55, 62), especially in the latter half (61). These patients may demonstrate chiasmal signs, in the case of suprasellar tumors, or with oculomotor palsies and scotomas when parasellar tumors are involved. Symptoms may disappear after term only to recur in successive pregnancies. Receptors for estrogen and progesterone on meningioma tumors have been thought to play a role in their growth during pregnancy (82).

Other

Rapid enlargement of craniopharyngiomas during pregnancy has been reported (65). Another rare pregnancy-related intracerebral event, which has been described in the last trimester of pregnancy, is an immune process called lymphocytic hypophysitis. It is characterized by diffuse lymphocytic infiltration of the pituitary gland and presents with a chiasmal syndrome as well as features of hypopituitarism (3, 4).

RECOVERY OF VISION WITH TREATMENT OF TUMOR

In general terms, the prognosis for visual recovery in patients who have lost visual acuity or field as a result of their tumor depends on the duration of symptoms, severity of visual loss, presence or absence of optic atrophy, age of the patient, and size of the tumor. Significant improvement of visual function occurs within 24 hrs of surgery in most patients. Further recovery may be documented for several months thereafter. The visual response after medical therapy is usually just as gratifying, but recovery with radiotherapy may take months.

Medical

Dopamine agonists have been established as an alternative to surgery for treatment of prolactinomas. Bromocriptine is the prototype in this class of drugs. Others include per-

golide, lisuride, metergoline, and cabergoline. These drugs usually cause a prompt reduction of serum prolactin levels (22) and, a decrease in the size of the tumor (68, 73), as demonstrated by the rapid improvement of visual field defects with treatment (25, 68), but not necessarily by neuroimaging. Problems associated with the use of bromocriptine include poor patient tolerance due to nausea, nasal congestion, hypotension, and sedation. Bromocriptine has a short halflife and is administered as an oral drug at a dosage of 2.5mg two or three times per day. Some investigators have treated patients with an injectable long-acting preparation with good effect (26, 48). Pergolide has the advantage of an extended halflife, which allows a once-daily therapy, and cabergoline may be administered once a week.

A long-acting, non-ergot-derived dopamine agonist, CV 205-502, has also been shown to be effective in both micro- (75) and macroadenomas (76). This drug acts on the D2 receptors to reduce serum prolactin and restore gonadal function. It is used once daily and, although side-effects have been reported in about 40% of patients, they usually diminish significantly within two weeks. Thus, although not recommended at this time for primary treatment of hyperprolactinemia, CV 205-502 may be a useful alternative for bromocriptine-intolerant individuals.

The role of bromocriptine in the management of other pituitary tumors is not as clearly defined. Reduction in the size of nonfunctioning pituitary tumors after treatment with bromocriptine has been documented (17, 80, 84), but it has been less dramatic than that achieved with prolactinomas. Rapid loss of vision has been seen upon withdrawal of bromocriptine used in the treatment of nonfunctioning pituitary tumors (11). Bromocriptine treatment has also been associated with pituitary apoplexy in both short-term (1) and long-term use (77, 86), but a direct causal relationship is unproven. The new long-acting somatostatin analogue, SMS 201-995, shows promise for the medical treatment of growth hormone- and thyrotropic-secreting adenomas (18, 79).

Cyproheptadine, a serotonin antagonist, has been reported to induce remissions in occasional patients with Cushing's disease and acromegaly caused by secreting pituitary adenomas.

Surgery

In most patients, prompt return of vision follows the uncomplicated surgical removal of the tumor. In the series reported by Hollenhorst and Young (33), visual field defects improved in 62% of patients after surgery and in 75% after surgery plus radiation therapy. In 15%, vision remained unchanged, and in 10%, it became worse after surgical removal. The results are even more impressive in a recent series of 100 patients who underwent transsphenoidal resection of the tumor (12). Improvement of visual acuity and visual field defects took place in nearly 80% of the patients, whereas worsening of the visual functions was observed in only 3%. In another study comprising 108 patients with macroadenomas (10), full recovery of vision was achieved postoperatively in 63%, and an improvement was achieved in 27%. The visual acuity and field, therefore, improved in 90% of the patients undergoing transsphenoidal surgery. The postoperative visual improvement did not depend on the size of the suprasellar tumor extension, the direction of its growth, the tumor consistency, or its invasiveness into the surrounding structures. However, total tumor removal was rarely possible in patients with a suprasellar extension greater than 2 cm. In this series, there were no instances of postoperative visual deterioration. The average incidence of recurrence was 12% and it occurred four to eight years postoperatively.

Recovery should begin with dramatic speed within a few days of surgery and continue through the ensuing weeks (39). In fact, if vision is worse or has not improved in the acute postoperative period, there should be concern about persistent visual pathway compression by hematoma, surgical pack, or residual tumor. There may also be direct injury to the chiasm or the optic nerve, or interference with their blood supply. Generally, maximum recovery takes place within four months, with little improvement expected beyond that period. Prognosis for recovery is better in patients with a short duration of visual loss preoperatively.

The recurrence of a tumor is always a major concern, especially in macroadenomas whose excision has been incomplete. The recurrence rate for non-secreting tumors causing visual loss depends to a great extent on the initial size of the tumor and the mode of treatment. Both bromocriptine and radiotherapy have been used effectively as adjuncts to surgery where recurrence was thought to be a significant possibility. The disadvantage of medical therapy is that it is invariably lifelong, and the danger of radiotherapy is late radiation necrosis (vasculitis), with subsequent optic atrophy.

Radiotherapy

For several decades, radiation therapy has played an important role in the treatment of pituitary tumors, either as primary or as adjunct therapy. The visual morbidity associated with radiotherapy must be weighed against the advantages of medical or surgical treatment. Radionecrosis of chiasmal and intracerebral visual pathways is a well described entity following treatment of pituitary and parasellar tumors (31, 32, 43). Visual deterioration after radiation therapy occurs with a peak incidence of eight to 18 months after treatment (66), but may occur up to three years later. Patients present with a fairly rapid onset of visual loss in one eye, followed shortly by the other eye. The course is progressively downhill. Visual field defects show a typical central scotoma, with or without arcuate defects (43). A chiasmal or optic tract pattern has also been described (66). The optic discs will initially appear normal unless there was a preexisting atrophy. By eight weeks after the onset, optic atrophy is established. Neuroimaging studies are important to differentiate the visual loss in radionecrosis from that due to a recurrent tumor, apoplexy, traction due to the empty sella syndrome, or chiasmal arachnoiditis. Magnetic resonance imaging, with the use of the intravenous paramagnetic agent gadolinium-diethylenetriaminepentaacetic acid (Gd-DTPA), has recently been helpful in this situation to demonstrate breakdown of the blood-brain barrier in delayed radiation-induced optic neuropathy (28).

The true incidence of radionecrosis is difficult to estimate because visual loss after radiotherapy may occur for other reasons. In a retrospective study of 25 patients with visual impairment treated with radiotherapy for macroadenoma (63), vision deteriorated in four patients due to recurrence of the tumor, tumor hemorrhage (apoplexy), possible optic nerve necrosis, and herniation of the optic chiasm into the pituitary fossa.

The pathological basis of radionecrosis in the central nervous system is primarily a vasculitis with intravascular thrombosis and secondary axonal ischemia. Based upon this observation, treatment with anticoagulants and hyperbaric oxygen has been attempted (29, 30). It would appear that the best results are obtained if hyperbaric oxygen is given within two days of visual loss. Treatment that is delayed until after two weeks following visual loss has been shown to be ineffective (60).

A rare complication of radiotherapy is induction neoplasia, which may occur five to 20 years after the initial treatment. Various types of sarcomas, as well as sarcomas mixed with recurrent pituitary adenomas, have been reported following radiotherapy to the parasellar region (53, 72).

CONCLUSION

Despite the fact that vision-related disorders from parasellar tumors may be on the decline due to earlier detection by sophisticated diagnostic techniques, it is nevertheless the responsibility of the physician who suspects the diagnosis of a parasellar tumor to pursue an enquiry related to the visual system. Referral for ophthalmic evaluation is part of the management of these patients in the early stage of diagnosis as well as in the long term care, whether it be medical, surgical, or inclusive of radiotherapy.

CASE ILLUSTRATIONS

Case 1.

A 46-year-old male was referred for visual assessment after being involved in a motor vehicle accident. On examination, his best corrected visual acuity was 20/20 OU with a bitemporal hemianopia (Fig. 12.1). Ocular motility and optic discs were normal. Serum testosterone and thyroid-stimulating hormone were below normal, but the patient was asymptomatic for endocrine disease. An MRI scan (Fig. 12.2) showed a large sellar and suprasellar mass with retention of the pituitary gland configuration (arrow). Transsphenoidal hypophysectomy confirmed the presence of a pituitary adenoma. Postoperatively, the visual field returned to normal.

Note:

1. Bitemporal hemianopia caused by pituitary adenoma.
2. Good visual outcome after transsphenoidal decompression.

Case 2.

A 32-year-old man complained of progressive loss of vision OD associated with diplopia over the past four years. He had also noted galactorrhea and an inability to maintain an erection or ejacu-

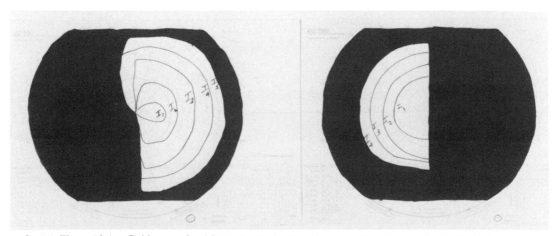

Case 1. Figure 12.1.   Goldmann visual field of patient with a bitemporal hemianopia due to pituitary adenoma.

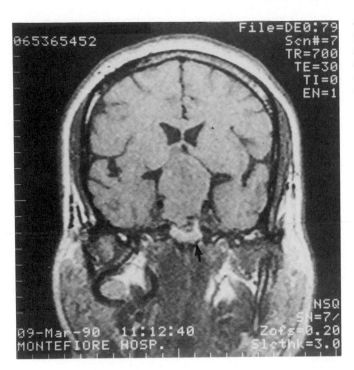

Case 1. Figure 12.2. MRI demonstrating coronal view of a large sellar mass with suprasellar extension, which proved to be a pituitary adenoma. The original "bean-shaped" pituitary configuration is indicated by the arrow.

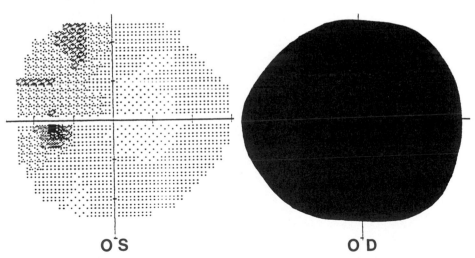

Case 2. Figure 12.3. Automated visual field of a patient with a junctional scotoma. There is a profound scotoma OD with no light perception vision, and a superotemporal field defect OS due to compression at Willebrand's knee.

late for two weeks prior to presentation. On examination, his visual acuity was no light perception OD, and 20/20 OS. The pupil OD was dilated and unresponsive to light (amaurotic). In addition, the right eye had a partial ptosis as well as adduction, elevation, and depression deficits, consistent with a III nerve palsy. The optic disc was markedly pale OD, and showed temporal pallor

OS. An automated threshold visual field obtainable in the left eye only, showed a supero-temporal field defect obeying the vertical midline (Fig. 12.3). An MRI revealed a large sellar mass that had suprasellar extension with more compression of the chiasm on the right than on the left side (arrow). In addition, there appeared to be bilateral extension into the cavernous sinuses. The bright

Case 2. Figures 12.4 & 12.5. Coronal and sagittal section of the MRI of a patient with a large sellar mass causing a compressive neuropathy at Willebrand's knee (arrow). In addition, there is cavernous sinus extension, which resulted in a III nerve palsy on the right side.

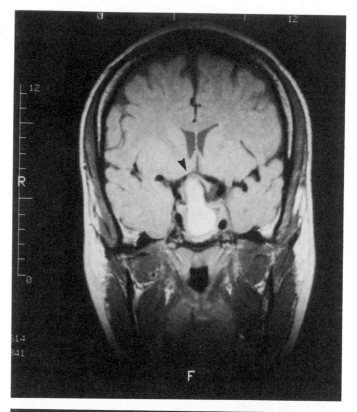

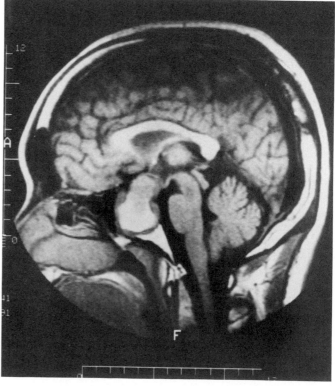

signal on the non-contrast enhanced T1 image is compatible with hemorrhage within the tumor (Figs. 12.4 and 12.5).

Note:

1. Junctional scotoma caused by a compressive optic neuropathy OD, and involvement of the contralateral inferonasal fibers at Willebrand's knee.
2. Cavernous sinus extention causing motility disorder (III nerve palsy).

Case 3.

A 32-year-old male presented with a two-week history of progressive left homonomous field loss associated with headache, photophobia, and scintillations in the field of visual loss. His best corrected visual acuity on initial presentation was 20/ 25 OD and 20/20 OS, but decreased to 20/80 OD and 20/30 OS two weeks later. He had an afferent pupillary defect and profound color visual loss on Ishihara color plates OD, as well as a left incongruous homonymous hemianopia (Fig. 12.6). The optic discs appeared normal. An MRI scan revealed a large suprasellar mass with posterior extension causing an obstructive hydrocephalus (Figs. 12.7 and 12.8). The CT scan showed this mass to be calcified. Endocrine studies were reportedly within normal limits. An initial biopsy was nondiagnostic, but a repeat craniotomy performed four months later confirmed the presence of a craniopharyngioma. By this time, the patient could only count fingers with the right eye, and was 20/50 OS, with chronic papilledema and bilateral sixth nerve palsies. Three months after definitive surgery, his vision remained "count fingers" in the temporal field OD and 20/50 OS, with

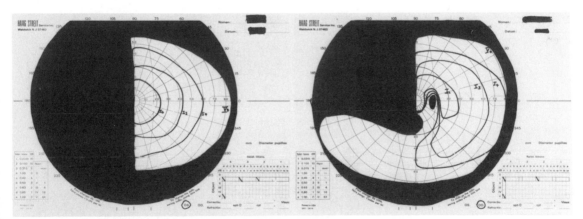

Case 3. Figure 12.6. Goldmann visual field of a patient with an incongruous left homonymous hemianopia due to a craniopharyngioma. The patient's vision was 20/25 OD and 20/20 OS.

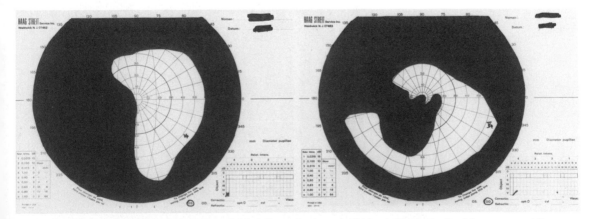

Case 3. Figure 12.7. Postoperative visual field performed seven months later. The patient's vision was count finger OD and 20/50 OS. Note that only the I_4 isopter is plotted, which reflects a poor central acuity.

Case 3. Figure 12.8. Coronal section of the MRI of the same patient with a large suprasellar craniopharyngioma.

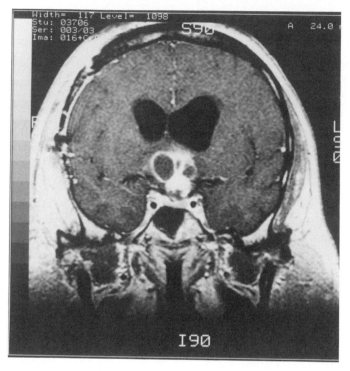

Case 3. Figure 12.9. Coronal section of the MRI demonstrating massive posterior extension of the tumor, as well as a dilated third ventricle due to an obstructive hydrocephalus.

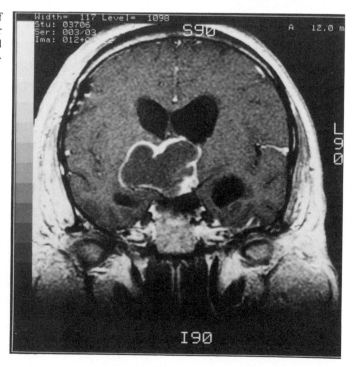

a persistent left homonymous hemianopia (Fig. 12.9), asymmetric optic atrophy, and a full range of ocular motility.

Note:

1. Symptoms of photophobia and scintillations associated with visual field loss.
2. An afferent pupillary defect associated with optic nerve compression in the right eye.
3. The initial visual field (Fig. 12.6) revealed a left homonymous hemianopia with all the isopters (I_2, I_3, I_4, V_4), which suggests good visual acuity at the time. However, the postoperative field (Fig. 12.9) was drawn with only the V_4 isopter, which implies poor acuity.

Case 4.

A 60-year-old woman with progressive loss of vision had consulted various optometrists for spectacles over the previous six months without enjoying visual improvement. She presented to an ophthalmologist for the first time with a visual acuity of hand movements bilaterally. Both pupils reacted poorly to light. Formal visual fields were unobtainable because of her poor vision, but a dense homonymous hemianopia was detected on confrontation fields. Her ocular motility was full but she had bilateral optic atrophy. An MRI scan showed a large suprasellar mass (Fig. 12.10). A CT scan demonstrated that the lesion was calcified (Fig. 12.11). An emergency transfrontal craniot-

omy was performed when she lost all light perception OS. Histology confirmed the preoperative diagnosis of a craniopharyngioma. On the first postoperative day, the patient's vision was count fingers OD and hand movements OS. Seven months later, she had 20/200 OD and 20/60 OS. Her visual field performed on a tangent screen showed a dense temporal hemianopia OS, and a central scotoma OD, with only a superotemporal island of vision remaining in that eye (Fig. 12.12).

Note:

1. Confrontation visual fields can be obtained despite profound loss of central acuity.
2. Return of vision from no light perception to 20/60 OS after prompt surgical decompression.

Case 5.

In 1984, a 51-year-old man was referred to a psychologist for decreased sexual performance in the absence of a galactorrhea. He developed an incidental bloody penile discharge that prompted further medical and neuroendocrine evaluation. He was diagnosed as having a craniopharyngioma with secondary hypopituitarism. He was managed conservatively, with serial visual field tests and neuroimaging studies and was given hormone supplements. An asymptomatic field defect was detected one year later. This defect was reportedly

Case 4. Figure 12.10. Sagittal section of MRI demonstrating a suprasellar mass that appeared calcified on an axial CT scan. (Fig. 12.11.)

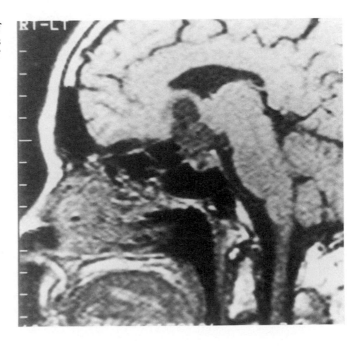

Case 4. Figure 12.11. Axial section of CT scan of the same patient demonstrating calcification of craniopharyngioma.

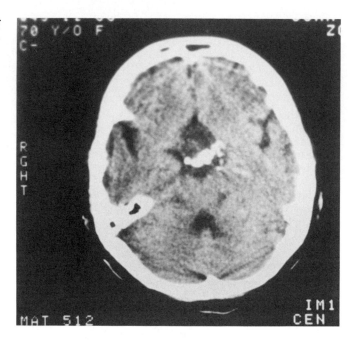

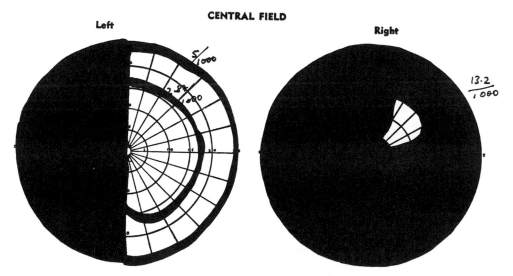

Case 4. Figure 12.12. Tangent screen visual field of a patient seven months after craniotomy for craniopharyngioma. The field shows a dense temporal defect OS with a central scotoma OD, and only a small island of vision remaining in the superotemporal field of that eye. The visual acuity at the time of this visual field was 20/200 OD and 20/60 OS, but it had been hand motions OD, and no light perception OS just prior to surgery.

stable over the next four years when, in 1989, the patient noted loss of vision to the right side. A cystic suprasellar tumor was found to be enlarging, causing a right homonymous hemianopia due to left optic tract compression. A frontal craniotomy was performed with subtotal excision of the tumor. Care was taken intraoperatively to avoid stripping the tumor from the optic tract and depriving the visual pathway of its vascular supply. Postoperatively, the patient achieved a visual acuity of 20/20 OU with a fixed right incongruous homonymous hemianopia one year later (Fig. 12.13). Significant residual tumor is present on MRI. (Figs. 12.14 and 12.15).

Note:

1. Sudden visual deterioration after a long period of apparent stability. On review of the patient's past visual fields, it was discovered that automated *suprathreshold* tests were performed that are essentially screening tests. A more appropriate test to detect early subtle field changes would have been an automated *threshold* test, such as the Humphrey program 24-2, or the Octopus program 30-2.

Case 6.

A 50-year-old female was treated for glaucoma for one year, but it was felt by her referring ophthalmologist that her optic discs and visual fields were not entirely consistent with the diagnosis of glaucoma. On examination, her visual acuity was 20/20 OD and 20/25 OS with a trace afferent defect OS. Goldmann visual fields revealed a full field OD and a temporal hemianopic defect that was more dense superiorly OS (Fig. 12.16). Fun-

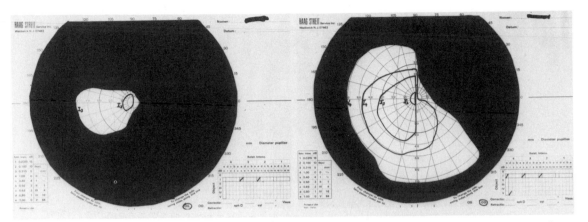

Case 5. Figure 12.13. Fixed right incongruous homonymous hemianopia one year after craniotomy for a craniopharyngioma. Visual acuity is 20/20 OU.

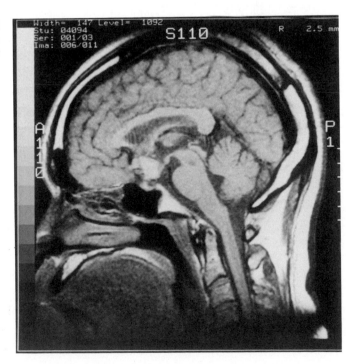

Case 5. Figures 12.14 and 12.15. Sagittal and coronal section of the MRI of a patient with residual tumor one year after craniotomy for craniopharyngioma.

Figure 12.15.

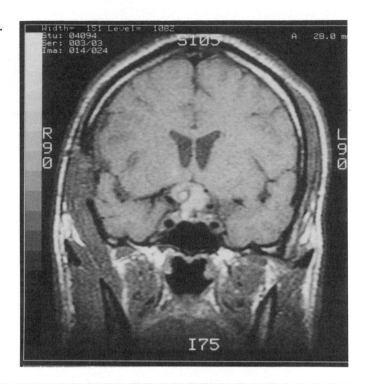

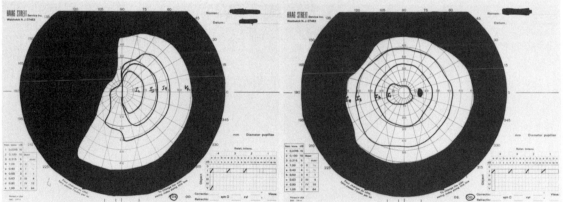

Case 6. Figure 12.16. Temporal field defect OS and a normal field OD on Goldmann perimetry. This visual field defect was not consistent with the patient's diagnosis of glaucoma, due to the sharp demarcation at the vertical meridian.

doscopy demonstrated asymmetrical glaucomatous cupping, that was more advanced on the left side, with a nasal wedge of pallor. An MRI study revealed a large sellar mass with suprasellar extension (Figs. 12.17 and 12.18). The patient was found to be hypercalcemic and was suspected of having Multiple Endocrine Neoplasia Type 1 on the basis of a nonsecreting pituitary adenoma and hyperparathyroidism. The patient underwent a transsphenoidal hypophysectomy and the visual

field recovered satisfactorily during the first postoperative week. (Fig. 12.19)

Note:

1. The distinction between glaucomatous cupping and optic atrophy may prove to be difficult.
2. The importance of correlating the optic disc appearance with the visual fields.

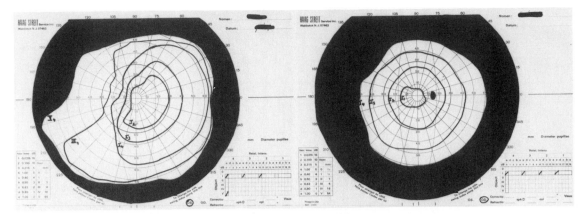

Case 6. Figure 12.17.   Recovery of field one week after surgery.

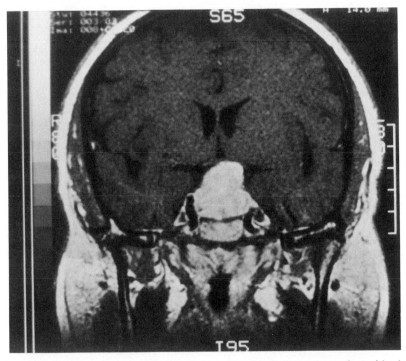

Case 6. Figures 12.18 and 12.19.   Sagittal and coronal views of the MRI of the same patient with a large sellar mass with suprasellar extension that produced a temporal field defect OS only (Fig. 12.16).

Case 7.

A 30-year-old para 0, gravida 1, woman of 24 weeks gestation developed frontal headaches associated with progressive loss of vision OS. Her visual acuity was 20/40 OD and 20/200 OS, with a marked pupillary afferent defect OS. She could identify 9/15 Ishihara color plates OD, and only the test plate OS. Automated threshold perimetry revealed a central scotoma OS, and a dense tem-poral defect OS respecting the vertical meridian (Fig. 12.20—first field). An MRI scan (Figs. 12.21 and 12.22) showed a large low-density suprasellar mass on T1-weighted image, with a normal pituitary gland. The radiological diagnosis was that of a meningioma. Treatment was initially nonoperative in order to maximize the condition of her fetus. Craniotomy was performed at 32 weeks' gestation due to progressive field loss. Figures

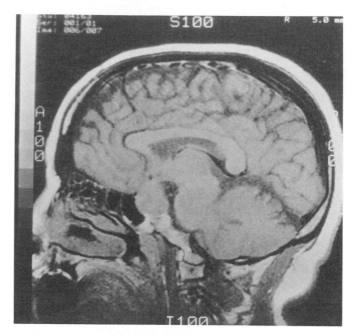

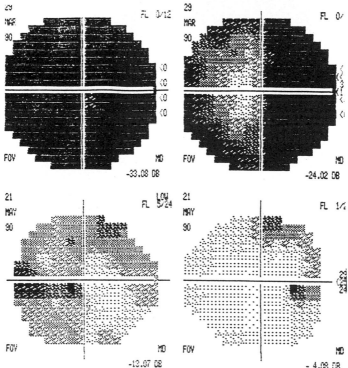

Case 7. Figures 12.20 and 12.21. Sequential automated threshold perimetry of a pregnant woman with a large suprasellar meningioma seen in sagital and coronal section on MRI in Figs. 12.22 and 12.23. The first visual field in Fig. 12.20 was recorded soon after presentation, when her visual acuity was 20/40 OD and 20/200 OS. The field shows a central scotoma OS and a dense temporal defect OD. The second field was recorded during the first week after craniotomy. The last field, in Fig. 12.21 was recorded four months after surgery, when her visual acuity was 20/20 OD and 20/40 OS.

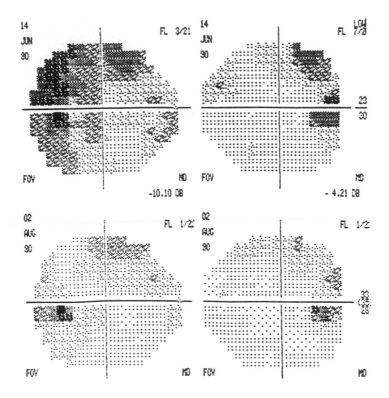

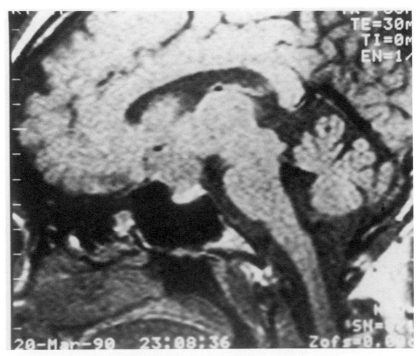

Case 7. Figures 12.22 and 12.23. Sagittal and coronal sections of the MRI scan performed on the pregnant woman with a suprasellar meningioma. Her visual fields are depicted in Fig. 12.20.

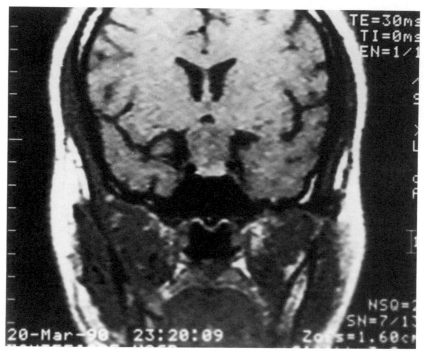

Figure 12.23.

12.20 and 12.23 demonstrate her sequential improvement on automated threshold perimetry over the ensuing four postoperative months. She achieved a visual acuity of 20/20 OD and 20/40 OS. The histopathology of the tumor was consistent with the diagnosis of meningioma. No estrogen receptor markers were performed on the specimen, which would have helped in the management of a recurrence during a subsequent pregnancy. At term, the patient gave birth to a healthy fetus by Cesarian section.

Note:

1. Enlargement of meningioma during pregnancy due to the presence of estrogen receptors.
2. The need for careful neuro-ophthalmic evaluation in such cases.

REFERENCES

1. Alhajje A., Lambert M., Crabbe J. Pituitary apoplexy in an acromegalic patient during bromocriptine therapy. J. Neurosurg., 63:288, 1985.
2. Anderson D., Faber P., and Maarcovitz S., et al. Pituitary tumors and the ophthalmologist. Ophthalmology, 90:1265, 1983.
3. Asa S.L., Bilbao J.M., Kovacs K., et al. Lymphocytic hypophysitis of pregnancy resulting in hypopituitarism: a distinct clinicopathologic entity. Ann. Int. Med., 95:166, 1981.
4. Baskin D.S.M., Townsend J.J., Wilson C.B. Lymphocytic hypophysitis of pregnancy simulating a pituitary adenoma: a distinct pathological entity. J. Neurosurg., 56:148, 1982.
5. Berg T., Nilius S.J., Enoksson, et al. Bromocriptine induced pregnancies in women with large prolactinomas. Clin. Endocrinol., 17:635, 1982.
6. Bergland R.M., Ray B.S., Torack R.M. Anatomic variations in the pituitary gland and adjacent structures in 225 human autopsy cases. J. Neurosurg., 28:93, 1968.
7. Bickerstaff E.R., Small J.M., Guest I.A. The relapsing course of certain meningiomas in relation to pregnancy and menstruation. J. Neurol. Neurosurg. Psychiat., 21:89, 1958.
8. Burrow G.N., Wortzman G., Rewcastle N.B., et al. Microadenomas of the pituitary and abnormal sellar tomograms in an unselected autopsy series. N. Eng. J. Med., 304:156, 1981.
9. Chamlin F., Davidoff L.M., Feiring E.H. Ophthalmologic changes produced by pituitary tumors. Am. J. Ophthal., 40:353, 1955.
10. Ciric I., Mikhael M., Stafford T., et al. Transsphenoidal microsurgery of pituitary macroadenomas with long-term follow-up results. J. Neurosurg., 59:394, 1983.
11. Clark J.D.A., Wheatley T., Edwards O.M. Rapid enlargement of non-functioning pituitary tumor following withdrawal of bromocriptine. J. Neurol. Neurosurg. Psychiatry, 48:287(letter), 1985.
12. Cohen A.R., Cooper P.R., Kupersmith M.J., et al. Visual Recovery after transsphenoidal removal of pituitary adenomas. Neurosurgery, 17:446, 1985.

13. Crosignani P., Ferrari C., Mattei A.M. Visual field defects and reduced visual acuity during pregnancy in two patients with prolactinoma: rapid regression of symptoms under bromocriptine. Case reports. Br. J. Obstet. Gynaecol., *91*:821, 1984.

14. Davidoff L.M. Studies in acromegaly. The anamnesis and symptomatology in one hundred cases. Endocrinology, *10*:461, 1926.

15. Dawson D.J., Enoch B.A., Shepherd D.I. Formed visual hallucinations with pituitary adenomas. Brit. Med. J., *289*:414, 1984.

16. de Lapersonne F., Cantonette A. Troubles visuals produits par les tumeurs de Phypophyse sans acromegalies. Arch. Ophthalmol., *30*:65, 1910.

17. D'Emden M.C., Harrison L.C. Rapid improvement in visual field defects following bromocriptine treatment of patients with non-functioning pituitary adenomas. Clin. Endocrinol. (Oxf.), *25*:697, 1986.

18. Ducasse M.C.R., Tauber J.P., Tourre A., *et al.* Shrinking of a growth hormone-producing pituitary tumor by continuous subcutaneous infusion of the somatostatin analog SMS 201-995. J. Clin. Endocrinol. Metab., *65*:1042, 1987.

19. Elkington S.G. Pituitary adenoma: Pre-operative symptomatology in a series of 260 patients. Br. J. Ophthalmol., *52*:322, 1968.

20. Erdheim J., Stumme E. Uber die Schwangerschaftsveranderung der Hypophuse. Beitr. Pathol. Anat. Allerg. Pathol., *46*:1, 1909.

21. Falconer M.A., Stafford-Bell M.A. Visual failure from pituitary and parasellar tumors occurring with favorable outcome in pregnant women. J. Neurol. Neurosurg. Psychiat., *38*:919, 1975.

22. Franks S., Jacobs H.S. Hyperprolactinaemia. Clin. Endocrinol. Metab., *12*:641, 1983.

23. Frohman L.J., Kupersmith M.J., Floyd W. The pituitary incidentaloma beyond the first year of follow-up. Letter J.A.M.A., *264*:2387, 1990.

24. Gemzell C., Wang F.W. Outcome of pregnancy in women with pituitary adenoma. Fertil. Steril., *31*:363, 1979.

25. Grimson B.S., Bowman Z.L. Rapid decompression of anterior visual pathways with bromocriptine. Arch. Ophthalmol., *101*:604, 1983.

26. Grossman A., Ross R., Wass J.A.H., *et al.* Depot bromocriptine treatment for prolactinomas and acromegaly. Clin. Endocrinol. (Oxf.), *24*:231, 1986.

27. Gutman I., Behrens M., Odel J. Bilateral central and centrocecal scotomata due to mass lesion. Br. J. Ophthalmol., *68*:336, 1984.

28. Guy J., Mancuso A., Quisling R.G., *et al.* Gadolinium-DTPA-enhanced magnetic resonance imaging in optic neuritis. Ophthalmology, *97*:592, 1990.

29. Guy J., Schatz N.J. Hyperbaric oxygen in the treatment of radiation-induced optic neuropathy. Ophthalmology, *93*:1083, 1986.

30. Guy J., Schatz N.J. Effectiveness of hyperbaric oxygen in treating radiation injury to the optic nerves and chiasm [Letter]. Ophthalmology, *97*:1246, 1990.

31. Hammer H.M. Optic chiasmal radionecrosis. Trans. Ophthalmol. Soc. U.K., *103*:208, 1983.

32. Harris J.R., Levene M.B. Visual complications following irradiation for pituitary adenomas and craniopharyngiomas. Radiology, *120*:167, 1976.

33. Hollenhorst R.W., and Young B.R. Ocular manifestations produced by adenomas of the pituitary gland: Analysis of 1000 cases. In: *Diagnosis and treatment of pituitary tumors*, p. 53. Edited by P.O. Kohler and G.T. Ross. New York, Elsevier, 1973.

34. Holness R.O., Ogundimu F.A. Langville R.A. Pituitary apoplexy following closed head trauma. Case report. J. Neurosurg., *59*:677, 1983.

35. Hoyt W.F. Correlative functional anatomy of the optic chiasm. Clin. Neurosurg., *17*:189, 1970.

36. Hoyt W.F., Lois O. The primate chiasm: details of visual fiber organization studied by silver impregnation techniques. Arch. Ophthalmol., *70*:69, 1963.

37. Hoyt W.F., Lois O. Visual fiber anatomy in the infrageniculate pathway of the primate. Uncrossed and crossed retinal fiber projection studied by Nauta silver stain. Arch. Ophthalmol., *68*:94, 1962.

38. Jain I.S., Gupta A., Khurana G.S., *et al.* Visual prognosis in pituitary tumor. Ann. Ophthalmol., *17*:392, 1985.

39. Kayan A., Earl C.J. Compressive lesions of the optic nerves and chiasm. Pattern of recovery following surgical treatment. Brain, *98*:13, 1975.

40. Kellen R.I., Burde R.M., Hodges F.J. Occult pituitary apoplexy associated with craniopharyngioma. J. Clin. NeuroOphthalmol., *8*:99, 1988.

41. Kennedy H.B., Smith R.J.S. Eye signs in craniopharyngiomas. Br. J. Ophthalmol., *59*:689, 1975.

42. Kirkham T.H. The ocular symptomatology of pituitary tumors. Proc. R. Soc. Med., *65*:517, 1972.

43. Kline L.B., Kim J.V., Ceballos R. Radiation optic neuropathy. Ophthalmology, *92*:1118, 1985.

44. Lloyd M.H., Belchetz P.E. The clinical features and management of pituitary apoplexy. Postgrad. Med. J., *53*:82, 1977.

45. Lundstrom M., Frisen L. Atrophy of optic nerve fibers in compression of the chiasm. Acta. Ophthalmol. (Copenh.), *54*:623, 1976.

46. Lundstrom M., Frisen L. Atrophy of optic nerve fibres in compression of the chiasm: prognostic implications. Acta. Ophthalmol. (Copenh.), *55*:208, 1977.

47. Lyle T.K., Clover P. Ocular symptoms and signs of pituitary tumors. Proc. R. Soc. Med., *54*:611, 1961.

48. Montini M., Pagani G., Gianola D., *et al.* Long-lasting suppression of prolactin secretion and rapid shrinkage of prolactinomas after a long-acting, injectable form of bromocriptine. J. Clin. Endocrinol. Metab., *63*:266, 1986.

49. Mueller G.L., McKenna T.J., Kelly G., *et al.* Papilledema in two patients with acromegaly and intrasellar pituitary tumors. Arch. Intern. Med., *141*:1491, 1981.

50. Muhr C., Bergstrom K., Grimelius L., *et al.* A parallel study of the roentgen anatomy of the sella turcica and the histopathology of the pituitary gland in 205 autopsy specimens. Neuroradiology, *21*:55, 1981.

51. Onetsi S.T., Wisniewski T., Post K.D. Clinical versus subclinical pituitary apoplexy: Presentation, surgical management, and outcome in 21 patients. Neurosurgery, *26*:980, 1990.

52. Ortiz-Suarez H., Erickson D.L. Pituitary adenomas of adolescents. J. Neurosurg., *43*:437, 1975.

53. Pieterse S., Dinning T.A.R., Blumberg P.C. Postir-

radiation sarcomatous transformation of a pituitary adenoma: a combined pituitary tumor. J. Neurosurg., *52*:283, 1982.

54. Ram Z., Findler G., Gutman I., *et al.* Visual hallucinations associated with pituitary adenoma. Neurosurgery, *20*:292, 1987.

55. Rand C.W. Two cerebral complications of pregnancy: brain tumor and subarachnoid hemorrhage. Clin. Neurosurg., *3*:104, 1957.

56. Reid R.L., Quigley M.E., Yen S.S.C. Pituitary apoplexy. A review. Arch. Neurol., *42*:712, 1985.

57. Reinecke M., Allolio B., Saeger W., *et al.* The "incidentaloma" of the pituitary gland: is neurosurgery required? J.A.M.A., *263*:2772, 1990.

58. Robert C.M. Jr., Feigenbaum J.A., Stern W.E. Ocular palsy occurring with pituitary tumors. J. Neurosurg., *38*:17, 1973.

59. Robinson J.L. Sudden blindness with pituitary tumors. J. Neurosurg., *36*:83, 1972.

60. Roden D., Bosley T.M., Fowble B., *et al.* Delayed radiation injury to the retrobulbar optic nerve and chiasm. Clinical syndrome and treatment with hyperbaric oxygen and corticosteroids. Ophthalmology, *97*:346, 1990.

61. Roelvink N.C.A., Kamphort W., van Alphen H.A.M., *et al.* Pregnancy-related primary brain and spinal tumors. Arch. Neurol., *44*:209, 1987.

62. Rucker C.W., Kearns T.P. Mistaken diagnosis in some cases of meningioma. Am. J. Ophthalmol., *51*:15, 1961.

63. Rush S.C., Kupersmith M.J., Lerch I., *et al.* Neuro-ophthalmological assessment of vision before and after radiation therapy alone for pituitary adenomas. J. Neurosurg., *72*:594, 1990.

64. Safran A.B., Kline L.B., Glaser J.S. Positive visual phenomena in optic nerve and chiasm disease: photopsias and photophobia. Neuro-opthalmology. Vol. X, edited by J.S. Glaser, St. Louis, The Mosby Co., p. 225, 1980.

65. Sachs B.P., Smith S.K., Casser J., *et al.* Rapid enlargement of craniopharyngioma during pregnancy. Br. J. Obstet. Gynaecol., *85*:557, 1978.

66. Schatz N.J., Lichstenstein S., Corbett J.J. Delayed radiation necrosis of the optic nerve and chiasm. In: *Neuro-ophthalmology: symposium of the University of Miami and the Bascom Palmer Eye Institute, edited by J.S. Glaser and J.L. Smith.*, *8*:131, St. Louis, C.V. Mosby, 1975.

67. Scheithauer B.W., Kovacs K.T., Young W.F., *et al.* The pituitary gland in pregnancy: a clinicopathologic and immunohistochemical study of 69 cases. Mayo Clin. Proc., *65*:461, 1990.

68. Spark R.F., Baker R., Bienfang C.D., *et al.* Bromocriptine reduces pituitary tumor size and hypersecretion. Requiem for pituitary surgery? J. Am. Med. Assoc., *247*:311, 1982.

69. Sunness J.S. The pregnant woman's eye. Major review. Surv. Ophthalmol., *32*:219, 1988.

70. Symon L., Jakubowshi J. Transcranial management of pituitary tumors with suprasellar extension. J. Neurol. Neurosurg. Psychiatry, *42*:123, 1979.

71. Symon L., Mohanty S. Hemorrhage in pituitary tumors. Acta. Neurochir., *65*:41, 1982.

72. Terry R.D., Hyams V.J., Davidoff L.M. Combined non-metastasizing fibrosarcoma and chromophobe tumor of the pituitary. Cancer, *12*:791, 1959.

73. Thorner M.O., Martin W.H., Rogol A.D., *et al.* Rapid regression of prolactinomas during bromocriptine treatment. J. Clin. Endocrinol. Metab., *51*:438, 1980.

74. Turkalj I., Braun P., Krupp P. Surveillance of bromocriptine in pregnancy. J.A.M.A., *247*:1589, 1982.

75. Vance M.L., Cragun J.R., Reirnnitz C., *et al.* CV 205-502 Treatment of hyperprolactinemia. J. Clin. Endocrinol. Metab., *68*:336, 1989.

76. Vance M.L., Lipper M., Klibanski A., *et al.* Treatment of prolactin-secreting pituitary macroadenomas with the long acting non-ergo dopamine agonist CV 205-502. Ann. Int. Med., *112*:668, 1990.

77. Wakai S., Fukushima T., Teramoto A., *et al.* Pituitary apoplexy: its incidence and clinical significance. J. Neurosurg., *55*:187, 1981.

78. Walsh F.B., Hoyt W.F. Clinical neuro-ophthalmology, Vol 3. Baltimore, Williams & Wilkins, 2141, 1969.

79. Warnet A., Timsit J., Chanson P., *et al.* The effect of somatostatin analogue on chiasmal dysfunction from pituitary macroadenomas. J. Neurosurg., *71*:687, 1989.

80. Wass J.A.H., Williams J., Charlesworthy M., *et al.* Bromocriptine in the management of large pituitary tumors. Br. J. Med., *284*:1908, 1982.

81. Weinberger L.M., Grant F.C. Visual hallucinations and their neuro-optical correlates. Arch. Ophthalmol., *23*:166, 1940.

82. Yu Z.Y., Wrange O., Haglund B., *et al.* Estrogen and progestin receptors in intracranial meningiomas. J. Steroid Biochem., *16*:451, 1982.

82. Weinberger L.M., Adler F.H., Grant F.C. Primary pituitary adenoma and the syndrome of cavernous sinus: a clinical and anatomical study. Arch. Ophthalmol., *24*:1197, 1940.

83. Wilson P., Falconer M.A. Patterns of visual failure with pituitary tumors. Clinical and radiological correlations. Brit. J. Ophthalmol., *52*:94, 1968.

84. Wollensen F., Andersen T., Karle A. Size reduction of extra-sellar pituitary tumors during bromocriptine treatment. Quantitation of effect on different types of tumors. Ann. Int. Med., *96*:281, 1982.

85. Wray S.H. Neuro-ophthalmologic manifestations of pituitary and parasellar lesions. Clin. Neurosurg., *24*:86, 1978.

86. Yamaji T., Ishibashi M., Kosaka K., *et al.* Pituitary apoplexy in acromegaly during bromocriptine therapy. Acta. Endocrinol. (Copenh.), *98*:171, 1981.

CHAPTER 13

Radiological Evaluation of Pituitary Lesions

JAMES HOFFMAN, M.D., and DANIEL L. BARROW, M.D.

The radiological diagnosis of lesions in the sellar and parasellar regions has undergone considerable change over the last several years. A number of rather inaccurate imaging modalities have given way to the more elegant imaging capabilities of computed tomography (CT) and magnetic resonance imaging (MRI). CT replaced plain films, polytomography, and pneumoencephalography for the diagnosis of these tumors and, more recently, MRI has become the primary imaging modality for diseases of the sellar and parasellar region. Plain skull films are still useful in assessing the contour and pneumatization of the sphenoid sinus for the surgeon planning a transsphenoidal operation. Cerebral angiography is necessary for accurate anatomical detail of the cerebral vasculature in planning surgical treatment of intracranial aneurysms. CT and/or MRI, however, provide images that allow one to create a well-defined differential diagnosis and plan surgical therapy for lesions in the sellar and parasellar areas. MRI has the additional advantage of being able to rule out the presence of an intracranial aneurysm that may mimic a pituitary adenoma.

NORMAL ANATOMY

On both CT and MRI, the normal pituitary gland can vary in size. In men, the normal gland measures 5–6 mm in height, whereas in women the gland tends to be much larger. The normal gland height in menstruating females can be as high as 9 mm (19). In men, the superior surface of the gland is flat to concave, whereas in women the superior surface of the gland may be concave, flat, or even convex in young females. Normally, the infundibulum is a midline structure, but, occasionally, it can be tilted or slightly off the midline.

On unenhanced MRI, the normal anterior pituitary gland (adenohypophysis) is isointense, with grey matter of the brain on all sequences, whereas the posterior pituitary (neurohypophysis) will demonstrate a high signal intensity or "posterior pituitary bright spot" (Fig. 13.1). There is some controversy regarding the etiology of this increased signal intensity (2,3). It has been suggested that phospholipid vesicles containing polypeptide hormones (vasopressin, oxytocin) bound to the carrier protein neurophysin account for this MRI property of the posterior pituitary (11). The "posterior pituitary bright spot" is not universally present but may be identified in over 60% of glands if both T1– and T2–weighted images are examined (3). On both CT and MRI, the pituitary gland will usually be enhanced homogeneously following the administration of contrast media, although in some patients the gland may have a somewhat mottled appearance. Following the administration of gadopentate dimeglumine, the MRI normally will demonstrate enhancement of other sellar and parasellar structures, including the dura of the cavernous sinus, the slowly flowing blood within the cavernous sinus, the infundibulum, and the median eminence of the hypothalamus. The latter structure is one of the circumventricular organs that lacks a blood-brain barrier.

Figure 13.1. Normal pituitary. (A) Sagittal MR demonstrates area of increased signal intensity in the posterior lobe (arrowhead). (B) Coronal T1–weighted MR demonstrates normal increased signal intensity in the posterior lobe (small arrowheads).

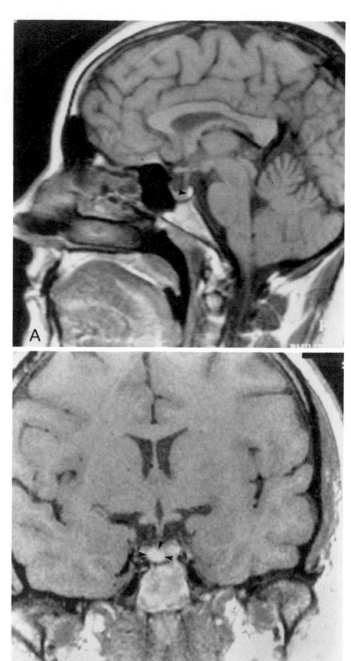

PITUITARY MICROADENOMAS

Pituitary adenomas are arbitrarily defined as microadenomas if they are smaller than 10 mm and as macroadenomas if they are 10 mm or larger. Most pituitary microadeno-

mas come to clinical attention by causing an endocrinopathy through the excessive secretion of one or more pituitary hormones. The most common hypersecretory adenomas secrete prolactin, growth hormone, or cortisol. The accuracy of both CT and MRI in detecting small pituitary tumors varies considerably in published studies. It has been shown that the detection rate for microadenomas with CT is less than 50% (4). Pituitary microadenomas are best illustrated on CT after the administration of intravenous contrast media and using slices 1–2 mm in thickness. Following infusion of contrast media, the normal pituitary gland will enhance immediately. Microadenomas, however, will not enhance immediately (Fig. 13.2) but may enhance approximately 30 min after an infusion of contrast media. If the CT study is delayed beyond 30 minutes after the administration of contrast, some microadenomas will become enhanced and may be missed with CT as they become indistinguishable from the normal pituitary gland. The typical CT appearance of a microadenoma following infusion of contrast media is a low density area located laterally in the anterior lobe of the pituitary gland. There may be some focal elevation of the diaphragma sellae with deviation of the pituitary infundibulum away from the lesion. Erosion of the floor of the sella is of little help since this can be a normal finding.

MRI has replaced CT as the primary imaging modality for pituitary tumors. The accuracy of MRI in detecting microadenomas, particularly when combined with the paramagnetic contrast agent, gadopentate dimeglumine, is better than CT and probably approaches 70% (12). A recent study has shown that unenhanced and enhanced T1-weighted sequences combined with three-dimensional low-angle shots resulted in a 90% success rate for identifying microadenomas, with a very low false-positive rate (8). The T1-weighted coronal sequence is the most useful since it provides good anatomical definition of the pituitary gland, carotid arteries, infundibulum, and optic chiasm. Without contrast media, small tumors will show up as areas of decreased signal intensity. On T2-weighted sequences, the tumor may have a higher signal intensity than the normal gland. In our experience, we have not found the T2-weighted sequences to be very helpful in the diagnosis of microadenomas and have discontinued the routine use of this sequence. The most definitive study using MRI consists of thin coronal slices, 1–2 mm in thickness, combined with paramagnetic contrast. The normal pituitary gland, cavernous sinus, and infundibulum will enhance immediately. On

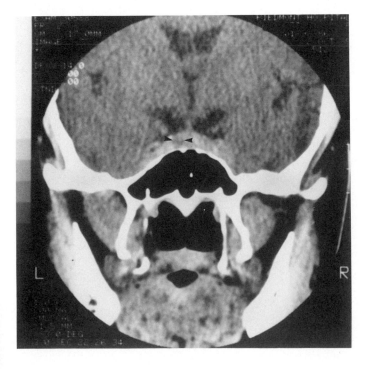

Figure 13.2. Microadenoma. Coronal CT scan following contrast infusion demonstrates a lucent area on the right side of the pituitary gland (arrowhead).

high-quality studies, the cranial nerves lying within the cavernous sinus can be identified. Microadenomas do not enhance immediately and, therefore, show up as areas of decreased signal intensity (Fig. 13.3). There may be a focal deformity of the diaphragma sellae with deviation of the pituitary infundibulum away from the tumor. The very small adenomas, frequently associated with Cushing's disease and acromegaly, (sometimes 3–4 mm) are the most difficult to diagnose on MRI because of their extremely small size (5).

PITUITARY MACROADENOMAS

Pituitary macroadenomas may present with an endocrinopathy due to excessive secretion of pituitary hormones or as a result of mass effect, primarily related to the optic nerves and chiasm. Hormonally inactive pituitary adenomas, or any other mass in the parasellar region, may cause hyperprolactinemia by compressing the pituitary stalk and interfering with the delivery of dopamine (the prolactin-inhibitory factor) to the gland. This results in the unrestrained release of

Figure 13.3. Microadenoma. (A) Noncontrast T1–weighted MRI demonstrates area of decreased signal intensity on the right side of the pituitary gland. (B) Contrast MRI demonstrates a focal area of decreased signal intensity on the right side of the gland. Note displacement of the pituitary infundibulum from right to left.

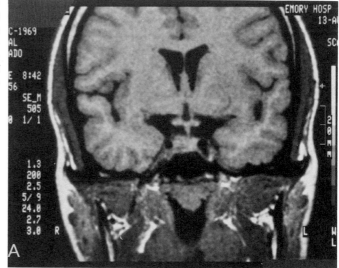

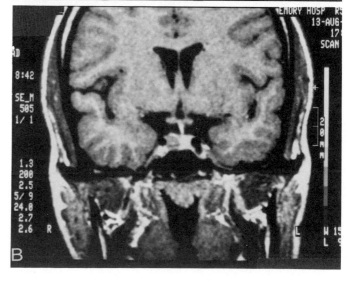

Figure 13.4. Macroadenoma. Coronal CT scan following intravenous administration of contrast media demonstrates a large intra- and suprasellar mass with a cystic component.

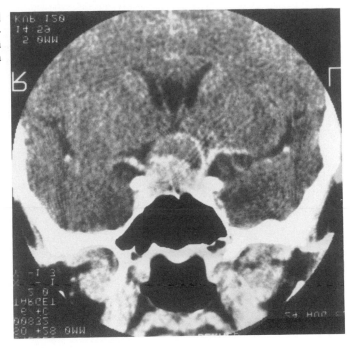

prolactin from normal lactotrophs in the pituitary gland.

Macroadenomas are readily detected by both CT and MRI. On CT, and after the administration of intravenous contrast media, these tumors may present as intrasellar and suprasellar masses with homogeneous enhancement (Fig. 13.4). Occasionally, hemorrhagic or cystic areas within tumors will not enhance. There may be erosion of the floor of the sella turcica with extension of the tumor into the sphenoid sinus.

MRI, with its improved resolution, has proven to be a more elegant imaging study than CT for these large tumors (9). MRI has the advantage of being able to demonstrate the relationship of the tumor to the optic chiasm and it will also rule out the presence of a large intrasellar or suprasellar aneurysm, thus eliminating the need for invasive carotid angiography. Large pituitary tumors can be diagnosed on both the noncontrast and the contrast MRI study. The T1-weighted sequence is the most useful study since it shows the anatomy to better advantage. On the noncontrast study, the large pituitary tumor will show up as a mass with a signal intensity that is isointense with the brain (Fig. 13.5). Following infusion of contrast media, there

is usually a homogeneous enhancement of the tumor unless there are areas of cyst formation or necrosis within the lesion. Hemorrhage can be better detected on MRI than CT. Acute hemorrhage within the tumor will show up as areas of high signal intensity on the T1-weighted sequence and with either high or low signal intensity on the T2-weighted sequence (Fig. 13.6). The areas of high signal intensity on the T1-weighted sequence will develop 48 to 72 hr after the hemorrhage.

Determination of invasion of the cavernous sinus by a pituitary adenoma is of practical importance as it may influence clinical decision-making. Cavernous sinus involvement may preclude complete surgical removal or make an attempt at total surgical excision too risky, such that medical or radiation therapy may be considered as alternatives or adjuncts to surgery. Unfortunately, determination of cavernous sinus invasion by pituitary adenomas with imaging techniques is inadequate. It is often impossible to be certain of the relationship between the lateral edge of a tumor and the cavernous sinus on CT.

Despite its improved resolution, MRI has not completely solved this problem because

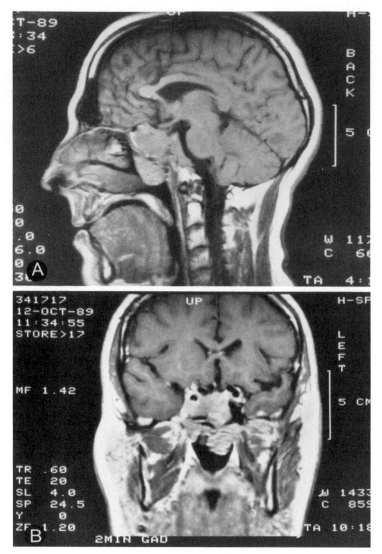

Figure 13.5. Macroadenoma. (A) Sagittal T1–weighted MRI without contrast demonstrates large intrasellar mass with erosion into the sphenoid sinus and destruction of the clivus. (B) Coronal MRI study following contrast infusion demonstrates a large enhancing mass with invasion of the cavernous sinus on the right side.

the medial wall of the cavernous sinus cannot be identified with certainty. If one can identify a tumor lateral to the carotid artery, there is certainly cavernous sinus invasion (Fig. 13.7). Some studies have suggested that MRI changes in signal intensity in the cavernous sinus will reliably determine invasion, but this has not proven to be very accurate. The use of contrast media may, in fact, make it more difficult to determine cavernous sinus invasion, since both the tumor

and the cavernous sinus will enhance with paramagnetic contrast media.

CRANIOPHARYNGIOMAS

Craniopharyngiomas are histologically benign tumors that arise from remnants of Rathke's pouch. There are two peak ages for occurrence of craniopharyngiomas. The first peak is the first to second decade, and the second peak is the fifth to sixth decade. These lesions are usually suprasellar in location but may extend into the third ventricle, posterior fossa, sella, or, occasionally, may be entirely intrasellar. A high percentage of craniopharyngiomas calcify, with the reported range of calcification from 70% to more than 90%. On CT, this type of tumor will usually present as a suprasellar mass with cystic changes and/or calcification within the tumor (Fig. 13.8). There may be little enhancement with contrast if the tumor is extensively calcified. There may be extensive bony erosion of the sella turcica and dorsum sellae if the tumor has been present for a long period of time.

MRI has replaced CT as the primary imaging modality for these tumors (15). The T1-weighted sequence images the tumor and associated anatomy better than the T2-weighted sequence. The appearance of craniopharyngiomas on MRI is somewhat variable. The neoplasm may present as areas of high or low signal intensity on T1-weighted sequences depending on the amount of cholesterol that is present in the tumor or on whether there has been hemorrhage within the tumor (Fig. 13.9). The tumor will present as a suprasellar mass that has mixed signal intensity either due to hemorrhage and/or to cholesterol content. Calcification can cause the tumor to have areas of decreased signal. On the T2-weighted sequence, the tumor will have a mixed signal intensity if it is calcified. The tumor will have areas of high signal intensity mixed with areas of low signal intensity or no signal intensity. Paramagnetic contrast is useful to illustrate better the extent of the tumor. The only advantage CT has over MRI is that the areas of calcification can be detected more accurately on the CT scan. These tumors may be difficult to differentiate from a Rathke's cleft cyst on MRI, since the latter can have a signal intensity similar to the craniopharyngioma. Rathke's cleft cysts, however, do not normally calcify.

MENINGIOMAS

Meningiomas are extraaxial tumors that arise from meningothelial cells that occur predominantly in the arachnoid villi. Basal meningiomas in the region of the pituitary may take their dural origin from the tuberculum sella, medial sphenoid wing, olfactory groove, optic nerve sheath, anterior clinoid, or anterior fossa over the roof of the orbit. Meningiomas in any of these regions may

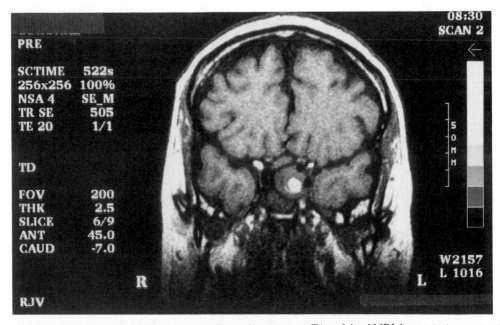

Figure 13.6.   Macroadenoma with hemorrhage. Coronal noncontrast T1–weighted MRI demonstrates an area of increased signal intensity compatible with acute hemorrhage.

Figure 13.7. Large pituitary adenoma. (A and B) Coronal MR following the administration of Gadolinium demonstrates tumor mass extending laterally to the carotid artery (arrowheads).

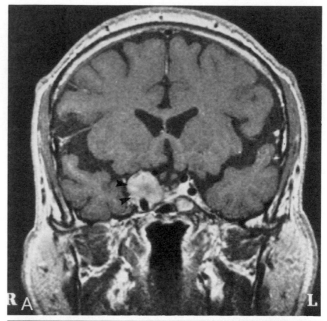

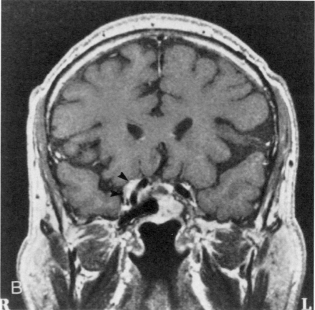

compress the pituitary gland and hypothalamus or infundibulum.

Meningiomas will present on CT as tumors with homogeneous enhancement following contrast administration, unless there is significant calcification within the tumor. One may also see an abnormality of the bone adjacent to the meningioma due to hyperostosis.

MRI, particularly when performed after the administration of contrast, defines the extent of these tumors better than CT (20). On the noncontrast MRI, using T1-weighted sequences, the tumor may have a signal intensity similar to normal brain, and, on T2-weighted sequences, the signal intensity may be similar to or slightly higher than brain. Gadolinium-DTPA is necessary to show the

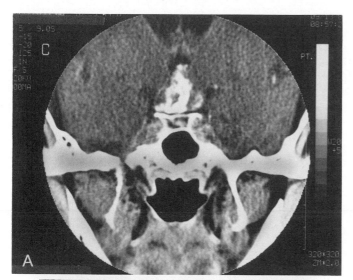

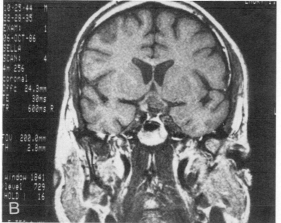

Figure 13.8. Craniopharyngioma. (A) Noncontrast CT scan demonstrating a large area of suprasellar calcification. (B) Coronal noncontrast MRI in the same patient demonstrates suprasellar mass with elevation of the optic chiasm.

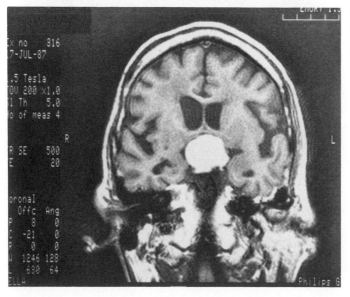

Figure 13.9. Craniopharyngioma. Coronal noncontrast T1–weighted MRI demonstrates a large suprasellar mass with increased signal intensity.

full extent of the tumor. Following infusion of this contrast media, meningiomas will show marked enhancement with smooth, regular margins (Fig. 13.10). There may be scattered areas of decreased signal intensity in the tumor due to areas of calcification. The hyperostosis of adjacent bone can be more difficult to detect on MRI than on CT.

Many neurosurgeons use angiography to evaluate the vascular supply of suspected meningiomas, determine the need for preoperative embolization, and assess the in-

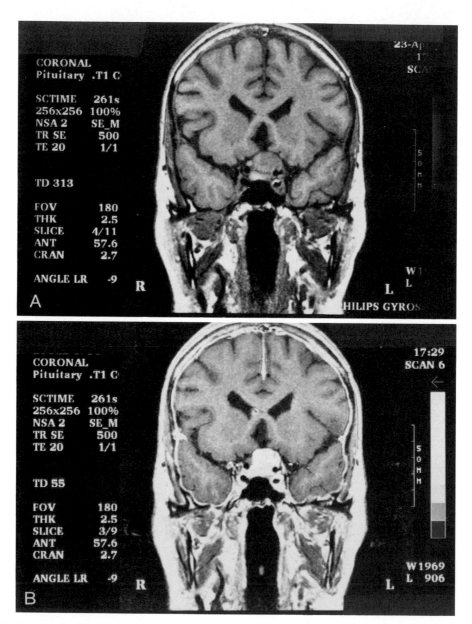

Figure 13.10. Suprasellar meningioma. (A) Noncontrast coronal T1–weighted MRI demonstrates suprasellar mass with involvement of the left carotid artery. (B) The contrast MRI in the same patient demonstrates a well-circumscribed, homogeneously-enhancing suprasellar mass. Notice normal enhancement of the cavernous sinus. There is also diffuse meningeal enhancement resulting from previous surgery.

Figure 13.11. Chordoma. Coronal non-contrast T1–weighted MRI demonstrates a mass lesion with destruction of the sellar floor and lateral extension involving the carotid artery and cavernous sinus on the left side.

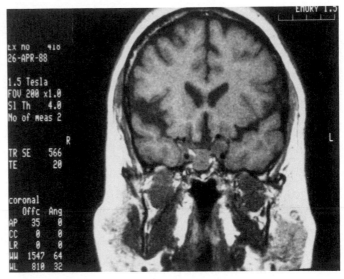

volvement of specific arteries and venous sinuses by the lesion. Meningiomas typically derive their vascular supply from meningeal vessels and usually have a characteristic blush that remains throughout the venous phase of the angiogram. Parasellar meningiomas are frequently supplied by the small meningeal vessels that arise from the cavernous portion of the internal carotid artery, and the meningohypophyseal trunk may be noticeably enlarged. The carotid siphon may be opened or closed and the supraclinoid portion of the artery may be displaced laterally or medially depending on the location of the tumor.

CHORDOMA

Chordomas are slow-growing, destructive, and locally-invasive tumors thought to arise from the remnants of the primitive notochord. These tumors are characteristically located either on the clivus or in the lower lumbar spine around the sacrum. Rostral growth from a clival chordoma with accompanying destruction of bone may involve the sella turcica, cavernous sinus, optic apparatus, and sphenoid sinus. When imaged with CT, a chordoma will present as a midline mass in the region of the clivus, with areas of calcification or bony destruction within the lesion. The tumor may show enhancement with intravenous contrast media.

MRI is the procedure of choice to evaluate these tumors since the relationship of the neoplasm to the optic chiasm, brainstem, cavernous sinus, and basilar artery can be better determined with MRI than CT (17). These tumors will have a signal intensity similar to brain on a T1-weighted MRI sequence (Fig. 13.11). On a T2-weighted sequence, they may have areas of high and low signal intensity within the lesion. Following infusion of contrast media, these tumors may show considerable enhancement. The hallmark of the chordoma is a lesion with areas of calcification that is destroying the clivus. The calcification may be difficult to detect on MRI, CT may be helpful in this situation (Fig. 13.12).

ANEURYSMS

Aneurysms arising from either the intracavernous or supraclinoid portion of the internal carotid artery may project into the suprasellar cistern and simulate a pituitary tumor. The CT scan with contrast media will demonstrate this lesion as a homogeneous enhancing mass, either in the suprasellar cistern or in the sella turcica. For this reason, angiography has been recommended in the past to differentiate certain pituitary tumors from aneurysms. However, since aneurysms have a fairly characteristic appearance on MRI, we believe that the use of angiography

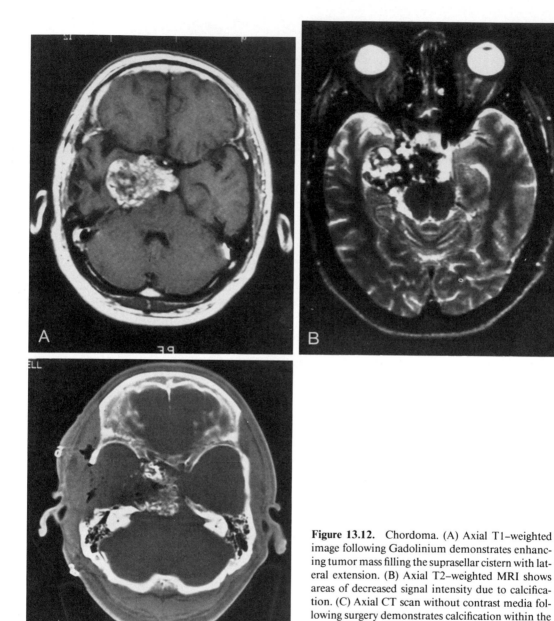

Figure 13.12. Chordoma. (A) Axial T1–weighted image following Gadolinium demonstrates enhancing tumor mass filling the suprasellar cistern with lateral extension. (B) Axial T2–weighted MRI shows areas of decreased signal intensity due to calcification. (C) Axial CT scan without contrast media following surgery demonstrates calcification within the tumor mass lying in the suprasellar cistern and on the clivus.

is no longer indicated for differentiating aneurysms from pituitary tumors (Fig. 13.13). Since aneurysms contain flowing blood, which does not normally give a signal on MRI, these lesions will show up as areas of decreased signal intensity on both T1– and T2–weighted sequences (13). Occasionally, the aneurysm may be partially thrombosed, in which case it would have areas of high signal intensity on the T1-weighted sequence and areas of decreased signal intensity on the T2-weighted sequence, depending on the age of the blood. If an aneurysm is identified on MRI, cerebral angiography is still necessary to clearly define its anatomy prior to surgical intervention.

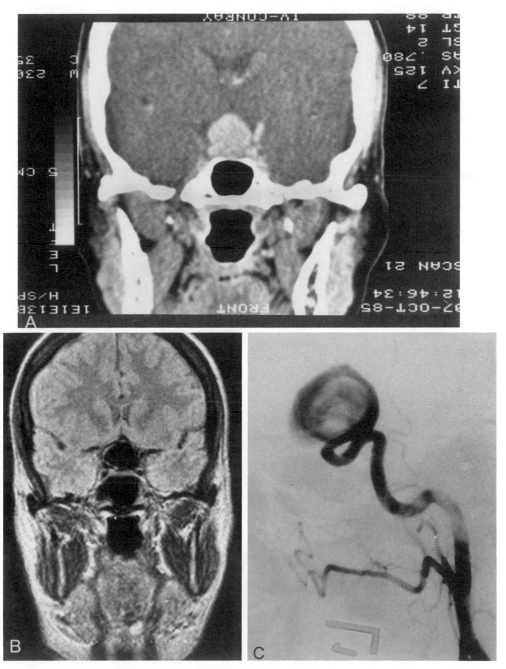

Figure 13.13. Suprasellar aneurysm. (A) Coronal contrast CT scan demonstrates a homogeneous-enhancing supra-sellar mass. (B) Coronal noncontrast MRI demonstrates large area of decreased signal intensity compatible with flow-ing blood. (C) Lateral view common carotid angiogram demonstrates a large suprasellar aneurysm.

RATHKE'S CLEFT CYSTS

Rathke's cysts are benign intrasellar cysts that originate from remnants of Rathke's pouch and are generally found in the pars intermedia. They are epithelial-lined cysts and contain mucoid material. Prior to modern imaging techniques, such as CT and MRI, these lesions were considered rare; however, recent literature reveals that more cases are being reported (18). When CT is used to image these cysts, they present as an intrasellar and/or suprasellar mass that has a density similar to CSF. They may rarely show calcification and, following administration of intravenous contrast media, one series reports that approximately half of the cases will show a ring-like enhancement pattern.

MRI characteristics of Rathke's cyst are variable, depending on the cyst contents (1). Most are hyperintense on both T1– and T2–weighted images but some lesions have a low signal intensity on T1-weighted images and a high signal intensity on T2-weighted images (Fig. 13.14); others, however, can demonstrate hyperintensity on T1-weighted sequences with the signal intensity diminishing on the T2-weighted sequences (Fig. 13.15).

Since these lesions have an appearance similar to craniopharyngiomas on imaging studies, they may be mistakenly diagnosed as a craniopharyngiomas or may be mistaken for necrotic pituitary adenomas.

EMPTY SELLA SYNDROME

Empty sella syndrome is characterized by the herniation of the subarachnoid space into the sella turcica. The condition may be divided into two types, primary and secondary. The primary type is due to a congenital defect in the diaphragma sella, resulting in herniation of the suprasellar cistern into the sella turcica. Secondary empty sella refers to those cases in which the extension of the suprasellar cistern into the sella occurs following surgery or irradiation of a large pituitary tumor.

Empty sella syndrome is usually an incidental finding, although, occasionally, it may be associated with endocrine abnormalities or visual field deficits. It is usually diagnosed because of enlargement of the sella turcica on plain films or seen as an incidental finding on CT or MRI. The CT appearance of empty sella syndrome is a low-density abnormality in the pituitary fossa, possibly with erosion of

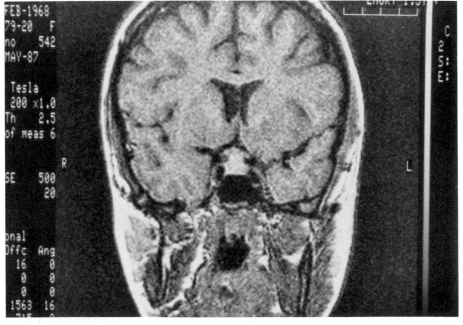

Figure 13.14. Rathke's cyst. Coronal noncontrast T1–weighted MRI demonstrates a suprasellar mass with compression of the optic chiasm.

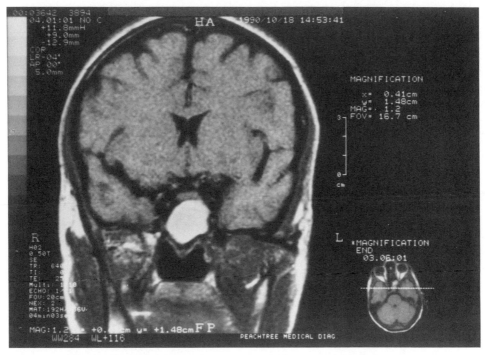

Figure 13.15.   Rathke's cyst. Coronal noncontrast T1–weighted MRI demonstrates large supra- and intrasellar mass with high signal intensity.

the floor of the sella turcica. Following infusion of contrast media, one should be able to identify enhancement of the pituitary infundibulum and, perhaps, of the normal pituitary gland, which is usually displaced posteriorly and inferiorly. It is best to obtain coronal views of these patients.

On MRI, empty sella will present as a decreased signal intensity in the sella turcica on the T1-weighted sequence and high signal intensity on a T2-weighted signal sequence (8). The signal intensity should be similar to CSF in the ventricular system or subarachnoid space (Fig. 13.16). The diagnosis of empty sella syndrome should not be considered unless one can identify the normal infundibulum and pituitary gland, which is inferiorly displaced. If the pituitary infundibulum cannot be identified, then the possibility of an intrasellar arachnoid cyst or a necrotic pituitary tumor should be considered.

PITUITARY ABSCESS

Pituitary abscess is an unusual condition and is usually associated with necrosis within a large pituitary adenoma. There are no specific diagnostic criteria for this abnormality. On CT, however, this may present as a low-density area in a large adenoma, and on MRI, it may present as an area of decreased signal intensity on the T1-weighted sequence and an area of high signal intensity on the T2-weighted sequence in a large pituitary adenoma (Fig. 13.17).

HISTIOCYTOSIS X

Histiocytosis X is a generic term for a group of disorders ranging from rather innocuous solitary eosinophilic granulomas of bone to lethal disseminated disorders of soft tissue. The etiology and pathophysiology of these disorders are poorly understood. Some forms of the disease have a pathological appearance and clinical course typical of an inflammatory condition, whereas others follow a neoplastic type of process. The solitary eosinophilic granuloma of the skull is almost always a self-limiting lesion that may be cured by excision. The eosinophilic granuloma can also be found in a variety of loca-

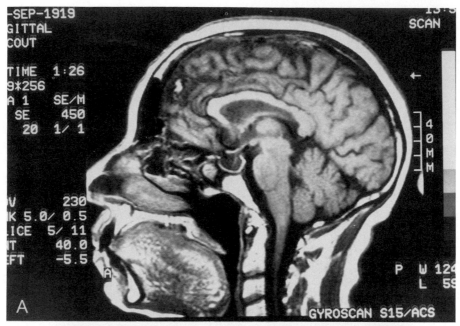

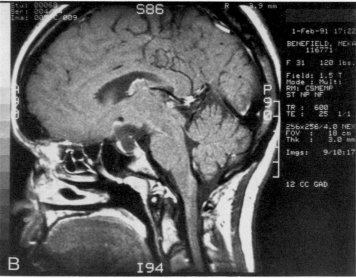

Figure 13.16.   Empty sella. (A) Sagittal T1–weighted MRI demonstrates CSF signal intensity in the sella turcica with the pituitary infundibulum displaced posteriorly. (B) Sagittal MRI on a different patient with an intrasellar and suprasellar arachnoid cyst—notice absence of pituitary infundibulum.

tions including the pituitary gland. Disseminated forms of histiocytosis X include Hand-Schuller-Christian and Letterer-Siwe diseases. The former refers to multifocal eosinophilic granulomas, which usually involve both the cranial vault and base of the skull. Lesions at the skull base may produce proptosis, growth retardation, diabetes insipi-

dus, and various forms of hypopituitarism. Localized masses involving the infundibular region and hypothalamus may produce obesity and hypogonadism in addition to diabetes insipidus. Various soft tissues may be affected by multifocal eosinophilic granuloma, including skin, lymph nodes, liver, lung, spleen, and bone marrow. Letterer-Siwe dis-

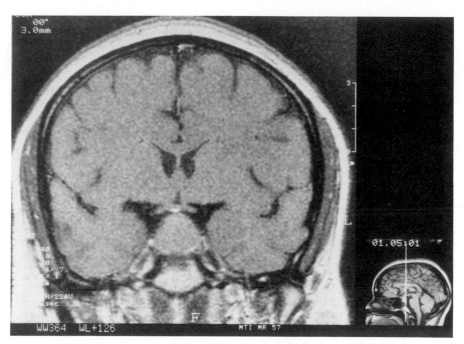

Figure 13.17. Pituitary abscess. Coronal T1–weighted noncontrast MRI demonstrates a supra- and intrasellar mass with isointense signal intensity. There is compression of the optic chiasm. Area of high signal intensity between the optic chiasm and mass represents compressed pituitary infundibulum.

ease is a disorder of young patients, usually infants, characterized by multiple histiolytic lesions, primarily of the skin.

On plain skull films, the eosinophilic granuloma appears as an area of rarefaction without surrounding sclerosis and with beveled margins on tangential views. When the disease occurs in the pituitary gland, it usually causes hypopituitarism. When imaged with CT following the administration of iodinated contrast, this lesion will present as a diffuse enlargement of the pituitary gland with enhancement (Fig. 13.18). This condition cannot be reliably differentiated from a pituitary adenoma. On MRI, the infundibulum is enlarged, demonstrates high signal intensity on T1-weighted images, and enhances with contrast (14).

SARCOIDOSIS

Sarcoidosis is an idiopathic granulomatous process that can involve almost any organ system in the body, including the lungs, liver, bone marrow, and brain. The nervous system is estimated to be involved in approximately 5% of cases. Sarcoidosis produces two types of lesions in the nervous system. The more common is a granulomatous leptomeningitis with a predilection for the base of the brain, particularly in the region of the hypothalamus and optic chiasm. Secondly, granulomas may occur in the brain or spinal cord parenchyma.

Hypothalamic involvement may be associated with seizures, psychiatric disturbances, hypothermia, diabetes insipidus, obesity, amenorrhea and galactorrhea, and sleep derangements. The lesion may simulate an optic nerve glioma and cause visual loss. Hypopituitarism is said to be uncommon, but its incidence may be underestimated.

When sarcoidosis involves the pituitary gland, imaging studies will show nonspecific enlargement of the pituitary gland and infundibulum (Fig. 13.19). There is no specific appearance of sarcoidosis of the pituitary gland on MRI (7). If there is leptomeningeal involvement, contrast enhanced MRI will demonstrate diffuse enhancement of the meninges over the convexity and base of the brain.

Figure 13.18. Histiocytosis X. Coronal CT scan following injection of water soluble contrast media in the subarachnoid space demonstrates enlargement of the pituitary gland with enlargement of the pituitary infundibulum.

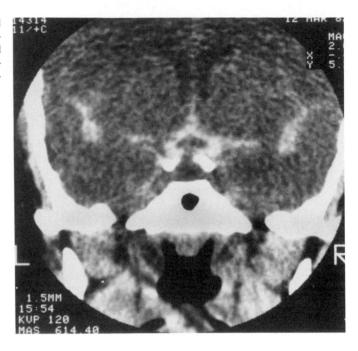

HYPOTHALAMIC GLIOMA

Astrocytomas can occur within the hypothalamus or optic pathways to produce a suprasellar mass with pituitary and visual dysfunction. The pilocytic astrocytoma is the most common type of astrocytoma to involve this area and characteristically arises in the walls of the third ventricle. There are two types of pilocytic astrocytomas, the juvenile and adult types, with the latter being somewhat more aggressive. Generally, these tumors are slow-growing and patients harboring these lesions may have a fairly long survival. Patients with hypothalamic gliomas present with a variety of clinical problems, including vision loss and hypothalamic and pituitary dysfunction. Optic chiasm gliomas may be found in patients with neurofibromatosis Type I. There is some controversy over the histology of these tumors. Some investigators believe that these tumors are hamartomas and have a benign course.

MRI is the best imaging study to show tumors involving the hypothalamus and optic chiasm (Fig. 13.20). CT is not as good in demonstrating the optic chiasm and hypothalamus and will require injection of contrast into the subarachnoid space to identify these structures. Although large tumors can be diagnosed on CT, small tumors will frequently be missed. Since hypothalamic tumors and optic chiasm gliomas can infiltrate and obstruct the third ventricle, the multiplanar imaging capability of MRI allows one to determine more accurately, the extent of these tumors. On the T1–weighted sequence, these tumors will have decreased signal intensity, and on the T2–weighted sequence, they will appear as increased signal intensity. Intravenous contrast media is helpful to illustrate the full extent of the neoplasm. If the tumor is confined to the optic nerve and chiasm, there may be little signal change in the tumor and one may see diffuse enlargement of the optic nerve and optic chiasm. In this case, the T1-weighted sequence would be the most diagnostic. When this tumor is suspected, both axial and coronal T1- and T2-weighted sequences should be performed.

MISCELLANEOUS LESIONS

A number of other lesions may occur in the suprasellar region; they may mimic the above lesions and are potential causes of hypothalamic or pituitary dysfunction.

A hypothalamic hamartoma often presents with precocious puberty. It is a pedunculated mass interposed between the mam-

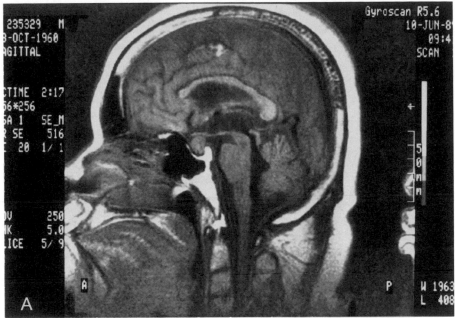

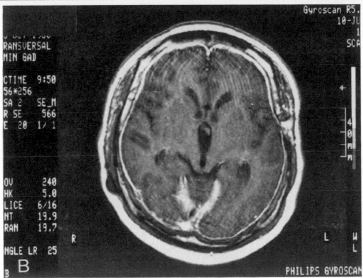

Figure 13.19. Sarcoidosis. (A) Sagittal noncontrast T1–weighted MRI demonstrates intra- and suprasellar mass. (B) Axial T1–weighted MRI following intravenous contrast media shows diffuse enhancement of the leptomeninges with abnormal enhancement of the tentorium.

illary bodies and the infundibulum. On MRI, these lesions are usually isointense with brain and so not enhance with contrast.

Lipomas of the infundibulum or hypothalamus and dermoid cysts will appear as hyperintense lesions on T1–weighted MRI (21).

Benshoff *et al.* reported on the MRI ap-

pearance of ectopia of the posterior pituitary (2). This entity occurs most often in pituitary dwarfism, but has been reported as a normal variant. In this situation, the "posterior pituitary bright spot" is not seen in its usual location but is located more cephalad, within the median eminence of the hypothalamus.

Lesions that are located entirely within the

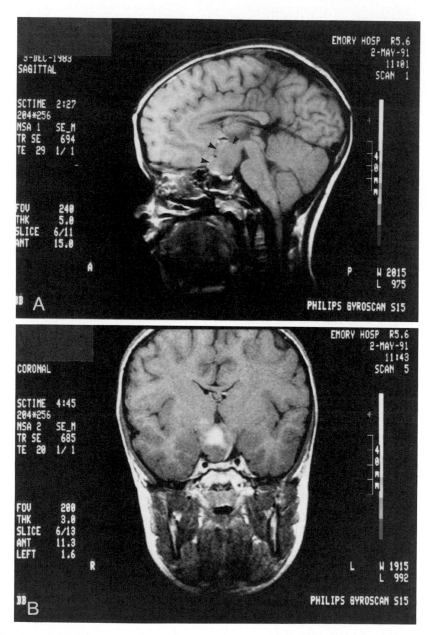

Figure 13.20. Hypothalamic glioma. (A) Sagittal noncontrast T1–weighted MRI demonstrates a large intra- and suprasellar mass (arrowheads). (B) Coronal T1–weighted MRI following intravenous contrast media demonstrates enhancement of this suprasellar mass with indentation of the third ventricle. The normal pituitary gland can be seen enhancing inferiorly through the mass. The linear structure between the mass and the pituitary gland represents the diaphragma sellae, which is displaced inferiorly.

pituitary stalk include choristomas (granular cell tumors), germinomas, lymphomas, and leukemic and other metastatic tumors. On MRI, these lesions will usually cause infundibular enlargement with enhancement similar to the MRI appearance of histiocytosis X and sarcoidosis.

REFERENCES

1. Asari S., Ito T., Tsuchida S. *et al.* MR apperance and cyst content of Rathke cleft cysts. J. Comput. Assist. Tomogr., *14*:532–535, 1990.
2. Benshoff E.R., Katz B.H., Ectopia of the posterior pituitary gland as a normal variant: Assessment with MR imaging. A.J.N.R., *11*:709–712, 1990.
3. Brooks, B.S., El Gammal, T., Allison, J.D. *et al.* Frequency and variation of the posterior pituitary bright signal on MR images. A.J.N.R., *10*:943–948, 1989.
4. Davis P.C., Hoffman J.C., Tindall G.T. *et al.* F. Prolactin-Secreting pituitary microadenomas: Inaccuracy of High-resolution CT imaging. A.J.R., *144*:151–156, 1985.
5. Doppman J.L., Frank J.A., Dwyer A.J. *et al.* Gadolinium DTPA enhanced MR imaging of ACTH-Secreting microadenomas of the pituitary gland. J. Comput. Assist. Tomogr. 1099; *12(5)*:727–735.
6. Fujisawa I., Nishimura K., Asato R. *et al.* Posterior lobe of the pituitary in diabetes insipidus: MR findings. J. Comput. Assist. Tomogr., *11*:221–225, 1987.
7. Hayes W.S., Sherman J.L., Stern B.J. *et al.* MR and CT evaluation of intracranial sarcoidosis. A.J.N.R., *8*:841–847, 1987.
8. Kaufman B., Tomsak R.L., Kaufman B.A. *et al.* Herniation of the suprasellar visual system and third ventricle into empty sellae: Morphologic and clinical considerations. A.J.N.R., *10*:65–76, 1989.
9. Kucharczyk W., Davis D.O., Kelly W.M. *et al.* Pituitary adenomas: High resolution MR imaging at 1.5 T^1. Radiology, *161*:761–765, 1986.
10. Kucharczyk J., Kucharczyk W. *et al.* Histochemical characterization and functional significance of the hyperintense signal on MR images of the posterior pituitary. A.J.N.R., *9*:1079–1983, 1988.
11. Kucharczyk W., Lenkinski R.E., Kucharczyk J. *et al.* The effect of phospholipid vesicles on the NMR relaxation of water: An explanation for the MR appearance of the neurohypophysis? A.J.N.R., *11*:693–700, 1990.
12. Newton D.R., Dillon W.P., Norman D. *et al.* Gd-DTPA-Enhanced MR imaging of pituitary adenomas. A.J.N.R., *10*:949–954, 1989.
13. Olsen W.L., Brant-Zawadzki M., Hodes J. *et al.* Giant intracranial aneurysms: MR imaging. Radiology, *163*:431–435, 1987.
14. Osborn A.G. MRI of the sellar/juxtasellar region. Part 1: Intrasellar and suprasellar masses. MRI Decisions (Nov-Dec); 19–30, 1991.
15. Pusey E., Kortman K.E., Flannigan B.D. *et al.* MR of craniopharyngiomas: Tumor delineation and characterization. A.J.N.R., *8*:439–444, 1987.
16. Stadnik T., Stenenaert A., Beckers A. *et al.* Pituitary microadenomas: Diagnosis with two- and three-dimensional MR imaging at 1.5 T before and after injection of gadolinium. Radiology, *176*:419–428, 1990.
17. Sze G., Uichanco L.S., Brant-Zawadzki M.N. *et al.* Chordomas: MR imaging. Radiology., *166*:187–191, 1988.
18. Voelker J.L., Campbell R.L., Muller J. Clinical, radiographic, and pathological features of symptomatic Rathke's cleft cysts. J. Neurosurg., *74*:535–544, 1991.
19. Wolpert S.M., Molitch M.E., Goldman J.A. *et al.* Size, shape, and appearance of the normal female pituitary gland. A.J.N.R., *5*:263–267, 1984.
20. Yeakley J.W., Kulkarni M.V., McArdie C.B. *et al.* High-Resolution MR imaging of juxtasellar meningiomas with CT and angiographic correlation. A.J.N.R., *9*:279–285, 1988.
21. Yousem D.M., Arrington J.A., Kumar A.J. *et al.* Bright lesions on sellar/parasellar T1-weighted scans. Clinical Imaging, *14*:99–105, 1990.

CHAPTER 14

Neuropathology of the Hypothalamus

SHOZO YAMADA, M.D., Ph.D., and TOSHIAKI SANO, M.D., Ph.D.

The hypothalamus is part of the diencephalon, which lies in the walls of the third ventricle below the hypothalamic sulci and is continuous across the floor of this ventricle.

Despite its small size, the hypothalamus contains many nuclei that consist of more or less functionally distinct cells, and it has complex and extensive afferent or efferent fiber connections. The activities of the hypothalamus can be divided roughly into endocrine functions mediated via neurosecretory pathways, and vegetative functions mediated through the limbic system. The details of the anatomy, physiology, and function of the hypothalamus have been reviewed well in other articles (35, 187, 192, 210).

This chapter addresses the pathology of the medical and surgical diseases affecting the hypothalamus. Please note that certain conditions will be described in Chapter 16 in relation to the target organs. In addition, since the hypothalamus forms a morphological and functional unit with the pituitary stalk and posterior pituitary, some conditions that chiefly affect the posterior pituitary and mainly arise in the sella turcica will be discussed in the next chapter.

CONGENITAL MALFORMATIONS AND HAMARTOMATOUS NEURONAL TUMORS OF THE HYPOTHALAMUS AND PITUITARY

Anencephaly

This is said to be the most severe and common fetal malformation of the head. The skull is grossly abnormal and the forebrain is replaced by a reddish irregular mass of vascular connective tissue with multiple cavities containing cerebrospinal fluid (CSF). In such infants, the hypothalamus, the posterior lobe, and the intermediate lobe are always missing, whereas a hypoplastic anterior lobe can be detected (108).

In anencephalic infants, the pituitary concentration of adrenocorticotropin (ACTH) and the blood level of growth hormone (GH) are both lower than in normal infants (7, 72). Immunohistochemical studies have demonstrated a varying number of somatotrophs, lactotrophs, thyrotrophs, and gonadotrophs, whereas immunorcactivity for ACTH or other proopiomelanocortin (POMC) derivatives is lacking in correspondence with the marked hypoplasia of the adrenal cortex (151). In contrast, the lactotrophs may be more numerous and have a greater cytoplasmic area than those in normal fetuses, suggesting that a stimulatory effect of the fetal hypothalamus is not essential for lactotroph development (22).

Septo-Optic Dysplasia

This is a relatively rare malformation of the brain midline structures that is of unknown etiology (43, 102, 137). The syndrome consists of two components: unilateral or bilateral hypoplasia of the optic nerves and chiasm, and a midline diencephalic malformation, including an abnormal septum pellucidum and hypoplasia of the hypothalamus and neurohypophysis. The former can result in visual disturbances, and the latter leads to a diencephalic-hypothalamic disorder associated with endocrinopathy.

The most common presentation is that of optic nerve hypoplasia and pituitary insufficiency. Most of these patients suffer from some form of endocrine dysfunction, such as hypothalamic hypopituitarism (most frequently GH-deficiency followed by ACTH-deficiency), hypoglycemia, hyperprolactinemia, and diabetes insipidus. Additional symptoms include vegetative dysfunction of the hypothalamus and precocious puberty.

Neuronal Tumors

The nature and origin of parasellar neuronal tumors is still controversial (12, 146, 167, 185). These lesions have variously been called hamartomas, choristomas, and gangliocytomas (12, 167, 185). They are considered to be hamartomatous rather than neoplastic because of their benign nature, slow growth, and histological resemblance to mature hypothalamic neuronal cells. In this chapter, such lesions are arbitrarily divided into hypothalamic neuronal hamartomas, intrasellar neuronal choristomas (gangliocytomas), and hamartoblastomas (Pallister–Hall syndrome).

Hypothalamic Neuronal Hamartomas

Hypothalamic neuronal hamartomas appear to be congenital malformations of normal neuronal elements and can be regarded as a manifestation of midline dysraphism. As associated cerebral malformations, corpus callosal defects or abnormalities of the optic apparatus have been reported in the literature (53).

Most of these lesions are asymptomatic and are only discovered incidentally at autopsy (194). They are usually small, ranging from a few millimeters to 1.5 cm in diameter (94). In contrast, the rare symptomatic hypothalamic hamartoma may vary in size from 1 to 5 cm in diameter. Such lesions are generally pedunculated and are attached to the ventral hypothalamus, anywhere from the tuber cinereum to the mamillary bodies, by a stalk containing myelinated fibers that hangs in the interpeduncular cistern (94, 170). Occasionally, they may have a wide attachment to the ventral surface or lie embedded within the hypothalamus, and they may even lie free in the interpeduncular cistern (187).

The disease manifests itself early in life and apparently occurs with equal frequency in both sexes (121), although it has sometimes been reported to be more frequent in males (225). The clinical features of hypothalamic hamartoma, both endocrinological and neurological, are as follows: isosexual precocious puberty (the most common presenting symptom); acromegaly (rare); diencephalic syndromes (very rare); and epileptic syndromes, including generalized tonic-clonic and gelastic (laughing) seizures (23). Other symptoms associated with hypothalamic hamartoma include mass effects, such as headaches or visual disturbances, or evidence of autonomic dysfunction, such as hyperphagia, hyperactivity, or somnolence, but such symptoms are also uncommon (20).

Isosexual true precocious puberty indicates abnormal early activation of the hypothalamic-pituitary-gonadal axis due to early elaboration of gonadotropins (see precocious puberty in Chapter 16). Approximately 70-90% of the patients with hypothalamic hamartoma develop precocious puberty (118, 225). However, the details of the pathogenesis of true isosexual precocious puberty due to such hamartomas is still uncertain. Immunohistochemical studies have demonstrated the presence of gonadotropin-releasing hormone (GnRH) within the hamartoma cells in some instances (46, 94, 159), but have failed to detect it in others (126). Furthermore, it is well established that other hormonally inactive mass lesions affecting the hypothalamus can also be associated with precocious puberty, i.e., hypothalamic astrocytoma, optic nerve glioma, craniopharyngioma, pinealoma, germ cell tumors, suprasellar cysts, polyostotic fibrous dysplasia, neurofibromatosis, and postinfectious states (126, 187, 190). In such instances, the lesions may interfere with the inhibitory effects of the posterior hypothalamus on the secretion of gonadotropins or stimulate the nuclei engaged in GnRH production. Alternatively, they may change the normal physiological pulsatile GnRH secretion from the hypothalamus, which inhibits the production and secretion of luteinizing hormone (LH) and follicle-stimulating hormone (FSH) (126, 187, 190).

In rare instances, acromegaly is associated

with a pituitary growth hormone cell adenoma that arises due to prolonged growth-
hormone-releasing hormone (GHRH) secretion from a hypothalamic hamartoma (11,
12, 185) (Fig. 14.1).

A complex diencephalic syndrome associated with disturbance of the water and calo-
ric balance, thermoregulation, and behavior
has been described in one reported case
(165).

Epilepsy is another common clinical feature. It usually commences in infancy (or
even in the neonatal period) and begins with
laughing attacks that often resemble normal
laughter, leading to a delay in the diagnosis
(23, 47, 130).

After a few years, however, the laughing attacks are accompanied by memory loss, facial myoclonus, and/or abnormal eye movements. Although psychomotor retardation is
found in some cases (20), the mental development is generally normal (47). In later
childhood or adolescence, secondary generalized epilepsy appears with multiple seizure
patterns, such as tonic-clonic, tonic, or
atonic seizures, and this is associated with
progressive cognitive impairment (23, 47).
The mechanism of the ictal laughter in these
patients is obscure. It has still not been defined whether such laughter is due to epileptic discharges within the hypothalamus itself
or whether it represents an automatism or release phenomenon, although generalized epileptic discharges are frequently observed in
the electroencephalograph during such seizures (23). The pathogenesis of associated
secondary generalized epilepsy is also uncertain. It is possible that other factors promoting cortical dysfunction need to be present
along with the hypothalamic hamartoma for
the epileptic syndrome and cognitive impairment to develop (23).

Microscopically, hypothalamic neuronal
hamartomas are primarily composed of mature neurons interspersed with glial cells (11,
12, 46, 94, 126, 146, 159, 185, 187). Neither
fibrous connective tissue nor vascular stroma
are prominent within these lesions. The ganglion cells vary in size and shape and resemble those of the normal hypothalamus or
tuber cinereum. These cells show neither
atypia nor mitotic activity and their cytoplasm usually contains aldehyde fuchsin-

positive membrane–bound secretory granules. Axonal processes are revealed by silver
staining and usually run irregularly, except
in some of the lesions attached to the hypothalamus via a pedicle (187). Immunohistochemical studies will detect GnRH (46, 94,
159), GHRH (11, 12, 185), and other hypothalamic neuropeptides, such as corticotropin-releasing factor (CRF), somatostatin
(SRIF), β-endorphin, oxytocin, and glucagon (12, 146). Electron microscopic studies
of such hamartomas are uncommon (11, 12,
94, 126, 146, 185, 187, 214), but, electron-
dense granules of about 100 nm in diameter
within the perikarya and nonmyelinated or
occasional myelinated neuronal processes
have been reported. Some of these granules
in the axons resemble dense–cored vesicles.
Synapse formation has also been noted. The
capillaries may or may not have fenestra-
tions.

Intrasellar Neuronal Choristoma

The pathogenesis of intrasellar neuronal
tumors is still enigmatic and the correct ter-
minology to describe these lesions is not even
defined, but all of these tumors are composed
of neurons resembling those of the hypothalamus, even though some have no direct
attachment to the hypothalamus itself.
Moreover, the presence of hypothalamic
neuropeptides in these neurons appears to be
proof of their hypothalamic origin. However,
intrasellar neuronal choristomas differ from
hypothalamic hamartomas in that they are
more frequently associated with pituitary adenomas and endocrine hyperfunction. In
fact, the vast majority of these tumors are
symptomatic, except for a few cases (103,
222).

Light microscopy shows that intrasellar
neuronal choristomas consist of mature ganglion cells of variable size that are either clus-
tered or scattered diffusely (12, 185, 187,
222). Small numbers of glial cells and nerve
fibers are also found (Fig. 14.2-A). These ganglion cells have large nuclei and contain Nissl
substance that is often located peripherally.
Ultrastructurally, the ganglion cells contain
numerous dense–cored secretory granules
that have an average diameter of 100 to 150
nm. These granules are also found in the cell

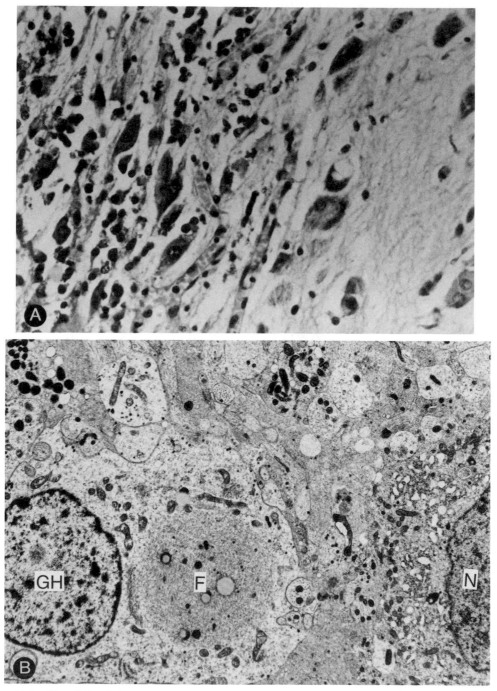

Figure 14.1. Hypothalamic hamartoma associated with a pituitary adenoma (GH-producing adenoma). Light microscopy shows border between hamartoma (right) and adenoma (left) (A). Original magnification × 80. Electron microscopy demonstrates a neuron (N), a neuropil, and a sparsely granulated GH cell (GH) having a characteristic fibrous body (F) (B) × 8470. (Reprinted with permission from Asa, S.L., Scheithauer, B.W., Bilbao, J.M., *et al.* A case of hypothalamic acromegaly: a clinicopathological study of six patients with hypothalamic gangliocytomas producing growth hormone releasing factor. J. Clin. Endocrinol. Metab., *58*:796–803, 1984.)

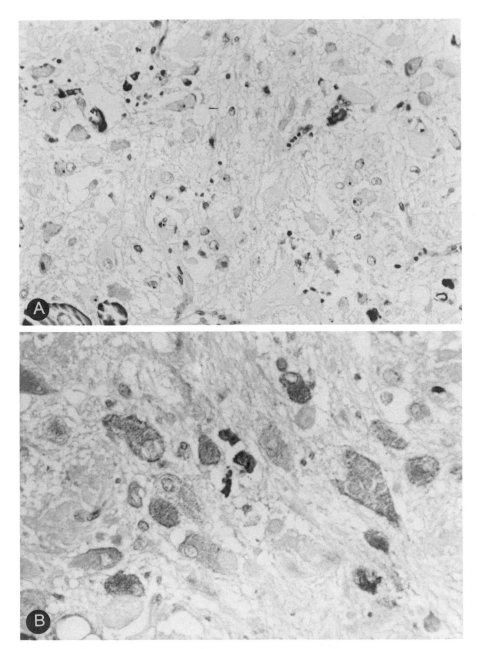

Figure 14.2. A case of intrasellar gangliocytoma. Light microscopy shows several nerve cells intermingled with glial cells and nerve fibers. Note the calcified deposits (A) × 340. Some nerve cells show immunoreactivity for galanin (B) × 250. The details of this case are described in Yamada *et al.* (222).

processes. The presence of numerous membrane–bound zebra–like bodies, which are common in gangliosidoses, has also been described (97). In the tumors associated with pituitary adenomas, intercellular junctions between the ganglion cells and adenoma cells can be demonstrated and neuronal processes

that run between the adenoma cells have also been found (187).

Immunohistochemical studies may reveal the presence of GHRH, SRIH, GnRH, CRF, vasoactive intestinal hormone, galanin, glucagon, serotonin, gastrin, neurophysin, oxytocin, β-endorphin, and β–lipotrophin in the cytoplasms of these neuronal cells (24, 222) (Fig. 14.2-B). Moreover, the presence of adenohypophyseal hormones, including prolactin (Prl), ACTH, and the α-subunit of glycoprotein hormones, has been confirmed immunohistochemically in some cases (116, 222). The associated pituitary lesion is a GH cell adenoma in most cases, but other possible lesions include nonfunctioning adenomas (116), Prl cell adenomas (116), corticotroph cell adenomas (116), and corticotroph cell hyperplasia (13).

The mechanism of the association between intrasellar neuronal choristoma and pituitary adenoma or hyperplasia remains uncertain. The most attractive hypothesis is that these adenomatous or hyperplastic lesions are attributable to increased stimulation of one pituitary cell type secondary to the excessive secretion of the corresponding releasing neuropeptides by the neuronal tumor, i.e., GHRH or vasoactive intestinal peptide in the case of GH cell adenoma (24, 116, 185), CRF in Cushing's disease (13), or vasoactive intestinal peptide in Prl cell adenoma (116). On the other hand, it is well known that neuronal tumors can occur in other parts of the central nervous system (CNS) and that they also show immunoreactivity for some releasing factors, but are usually unassociated with endocrinopathy (143). This suggests the importance of a direct circulatory pathway from such neuronal tumors to the pituitary in the development of pituitary lesions. However, some intrasellar neuronal choristomas that demonstrate the presence of immunoreactive adenohypophysiotropic peptides, are not associated with any evidence of pituitary dysfunction (143, 222). Conversely, in some cases, the corresponding adenohypophysiotropic peptides cannot be demonstrated immunohistochemically despite the presence of a pituitary adenoma (12, 116). Hence, no satisfactory explanation can be provided yet for the coexistence of intrasellar neuronal choristoma and pituitary adenoma or hyperplasia.

Hypothalamic Hamartoblastoma Syndrome (Pallister-Hall Syndrome)

This rare congenital disorder was first reported as a distinct entity by Hall *et al.* in 1980 (70). It consists of hypothalamic hamartoblastoma in association with craniofacial anomalies, limb anomalies, multiple organ anomalies, and multiple endocrine abnormalities. These anomalies are reviewed well in a recent paper (86). The multiple endocrine abnormalities include panhypopituitarism, hypothyroidism, hypoadrenalism, and cryptorchidism with micropenis, which is due to hypoplasia or dysplasia of the corresponding organ (86).

Light microscopy usually shows small, uniform cells of variable density, resembling primitive, undifferentiated germinal cells or it may show mature gray matter. The former features suggest a neoplastic potential for this lesion (38), whereas the latter support the hypothesis that such tumors retain the ability to mature with time (67). Neither nuclear atypia nor mitoses are generally noted. Ultrastructually, the presence of unusual pleomorphic vesicles has been reported (86). Based on these histological studies, it has been suggested that hypothalamic hamartoblastomas arise from the hypothalamic plate during or prior to the fifth week of gestation (38, 67).

CYSTIC LESIONS OF THE HYPOTHALAMUS AND PARASELLAR REGION

A great variety of cystic lesions can occur in the region of the sella and the hypothalamus. These lesions are often difficult to diagnose accurately only on the basis of clinical or radiological findings, and their differentiation is usually only possible by histological studies. Pituitary adenomas can also become cystic (cystic adenoma) (83), but most of these cystic lesions are considered to be primary. Some of them are neoplastic, including epidermoid or dermoid cysts, Rathke's cleft cyst, and craniopharyngioma, whereas others are not neoplastic, i.e., arachnoid cysts (157), colloid cysts of the third ventricle (206), mucoceles (63), abscesses (114), and parasitic cysts (152, 161). This section discusses the more common lesions that are considered to have endocrinologic consequences; Rathke's cleft cysts are reviewed in the next chapter.

Epidermoid and Dermoid Cysts

These cysts are histologically benign congenital tumors that result from aberrant closurc of the dorsal neural tube (19). They are uncommon and comprise approximately 1% of all intracranial neoplasms (19, 223). The epidermoid cyst is about 10 times more common than the dermoid cyst. Epidermoid cysts have a slight male predominance and, most often, become symptomatic between the ages of 20 and 50 years, whereas dermoid cysts have no sex preference and are most frequently diagnosed in childhood (40, 173). Epidermoid cysts are most often found in the cerebellopontine angle, followed by the parasellar region and the diploe. In contrast, dermoid cysts tend to lie along the midline and only infrequently involve the parasellar region. Epidermoid cysts grow as a result of the accumulation of keratin and cholesterol following the desquamation of epithelial cells, whereas dermoid cysts enlarge by glandular secretion as well as by desquamation (19). This active glandular secretion may contribute to the more rapid growth of dermoid cysts compared with epidermoid cysts (187). Symptoms and signs vary according to the site of the lesion; the most common sequelae of parasellar epidermoid or dermoid cysts are

visual disturbances, including visual impairment, primary optic atrophy, and bitemporal hemianopia (40, 136, 150). Hypothalamic or hypophyseal disturbance may or may not be apparent (123, 168, 221), and diabetes insipidus may occur occasionally. These lesions are usually not confined to the suprasellar region, but, instead, extend in various directions. Some parasellar cysts are associated with epileptic seizures when they expand under the temporal lobe (40), and rupture can produce dramatic clinical consequences, such as death, aseptic meningitis, convulsions, hydrocephalus, and transient cerebral ischemia (110, 221).

Microscopically, epidermoid cysts are composed of a thin layer of stratified, keratinized squamous epithelium that is supported by a thin outer layer of connective tissue. Dermoid cysts additionally contain a variety of skin appendages, such as sweat glands, sebaceous glands, and hair follicles (Fig. 14.3). Sometimes bone and cartilage are found in the cyst wall. A lack of endodermal elements distinguishes dermoid cysts from teratomas. Epidermoid cysts are characteristically filled

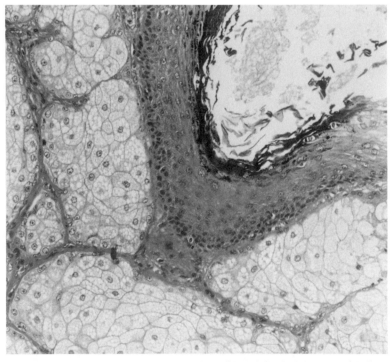

Figure 14.3. Suprasellar dermoid cyst. This tumor consists of keratinized squamous epithelium associated with abundant sebaceous glands. × 250.

with a silvery material that consists of keratin and cholesterol crystals derived from the desquamation and breakdown of keratin from the cyst wall. In contrast, the contents of a dermoid cyst is buttery yellow due to the presence of sebum and hair as well as the relatively low cholesterol content. Pericystic fibrosis or a foreign body reaction to cholesterol occurs if the cyst contents escape into the surrounding subarachnoid space. Malignant change to squamous cell carcinoma has also occasionally been reported (115).

Craniopharyngioma

Craniopharyngioma is a well-known cystic tumor that is located in the suprasellar region close to the pituitary stalk. These lesions comprise approximately 2.5% to 4% of intracranial neoplasms (34), and, in children, they account for 6% to 9% of brain tumors and 14% of supratentorial tumors (81, 129). They are thus much more common in children, with the peak incidence being from 10 to 20 years of age (17), but an appreciable proportion of patients first develop symptoms after 40 years of age (180). In addition, cases occurring in senescence as well as in the neonatal period have been reported (84, 112). These tumors seem to occur with equal frequency in both sexes (34).

The general clinical, diagnostic, and therapeutic aspects of craniopharyngiomas have been reviewed well in recent papers (3, 34, 81, 224). The principal symptoms consist of visual disturbances, increased intracranial pressure (headache, papilledema), endocrine dysfunction (varying degrees of hypopituitarism, hyperprolactinemia, and diabetes insipidus), cranial nerve palsies, and psychiatric abnormalities. It should be noted that these clinical symptoms and signs differ in incidence between younger and older patients (17, 34, 180).

Craniopharyngiomas are usually localized in the suprasellar region, but are occasionally located entirely within the third ventricle (61) or inside the sella turcica (77). Rare cases have also been reported in the optic chiasm (29), infrasellar region (5), and cerebellopontine angle (8). These tumors are often partly solid with cystic areas, but, usually, the cystic component predominates and, sometimes, the tumors are wholly cystic. Only 14% have no cystic component (17). They vary greatly in size and extent, but, generally, grow large enough to displace the neighboring tissues, affecting the optic chiasm anteriorly, the diaphragma sella and pituitary gland inferiorly, and the third ventricle superiorly (Fig. 14.4).

In almost all cystic craniopharyngiomas, the cyst walls are either smooth or they show papillary–like protrusions, and are lined by stratified squamous epithelium that is supported by a collagenous basement membrane. A few tumors (4%) have only a single layer of cuboidal or columnar cells, often associated with ciliated or goblet cells, which is a picture similar to that of Rathke's cleft cyst (17). The cyst fluid may be yellow, light tan, greenish, dark brown (like motor or machine oil), or, rarely, bright red when it results from recent hemorrhage. Its viscosity varies from watery to sludge–like. Cyst fluid is generally rich in cholesterol crystals.

In contrast, the solid portion of the craniopharyngioma is composed of trabeculae of epithelial cells with an intervening loose connective stroma (Fig. 14.5-A). These epithelial trabeculae contain mainly polygonal or elongated cells and are often associated with foci of keratinization. The periphery of the epithelial mass is lined by a single layer of dark–staining cuboidal or columnar cells. In the central zones of such epithelial masses, so called "stellate cells" can be found. These have long processes binding numerous microcystic spaces and may be produced by a primary degenerative or liquefactive process or by massive expansion of the extracellular space (Fig. 14.5-B). On histological examination, the stellate cells seem to resemble connective tissue cells, but they are now recognized to be epithelial cells. These structures, the epithelial nests and the central reticulated zones, have some resemblance to the developing enamel organ, so this type of tumor has been called an adamantinomatous craniopharyngioma (17, 34, 64, 178, 187).

Calcification or bone formation can occur as a regressive change in the epithelial cells. The calcification can be detected not only microscopically but radiologically as well and its presence is generally confirmed microscopically in almost all younger patients

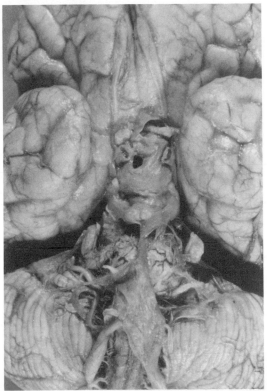

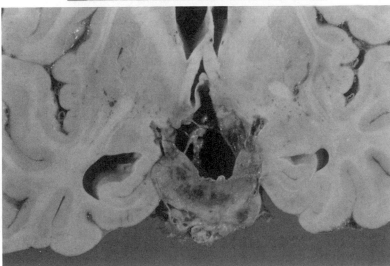

Figure 14.4. An autopsy case of craniopharyngioma shows large suprasellar mass lesion (A) extending into the third ventricle (B).

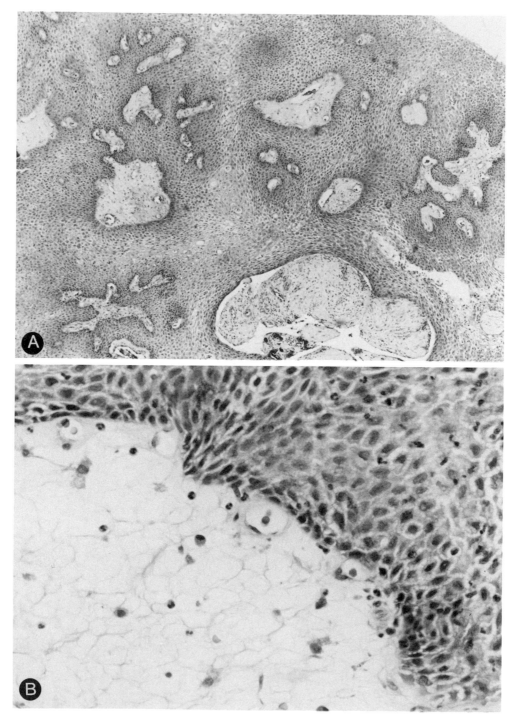

Figure 14.5. A typical microscopic appearance of an adamantinomatous type of craniopharyngioma (A) × 80. The central zones of these epithelial masses consist of "stellate cells" that have long processes binding numerous microcystic spaces (B) × 500.

and in approximately half of older patients (17).

The border between the tumor and the adjacent brain is well defined grossly, but is often irregular microscopically, and intense reactive gliosis with the formation of Rosenthal fibers may occur (17, 34, 64, 178, 187) (Fig. 14.6). Some authors have stated that forcible removal of the tumor, which is attached firmly to the hypothalamus, produces hypothalamic damage and that complete resection is therefore impossible (17, 100). Others have claimed that such a "glial reaction" may well constitute a safe resection margin between the tumorous epithelial cells and the functioning hypothalamic neurons (205). On the other hand, it has been reported that tumor remaining after surgery is more likely to be adherent to a major artery than to the hypothalamus or the optic chiasm (33). This may be because the mesenchymal reaction of vessel walls is more prominent and produces tougher fibrosis than that due to reactive gliosis.

Electron microscopy shows the presence of desmosomes and tonofilaments in addition to varying numbers of glycogen granules and other organelles. Tonofilaments are commonly seen in bundles and often connect with the desmosomes; they rarely aggregate with each other and appear to be like the electron–dense bodies that correspond to the microscopically identifiable keratohyaline granules in epithelial cells (64).

Some craniopharyngiomas may be aggressive and show rapid growth, with bony invasion and compression of the surrounding structures. However, these aggressive tumors do not show any histological differences from the more indolent lesions (122). Malignant transformation of craniopharyngioma after radiotherapy has also been reported (141).

The relationship of craniopharyngioma to epidermoid cyst, adamantinoma, and Rathke's cleft cysts is quite complicated (64, 142, 178). The morphologic appearances of craniopharyngiomas in many ways resemble that of suprasellar epidermoid cysts, adamantinomas of the jaw, or Rathke's cleft cysts. This is perhaps not surprising when

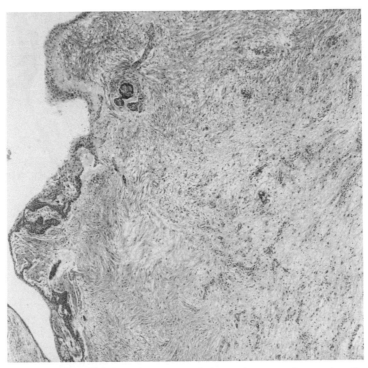

Figure 14.6. The border between the tumor and the hypothalamus shows massive reactive gliosis × 65. (Courtesy of Matsushita, H., Toranomon Hospital, Tokyo, Japan.)

taking into account their common embryological origin, since craniopharyngiomas are
considered to be congenital tumors arising
from the epithelial remnants of Rathke's
pouch.

BENIGN NEOPLASMS

Meningiomas

Meningiomas that are mainly localized to
the suprasellar region are conventionally
called suprasellar meningiomas and usually
arise in the tuberculum sella, planum sphe-
noidale, or diaphragma sella. They represent
4% of surgically treated intracranial meningiomas and 13% of those found incidentally
at necropsy (199, 220) and they show a
marked adult female preponderance. The
clinical presentation and surgical management of these lesions have been discussed
thoroughly in recent papers (27, 199). Visual
disturbance is the most common symptom,
and varying degrees of hypopituitarism or
hyperprolactinemia may also be detected.
Meningiomas arising from the diaphragma
sella do not cause hyperostosis and may enlarge the sella, thus leading to misdiagnosis as
a pituitary adenoma (131). The histological
spectrum of meningiomas is well known
(178) and, since these tumors are identical to
meningiomas occurring at other sites, their
histology will not be described here. However, it is important to remember that the
histological subtype of meningioma, except
for angioblastic meningioma, does not usually correlate with the biological behavior of
the tumor or its potential for recurrence
(101).

Lipomas

Intracranial lipomas are very rare, accounting for less than 0.5% of all intracranial
tumors, and have generally been considered
to be hamartomatous lesions of ectodermal
origin rather than true neoplasms. They affect the corpus callosum in half of the cases,
but may also be found at other sites, such as
the suprasellar region (Fig. 14.7); the ambi-
ent, quadrigeminal, and cerebellopontine
cisterns; or the sylvian fissure (98). Some of
them are asymptomatic and may be incidental or postmortem findings. Most of the

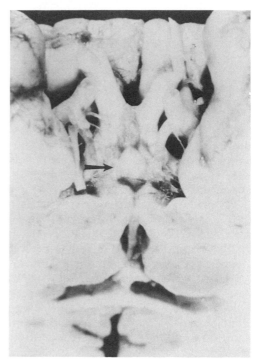

Figure 14.7. A whitish-yellow, mainly suprasellar-lo-
cated lipoma is shown (arrow). (Courtesy of Bilbao,
J.M., St Michael's Hospital, Toronto, Canada.)

symptomatic lipomas arise in the corpus callosum and are often associated with agenesis
of the corpus callosum. Lipomas of the hypothalamic region may cause varying degrees of hypopituitarism or hyperprolactinemia (56, 60, 98).

Histologically, they are composed of adipose tissue that may often contain mesoder-
mal derivatives, such as cartilage and bone
(56). Although they are benign and slow–
growing lesions, they usually adhere tightly
to the surrounding nervous tissue, so that
complete resection is rarely possible (98).

MALIGNANT NEOPLASMS

Gliomas

Gliomas of the hypothalamus are usually
reported as a single entity, but we often en-
counter difficulty in determining the precise
origin of these tumors, which frequently arise
in the retroorbital optic nerve and chiasm or
in the brain parenchyma surrounding the hypothalamus and extend into the hypothala-

mus, or vice versa (187). Hence, these tumors have also been classified as diencephalic gliomas or optico–hypothalamic gliomas (6, 145, 171). Indeed, it has been reported that 70% of diencephalic gliomas involve the third ventricle and hypothalamus, while 60% of optic pathway gliomas involve the chiasm and hypothalamus (6, 207). These hypothalamic gliomas comprise 2% of all parasellar lesions presenting with visual disturbance (65) and represent 6% of the low–grade astrocytomas and 1% of the malignant astrocytomas detected in childhood (21).

Hypothalamic gliomas are more frequent in children and predominantly affect males (65). They are generally low–grade astrocytomas called pilocytic astrocytomas, although malignant astrocytomas and gangliogliomas can also occur and may be associatcd with neurofibromatosis (6, 65, 92, 171).

The presenting manifestations are related to the patient's age, but usually include endocrine disorders due to involvement of the hypothalamic nuclei and/or hypothalamo–pituitary pathways; visual disturbance secondary to compression or infiltration of the adjacent optic pathways and/or intracranial hypertension; or hydrocephalus resulting from obstruction of the third ventricle (65, 171). The endocrinological manifestations include a well–known disorder termed "diencephalic syndrome" or "Russell's syndrome" (177), which occurs primarily in young children. This syndrome is characterized by the presence of severe emaciation and a marked increase of the serum GH level in infancy and early childhood (see Chapter 16). The mechanism of this syndrome is still unknown, although several possibilities have been proposed (41, 127, 139), but it seems conceivable that it may due to the slowly progressive disturbance of an immature anterior hypothalamus when taking into account its rarity in children more than two years old or in association with tumors other than benign gliomas. Most lesions causing the diencephalic syndrome are low–grade gliomas in the anterior hypothalamus, but, in rare cases, they may be malignant gliomas (215), ependymomas (4), germinomas (30), or gliomas associated with neurofibromatosis (215).

Pilocytic astrocytoma is the most common histological type in this group; such lesions generally show a predilection for the optic nerves and chiasm, the basal ganglia, the cerebellum, and (less often) the cerebral white matter. Two variants of this tumor are recognized, the adult type and the juvenile type (termed "juvenile pilocytic astrocytoma" (178)), with the juvenile type being far more common. They are soft, lobulated, gray–tan, solid lesions and attain a considerable size. Cystic and calcified degeneration can often be found, especially in tumors located in the walls of the third ventricle. Microscopically, these tumors are composed of uniform bipolar cells with stiff, elongated processes containing abundant glial fibers that show strong staining with phosphotungstic acid and hematoxylin (PATH), as well as immunopositivity for glial fibrillary acid protein (GFAP). Rosenthal fibers may well be noted; these are intracytoplasmic hyaline eosinophilic bodies that stain dense blue with PATH, show variable GFAP immunoreactivity, and are thought to be derived from degenerating glial fibrils (54). They are peculiar to glial filament–producing cells and are a helpful histological feature for the diagnosis of these tumors, although such bodies are not specific to pilocytic astrocytoma and can also be found in lesions causing chronic reactive gliosis, i.e., craniopharyngiomas.

Juvenile pilocytic astrocytomas have essentially the same biological behavior as ordinary pilocytic astrocytomas, but microcysts are found more commonly (Fig. 14.8). In the areas containing microcysts, the cells are not piloid but are predominantly fibril–poor protoplasmic astrocytes. Atypia and mitotic figures are rare or absent. Vascular proliferation is often found but should not be interpreted as having a malignant connotation, as it does in the case of fibrillary astrocytomas of the cerebral hemispheres or brainstem. Electron microscopy demonstrates long cell processes filled with glial filaments, whereas those of protoplasmic astrocytes contain few filaments (186). Rosenthal fibers are seen as dense amorphous structures lying among the glial fibrils (54).

These tumors are histologically benign and grow slowly, although malignant transformation may occur in rare cases (145). Thus, their relatively poor prognosis is pri-

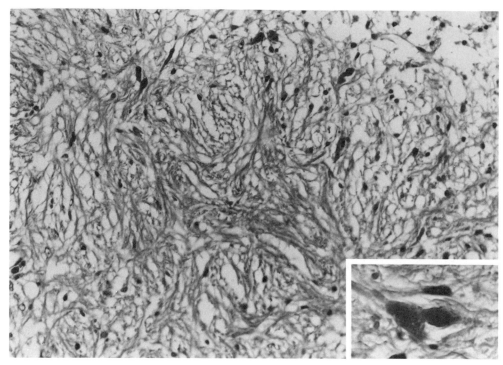

Figure 14.8. A juvenile pilocytic astrocytoma of the hypothalamus. This tumor is composed of bipolar fibrillated astrocytes associated with microcystic components (A) × 330. Inset shows Rosenthal fibers. (B) × 1000.

marily due to the surgically inaccessible deep–seated location in the hypothalamus.

In rare instances, astrocytomas can also originate in the pituitary stalk and in the posterior pituitary gland (Fig. 14.9). Historically, they were called "pituicytomas," but there has been some confusion over the use of this term because it has also been used for granular cell tumors (see Chapter 15) since it was first mentioned by Liss & Kahn (120). Hence, it is now considered that "pituicytoma" should be used to designate only neurohypophyseal tumors clearly derived from astrocytes (172), or that vague terms like this and infundibuloma (158) should be abandoned and that such tumors should simply be called astrocytomas of the infundibulum or posterior pituitary (187).

Most such astrocytomas appear to arise in the infundibulum and grow down the pituitary stalk, but, rarely, they may originate in the posterior pituitary. These tumors may be associated with visual disturbance, hyperprolactinemia, or varying degrees of hypopituitarism (172). Their microscopic and ultra-

structural appearance is basically the same as that of the pilocytic astrocytomas found in other parts of the CNS (172, 188).

Germ Cell Tumors

Intracranial germ cell tumors are rare lesions that comprise 0.3% to 3.4% of primary intracranial tumors and reach a higher incidence of up to 10% in Japan (10, 25, 89, 208). The majority of these tumors occur before 30 years of age, with a peak incidence in the second decade, and they affect males more frequently (approximately 2:1) (25, 90, 216). They are assumed to arise from the antecedent presence of germ cells, although it is still uncertain whether this occurs due to malmigration, embryonic cell nests, or a localized hamartomatous or dysplastic process (69, 90, 197). Most intracranial germ cell tumors originate in the midline and affect the pineal region (58%), the suprasellar area (40%), or both sites either sequentially or simultaneously (10%) (90).

The spectrum of intracranial germ cell tumors is the same as that of such lesions in the gonads, retroperitoneum, and mediastinum (25, 138), and they can be categorized into germinomas (61% to 65%) teratomas (immature and malignant) (18% to 33%), embryonal carcinomas (3% to 5%), endodermal sinus tumors (yolk sac tumors) (1% to 7%), and choriocarcinomas (1% to 5%) (25, 90) (Fig. 14.10). Mixed tumors having more than two different kinds of germ cell elements account for 10% to 50% of these lesions (25, 176). The detailed histological appearance of these tumors is outside the scope of this chapter, but the following points should be noted. Nongerminomatous germ cell tumors affect males more frequently (3:1) when compared with germinomas (2:1) (90). Germinomas are more common lesions (58% to 73%) and are more predominant in females (1 to 2:1) in the suprasellar region when compared to the pineal region (25, 80, 90, 113). Nongerminomatous germ cell tumors are more frequently encountered in the first decade of life than germinomas (25, 90). The prognosis is much better for germinomas than for the other types of germ cell tumors (25, 90), and it appears to be worse for suprasellar germinomas than for pineal germinomas (80), although a similar prognosis for both locations has also been reported (113). CSF metastases

occur in 5% to 57% of germinomas and are generally reported to be more frequent in suprasellar than in pineal germinomas (90, 113). Although α-fetoprotein, human chorionic gonadotropin (hCG), and carcinoembryonic antigen levels in both serum and CSF have been used as markers for making a differential diagnosis of germ cell tumors and monitoring the therapeutic response, it should be noted that there are often discrepancies between the results of immunohistochemical staining of tumors for these markers and their serum or CSF levels (195).

In the suprasellar region, germinomas are the most common histological type, although other germ cell tumors can also arise here (90). These tumors (whether primary or secondary) are usually quite large, have no capsule, and affect the hypothalamus, pituitary stalk, and optic nerves. The pituitary gland, primarily the neurohypophysis, is also involved by 20% of these tumors (148). Although they are rare, primary intrasellar germinomas have also been reported (148). The clinical presentation of a suprasellar germinoma is related to the tumor's anatomical location (80). The interval until diagnosis is generally longer for germinomas of the suprasellar region than for pineal lesions. Dia-

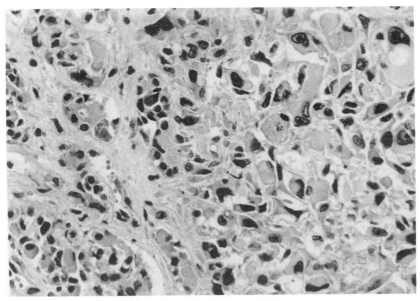

Figure 14.9. A gemistocytic astrocytoma of the posterior pituitary gland. Note the anterior pituitary gland (left) × 800. (Courtesy of Kovacs, K., St Michael's Hospital, Toronto, Canada.)

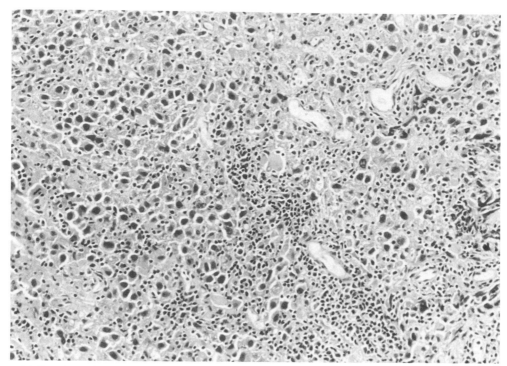

Figure 14.10.   A germinoma arising from the hypothalamus showing large polygonal or spheroidal germinal cells and conspicuous lymphoid infiltrate × 250.

betes insipidus, visual disturbances, and hypopituitarism are the well-known clinical triad of symptoms caused by suprasellar germinomas, and approximately half of these tumors are associated with the triad (87). Diabetes insipidus due to compression or destruction of the hypothalamus and pituitary stalk is the earliest and most prominent symptom, with a reported frequency ranging from 40% to 95% (90, 174). According to an epidemiological survey of 713 cases of diabetes insipidus in Japan, 27% were due to intracranial tumors, and 42% of these tumors were germinomas (9). Visual disturbance related to compression or infiltration of the optic nerves, chiasm, and tracts occurs in 30% of the patients (174) and is the most common symptom causing patients to seek medical attention (174, 197). Primary optic atrophy without papilledema and visual field defects (bitemporal hemianopia) are the most common findings (197). Varying degrees of hypopituitarism are noted in approximately 20% of cases (187), and precocious puberty is also found in rare cases. This may

be due either to hypothalamic destruction resulting in the loss of neural influences that tonically inhibit gonadotropin production (174), or to hCG production by the tumor itself. Precocious puberty primarily affects males, since hCG stimulates testosterone production, but has no similar effect on the ovaries (219). Other rare symptoms include hydrocephalus, ophthalmoplegia, and various signs of hypothalamic dysfunction, such as hypodypsia, adipsia, pyrexia, anorexia, hyperphagia and obesity, electrolytic imbalances, amnesia, irritability, drowsiness, and somnolence (39, 51, 87, 174, 197).

Chordomas

Chordomas are histologically benign tumors that are generally considered to arise from intraosseus notochordal remnants. These lesions arise along the craniospinal axis and are most commonly found in the sacrococcygeal area (50%), followed by the skull base (35%) and the vertebral bodies (10%) (76). Cranial chordomas have a slight male predominance and affect all age groups, but are most common in the fourth and fifth decades (164). Cranial chordomas may be divided into two broad categories based on their anatomical location; i.e., basisphenoidal (upper clivus) or basioccipital (lower clivus) (162). The clinical manifestations of these tumors vary depending on the location; upper cranial nerve involvement (including visual disturbance and cavernous sinus syndrome) and endocrine disturbances are associated with basisphenoidal lesions (111, 162). The very rare occurrence of ectopic intrasellar chordomas has also been reported (128).

Chordoma is a soft, jelly–like, lobulated tumor that is often associated with hemorrhage, calcification, or cystic change. Histologically, the tumor is made up of cells arranged in cords, syncytia, and clusters that are surrounded by a mucinous or chondroid stroma that often contains scattered lymphocytes. The tumor cells are called "physaliferous" cells and they feature intracellular vacuoles containing PAS– and mucicarmine–positive mucin and glycogen granules (Fig. 14.11). These cells sometimes resemble the "signet–ring" cells found in adenocarcinomas. In such instances, reticulin staining may be useful to differentiate chordoma from adenocarcinoma (169). These vacuoles can be found not only intracellularly but also extracellularly (198). Ultrastructural features, i.e., the accumulation of mitochondria and endoplasmic reticulum, may be useful to differentiate these lesions from chondrosarcomas or chordoid sarcomas, which appear similar to chordomas by light microscopy (154). Although they are slow–growing and histologically benign, they have been regarded clinically as malignant because of their critical location, locally aggressive nature, and extremely high recurrence rate. However, there is generally no correlation between the histological features (cellular pleomorphism, mitotic figures, or hyperchromatic nuclei are rarely found) and patient survival (169), although it should be noted that chondroid chordoma (a subtype containing chondroid elements) has been reported to have a better prognosis than chor-

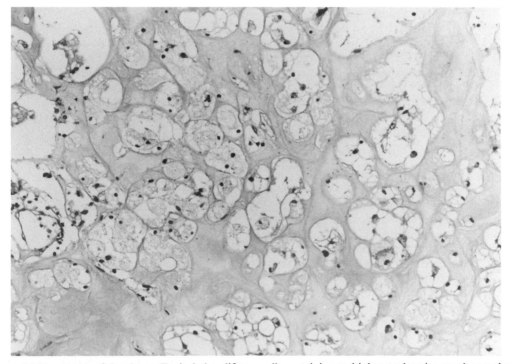

Figure 14.11.   A case of chordoma. Typical physaliferous cells containing multiple cytoplasmic vacuoles are shown within a matrix × 250.

doma without chondroid elements (73, 162, 169). It is well known that metastasis to bone, lymph nodes, the lungs, and the skin can occur in patients with chordoma, especially in the late stages, and 10% to 47% of patients will develop metastases (36, 73, 76). However, metastases arising from intracranial chordomas are very rare (162).

Lymphoma, Plasmacytoma, and Leukemia

Central nervous system lymphoma can be both primary and secondary (74, 79, 124). It is quite rare and accounts for approximately 1% of all brain tumors (91). However, CNS lymphoma has increased in frequency in the last 10 years and has been well reviewed in some recent papers (74, 79, 91). Various subtypes exist, and non-Hodgkin's lymphoma is the most common histological type; it is composed of histiocytic cells or large immunoblastic cells with B cell surface markers (79). The primary lymphoma is an intrinsic cerebral neoplasm whereas the secondary lymphoma more frequently affects the meninges and less often involves the cerebral parenchyma (74).

The third ventricle or hypothalamus are involved by less than 10% of such tumors (187). The lesion is usually diffuse, infiltrative, and extends down the pituitary stalk to affect the neurohypophysis (187). In such instances, diabetes insipidus, varying degrees of hypopituitarism, weight loss, and somnolence can occur (15, 78, 156, 189). Although it is very rare, lymphoma arising in or mainly located in the hypothalamic region has also been reported (78, 156, 189).

In rare instances, a solitary plasmacytoma develops in the skull, the meninges, or the brain (125). It may be the first manifestation of multiple myeloma. Rare cases arising in an intrasellar location or in the hypothalamus itself have also been reported (42, 213). Plasma cell granulomas and meningiomas containing a plasma cell-lymphocytic component (82) must be considered in the differential diagnosis (125). Immunohistochemical studies can confirm monoclonal immunoglobulin production by the cells and are very useful for making a definite diagnosis of this type of tumor (125).

Involvement of the CNS by leukemia has also been reported, and most cases involve leukemic infiltration of the spinal nerve roots or leukemic meningitis, with mass lesions in the brain being very unusual (62). There are various histological types, including acute or chronic myelocytic or lymphocytic leukemia. The hypothalamus or hypophysis can be affected by leukemic infiltration and/or thrombosis of the small vessels due to leukemic cell aggregates (93). In such instances, diabetes insipidus is the most common endocrinological feature (93, 132), and, on rare occasions, this may precede any other symptoms of leukemia (160). It has been reported that up to 15% of leukemia–associated diabetes insipidus is vasopressin-resistant (106).

Metastatic Tumors

The pituitary gland, especially the neurophypophysis, is one of the favored sites for metastatic brain tumors (see Chapter 15). A few such patients show involvement of the tuber cinereum and/or various parts of the hypothalamus as well as the proximal pituitary stalk, which results in diabetes insipidus (55). Thus, in the majority of these patients, the hypothalamus is affected by the invasion of a nearby metastatic tumor or by compression as the metastasis enlarges (187). One interesting case has been reported in which Cushing's disease developed secondary to corticotroph cell hyperplasia caused by CRF secretion from a median eminence metastasis of a prostatic carcinoma (32) (Fig. 14.12).

The metastatic tumors are usually carcinomas, rarely lymphomas or leukemias, and very occasionally sarcomas.

INFLAMMATORY DISORDERS

Sarcoidosis

Sarcoidosis is a systemic, noncaseating granulomatous disease of unknown origin. It may affect any organ system, but usually involves the lungs, lymph nodes, skin, eyes, spleen, and liver. Involvement of the CNS by sarcoidosis is relatively uncommon, affecting 3.5% to 5.0% of the patients with this disease (52, 155). Pituitary-hypothalamic involvement is quite rare, at less than 1%, but is more frequent than the involvement of any other endocrine organ (200). Most sarcoido-

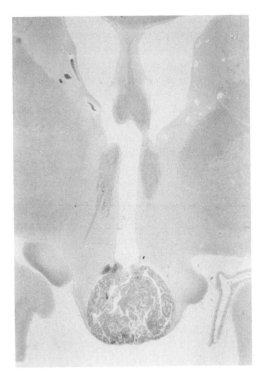

Figure 14.12. A coronal section of a hypothalamic metastasis of a prostatic carcinoma. (Courtesy of Bilbao, J.M., St Michael's Hospital, Toronto, Canada.)

ing degrees of hypopituitarism, in which gonadotropins, thyrotropin-stimulating hormone (TSH), and ACTH are most often affected (218), may be due to hypothalamic or pituitary involvement in this disease. In the majority of these cases, a hypothalamic disorder is assumed to cause the hypopituitarism, because more than 90% of patients retain pituitary responsiveness to the corresponding hypothalamic releasing factors (203). Hyperprolactinemia is not uncommon, and it may develop without any other evidence of pituitary dysfunction (212).

Light microscopy shows discrete noncaseating granulomas containing multinucleated giant cells. Such granulomas are often surrounded by a lymphocytic infiltration and may contain an intercellular reticulum. Appreciable areas of necrosis cannot be found in these granulomas, unlike those due to infectious diseases, but the histological features of some granulomas may be indistinguishable from those of infectious origin, apart from the absence of organisms. Thus, special stains for organisms such as fungi, treponema, and tubercle bacilli are important in the differential diagnosis of sarcoidosis. Making the issue more complex, the histological features depend mainly on the stage of development and range from typical granulomas to fibrous scarring with or without calcification. Electron microscopy (211) generally has no role in the diagnosis of this condition (187).

Histiocytosis X

Histiocytosis X is a systemic disorder of unknown etiology that can affect almost every organ by the pathological proliferation of reticuloendothelial cells. Historically, it was divided into three subtypes, i.e., eosinophilic granuloma, Hand–Schüller–Christian disease, and Letterer–Siwe disease. However, the distinction among these subtypes is not always clear–cut and transitional cases are not uncommon, although some cases certainly have clinical features distinct enough for classification into one of these three categories. Therefore, use of the general term "histiocytosis X" is preferable and the three categories are better considered as representing parts of the spectrum of a single disease entity (117). This disease can vary in presen-

sis patients with pituitary–hypothalamic lesions have obvious manifestations of systemic sarcoidosis, although pituitary-hypothalamic sarcoidosis as the sole manifestation of this disease has also been reported (109).

Granulomatous leptomeningitis that also involves the hypothalamic–pituitary region is the most common pattern of CNS sarcoidosis.

The clinical signs of pituitary-hypothalamic involvement are varied, including diabetes insipidus, somnolence, obesity, abnormal temperature and vascular regulation, hypopituitarism, and hyperprolactinemia. Diabetes insipidus, which may be due to sarcoidosis invading the supraoptic nucleus of the hypothalamus, appears to be the most common finding in CNS sarcoidosis. It should be noted, however, that polydipsia and polyuria caused by a primary thirst disorder may be more common than true diabetes insipidus in such instances (202). Vary-

tation from a benign solitary bone lesion to widely disseminated multiple-organ involvement, so the clinical manifestations and prognosis are extremely variable (196). Skin, lymph nodes, lung, liver, kidney, stomach, thymus, spleen, bone marrow, and the CNS can all be affected. Involvement of the CNS is not uncommon in patients with disseminated disease, and there is an apparent predilection of the lesion for the hypothalamus and posterior pituitary. Diabetes insipidus and GH-deficiency are well recognized consequences of hypothalamic involvement (26). Other endocrinopathies, such as hypoadrenalism, hypothyroidism, hypogonadism, and hyperprolactinemia may also be found, but these are less common (26, 66). Hypothalamic or pituitary-stalk dysfunction can be produced by a primary lesion or result from the extension of bone lesions. A few cases of diabetes insipidus show all the features of Hand-Schüller-Christian disease, but it should be noted that the hypothalamus or pituitary gland can be affected primarily by histiocytosis X (144, 147), and that endocrinopathy may be found in the absence of abnormal radiological findings in the initial stage (183).

Light microscopy shows tissue destruction and infiltration of foamy histiocytes, macrophages, lymphocytes, plasma cells, and eosinophils in the active stage (Fig. 14.13). In some cases, especially after irradiation, fibrosis is a prominent feature and makes diagnosis difficult. Immunohistochemical studies demonstrate immunopositivity for S–100 antigen in the histiocytes, suggesting that they may represent the proliferation of epidermal Langerhans cells. Ultrastructural examination demonstrates cytoplasmic Birbeck granules, which are the hallmark of this disease (57) (Fig. 14.13). The etiology of histiocytosis X is still controversial. Recent studies have suggested that the disease is associated with a deficiency of circulating suppressor (T_8) lymphocytes and an increased helper (T_4)/suppressor (T_8) ratio (28). However, it still remains uncertain whether the deficiency of suppressor cells is a cause of histiocytosis X, an effect of the disease, or simply a "paraphenomenon" (28).

Other Inflammatory Disorders

In the literature, giant cell granulomas and plasma cell granulomas have been reported as distinct clinicopathological entities. Giant cell granulomas are mainly a disease of the pituitary gland and, histologically, show

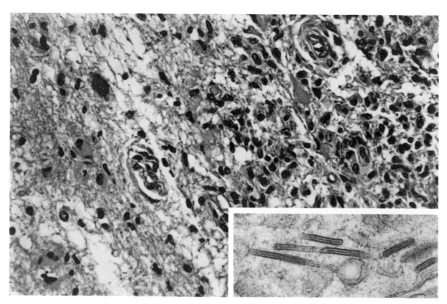

Figure 14.13.   A histiocytosis X of the hypothalamus. Light microscopy demonstrates abundant histiocytes (right) and hypothalamic neuron (left) × 400. Inset showing Birbeck granules × 42000. (Courtesy of Bilbao, J.M., St Michael's Hospital, Toronto, Canada.)

giant cells plus histiocytes, lymphocytes, and plasma cells. In contrast, plasma cell granulomas can be found in the hypothalamus as well as in other parts of the CNS. They contain lymphocytes and plasma cells without any histiocytes or giant cells.

The etiology and pathogenesis of these rare granulomatous disorders remains obscure, and other kind of inflammatory or infectious disorders must be carefully ruled out to confirm their diagnosis. Both conditions are reviewed well in the recent literature (59, 184).

Lymphocytic adenohypophysitis is another condition belonging to this category, but it will be discussed in Chapter 15.

INFECTIOUS DISEASES

A great variety of infectious agents can affect the hypothalamo–pituitary region as a consequence of either direct infiltration or secondary vascular damage (hemorrhage or infarction). Such infections are associated with hypothalamic and pituitary dysfunction, which varies in its time of onset, its duration, and its severity. The causative organisms include bacteria (1, 2, 58, 135, 153), fungi (187, 210), protozoa and metazoa (133, 140), and viruses (16, 31, 85, 105, 119, 204).

Tuberculosis

In tuberculous meningitis, the hypothalamus and pituitary may be affected and hypothalamo–pituitary dysfunction may develop as a result (Fig. 14.14). Diabetes insipidus is the more common sequel, but hypopituitarism can also occur. In the acute stage, this disease is characterized by caseating granulomas and a fibroinflammatory reaction, and the histological diagnosis can easily be made. In contrast, dystrophic calcification is common in the chronic stage, and secondary endarteritis often causes infarction of the hypothalamus or pituitary stalk. One variant of this disease presents as massive encapsulated granulomatous necrosis containing cholesterol deposits and small foci of calcification inside the sella. In such instances, hypopituitarism develops as a consequence of pituitary gland destruction. However, it should be noted that a similar state may also be found due to gumma, abscess, or craniopharyngioma (14, 135, 193).

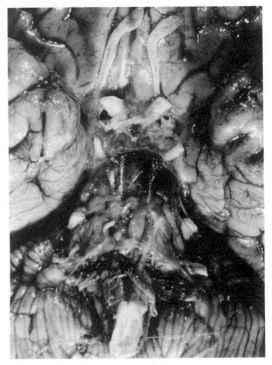

Figure 14.14. Tuberculous meningitis shows dense inflamation and fibrosis, particularly in basal leptomeninges.

VASCULAR DISEASES

Vascular lesions of the hypothalamus are usually found in the setting of generalized cerebrovascular disease (99), but they can also occur in association with primary intracranial vascular disease (Fig. 14.15), hypotensive shock, intracranial hypertension, hematological disease, infectious disease, or trauma (68, 99, 134, 149, 179, 191, 201). The lesions produced may result in varying degrees of hypothalamic and pituitary dysfunction.

ANEURYSMS

It is well–known that some giant cerebral aneurysms, arising most often from the internal carotid artery, can produce a clinical picture resembling that of an intrasellar or suprasellar tumor. Considering the close relationship of the circle of Willis to the pituitary and hypothalamus, it is obvious that a large aneurysm originating from the internal

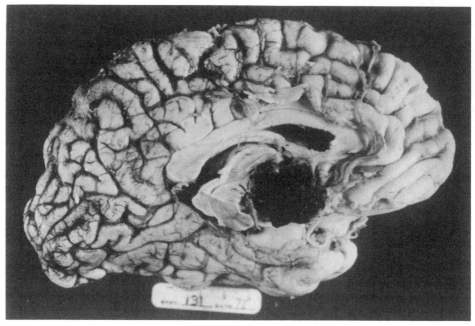

Figure 14.15. A 32-year-old man with a history of delayed puberty and obesity was seen, initially, with bitemporal hemianopia and headache, which were followed by slowly progressive memory loss and intellectual impairment. Mid-sagittal section shows large cavernous angioma involving diencephalon and anterior third ventricle. (Reprinted with permission from Mizutani T., Goldberg, H.I., Kerson, L.A., *et al.* Cavernous hemangioma in the diencephalon. Arch. Neurol., 38:379–382, 1981.)

carotid artery or the anterior communicating artery can cause compression of these structures, which may result in hypothalamo–hypophyseal dysfunction (163, 182, 217). The incidence of aneurysms mimicking hypophyseal tumors has been reported as being approximately 1.4% of all intracranial aneurysms (217).

Such hypothalamic lesions can also arise not by the mass effect of an unruptured giant aneurysm but by subsequent aneurysmal rupture. Crompton reported that 61% of 106 consecutive patients dying from a ruptured aneurysm had hypothalamic lesions, which were most often found in those patients with aneurysms of the anterior and posterior communicating arteries (44). These lesions consisted of three types: a) zones of ischemic necrosis of up to 5 mm in size; b) microhemorrhages around perforating arteries or selective microhemorrhage into the paraventricular and supraoptic nuclei; and c) massive hemorrhage due to blood escaping from a ruptured aneurysm. The pathogenesis of ischemic necrosis and microhemorrhages

may be related to either intense vasoconstriction or venous back pressure produced by the subarachnoid hemorrhage. However, there is a considerable discrepancy between postmortem hypothalamic involvement and the clinical recognition of symptoms attributable to this region.

TRAUMA

Morphological studies in head trauma have shown a high prevalence of hypothalamo–pituitary lesions, varying from massive infarction of the anterior pituitary to diffuse hemorrhage in the hypothalamus (45, 50, 71, 104). However, in many cases, the symptoms related to these lesions are masked by those of other concomitant lesions. In the hypothalamus, the anterior part is the most commonly affected site in head trauma, due to disruption or vascular damage including vasospasm (175). Such lesions are often associated with optic pathway damage resulting from avulsion of the optic chiasm or deceleration injury (187, 192, 209). In such instances, hypothalamic dysfunction including diabetes insipidus can occur (175). In contrast, the part of the hypothalamus behind the infundibulum is usually not involved (175). The pituitary stalk can also be interrupted by shearing or avulsion due to head trauma. This is usually associated with disturbance of the blood supply to the gland and results in infarction of the anterior pituitary and hemorrhage into the posterior pituitary. Such cases are more commonly encountered than direct pituitary injury due to sellar floor fractures (209). The diabetes insipidus that occurs in these patients is usually transient, because the hemorrhagic involvement of the posterior pituitary is not so extensive (50, 104). However, more severe diabetes insipidus can occur as a result of high stalk transection or infundibular or inferior hypothalamic infarction.

Post-traumatic hypopituitarism can also develop in either the acute or chronic stage and, in the latter case, hypogonadism may precede panhypopituitarism by months or even years (37).

HYDROCEPHALUS

Chronic hydrocephalus of either the noncommunicating or communicating type may be complicated by a variety of endocrine disturbances, including hypopituitarism, amenorrhea, diabetes insipidus, and precocious puberty (18, 75, 88, 95). The hypopituitarism seems to result from damage to the hypothalamus rather than to the pituitary gland or its stalk, and presumably is secondary to enlargement of the third ventricle affecting the hypothalamus. Damage to the hypothalamic nuclear architecture with gliosis or neuronal loss has been noted at autopsy (75).

MISCELLANEOUS CONDITIONS AFFECTING THE HYPOTHALAMUS

Certain generalized diseases of the CNS may affect the hypothalamus and produce hypothalamic and pituitary dysfunction. Wernicke's encephalopathy, a metabolic disease developing in the setting of chronic alcoholism, occasionally involves the mammillary bodies, and hypothalamic nuclei, resulting in Korsakoff's syndrome. Small

hemorrhages are typically seen in the affected areas in this disease (166). Demyelination of the lateral hypothalamus in multiple sclerosis can produce aphagia and cachexia (96). The presence of Lewy neuronal inclusion bodies in the hypothalamic nuclei has been noted in Parkinson's disease (107). In addition, a recent review article describes dysautonomia, temperature intolerance, a decreased hypothalamic dopamine content, abnormal GH dynamics, and abnormal levels of melanocyte-stimulating hormone, β–endorphin, and SRIF in the CSF as an endocrinopathy associated with Parkinson's disease (181).

Transection of the pituitary stalk, either for the treatment of breast cancer or diabetic retinopathy, or as a complication of the surgical treatment of sellar tumors, can produce some considerable changes not only in the pituitary gland and stalk, but also in the hypothalamus. The extent or severity of the lesion generally depends on the level at which the stalk is transected. Characteristic findings have been described well in some reports (48, 49). Complete stalk transection leads to hypopituitarism in the order of gonadotropic, corticotropic, or thyrotropic secretion, whereas GH secretion may remain normal and hypersecretion of prolactin may occur. Diabetes insipidus is another important sequel of hypophysectomy or stalk transection. It is well known that the pattern of diabetes insipidus depends on the level at which the stalk is transected, but it should be also noted that the degree of diabetes insipidus can be modified by the degree to which anterior pituitary hormones are also involved, or the extent to which glucocorticoids are replaced.

REFERENCES

1. Abramsky O., Soffer D., and Marks E.S. Diabetes insipidus as a complication of pneumococcal meningitis. J. Am. Geriatr. Soc., 21:232–234, 1973.
2. Adams M., Rhyner P.A., Day J., et al. Whipple's disease confined to the central nervous system. Ann. Neurol., 21:104–108, 1987.
3. Adamson T.E., Wiestler O.D., Kleihues P., et al. Correlation of clinical and pathological features in surgically treated craniopharyngiomas. J. Neurosurg., 73:12–17, 1990.
4. Addy D.P., and Hudson F.P. Diencephalic syndrome of infantile emaciation. Analysis of literature and report of 3 cases. Arch. Dis. Child., 47:338–343, 1972.

5. Akimura T., Kameda H., Abiko S., *et al.* Infrasellar craniopharyngioma. Neuroradiology, *31:*180–183, 1989.
6. Albright A.L., Price R.A., and Guthkelch A.N. Diencephalic gliomas of children. A clinicopathologic study. Cancer, *55:*2789–2793, 1985.
7. Allen J.P., Greer M.A., MacGilvra R., *et al.* Endocrine function in an anencephalic infant. J. Clin. Endocrinol. Metab., *38:*94–98, 1974.
8. Altinors N., Senveli E., Erdogan A., *et al.* Craniopharyngioma of the cerebellopontine angle. J. Neurosurg., *60:*842–844, 1984.
9. Annual Report of the Ministry of Health and Welfare Pituitary Dysfunction Research Committee [in Japanese]. 34–42, 1975.
10. Araki C., and Matsumoto S. Statistical reevaluation of pinealoma and related tumors in Japan. J. Neurosurg., *30:*146–149, 1967.
11. Asa S.L., Bilbao J.M., Kovacs K., *et al.* Hypothalamic neuronal hamartoma associated with pituitary growth hormone cell adenoma and acromegaly. Acta. Neuropathol. (Berl.), *52:*231–234, 1980.
12. Asa S.L., Scheithauer B.W., Bilbao J.M., *et al.* A case for hypothalamic acromegaly: a clinicopathological study of six patients with hypothalamic gangliocytomas producing growth hormone releasing factor. J. Clin. Endocrinol. Metab., *58:*796–803, 1984.
13. Asa S.L., Kovacs K., Tindall G.T., *et al.* Cushing's disease associated with an intrasellar gangliocytoma producing corticotropin-releasing factor. Ann. Intern. Med., *101:*789–793, 1984.
14. Asherson R.A., Jackson W.P.U., and Lewis B. Abnormalities of development associated with hypothalamic calcification after tuberculous meningitis. BMJ, *2:*839–843, 1965.
15. Ashworth B. Cerebral histiocytic lymphoma presenting with loss of weight. Neurology, *32:*894–896, 1982.
16. Baker A.B., Cornwell S., and Brown I.A. Poliomyelitis. VI. The hypothalamus. Arch. Neurol. Psychiatry, *68:*16–36, 1952.
17. Banna M. Craniopharyngioma: based on 160 cases. Brit. J. Rad., *49:*206–223, 1976.
18. Barbar S.G., and Garvan N. Hypopituitarism in normal-pressure hydrocephalus. BMJ, *1:*1039–1041, 1979.
19. Baxter J.W., and Netsky M.G. Epidermoid and dermoid tumors: pathology. In: *Neurosurgery, vol 1.* pp. 655–661, edited by R.H. Wilkins and S.S. Rengachary, New York, McGraw-Hill Company, 1985.
20. Beal M.F., Kleinman G.M., Ojemann R.G., *et al.* Gangliocytoma of third ventricle: hyperphagia, somnolence, and dementia. Neurology, *31:*1224–1228, 1981.
21. Becker L.E., and Yates A.J. Astrocytic tumors in children. Major Prob. Pathol., *18:*373–396, 1986.
22. Begeot M., Dubois M.P., and Dubois P.M. Evolution of lactotropes in normal and anencephalic human fetuses. J. Clin. Endocrinol. Metab., *58:*726–730, 1985.
23. Berkovic S.F., Andermann F., Melanson D., *et al.* Hypothalamic hamartomas and ictal laughter: evolution of a characteristic epileptic syndrome and diagnostic value of magnetic resonance imaging. Ann. Neurol., *23:*429–439, 1988.
24. Bevan J.S., Asa S.L., Rossi M.L., *et al.* Intrasellar gangliocytoma containing gastrin and growth hormone-releasing hormone associated with a growth hormone-secreting pituitary adenoma. Clin. Endocrinol. (Oxf.), *30:*213–224, 1989.
25. Bjornsson J., Scheithauer B.W., Okazaki H., *et al.* Intracranial germ cell tumors: pathobiological and immunohistochemical aspects of 70 cases. J. Neuropathol. Exp. Neurol., *44:*32–46, 1985.
26. Braunstein G.D., and Kohler P.O. Pituitary function in Hand-Schüller-Christian disease. Evidence for deficient Growth-hormone release in patients with short stature. N. Engl. J. Med., *286:*1225–1229, 1972.
27. Brihaye J., and VanGeertruyden M.B. Management and surgical outcome of suprasellar meningiomas. Acta. Neurochir. (suppl), *42:*124–129, 1988.
28. Broadbent V., and Pritchard J. Histiocytosis X - current controversies. Arch. Dis. Child., *60:*605–607, 1985.
29. Brodsky M.C., Hoyt W.F., Barnwell S.L., *et al.* Intrachiasmatic craniopharyngioma: a rare cause of chiasmal thickening. J. Neurosurg., *68:*300–302, 1988.
30. Burr I.M., Slonim A.E., Danish R.K., *et al.* Diencephalic syndrome revisited. J. Pediatr., *88:*439–444, 1976.
31. Caplan R.H., Glasser J.E., and Rodman C.A. Partial hypothalamic insufficiency resulting from herpes simplex encephalitis: report of a probable case. Minn. Med., *65:*341–344, 1982.
32. Carey R.M., Varma S.K., Drake C.R. Jr., *et al.* Ectopic secretion of corticotropin-releasing factor as a cause of Cushing's syndrome: a clinical, morphologic, and biochemical study. N. Engl. J. Med., *311:*13–20, 1984.
33. Carmel P.W., Antuness J.L., and Chang C.H. Craniopharyngiomas in children. Neurosurgery, *11:*382–389, 1982.
34. Carmel P.W. Craniopharyngiomas. In: *Neurosurgery,* vol. 1, edited by R.H. Wilkins, and S.S. Rengachary, pp. 905–916, New York, McGraw-Hill Book Company, 1985.
35. Carpenter M.B. *Core Textbook of Neuroanatomy,* 2nd ed. pp. 216–235, Baltimore, Williams & Wilkins, 1978.
36. Chambers P.W., and Schwinn C.P. Chordoma: a clinicopathological study of metastasis. Am. J. Clin. Pathol., *72:*765–776, 1979.
37. Clark J.D.A., Raggatt P.R., and Edwards O.M. Hypothalamic hypogonadism following major head injury. Clin. Endocrinol. (Oxf.), *29:*153–165, 1988.
38. Clarren S.K., Alvord E.C., and Hall J.G. Congenital hypothalamic hamartoblastoma, hypopituitarism, imperforate anus, and postaxial polydactyly—A new syndrome? Part II: Neuropathological consideration. Am. J. Med. Genet., *7:*75–83, 1980.
39. Coffey R.J. Hypothalamic and basal forebrain germinoma presenting with amnesia and hyperphagia. Surg. Neurol., *31:*228–233, 1989.

40. Conley F.K. Epidermoid and dermoid tumors: clinical features and surgical management. In: *Neurosurgery,* vol 1, edited by R.H. Wilkins, and S.S. Regachary, pp. 668–673, New York, Mc-Graw-Hill Company, 1985.

41. Connors M.H., and Sheikholislam B.M. Hypothalamic symptomatology and its relationship to diencephalic tumor in childhood. Childs Brain, *3:*31–36, 1977.

42. Coryachkina G.P. Solitary plasmacytoma of the hypothalamus. Arkh. Pathol., *41:*53–57, 1979.

43. Costin G., and Murphree A.L. Hypothalamic-pituitary function in children with optic nerve hypoplasia. Am. J. Dis. Child., *139:*249–254, 1985.

44. Crompton M.R. Hypothalamic lesions following the rupture of cerebral berry aneurysms. Brain, *86:*301–314, 1963.

45. Cromptom M.R. Hypothalamic lesions following closed head injury. Brain, *94:*165–172, 1971.

46. Culler F.L., James H.E., Simon M.L., *et al.* Identification of gonadotropin-releasing hormone in neurons of a hypothalamic hamartoma in a boy with precocious puberty. Neurosurgery, *17:*408–412, 1985.

47. Curatolo P., Cusmai R., Finocchi G., *et al.* Gelastic epilepsy and true precocious puberty due to hypothalamic hamartoma. Dev. Med. Child. Neurol., *26:*509–527, 1984.

48. Daniel P.M., and Prichard M.M.L. The human hypothalamus and pituitary stalk after hypophysectomy or pituitary stalk section. Brain, *95:*813–824, 1972.

49. Daniel P.M., and Prichard M.M.L. Studies of the hypothalamus and the pituitary gland: with special reference to the effects of transection of the pituitary stalk. Acta. Endocrinol. (Copenh.) [Suppl], *201:*1–216, 1975.

50. Daniel P.M., and Treip C.S. Lesions of the pituitary gland associated with head injuries. In: *The Pituitary Gland,* edited by G.W. Harris and B.T. Donovan, pp. 519–534, Berkeley, University of California Press, 1966.

51. Dariano J.A.F., Furlanetto T.W., Costa S.S., *et al.* Suprasellar germinoma: an unusual clinical presentation. Surg. Neurol., *15:*294–297, 1981.

52. Delaney P. Neurological manifestations in sarcoidosis. Ann. Intern. Med., *87:*336–345, 1977.

53. Diebler C., and Ponsot G. Hamartomas of the tuber cinereum. Neuroradiology, *25:*93–101, 1983.

54. Dinda A.K., Sarkar C., and Roy S. Rosenthal fibers: an immunohistochemical, ultrastructural and immunoelectron microscopic study. Acta. Neuropathol. (Berlin), *79:*456–460, 1990.

55. Duchen L.W. Metastatic carcinoma in the pituitary gland and hypothalamus. J. Path. Bacteriol., *91:*347–355, 1966.

56. Esposito S., and Nardi P. Lipoma of the infundibulum. J. Neurosurg., *67:*304–306, 1987.

57. Favara B.E., McCarthy R.C., and Mierau G.W. Histiocytosis X. In: *Pathology of Neoplasia in Children and Adolescents,* edited by M. Finegold, pp. 126–144, Philadelphia, W.B. Saunders, 1986.

58. Fenton L.J., and Kleinman L.I. Transient diabetes insipidus in a newborn infant. J. Pediatr., *85:*79–81, 1974.

59. Ferrer I., Garcia Back M., *et al.* Plasma cell granuloma of the hypothalamic region. Acta. Neurochir. (Wien), *99:*152–156, 1989.

60. Friede R.L. Osteolipomas of the tuber cinereum. Arch. Pathol. Lab. Med., *101:*369–372, 1977.

61. Fukushima T., Hirakawa K., Kimura M., *et al.* Intraventricular craniopharyngioma: its characteristics in magnetic resonance imaging and successful total removal. Surg. Neurol., *33:*22–27, 1990.

62. Garofalo M. Jr., Murali R., Halperin I., *et al.* Chronic lymphocytic leukemia with hypothalamic invasion. Cancer, *64:*1714–1716, 1989.

63. Gerlings P.G. Sphenoidal sinus mucocele presenting as hypophyseal tumour. Acta. Neurochir. (Wien), *61:*167–171, 1982.

64. Ghatak N.R., Hirano A., and Zimmerman H.M. Ultrastructure of a craniopharyngioma. Cancer, *27:*1465–1475, 1971.

65. Gillett G.R., and Symon L. Hypothalamic glioma. Surg. Neurol., *28:*291–300, 1987.

66. Goodman R.H., Post K.D., Molitch M.E., *et al.* Eosinophilic granuloma mimicking a pituitary tumor. Neurosurgery, *5:*723–725, 1979.

67. Graham J.M. Jr., Saunders R., Fratkin J., *et al.* A cluster of Pallister-Hall syndrome cases, (congenital hypothalamic hamartoblastoma syndrome). Am. J. Med. Genet. [suppl], *2:*53–63, 1986.

68. Graus F., Rogers L., and Posner J. Cerebrovascular complications in patients with cancer. Medicine, *64:*16–35, 1985.

69. Grote E., Lorenz R., and Vuia O. Clinical and endocrinological findings in ectopic pinealoma and spongioblastoma of the hypothalamus. Acta. Neurochir. (Wien), *53:*87–98, 1980.

70. Hall J.G., Pallister P.D., Clarren S.K., *et al.* Congenital hypothalamic hamartoblastoma, hypopituitarism, imperforate anus, and postaxial polydactyly - A new syndrome? Part I: Clinical, causal, and pathogenetic consideration. Am. J. Med. Genet., *7:*47–74, 1980.

71. Harper C.G., Doyle D., Adams J.H., *et al.* Analysis of abnormalities in pituitary gland in non-missile head injury: study of 100 consecutive cases. J. Clin. Pathol., *39:*769–773, 1986.

72. Hayek A., Driscoll S.G., and Warshaw J.B. Endocrine studies in anencephaly. J. Clin. Invest., *52:*1636–1641, 1973.

73. Heffelfinger M.J., Dahlin D.C., MacCarty C.S., *et al.* Chordomas and cartilaginous tumors at the skull base. Cancer, *32:*410–420, 1973.

74. Helle T.L., Britt R.H., and Colby T.V. Primary lymphoma of the central nervous system. Clinicopathological study of experience at Stanford. J. Neurosurg., *60:*94–103, 1984.

75. Hier D.B., and Wiehl A.C. Chronic hydrocephalus associated with short stature and growth hormone deficiency. Ann. Neurol., *2:*246–248, 1977.

76. Higinbotham N.L., Phillips R.F., Farr H.W., *et al.* Chordoma—thirty-five-year study at Memorial Hospital. Cancer, *20:*1841–1850, 1967.

77. Hiramatsu K., Takahashi K., Ikeda A., *et al.* A case of intrasellar craniopharyngioma. Tokai J. Exp. Clin. Med., *12:*135–140, 1987.

78. Hirata K., Izaki A., Tsutsumi K., *et al.* A case of primary hypothalamic malignant lymphoma with diabetes insipidus. No Shinkei Geka (English abstract), *17*:461–466, 1989.

79. Hochberg F.H., and Miller D.C. Primary central nervous system lymphoma. J. Neurosurg., *68*:835–853, 1988.

80. Hoffman H.J. Suprasellar germinomas. In: *Pediatric Neurosurgery,* pp. 487–491, Philadelphia, Grune & Stratton, 1982.

81. Hoffman H.J. Craniopharyngiomas. Prog. Exp. Tumor Res., *30*:325–334, 1987.

82. Horten B.G., Urich H., and Stefoski D. Meningiomas with conspicuous plasma cell-lymphocytic components. A report of five cases. Cancer, *43*:258–264, 1979.

83. Horvath E., and Kovacs K. The adenohypophysis. In: *Functional Endocrine Pathology,* Vol 1, edited by K. Kovacs, and S.L. Asa, pp. 245–281, Boston, Blackwell Scientific Publication, 1990.

84. Hurst R.W., McIlhenny J., Park T.S., *et al.* Neonatal craniopharyngioma: CT and ultrasonographic features. J. Comput. Assis. Tomogr., *12*:858–861, 1988.

85. Hägg E., Aström L., and Steen L. Persistent hypothalamic-pituitary insufficiency following acute meningoencephalitis. Acta. Med. Scand., *203*: 231–235, 1978.

86. Iafolla K., Fratkin J.D., Spiegel P.K., *et al.* Case report and delineation of the congenital hypothalamic hamartoblastoma syndrome (Pallister-Hall syndrome). Am. J. Med. Genet., *33*:489–499, 1989.

87. Izquierdo J.M., Sanz F., Val Bernal F., *et al.* Pinéalomes ectopiques de la région opto-chiasmatique (disgerminomes suprasellaires). Neurochirurgie, *20*:409–420, 1974.

88. Jacob L. Diabetes mellitus in normal pressure hydrocephalus. J. Neurol. Neurosurg. Psychiat., *40*:331–335, 1977.

89. Jellinger K. Primary intracranial germ cell tumours. Acta. Neuropathol. (Berl.), *25*:291–306, 1973.

90. Jennings M.T., Gelman R., and Hochberg F. Intracranial germ-cell tumors: natural history and pathogenesis. J. Neurosurg., *63*:155–167, 1985.

91. Jiddane M., Nicoli F., Diaz P., *et al.* Intracranial malignant lymphoma. Report of 30 cases and review of the literature. J. Neurosurg., *65*:592–599, 1986.

92. Johannsson J.H., Rekata H.L., and Roessmann U. Gangliogliomas: pathological and clinical correlation. J. Neurosurg., *54*:58–63, 1981.

93. Juan D., Hsu S.D., and Hunter J. Case report of vasopressin-responsive diabetes insipidus associated with chronic myelogenous leukemia. Cancer, *56*:1468–1469, 1985.

94. Judge D.M., Kulin H.E., Page R., *et al.* Hypothalamic hamartoma: a source of luteinizing hormone-releasing factor in precocious puberty. New Engl. J. Med., *296*:7–10, 1977.

95. Kahana L., Lebovitz H., Lush W., *et al.* Endocrine manifestations of intracranial extrasellar lesions. J. Clin. Endocrinol. Metab., *22*:304–324, 1962.

96. Kamalian N., Keesey R.E., and ZuRhein G.M. Lateral hypothalamic demyelination and cachexia in a case of 'malignant' multiple sclerosis. Neurology, *25*:25–30, 1975.

97. Kamel O.W., Horoupian D.S., and Silverberg G.D. Mixed gangliocytoma-adenoma: a distinct neuroendocrine tumor of the pituitary fossa. Hum. Pathol., *20*:1198–1203, 1989.

98. Kazner E., Stochdorph O., Wende S., *et al.* Intracranial lipoma. Diagnostic and therapeutic considerations. J. Neurosurg., *52*:234–245, 1980.

99. Kelemen J., and Becus T. Histopathologic changes of the human hypothalamus in systemic atherosclerosis. A clinicopathological study. Neurol. Psychiatr. (Bucur), *15*:65–72, 1977.

100. Kempe L.G. *Operative Neurosurgery. Cranial, Cerebral and Intracranial Vascular Disease.* Vol 1, pp. 90–93, New York, Springer-Verlag, 1968.

101. Kepes J.J. *Meningiomas: Biology, Pathology, and Differential Diagnosis,* 1st ed., pp. 116–149, New York, Masson Publishing, 1982.

102. Kewitz G., Girard J., Probst A., *et al.* Septo-optic pituitary dysplasia. Helv. Paediat. Acta., *39*:355–364, 1984.

103. Kiyono H. Die histopathologie der hypophyse. Virchows Arch [A], *259*:388–465, 1926.

104. Kornblum R.N., and Fisher R.S. Pituitary lesions in craniocerebral injuries. Arch. Pathol., *88*:242–248, 1969.

105. Kupari M., Pelkonen R., and Valtonen V. Post-encephalitic hypothalamic-pituitary insufficiency. Acta Endocrinol. (Copenh.), *94*:433–438, 1980.

106. Laakso W.B. Diabetes insipidus secondary to acute leukemia: a case report. Am. J. Med. Sci., *247*:451–456, 1964.

107. Langston J.W., and Forno L.S. The hypothalamus in Parkinson disease. Ann. Neurol., *3*:129–133, 1978.

108. Larroche J.C. Malformations of the nervous system. In: *Greenfield's Neuropathology,* edited by W. Blackwood and J.A. Carselis, pp. 385–450, London, Edward Arnold, 1976.

109. Larvton F.G., Beardwell C.G., Shalet S.M., *et al.* Hypothalamic-pituitary disease as the sole manifestation of sarcoidosis. Postgrad. Med. J., *58*:771–772, 1982.

110. Laster D.W., Moody D.M., and Ball M.R. Epidermoid tumors with intraventricular and subarachnoid fat: report of two cases. A.J.R., *128*:504–507, 1977.

111. Laws E.R., Jr. Cranial chordomas. In: *Neurosurgery,* Vol 1, edited by R.H. Wilkins, and S.S. Rengachary, pp. 927–930, New York, McGraw-Hill, 1985.

112. Lederman G.S., Recht A., Leoffler J.S., *et al.* Craniopharyngioma in an elderly patient. Cancer, *60*:1077–1080, 1987.

113. Legido A., Packer R.J., Sutton L.N., *et al.* Suprasellar germinomas in childhood. A reappraisal. Cancer, *63*:340–344, 1989.

114. Lerama O.B., and Char G. Intrasellar abscess simulating a pituitary tumour. W. Indian Med. J., *38*:171–175, 1989.

115. Lewis A.J., Cooper P.W., Kassel E.E., *et al.* Squamous cell carcinoma arising in a suprasellar epidermoid cyst: case report. J. Neurosurg., *59*:538–541, 1983.

116. Li J.Y., Racadot O., Kujas K., *et al.* Immunocytochemistry of four mixed pituitary adenomas and intrasellar gangliocytomas associated with different clinical syndromes: acromegaly, amenorrheagalactorrhea, Cushing's disease and isolated tumoral syndrome. Acta Neuropathol. (Berl.), *77*:320–328, 1989.

117. Lichtenstein L. Histiocytosis X. Integration of eosinophilic granuloma of bone, Letterer Siwe disease and Schüller Christian disease as related manifestations of a single nosologic entity. Arch. Pathol., *56*:84–102, 1953.

118. Lin S.R., Bryson M.M., Gobien R.P., *et al.* Neuroradiologic study of hamartomas of the tuber cinereum and hypothalamus. Neuroradiology, *16*:17–19, 1978.

119. Lipsett M.B., Dreifuss F.E., and Thomas L.B. Hypothalamic syndrome following varicella. Am. J. Med., *32*:471–475, 1962.

120. Liss L., and Kahn E.A. Pituicytoma. Tumor of the sella turcica. A clinicopathological study. J. Neurosurg., *15*:481–488, 1958.

121. List C.F., Dowmann C.E., Bagchi B.K., *et al.* Posterior hypothalamic hamartomas and gangliogliomas causing precocious puberty. Neurology, *8*:164–174, 1958.

122. Liszczak T., Richardson E.P., Phillips J.P., *et al.* Morphological, biochemical, ultrastructural, tissue culture and clinical observations of typical and aggressive craniopharyngiomas. Acta Neuropathol. (Berl.), *43*:191–203, 1978.

123. MaCarty C.S., Leavens M.E., Love J.G., *et al.* Dermoid and epidermoid tumors in the central nervous system of adults. Surg. Gynecol. Obstet., *108*:191–198, 1959.

124. Mackintosh F.R., Colby T.V., Podolsky W.J., *et al.* Central nervous system involvement in non-Hodgkin's lymphoma: an analysis of 105 cases. Cancer, *49*:586–595, 1982.

125. Mancardi G.L., and Mandybur T.I. Solitary intracranial plasmacytoma. Cancer, *51*:2226–2233, 1983.

126. Markin R.S., Leibrock L.G., Huseman C.A., *et al.* Hypothalamic hamartoma: a report of 2 cases. Pediat. Neurosci., *13*:19–26, 1987.

127. Maroon J.C., and Albright L. "Failure to thrive" due to pontine glioma. Arch. Neurol., *34*:295–297, 1977.

128. Mathews W., and Wilson C.B. Ectopic intrasellar chordoma. J. Neurosurg., *39*:260–263, 1974.

129. Matson D.D. *Neurosurgery of Infancy and Childhood.* 2nd ed. pp. 544–574, Springfield, Charles C. Thomas, 1969.

130. Matustik M.C., Eisenberg H.M., and Meyer W.J. Gelastic (laughing) seizures and precocious puberty. Am. J. Dis. Child., *135*:837–838, 1981.

131. Michael A.S., and Paige M.L. MR imaging of intrasellar meningiomas simulating pituitary adenomas. J. Comput. Assist. Tomogr., *12*:944–946, 1988.

132. Miller V.I., and Campbell W.G. Jr. Diabetes insipidus as a complication of leukemia: a case report with a literature review. Cancer, *28*:666–673, 1971.

133. Milligan S.A., Katz M.S., Craven P.C., *et al.* Toxoplasmosis presenting as panhypopituitarism in a patient with the acquired immune deficiency syndrome. Am. J. Med., *77*:760–764, 1984.

134. Mishra S.K. Thrombotic thrombocytopenic purpura. Semin. Neurol., *5*:317–320, 1985.

135. Mohr P.D. Hypothalamic-pituitary abscess. Postgrad. Med. J., *51*:468–471, 1975.

136. Mori K., Handa H., Moritake K., *et al.* Suprasellar epidermoid. Neurochirurgia (Stuttg.), *25*:138–142, 1982.

137. Morishima A., and Aranoff G.S. Syndrome of septo-optic-pituitary dysplasia: the clinical spectrum. Brain Dev., *8*:233–239, 1986.

138. Mostofi F.K. Pathology of germ cell tumors of testis. A progress report. Cancer, *45*:1735–1754, 1980.

139. Namba S., Nishimoto A., and Yagyu Y. Diencephalic syndrome of emaciation (Russell's syndrome). Long-term survival. Surg. Neurol., *23*:581–588, 1985.

140. Navia B.A., Petito C.K., Gold J.W.M., *et al.* Cerebral toxoplasmosis complicating the acquired immune deficiency syndrome: clinical and neuropathological findings in 27 patients. Ann. Neurol., *19*:224–238, 1986.

141. Nelson G.A., Bastian F.O., Schlitt M., *et al.* Malignant transformation in craniopharyngioma. Neurosurgery, *22*:427–429, 1988.

142. Netsky M.G. Epidermoid tumors. Review of the literature. Surg. Neurol., *29*:477–483, 1988.

143. Nishio S., Takei Y., and Fukui M. Immunoreactivity with hypothalamic neuropeptides in neuronal neoplasms of the central nervous system. Neurol. Med. Chir. (Tokyo), *27*:105–109, 1987.

144. Nishio S., Mizuno J., Barrow D.L., *et al.* Isolated histiocytosis X of the pituitary gland: case report. Neurosurgery, *21*:718–721, 1987.

145. Nishio S., Takeshita I., Fukui M., *et al.* Anaplastic evolution of childhood optico-hypothalamic pilocytic astrocytoma: report of an autopsy case. Clin. Neuropathol., *7*:245–258, 1988.

146. Nishio S., Fujiwara S., Aiko Y., *et al.* Hypothalamic hamartoma. J. Neurosurg., *70*:640–645, 1989.

147. Ober K.P., Alexander E. Jr., Challa V.R., *et al.* Histiocytosis X of the hypothalamus. Neurosurgery, *24*:93–95, 1989.

148. Oishi M., Iida T., Koide M., *et al.* Primary intrasellar microgerminoma detected by magnetic resonance imaging: case report. Neurosurgery, *25*:457–462, 1989.

149. Oka K., Yamashita M., Sadoshima S., *et al.* Cerebral haemorrhage in moyamoya disease at autopsy. Virchows Arch. [A], *392*:247–261, 1981.

150. Olivecrona H. On suprasellar cholesteatomas. Brain, *55*:122–134, 1932.

151. Osamura R.A. Functional prenatal development of anencephalic and normal anterior pituitary glands in human and experimental animals stud-

ied by peroxidase-labeled antibody method. Acta. Pathol. Jpn., *27*:495–509, 1977.

152. Ozgen T., Bertan V., Kansu T., *et al.* Intrasellar hydatid cyst: case report. J. Neurosurg., *60*:647–648, 1984.

153. Pai K.G., Rubin H.M., Wedemeyer P.P., *et al.* Hypothalamic-pituitary dysfunction following group B beta hemolytic streptococcal meningitis in a neonate. J. Pediatr., *88*:289–291, 1976.

154. Pardo-Mindan F.J., Guillen F.J., and Villas C. A comparative ultrastructure study of chondrosarcoma, chordoid sarcoma, and chordoma. Cancer, *47*:2611–2619, 1981.

155. Pentland B., Douglas-Mitchell J., Cull R.E., *et al.* Central nervous system sarcoidosis. Q. J. Med., *56*:457–465, 1985.

156. Peters F.T.M., Keuning J.J., and DeRooy H.A.M. Primary cerebral malignant lymphoma with endocrine defect. Case report and review of the literature. Neth. J. Med., *29*:406–410, 1986.

157. Pierre-Kahn A., Capelle L., Brauner R., *et al.* Presentation and management of suprasellar arachnoid cysts, review of 20 cases. J. Neurosurg., *73*:355–359, 1990.

158. Posener L., Mitchener J.W., and Skwarok E.W. Infundibuloma: a case report with a brief review of the literature. J. Neurosurg., *14*:680–684, 1957.

159. Price R.A., Lee P.A., Albright L., *et al.* Treatment of sexual precocity by removal of a luteinizing hormone-releasing hormone secreting hamartoma. J.A.M.A., *251*:2247–2249, 1984.

160. Puolakka K., Korhonen T., and Lahtinen R. Diabetes insipidus in preleukaemic phase of acute myeloid leukemia in 2 patients with empty sella turcica. Scand. J. Haematol., *32*:364–366, 1984.

161. Rafael H., and Gómez-Llata S. Intrasellar cysticercosis: case report. J. Neurosurg., *63*:975–976, 1985.

162. Raffel C., Wright D.C., Gutin P.H., *et al.* Cranial chordomas: clinical presentation and results of operative and radiation therapy in twenty-six patients. Neurosurgery, *17*:703–710, 1985.

163. Raymond L.A., and Tew J. Large suprasellar aneurysms imitating pituitary tumour. J. Neurol. Neurosurg. Psychiat., *41*:83–87, 1978.

164. Reddy E.R., Mansfield C.M., and Hartman G.V. Chordoma. Int. J. Radiation Oncol. Biol. Phys., *7*:1709–1711, 1981.

165. Reeves A.G., and Plum F. Hyperphagia, rage and dementia accompanying a ventromedial hypothalamic neoplasm. Arch. Neurol., *20*:616–624, 1969.

166. Reuler J.B., Girard D.E., and Cooney T.G. Current concepts. Wernicke's encephalopathy. N. Engl. J. Med., *312*:1035–1039, 1985.

167. Rhodes R.B., Dusseau J.J., Boyd A.S., *et al.* Intrasellar neuraladenohypophyseal choristoma. A morphological and immunocytochemical study. J. Neuropathol. Exp. Neurol., *41*:267–280, 1982.

168. Rhodes R.H., Davis R.L., Beamer Y.B., *et al.* A suprasellar epidermoid cyst with symptoms of hypothalamic involvement: case report and a review of pathogenetic mechanisms. Bull. Los Angeles Neurol. Soc., *46*:26–32, 1981.

169. Rich T.A., Schiller A., Suit H.D., *et al.* Clinical and pathologic review of 48 cases of chordoma. Cancer, *56*:182–187, 1985.

170. Richter P.B. True hamartoma of the hypothalamus associated with pubertas praecox. J. Neuropathol. Exp. Neurol., *10*:368–383, 1951.

171. Rodriguez L.A., Edwards M.S.B., and Levin V.A. Management of hypothalamic gliomas in children: an analysis of 33 cases. Neurosurgery, *26*:242–247, 1990.

172. Rossi M.L., Bevan J.S., Esiri M.M., *et al.* Pituicytoma (pilocytic astrocytoma). J. Neurosurg., *67*:768–772, 1987.

173. Rubin G., Scienza R., Pasqualin A., *et al.* Craniocerebral epidermoids and dermoids. A review of 44 cases. Acta Neurochir. (Wien), *97*:1–16, 1989.

174. Rubin P., and Kramer S. Ectopic pinealoma: a radiocurable neuroendocrinologic entity. Radiology, *85*:512–523, 1965.

175. Rudelli R., and Deck J.H.N. Selective traumatic infarction of the human anterior hypothalamus. J. Neurosurg., *50*:645–654, 1979.

176. Rueda-Pedraza M.E., Heifetz S.A., Sesterhenn I.A., *et al.* Primary intracranial germ cell tumors in the first two decades of life: a clinical, light-microscopic, and immunohistochemical analysis of 54 cases. Perspect. Pediatr. Pathol., *10*:160–207, 1987.

177. Russell A. A diencephalic syndrome of emaciation in infancy and childhood. Arch. Dis. Child., *26*:274–280, 1951.

178. Russell D.S., and Rubinstein L.J. *Pathology of Tumours of the Nervous System.* Fifth ed., pp. 1–1012, London, Edward Arnold, 1989.

179. Russell J.D., and Wise P.H. Vascular malformation of hypothalamus: a case of isolated growth hormone deficiency. Pediatrics, *66*:306–309, 1980.

180. Russell R.W.R., and Pennybacker J.B. Craniopharyngioma in the elderly. J. Neurol. Neurosurg. Psychiat., *24*:1–13, 1961.

181. Sandyk R., Iacono R.P., and Bamford C.R. The hypothalamus in Parkinson's disease. Ital. J. Neurol. Sci., *8*:227–234, 1987.

182. Sarwar M., Batniktzky S., and Schechter M.M. Tumorous aneurysms. Neuroradiology, *12*:79–97, 1976.

183. Sawhny B.S., and Dohn D.F. Neuroendocrinological aspects of histiocytosis X of the central nervous system. Surg. Neurol., *14*:237–239, 1980.

184. Scanarini M., d'Avella D., Rotilio A., *et al.* Giant-cell granulomatous hypophysitis: a distinct clinicopathological entity. J. Neurosurg., *71*:681–686, 1989.

185. Scheithauer B.W., Kovacs K., Randall R.V., *et al.* Hypothalamic neuronal hamartoma and adenohypophyseal neuronal choristoma: their association with growth hormone adenoma of the pituitary gland. J. Neuropathol. Exp. Neurol., *42*:64, 1983.

186. Scheithauer B.W., and Bruner J.M. The ultrastructural spectrum of astrocytic neoplasms. Ultrastruct. Pathol., *11*:535–581, 1987.

187. Scheithauer B.W. The hypothalamus and neurohypophysis. In: *Functional Endocrine Pathology,* Vol 1, edited by K. Kovacs and S.L. Asa, pp. 170–244, Boston, Blackwell Scientific Publications, 1990.

188. Scothorne C.M. A glioma of the posterior lobe of the pituitary gland. J. Pathol. Bacteriol., *69:*109–112, 1955.

189. Scully R.E., Mark E.J., and McNeely B.U. Case records of the Massachusetts general hospital. Case 31–1982. N. Engl. J. Med., *307:*359–368, 1982.

190. Sharma R.R. Hamartoma of the hypothalamus and tuber cinereum: a brief review of the literature. J. Postgrad. Med., *33:*1–13, 1987.

191. Sheehan H.L., and Whitehead R. The neurohypophysis in post-partum hypopituitarism. J. Pathol. Bacteriol., *85:*145–169, 1963.

192. Sheehan H.L., and Kovacs K., Neurohypophysis and hypothalamus. In: *Endocrine Pathology, General and Surgical,* edited by J.M.B. Bloodworth Jr., pp. 45–99, Baltimore, Williams & Wilkins, 1982.

193. Sherman B.M., Gorden P.H., and DiChiro G. Postmeningitic selective hypopituitarism with suprasellar calcification. Arch. Intern. Med., *128:*600–604, 1971.

194. Sherwin R.P., Grassi J.E., and Sommers S.C. Hamartomatous malformations of the posterolateral hypothalamus. Lab. Invest., *11:*89–97, 1962.

195. Shokry A., Janzer R.C., Von Hochstetter A.R., et al. Primary intracranial germ-cell tumors. A clinico-pathological study of 14 cases. J. Neurosurg., *62:*826–830, 1985.

196. Sims D.G. Histiocytosis X. Follow-up of 43 cases. Arch. Dis. Child., *52:*433–440, 1977.

197. Simson L.R., Lampe I., and Abell M.R. Suprasellar germinomas. Cancer, *22:*533–544, 1968.

198. Sirikulchayanonta V., and Sriurairatna S. Ultrastructure of chordoma. A case report. Acta. Pathol. Jpn., *35:*1233–1239, 1985.

199. Solero G.L., Giombini S., and Morello G. Suprasellar and olfactory meningiomas. Report on a series of 153 personal cases. Acta. Neurochir. (Wien), *67:*181–194, 1983.

200. Stern B.J., Krumholz A., Johns C., et al. Sarcoidosis and its neurological manifestations. Arch. Neurol., *42:*909–917, 1985.

201. Stone W.M., Toledo J.D., and Romanul F.C.A. Horner's syndrome due to hypothalamic infarction. Clinical, radiological, and pathological correlations. Arch. Neurol., *43:*199–200, 1986.

202. Stuart C.A., Neelson F.A., and Lebovitz H.E. Disordered control of thirst in hypothalamic-pituitary sarcoidosis. N. Engl. J. Med., *303:*1078–1082, 1980.

203. Stuart C.A., Nulon E.A., and Lebovitz H.E. Hypothalamic insufficiency: the cause of hypopituitarism in sarcoidosis. Ann. Intern. Med., *88:*589–593, 1978.

204. Sung J.H., Hayano M., Mastri A.R., et al. A case of human rabies and ultrastructure of the Negri body. J. Neuropathol. Exp. Neurol., *35:*541–559, 1976.

205. Sweet W.H. Recurrent craniopharyngioma: therapeutic alternatives. Clin. Neurosurg., *27:*206–229, 1980.

206. Symon L., Pell M., Yasargil M.G., et al. Surgical techniques in the management of colloid cysts of the third ventricle. Adv. Tech. Stand. Neurosurg., *17:*121–157, 1990.

207. Tenny R.T., Laws E.R., Younge B.R., et al. The neurosurgical management of optic glioma. Results in 104 patients. J. Neurosurg., *57:*452–458, 1982.

208. The committee of the Brain Tumor Registry in Japan: Brain tumor registry in Japan. Shinkei Kenkyu No Shinpo, *22:*5–14, 1978.

209. Treip C.S. Hypothalamic and pituitary injury. J. Clin. Pathol., *23*(Suppl 4):178–186, 1970.

210. Treip C.S. The hypothalamus and pituitary gland. In: *Greenfield's Neuropathology,* vol. 1, edited by W. Blackwood, and J.A. Carselis, Lp. 170–244, London, Edward Arnold, 1976.

211. Trombley I.K., Mirra S.S., and Miles M.L. An electron microscopic study of central nervous system sarcoidosis. Ultrastruct. Pathol., *2:*257–267, 1981.

212. Turkington R.W., and Macindae J.H. Hyperprolactinemia in sarcoidosis. Ann. Intern. Med., *76:*545–549, 1972.

213. Urbanski S.J., Bilbao J.M., Horvath E., et al. Intrasellar solitary plasmacytoma terminating in multiple myeloma. A report of a case including electron microscopical study. Surg. Neurol., *14:*233–236, 1980.

214. Vaquero J., Carrillo R., Oya S., et al. Precocious puberty and hypothalamic hamartoma. Report on a new case with ultrastructural data. Acta. Neurochir. (Wien), *74:*129–133, 1985.

215. Waga S., Shimizu T., and Sakakura M. Diencephalic syndrome of emaciation (Russell's syndrome). Surg. Neurol., *17:*141–146, 1982.

216. Wara W.M., Jenkin D.T., Evans A., et al. Tumors of the pineal and suprasellar region: children's cancer study group treatment results 1960–1975. A report from children's cancer study group. Cancer, *43:*698–701, 1979.

217. White J.C. Aneurysms mistaken for hypophyseal tumors. Clin. Neurosurg., *10:*224–250, 1964.

218. Winnacker J.L., Bechen K.L., and Katz S. Endocrine aspects of sarcoidosis. N. Engl. J. Med., *278:*483–493, 1968.

219. Winter J.S.D., Taraska S., and Faiman C. The hormonal response to HCG stimulation in male children and adolescents. J. Clin. Endocrinol. Metab., *34:*348–353, 1972.

220. Wood M.W., White R.J., and Kernohan J.W. One hundred intracranial meningiomas found incidentally at necropsy. J. Neuropathol. Exp. Neurol., *16:*337–340, 1957.

221. Yamada S., Aiba T., Shishiba Y., et al. CT and MR appearance of multiple intracranial lesions associated with suprasellar dermoid cyst. Radiat. Med., *7:*261–264, 1989.

222. Yamada S., Stefaneanu L., Kovacs K., et al. Intrasellar gangliocytoma with multiple immunoreactivities. Endocr. Pathol., *1:*58–63, 1990.

223. Yasargil M.G., Abernathy C.D., and Sarioglu A.C. Microneurosurgical treatment of intracranial dermoid and epidermoid tumors. Neurosurgery, *24:*561–567, 1989.

224. Yasargil Y.G., Curcic M., Kis M., *et al.* Total removal of craniopharyngiomas. Approaches and long-term results in 144 patients. J. Neurosurg., *73:*3–11, 1990.

225. Zúñiga O.F., Tanner S.M., Wild W.O., *et al.* Hamartoma of CNS associated with precocious puberty. Am. J. Dis. Child., *137:*127–133, 1983.

CHAPTER 15

Neuropathology of the Pituitary

SHOZO YAMADA, M.D., Ph.D., and TOSHIAKI SANO, M.D., Ph.D.

The sella turcica contains many different kinds of tissues in close proximity that can give rise to a great variety of tumors and tumorlike conditions, which are listed in Table 15.1.

The majority of the tumors of the sella turcica are pituitary adenomas, which are histologically benign tumors derived from adenohypophyseal cells, and many of the other lesions affecting this region are quite rare. Some of them are of considerable clinical significance, whereas others are only incidental autopsy findings. This chapter focuses on the pathology of diseases that are unique to the sella turcica, since the histological features of lesions also occurring in other regions are basically identical in all locations. In addition, certain conditions that were described in Chapter 14 have also been excluded from this chapter, as have certain anomalies and circulatory disorders that are reviewed in Chapter 16.

PITUITARY ADENOMAS

Pituitary adenomas are benign tumors consisting of and arising from adenohypophyseal cells. They account for approximately 10% of intracranial tumors and are found to be present in 2.7% to 27% of unselected routine adult autopsies (35, 73, 216, 322). These tumors occur in both sexes and affect all age groups. They vary in size, growth rate, clinical symptoms, endocrine function, radiological findings, cellular composition, and morphological features.

Pituitary adenomas grow either by expansion or invasion and the pattern of growth is not necessarily related to the size of the tumors. Most of these lesions are histologically benign, grow slowly, and remain confined to the sella turcica. They usually have distinct borders, but are not truly encapsulated by a fibrous capsule and are, instead, surrounded by a "pseudocapsule" consisting of compressed adenohypophyseal cells and the condensed reticulin fibers of the adjacent nontumorous anterior lobe. The interface with the surrounding dura is also usually discrete. In contrast, some adenomas have a more rapid growth rate despite their fundamentally benign character and can reach a considerable size. Such tumors tend to invade the surrounding tissues, damage the cranial nerves, and spread outside the sella turcica, thus producing symptoms of local compression such as visual disturbance, headache, and various degrees of hypopituitarism.

Pituitary adenomas can be classified in various ways, including, according to their size, radiological appearance, endocrine function, morphology, and cytogenesis. The classification of pituitary adenomas on the basis of their morphological features has undergone substantial changes. Traditionally, they were categorized by their staining properties into acidophilic, basophilic, and chromophobic adenomas. Although simple, this classification was of limited usefulness, because it failed to consider hormone production, structure–function relationships, and tumor cytogenesis. For instance, acidophilic adenomas were once thought to secrete growth hormone in excess and to be associated with gigantism and/or acromegaly, but it is now known that they can also pro-

TABLE 15.1.
Tumors and Tumorlike Lesions in the Sella Turcica

Tumors arised from adenohypophyseal cells
  Pituitary adenoma
  Pituitary carcinoma
Other primary tumors
  Angioma and angiosarcoma
  Chordoma
  Craniopharyngioma
  Fibroma and fibrosarcoma
  Glioma
  Granular cell tumor
  Germinoma (ectopic pinealoma)
  Meningioma
  Neuronal tumor
  Sarcoma
  Teratoma
Metastatic tumor
  Carcinoma
  Sarcoma, leukemia, lymphoma, melanoma
Tumorlike conditions
  Inflammatory
    Infectious
    Lymphocytic adenohypophysitis
    Sarcoidosis, histiocytosis X, Giant cell granuloma
  Metabolic
    Amyloidosis
    Hemochromatosis
    Mucopolysaccharidosis
  Vascular
    Giant aneurysm
  Other
    Rathke's cleft cyst
    Empty sella syndrome

duce prolactin or may even be endocrinologically nonfunctioning.

Advances in methodology, especially the introduction of immunohistochemical techniques and electron microscopy, have contributed much new information regarding the functional behavior of pituitary adenomas, and have led to a new classification based on hormone content, cellular composition, ultrastructural features, and cytogenesis (90, 102, 106, 134). This new classification system is summarized in Table 15.2. Moreover, the recent application of sophisticated methods, including immunoelectron microscopy (24), tissue culture (9), reverse hemolytic plaque assay (314), and hybridization histochemistry (162), as well as the application of nonhormonal immunohistochemical markers (316), has provided further important data and has opened up various avenues towards the better understanding of the structure–function correlations of these tumors.

In the following pages, some details of the morphological aspects of pituitary adenomas are described with respect to their cellular derivation and their clinical correlations.

Growth Hormone (GH) Cell Adenomas

GH-cell adenomas arise from and consist of GH-cells and are accompanied clinically by gigantism and/or acromegaly (135, 191). Light microscopy shows such tumors to be acidophilic or chromophobic as well as PAS-negative (102, 106, 134). Electron microscopy reveals two morphologically distinct subtypes, which are the densely-granulated and the sparsely-granulated GH-cell adenoma (102, 106, 133–135, 191). These variants occur with approximately equal frequency, but about 10% of tumors show a mixture of both cell types (259).

Densely-granulated GH-cell adenomas are composed of adenomatous GH cells that are similar to normal GH cells (Fig. 15.1). They are acidophilic by conventional stain-

TABLE 15.2.
Classification of Pituitary Adenomas

Tumor type	Incidence (%)[a]	
Growth-hormone (GH) cell adenoma	14.0	
densely-granulated		6.7
sparsely-granulated		7.3
Prolactin- (PRL) cell adenoma	27.2	
GH-PRL-cell adenoma	8.4	
Mixed GH-cell-PRL-cell adenoma		4.8
Mammosomatotroph-cell adenoma		1.4
Acidophil stem-cell adenoma		2.2
Corticotroph-cell adenoma	8.1	
Thyrotroph-cell adenoma	1.0[b]	
Gonadotroph-cell adenoma	6.4[c]	
Clinically-nonfunctioning adenoma	31.2	
Silent somatotroph-cell adenoma		Very rare
Silent corticocotroph-cell adenoma		6.0[d]
subtype-1 silent adenoma		
subtype-2 silent adenoma		
Silent thyrotroph-cell adenoma		
Silent gonadotroph-cell adenoma		
Silent subtype-3 adenoma		
Null-cell adenoma		16.3
Oncocytoma		8.9
Unclassified plurihormonal adenoma	3.7	

[a]Cited from Ref. No 103
[b]Including silent thyrotroph cell adenoma
[c]Including silent gonadotroph cell adenoma
[d]Including silent subtype 3 adenoma

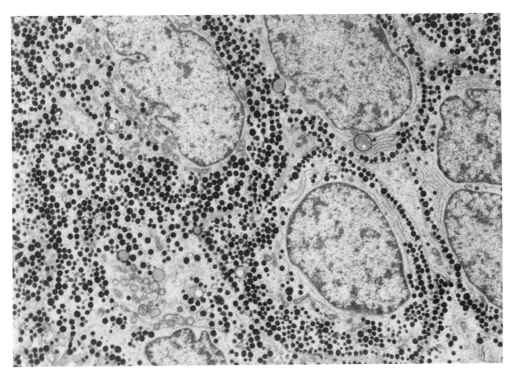

Figure 15. 1.   Electron micrograph of a densely granulated GH-cell adenoma. The tumor consists of closely-apposed middle-sized cells, with spherical or slightly irregular nuclei. The cytoplasm is well differentiated and contains numerous secretory granules, ×6000.

ing methods and have a trabecular, sinusoidal, or diffuse histological appearance. This type of adenoma shows strong GH immunopositivity of the entire cytoplasm by the avidin–biotin–peroxidase complex (ABC) method (78, 79, 130). Many of these adenomas also show scattered immunopositivity for prolactin (Prl) (16) and one or more of the glycoprotein hormones, or especially for the α-subunit of such glycoprotein hormones (156, 214, 231). Electron microscopy demonstrates that densely-granulated GH-cell adenomas consist of cells characterized by well–developed rough endoplasmic reticulum (RER), prominent Golgi complexes, and numerous even, spherical, electron-dense secretory granules ranging from between 150 and 600 nm in diameter, with the majority being from 400 to 500 nm (90, 102, 106, 134, 146, 259, 292).

Sparsely-granulated GH-cell adenomas are chromophobic or slightly acidophilic and exhibit a diffuse histological pattern. By the ABC method, immunopositivity for GH is

evident in the cytoplasm in the form of streaks, crescents, or ring-like structures (130), but it is generally not as prominent as in the densely-granulated adenomas. The ultrastructural features of sparsely-granulated GH-cell adenomas show no resemblance to those of normal GH cells (Fig. 15.2) (90, 102, 106, 134, 146, 259, 292). They have irregular nuclei, widely dispersed RER, tubular smooth endoplasmic reticulum (SER), conspicuous Golgi complexes, several centrioles and cilia, and also possess fibrous bodies. The fibrous bodies consist of spherically-arranged type-2 filaments and are the most conspicuous morphologic marker of this type of adenoma (36, 92, 267). They can be identified as structures that are positive for cytokeratin by conventional immunohistochemical methods (Fig. 15.3) (156, 190, 205).

As associated features, endocrine amyloid deposits (153, 193) and tubuloreticular inclusions (102, 106, 134, 147) are commonly noted in both types of GH-cell adenoma. Moreover, scattered acidophil stem cells

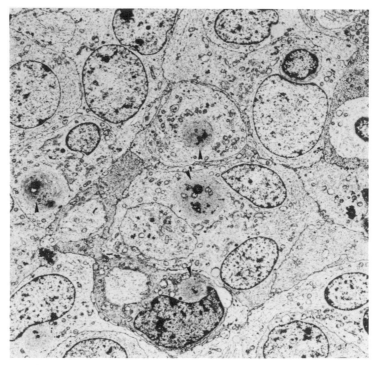

Figure 15.2. Electron micrograph of a sparsely-granulated GH-cell adenoma. The secretory granules are small and scarce. Note the high frequency of fibrous bodies (arrowheads) ×3600.

(134) or mammosomatotroph cells (163, 236) can also be found in some of these adenomas.

Such tumor-cell heterogeneity may suggest different phases of differentiation of the adenoma cells or, alternatively, a multiclonal derivation for such adenomas. In adenomas with heterogeneous cell populations, the diagnosis has to be determined from the predominant cell type.

Both types of GH-cell adenomas are regarded as variants of the same tumor (133) and they do not differ in endocrine function, so there is no correlation between adenoma type and the serum GH level or effect of GHRH in vitro (119, 134, 292). However, from the clinical standpoint, the separation of these two variants is important, since their prognosis is different. Densely-granulated GH-cell adenomas are usually slowly expanding tumors that remain confined to the sella for a long time and have a high surgical cure rate. In contrast, sparsely-granulated GH-cell adenomas usually present at an earlier age, have a faster growth rate, are more likely to be invasive tumors or macroadenomas (with or without associated visual disturbance), and have a lower surgical cure rate (134, 234, 275). Postoperative irradiation may, therefore, be indicated for the patients with sparsely-granulated GH-cell adenomas if the initial surgery is unsuccessful.

Bromocriptine, a dopaminergic agonist, and SMS 201-995, a long-acting somatostatin analogue, have both been used to reduce serum GH levels and the size of such tumors (86, 191, 220). Such medical treatment may result in significant morphological changes of these tumors. The only conspicuous change noted in GH adenoma cells treated with bromocriptine is an increase of lysosomes (102, 103, 212), while morphometric analysis (a precise and quantitative method of demonstrating minute changes in cellular components) has shown that the number and size of the secretory granules is greater in SMS 201–995–treated tumors than in untreated tumors (68, 154). However, in the majority of tumors treated with SMS 201-995 no morphological alterations can be found (20). Thus, it seems likely that both these agents act on GH adenoma cells at a post-translational level due to inhibition of the secretory process, rather than via the direct suppression of hormone synthesis.

Prolactin- (Prl) Cell Adenomas

Prl-cell adenomas are associated with hyperprolactinemia, which is manifested clinically as amenorrhea or galactorrhea in women and as decreased libido, impotence, and oligospermia in men. In other cases, especially in postmenopausal women and in some men, Prl-cell adenomas may not be associated with any specific clinical signs and symptoms, leading to delays in their diagnosis and treatment (113).

These adenomas are also either densely granulated or sparsely granulated. Unlike GH-cell adenomas, no correlation exists between the secretory granule density and either the serum Prl level or the clinical characteristics (178). It is well known that some

Prl-cell adenomas never become macroadenomas, while others rapidly undergo suprasellar extension or invade adjacent tissues (265). Such differences in the biological behavior of these tumors are not reflected in their known morphological features, and further studies are needed to determine which findings can actually predict the growth rate of Prl-cell adenomas.

Densely-granulated Prl-cell adenomas are very rare; they are acidophilic by conventional staining, have a trabecular pattern, and show strong diffuse cytoplasmic immunopositivity for Prl (100, 134). Electron microscopy shows that the ultrastructural features of these densely-granulated Prl cells have a considerable resemblance to those of densely-granulated GH adenoma cells. They possess well–developed RER, have prominent Golgi complexes containing immature secretory granules, and also have numerous spherical, oval, or irregular secretory granules of up to 600–700 nm in diameter. Some

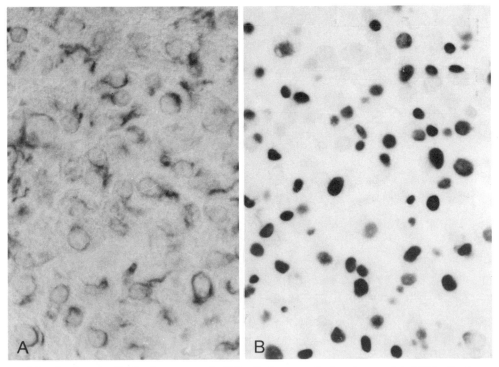

Figure 15.3. Cytokeratin distribution patterns in GH-cell adenomas. In densely-granulated GH-cell adenoma, cytokeratin immunoreactivity is demonstrated in the perinuclear zone (A), while in sparsely-granulated GH-cell adenoma, it exhibits as a spherical mass that is identical to a fibrous body defined by electron microscopic observation (B) ×1000.

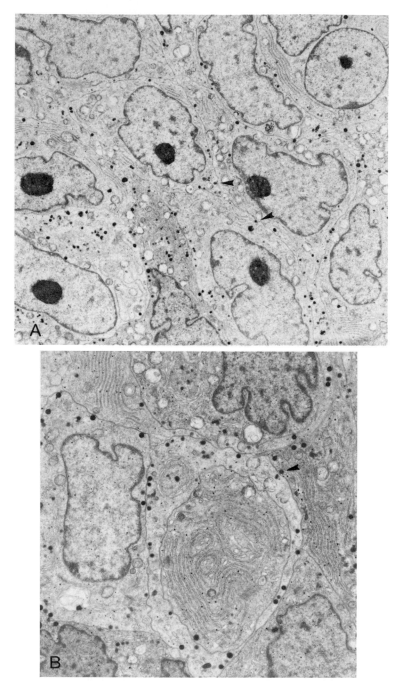

Figure 15.4. Electron micrographs of a sparsely-granulated Prl-cell adenoma. The cells contain oval or irregular nuclei with light chromatin substance and marked dark nucleoli. The abundant cytoplasm possesses well-developed RER and Golgi apparatus (A) ×4500. Extensively developed RER and large Golgi apparatus harboring secretory granules are well shown in this case (B). In both cases, secretory granules are scarce and granule extrusions are found (arrowheads) ×6600.

of these secretory granules undergo misplaced exocytosis (134, 146, 149). Sparsely-granulated Prl-cell adenomas are far more common and are actually the most frequent tumor arising in the human pituitary (102, 134). Histologically, this type of adenoma is chromophobic or slightly acidophilic, with erythrosin and carmoisin staining usually revealing a few small secretory granules in the cytoplasm of the adenoma cells. Immunohistochemistry is of fundamental importance in the diagnosis of this type of tumor, since Prl immunostaining is strong in the Golgi sacculi despite the paucity of secretory granules. The areas of immunopositivity are ring–like, crescent–shaped, or streaked (55, 100, 102, 116, 134, 190, 244, 259). This characteristic "Golgi pattern" seems to be restricted to these adenoma cells and has not been observed in other adenohypophyseal cells. The ultrastructural features are similar to those of stimulated nontumorous Prl cells and include conspicious RER, which often forms whorls, termed Nebenkerns; prominent Golgi complexes; and sparsely distributed spherical, oval, or irregularly shaped, evenly electron–dense secretory granules of 150–

300 nm in diameter (Fig. 15.4). A characteristic ultrastructural marker of Prl-cell adenomas is the presence of misplaced exocytosis, which means the extrusion of secretory granules through the lateral cell membranes. The frequency of such granule extrusion varies from tumor to tumor and even from cell to cell within a single lesion (55, 100, 102, 116, 134, 146, 197, 245, 259).

Calcification and endocrine amyloid deposition are seen in some Prl-cell adenomas (Fig. 15.5) (28, 148, 196, 233, 301). In rare cases, the calcification may be so extensive that it produces a "pituitary stone" that can be recognized by radiological studies (228). Such changes are most frequently associated with this type of adenoma, but they are not pathognomonic and may also be found in other types of adenoma. It is still unknown why these changes more frequently accompany Prl-cell adenomas.

Bromocriptine is a dopaminergic agonist that has been used extensively for the treatment of Prl-cell adenomas. It is now well established that the administration of this drug can rapidly decrease the serum Prl level (288) and can cause a dramatic reduction in the

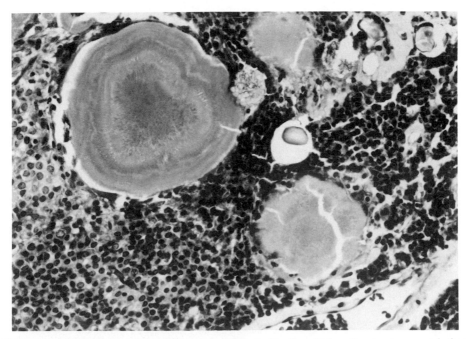

Figure 15.5. Amyloid deposition in a Prl-cell adenoma. Spherical bodies with lamellar structure contain fine needle-like substance radiating concentrically, ×360.

volume of large Prl-cell adenomas (41, 185, 287). Many in vivo and in vitro morphological studies (including morphometric analysis) have been performed to investigate the effects of bromocriptine on human Prl-cell adenomas (3, 14, 53, 83, 151, 230, 247, 290). The marked changes in morphology noted include changes in the nuclear chromatin pattern, a reduction in cell size largely attributable to a reduced cytoplasmic volume, and a significant decrease in the volume density of the endoplasmic reticulum and Golgi complexes (Fig. 15.6). These findings suggest that the drug acts at the transcriptional level and confirm that tumor shrinkage due to bromocriptine is the result of a reduction in cell size and is not secondary to vascular alterations or changes in the tumor milieu. The effects of bromocriptine are reversible and, when it is discontinued, the adenoma usually increases in size and there is a simultaneous rise in the serum Prl level. However, electron microscopy has suggested that the changes

induced by bromocriptine may persist focally in some Prl-cell adenomas (100). In addition, the long–term treatment (several months or more) of Prl-cell adenoma is accompanied by an increase of fibrosis and regressive changes. These alterations may cause subsequent surgery to yield unfavorable results (27, 56, 67, 152).

It is important to emphasize that hyperprolactinemia, especially at levels of less than 200 ng/ml, can be secondary to many other sellar lesions, such as other types of pituitary adenoma, the empty sella syndrome, lymphocytic adenohypophysitis, metastatic carcinoma, and craniopharyngioma (47, 302). In these cases, the growing lesions compress or damage the hypothalamus or the pituitary stalk, thereby inhibiting the production, release, and/or transport of hypothalamic Prl-inhibiting factors and leading to mild hyperprolactinemia. In some cases, hormonal, clinical, and conventional histological studies are not sufficient to definitely distinguish

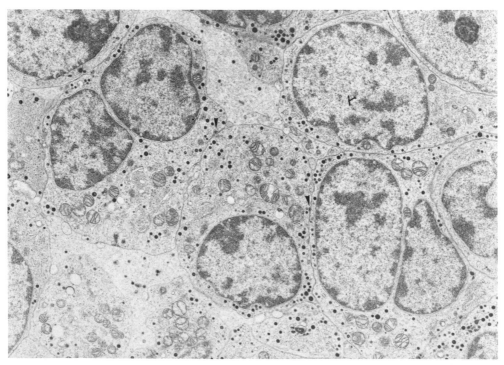

Figure 15.6.   Electron micrograph of a sparsely-granulated Prl-cell adenoma treated with bromocriptine. The cells have hyperchromatic nuclei and inconspicuous nucleoli. The volume densities of RER and Golgi apparatus are clearly reduced in the markedly diminished cytoplasm. Granule extrusions still can be found (arrowheads) ×6000.

between these different forms of hyperprolactinemia. Therefore, in order to confirm these diagnoses of Prl-cell adenoma, immunohistochemical and ultrastructural techniques are indispensable (95, 232, 315).

GH–Prl-Cell Adenomas

It has been shown that approximately 30% of GH-cell adenomas are accompanied by hyperprolactinemia (143, 269). These tumors represent the most frequent type of plurihormonal adenoma (see plurihormonal adenomas), and recent immunohistochemical studies have demonstrated the presence of Prl-immunopositivity in half of the tumors causing acromegaly (15). Moreover, the frequency of detection of Prl in GH-cell adenomas is much higher in the studies using Prl mRNA analysis than in those using conventional immunohistochemistry (164, 201). These tumors have been divided into three morphologically distinct adenoma types: mixed GH-cell–Prl-cell adenomas, mammosomatotroph-cell adenomas, and acidophil-stem-cell adenomas (102, 106, 134).

Mixed GH-Cell–Prl-Cell Adenomas

Mixed GH-cell–Prl-cell adenomas are fairly common and are associated with high blood GH levels and varying degrees of hyperprolactinemia (23, 46, 102, 117, 134, 160). They are bimorphous tumors consisting of densely or sparsely granulated GH cells and Prl cells, with the most common combination being that of densely granulated GH cells and sparsely granulated Prl cells (Fig. 15.7-A). The preponderance of one of the cell types determines the tumors' staining properties as acidophilic or chromophobic, or as a mixture of these two types. Although the immunostaining pattern and intensity varies depending on the granularity of the cells, immunohistochemical studies reveal the presence of GH and Prl in different cells. The number and distribution of the GH- and Prl-immunopositive cells varyies from case to case, and they often show an uneven distribution within a single tumor. In some tumors, the existence of cells containing both GH and Prl (bihormonal mammosomatotroph cells) can be identified using immunoelectron microscopy (15, 16, 80, 89, 236).

Mammosomatotroph-Cell Adenomas

Mammosomatotroph-cell adenomas are also bihormonal and monomorphous. They may derive from mammosomatroph cells that are well differentiated and capable of producing both GH and Prl (97). Unlike acidophil-stem-cell adenomas, these tumors are usually slow-growing and benign. Patients with this type of tumor show a long history of gigantism or acromegaly that may or may not be accompanied by hyperprolactinemia. By conventional staining, these tumors are intensely acidophilic. Immunohistochemical staining demonstrates the presence of GH and Prl in the same adenoma cells, but immunostaining for Prl is frequently weak or undetectable at the microscopic level. GH- and Prl-immunopositivity can be demonstrated in the same or in separate secretory granules by immunoelectron microscopy (Fig. 15.7-C) (60, 87, 236). The electron microscopic features of these tumors strikingly resemble those of well differentiated, massively granulated GH adenoma cells (Fig. 15.7-B). The secretory granules are often irregular, evenly electron-dense, or have a mottled appearance and measure from 200 to 2,000 nm in diameter. Misplaced exocytosis and large extracellular deposits of secretory material, which are usually not found in GH-cell adenomas, are typical ultrastructural features of these adenomas (97, 102, 106, 134). Electron microscopy is the only reliable tool for the diagnosis of this type of adenoma.

Acidophil-Stem-Cell Adenomas

Acidophil-stem-cell adenomas are bihormonal but monomorphous tumors. They are assumed to derive from common progenitor cells capable of differentiating into either GH–or Prl–secreting cells or into cells producing both GH and Prl. Clinically, these tumors are commonly associated with varying degrees of hyperprolactinemia, but are hormonally less active compared to well–differentiated Prl-cell adenomas of a comparable size (91, 94, 102, 134).

Acromegaly may develop in some cases, but it is not always associated with the elevation of serum GH levels. These adenomas are characteristically aggressive, invasive,

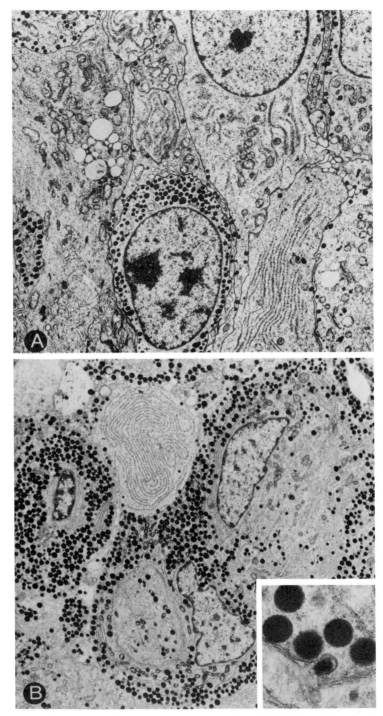

Figure 15.7. Electron micrographs of GH-Prl-cell adenomas. Mixed GH-cell and Prl-cell adenoma consisting of densely-granulated GH cells and sparsely-granulated Prl cells (A) ×4500. Mammosomatotroph cell adenoma resembling densely granulated GH-cell adenoma (B) ×4500. Inset shows granule extrusion, ×45000. Double immuno-

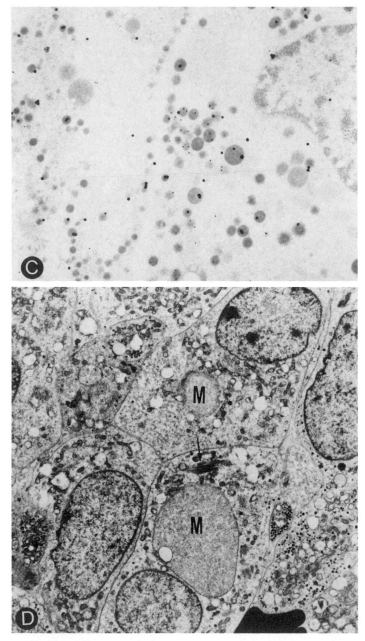

staining of a mammosomatotroph-cell adenoma. One cell (left) contains only Prl (40-nm gold particles) in the secretory granules. The other cell (right) shows Prl in most secretory granules and GH (15-nm gold particles) in a few secretory granules (C) ×18500. Acidophil stem cell adenoma resembling sparsely granulated GH-cell adenoma. Note mitochondrial gigantism (M) and dense tubular structure (arrow) (D) ×3600.

and rapidly-growing tumors (91, 94, 102, 134). On light microscopy, acidophil-stem-cell adenomas show a diffuse pattern and are chromophobic or slightly acidophilic due to oncocytic change, which is one of the morphological characteristics of this type of adenoma. Immunohistochemical studies reveal both GH and Prl in the cytoplasm of the same cells but, in some cases, the GH-immunoreactivity is weak, focal, or even absent at the microscopic level (Fig. 15.8). Ultrastructural studies are needed for making the definitive diagnosis of this tumor, since its features at this level are obviously different from those of any of the known types of adenohypophyseal cells or other types of adenomas, although some features are reminiscent of adenomatous, sparsely-granulated GH cells (fibrous bodies) and Prl cells (misplaced exocytosis). Electron microscopy shows these adenomas to be composed of closely–apposed elongated cells with irregular nuclei and abundant cytoplasm containing scattered RER; moderately or poorly de-

veloped Golgi complexes; and often fibrous bodies, centrioles, and cilia. The secretory granules are small and sparse, measure from 100 to 300 nm in diameter, and are generally located in the cell periphery. Misplaced exocytosis can also be found, but it is rare in general. Other characteristic ultrastructural features are oncocytic change and mitochondrial gigantism (Fig. 15.7-D). This latter peculiar form of mitochondria can also be observed as cytoplasmic vacuolization at the light microscopic level (91, 94, 134).

Corticotroph (ACTH) Cell Adenomas

Corticotroph cell adenomas produce ACTH, β–lipotropin, endorphins, and other related peptides that are the derivatives of the hormone called proopiomelanocortin (POMC). Clinically, they are associated with Cushing's disease or Nelson's syndrome (102, 134, 190). Almost all of the adenomas found in patients with Cushing's disease are microadenomas, and often no tumor is found at surgery (187), whereas the adeno-

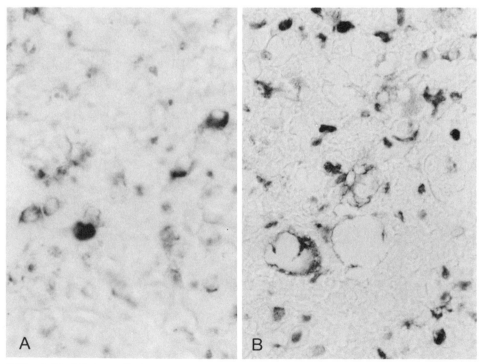

Figure 15.8. Acidophil stem cell adenoma. Tumor cells are faintly positive for GH and only a few cells are strongly positive (A). In contrast, Prl-immunoreactivity showing Golgi pattern is prominent in many cells (B). Some vacuolated areas are also positive for Prl, $\times 720$.

mas in Nelson's syndrome patients (who have previously undergone bilateral adrenarectomy to control preexisting hypercortisolism) are usually large, aggressive, invasive, and difficult to operate (61).

It has been reported that a significant number of corticotroph-cell adenomas lie in the central part of the pituitary gland, which would be consistent with the evidence that the vast majority of corticotroph cells in the normal pituitary gland are present in the median wedge (81, 218). Others claim that, more often, they are located in lateral wings on each side (30, 39, 140). This contradiction may reflect differences in the definition of "lateral" and "medial," but it seems likely that most of these tumors do not occur precisely in the midline. Lamberts *et al.* have divided corticotroph-cell adenomas into two groups based on their histological and biochemical features, i.e., those of anterior-lobe or intermediate-lobe origin (142). However, subsequent morphological and immunohistochemical studies have not supported an intermediate-lobe origin of these adenomas (188, 189).

Histologically, most corticotroph-cell adenomas are intensely basophilic with varying degrees of aniline blue, PAS, and lead hematoxylin staining. The growth pattern of these tumors is often sinusoidal and follicle formation is also found in some cases. The adenoma cells resemble normal corticotroph cells (40, 106, 161, 187, 235, 242) so, occasionally it is difficult to distinguish small adenomas from nodular foci of corticotroph-cell hyperplasia (see the section on hyperplasia). Immunohistochemical studies reliably show the presence of ACTH, β-lipotropin, and endorphins in the cytoplasm of the adenoma cells, with immunopositivity for other POMC-related peptides often being less conspicuous than that for ACTH. By electron microscopy (134, 146, 187, 235, 242), these basophilic adenomas are well–differentiated, densely granulated tumors consisting of medium–sized, angular cells with round to oval nuclei. The cytoplasm possesses abundant short strands of RER, prominent Golgi complexes, scattered polyribosomes, and numerous, slightly indented or spherical secretory granules, which are often more numerous at the cell periphery and measure 200–450 nm

in diameter. As do normal corticotroph cells, the adenoma cells usually contain cytoplasmic (mainly perinuclear) bundles of type 1 filaments, which are a hallmark of this type of adenoma (Fig. 15.9). A heavy deposit of type 1 filaments that often enlarges the cell and displaces other organelles towards the periphery or the nucleus is the ultrastructural equivalent of Crooke's hyalinization (59, 96, 102, 134). This feature can also be observed at the light microscopic level as a ring–like chromophobic or slightly acidophilic coloration in the perinuclear area (Fig. 15.10). Crooke's hyalinization is found in the cytoplasm of nontumorous corticotroph cells in the presence of hypercortisolism due to any endogenous or exogenous cause. This finding indicates an increase in negative feedback by elevated glucocorticoid levels and the lack of such a change signifies no responsiveness to such negative feedback. Therefore, massive Crooke's hyalinization is not exhibited in corticotroph-cell adenomas, except in a few cases (59). The functional significance of these "Crooke's-cell adenomas" is unclear, but it may suggest the possibility that hormone production in the adenoma is not fully autonomous.

Only a few of the endocrinologically active corticotroph cell adenomas are chromophobic and contain a few fine PAS–positive cytoplasmic granules (102, 134). Immunohistochemistry generally reveals positivity for ACTH and related peptides, but there is only slight positivity in some cells and even no staining at all in others. Electron microscopy shows that chromophobic corticotroph-cell adenomas are sparsely granulated tumors. They are less differentiated, larger, and more aggressive (recur more frequently) than the basophilic tumors, which are usually small microadenomas (102).

Nelson's syndrome consists of the development of a corticotroph-cell adenoma in a patient who has previously undergone bilateral or subtotal adrenalectomy (61). As the corticosteroid feedback mechanism is lost, a rapidly-proliferating adenoma that secretes ACTH becomes manifest clinically by an abnormally elevated serum ACTH level and hyperpigmentation caused by the secretion of either β–lipotropin or β-melanocyte-stimulating hormone (or both) (260). Most of the

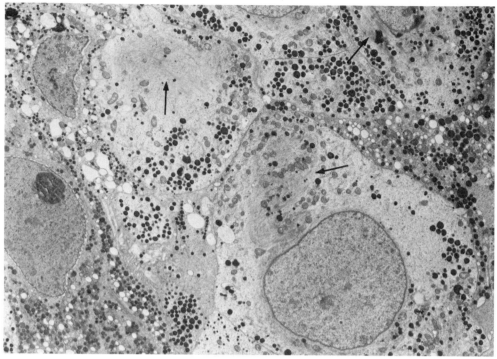

Figure 15.9. Electron micrograph of a densely granulated corticotroph-cell adenoma. The tumor consists of elongated and angular cells having a large number of secretory granules that vary in number, size, shape, and electron density. Note bundles of type-1 filaments (arrows) ×4800.

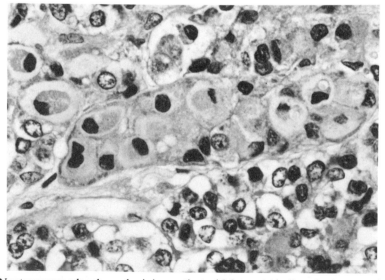

Figure 15.10. Nontumorous adenohypophysis in a patient with hypercortisolinemia. A group of corticotroph cells exhibit Crooke's hyaline change, in which a clear ring-like halo is present ×720.

adenomas found in patients with Nelson's syndrome are basophilic and PAS-positive. Immunostaining also demonstrates the presence of ACTH and related peptides in the cytoplasm of these tumors and their ultrastructural features are similar to those of Cushing's disease, with the exception that type I filaments are inconspicuous or absent (102, 134, 260).

Thyrotroph-Cell Adenomas

Thyrotroph-cell adenomas are very rare. Several published cases were insufficiently documented and the diagnosis has been based largely on indirect evidence with no detailed histological investigations of these tumors. Thus, these uncommon adenomas are still incompletely defined.

Thyrotroph-cell adenomas occur mainly under two sets of circumstances. The vast majority of these tumors originate in patients with a long history of untreated or insufficiently managed hypothyroidism (58, 118, 249, 304), which is consistent with the view that a lack of negative feedback by thyroid hormone stimulates the pituitary thyrotroph cells and leads to their hyperplasia and subsequent adenomatous change (261). These tumors are likely to be large and associated with visual disturbance by the time they are diagnosed. In patients with a thyroid that is normally capable of hormone production, thyrotroph cell adenomas are accompanied by hyperthyroidism (elevated TSH, T_3, and T_4 levels) (2, 75, 173, 181, 295) or euthyroidism (71, 243, 255, 295). In addition, it was suggested in one patient with a thyrotroph cell adenoma that hyperthyroidism resulted from low levels of serum TSH with enhanced biologic activity (22). Moreover, it must be noted that these differences of thyroid function in thyrotroph-cell adenomas cannot be distinguished on a morphological basis.

Microscopically, thyrotroph-cell adenomas are usually well vascularized, chromophobic tumors exhibiting a prominent sinusoidal growth pattern and they show only weak PAS or aldehyde-threonine positivity. Immunohistochemical studies may show TSH- and/or the α-subunit of glycoprotein-hormone immunopositivity in the cytoplasm of these adenoma cells. However, strong positivity for TSH or the α-subunit is a rare finding, and only scattered TSH-immunopositive cells or even no such cells are demonstrated in some adenomas. The reason for such immunonegativity often being found in thyrotroph-cell adenomas is not well understood, but several possibilities have been proposed, e.g., immunonegativity may be due to rapid hormone release or the loss of hormone during tissue fixation and processing. Alternatively, it is possible that an abnormal TSH is synthesized that lacks TSH immunoreactivity but still has bioactivity. Hence, electron microscopic studies are necessary in the morphological diagnosis of this type of adenoma. Electron microscopy shows that thyrotroph-cell adenomas consist of well–differentiated cells that resemble normal thyrotrophs cells, or of poorly-differentiated cells that are rather similar to those found in null-cell adenomas (71, 102, 106, 118, 134, 173, 234, 243, 260). In the former type of adenoma, the cells are elongated or angular, with long cytoplasmic processes, and have ovoid or irregular nuclei with little heterochromatin, prominent nucleoli, abundant RER, prominent Golgi complexes, and varying numbers of secretory granules measuring 150–250 nm in diameter. The secretory granules are spherical, often have lucent halos, and tend to line up along the cell membrane and accumulate in the cytoplasmic processes (Fig. 15.11).

Although these ultrastructural features of thyrotroph-cell adenomas are different from those of thyroidectomy cells (32), thyroidectomy cells can also occasionally be identified in some thyrotroph-cell adenomas (Fig. 15.11). These cells are large and vacuolated and often have large intensely PAS–positive granules. Ultrastructurally, these cells are characterized by the presence of markedly dilated endoplasmic reticulum. The occurrence of thyroidectomy cells indicates that the adenoma cells are responsive to thyroid hormone deficiency.

Gonadotroph Cell Adenomas

Gonadotroph-cell adenomas are found more often in older patients and actually occur more frequently than was previously suspected.

The pathogenesis of these adenomas is obscure, but it has become generally accepted

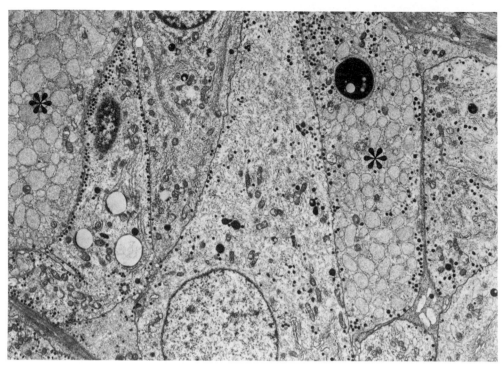

Figure 15.11.   Electron micrograph of a thyrotroph-cell adenoma. The tumor consists of well–differentiated polar cells with sparse, and small secretory granules often lining up along the cell membrane. In this case thyroidectomy cells, which are characterized by the presence of markedly dilatated endoplasmic reticulum, can be seen (asterisks) × 6000.

that they arise spontaneously (276, 278, 279) rather than in response to preceding primary hypogonadism, despite some reports of gonadotroph-cell adenomas associated with long–standing primary hypogonadism (128, 206, 284). Clinically, some of these adenomas are associated with hypogonadism (207, 279) or, rarely, with supranormal serum testosterone levels (276, 307, 321). Most gonadotroph-cell adenomas, however, seem to be clinically silent, with a history of normal pubertal development and normal fertility (279). Gonadotroph-cell adenomas have been reported chiefly in middle-aged males (279). In contrast, the diagnosis of gonadotroph cell adenoma is difficult to make in women, probably because these adenomas often present after the menopause when serum gonadotropin levels are normally high anyway (99, 207, 279). Nevertheless, these adenomas are being increasingly recognized by morphological studies and some authors report that 10% to 17% of pituitary adenomas are gonadotroph-cell adenomas (63).

The most common hormonal characteristic is the hypersecretion of FSH (279), which is often accompanied by hypersecretion of the α-subunit (33, 49, 277, 298) and, less often, by the hypersecretion of LH (44, 49, 99, 276, 307, 321). Other hormonal characteristics include an exaggerated response of gonadotropins, including the α-subunit, to GnRH (7, 64, 144), an abnormal response to TRH (144, 278), and an erratic suppression response to gonadal steroids (7, 217). Snyder suggests that pituitary adenomas with hypersecretion of the α-subunit alone (121) may be gonadotroph-cell adenomas (279).

Light microscopy shows that gonadotroph-cell adenomas are chromophobic and may have a few fine PAS–positive cytoplasmic granules. The cells are small to medium–sized and polygonal or elongated, with a prominent sinusoidal growth pattern and frequent pseudorosette formation around vessels (33, 99, 102, 106, 127, 128, 134, 260, 293, 294). In some tumors (especially in men), follicle formation is seen and the lumens are filled with a homogenous intensely PAS–positive substance (99, 102, 134). Immunohistochemical studies demonstrate the α-subunit, TSH, FSH and LH in combination or, more rarely, show FSH, the α–subunit, or LH alone (99, 102, 134, 192, 215, 293, 294, 315). Since both LH and FSH are supposed to be produced by the same cell, the presence of only one hormone suggests that certain tumors may arise from clones secreting only FSH or LH; alternatively, these adenomas may lose their potential to produce both FSH and LH, while proliferating. A diffuse, strong immunopositivity for FSH, LH, or the α-subunit is very rare. Instead, scattered positive cells that occur singly or in clumps and present an uneven distribution within the tumor are commonly found. Gonadotroph-cell adenomas in males usually reveal some immunoreactivity, whereas some of the tumors in females are immunonegative. We have no definite answers to explain this lack of immunoreactivity, but it may be that an abnormal FSH/LH/α-sub-

unit molecule is produced by these tumors that is not immunoreactive. Alternatively, the hormone may be lost during fixation or embedding, or it may be bound to a large protein molecule that blocks immunoreactivity (315).

By electron microscopy (33, 99, 102, 127, 128, 134, 192, 260, 293, 294, 315), sexual dichotomy is noted. In men, adenoma cells vary in their degree of differentiation, but are commonly less differentiated than those seen in women. They consist of polar, polyhedral, and elongated cells with ovoid nuclei. The cytoplasm contains sparse RER, moderately developed Golgi complexes, many microtubules, and sparse spherical secretory granules. These secretory granules measure up to 200 nm in diameter and tend to line up along the plasma membrane or accumulate in the cytoplasmic processes (Fig. 15.12). Some less differentiated adenomas appear to have ultrastructural features rather similar to those of null-cell adenomas. In women, these tumors are well differentiated and the cells re-

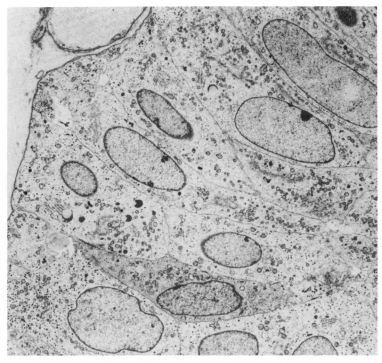

Figure 15.12. Electron micrograph of a gonadotroph-cell adenoma (male type). The tumor consists of elongated polar cells with uniform nuclei. Small secretory granules are unevenly distributed in the moderately differentiated cytoplasm, ×3000.

semble nontumorous gonadotroph cells, except for the small size of the secretory granules (50-150 nm). Secretory granules also tend to accumulate in the cell processes in tumors in women. Marked dilation of the Golgi complexes, termed the honeycomb Golgi, is a striking feature of gonadotroph-cell adenomas in women (99, 106). This peculiar structure of the Golgi complex has only been seen in females; they are composed of nearly perfect spheres of various sizes that contain a homogenous, electron–lucent substance, and there are hardly any developing secretory granules (Fig. 15.13).

Clinically Nonfunctioning Adenomas

Approximately one–fourth of surgically removed pituitary adenomas have no clinical or biochemical evidence of hypersecretion of any known adenohypophyseal hormones and are variously called silent, nonsecreting, or nonfunctioning adenomas (29, 134, 260). They usually present with symptoms related to their mass effect, such as headache and visual disturbance, or with symptoms of hypopituitarism, because of their lack of a characteristic clinical syndrome or serum hormone marker.

These tumors have been classified morphologically as null-cell adenomas or oncocytomas (102, 106, 134). Recent studies, however, indicate that these clinically nonfunctioning adenomas represent a morphologically heterogeneous group that can be fitted largely into two categories based on their immunohistochemical and ultrastructural features (102, 106). One group includes the tumors comprised of cells that have immunohistochemical and ultrastructural features of the established adenohypophyseal cell types, including silent somatotroph-, corticotroph-, thyrotroph-, and gonadotroph-cell adenomas. As demonstrated by immunohistochemical (82, 93, 102, 134, 137, 227, 293) and in situ hybridization studies (137, 200), these silent adenomas contain and produce one or more of the known adenohypophyseal hormones and express the mRNA of the corresponding hormone, indicating that gene expression occurs. Although several theories

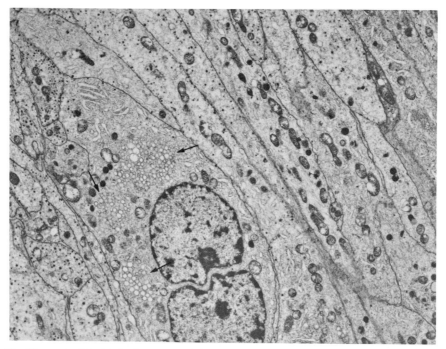

Figure 15.13. Electron micrograph of a gonadotroph-cell adenoma (female type). The tumor consists of markedly polar cells with long attenuating processes. RER are slightly dilated and secretory granules are scarce, small, and often accumulate in the cell processes. Note the characteristic honeycomb Golgi apparatus (arrows) ×4500,

have been proposed to explain the discrepancy between these morphological features and the clinical–biochemical presentation, no definite answers have been obtained so far and the mechanism underlying the silence of these tumors is still elusive (93, 137, 227).

The second group includes tumors consisting of cells having none of the specific characteristics of the five known adenohypophyseal cell types and possessing neither morphological nor immunohistochemical markers that indicate their cytogenesis or direction of differentiation. They are variously known as null-cell adenomas, oncocytomas, or silent subtype-3 adenomas.

From the clinical standpoint, it should be noted that the incidence of the different tumor types varies depending on the patient's age. For example, null-cell adenomas and oncocytomas, which are the most common types of nonfunctioning adenomas, usually occur in older patients and only rarely become clinically manifest before the 5th decade (134, 170, 317). In contrast, silent subtype-3 adenomas and silent corticotroph-cell adenomas predominate in patients less than 40 years of age, and this trend is even more obvious in patients under the age of 30 (317). It is still unclear whether these various morphologically distinct tumor types differ in their biological behavior, growth rate, invasiveness, recurrence rate, and therapeutic responsiveness. However, it is generally considered that null-cell adenomas and oncocytomas are slowly growing tumors, whereas some silent corticotroph-cell adenomas have a more rapid growth rate, are more likely to undergo apoplexy, and demonstrate more frequent recurrence (93, 104, 257). Therefore, all clinically nonfunctioning adenomas should be examined not only by conventional light microscopy but also by immunohistochemistry and electron microscopy to achieve a correct morphological diagnosis, which may provide useful information to aid the neurosurgeon in assessing the prognosis and making decisions regarding treatment.

Silent Somatotroph-Cell Adenomas.

Patients with silent somatotroph-cell adenomas have normal or slightly elevated serum GH levels, but show no clinical evidence of acromegaly (123, 137, 291). The ad-

enoma cells appear to be similar to sparsely-granulated GH adenoma cells on electron microscopy and contain fibrous bodies, but immunohistochemical studies demonstrate a variable GH content (none to moderate amounts) in the cytoplasm of the adenoma cells (Fig. 15.4). Tissue culture studies disclose a low initial rate of in vitro GH secretion with a spontaneous rise after several days and increased GH release after exposure to GHRH. In situ hybridization studies reveal GH mRNA expression by the adenoma cells (137). Thus, no definite answer can be offered as to the clinical silence of these tumors, but the secretion of GH or IGF-I lacking bioactivity has been suggested as the cause of the silence of these tumors associated with slightly elevated serum GH levels (123).

Silent Corticotroph-Cell Adenomas

Silent corticotroph-cell adenomas are characterized by the presence of immunopositive ACTH or related peptides in the adenoma cells without any symptoms of Cushing's disease (82, 93, 102, 106, 126, 134, 227). Serum ACTH and cortisol levels are generally normal, although an occasional patient may have high serum ACTH levels that are unassociated with hypercortisolism (199, 229). Although the pathophysiology of the clinical silence of these tumors is unclear, the synthesis of hormone lacking bioactivity (310) or its destruction within the adenoma cells (126) have been proposed as mechanisms. Recent studies of POMC gene expression have suggested that the absence of symptoms of Cushing's disease in patients with silent corticotroph-cell adenomas is due to an abnormality that is not in the coding sequence of the POMC gene or of its RNA processing, but rather lies at or after the translational steps (260). These tumors can be divided into two subtypes according to their ultrastructural features (102, 104, 106).

Subtype-1 Silent Corticotroph-Cell Adenomas. These are basophilic, strongly PAS-positive adenomas, containing immunoreactive ACTH and related peptides, and exhibiting ultrastructural features corresponding to those of well–differentiated corticotroph-cell adenomas in Cushing's disease (93, 102, 104, 134). In some tumors, lyso-

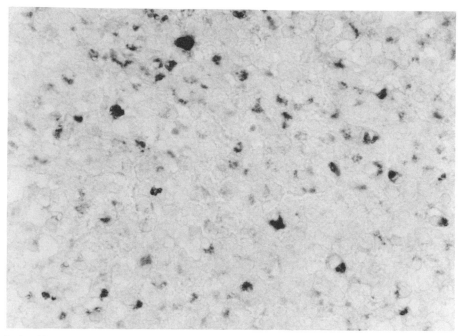

Figure 15.14.   Silent somatotroph-cell adenoma. Some tumor cells show varying degrees of GH-immunoreactivity, but they are small in number ×720.

somal activity and crinophagy may be increased (126).

Subtype-2 Silent Corticotroph-Cell Adenomas. These tumors are chromophobic or slightly basophilic and often show a sinusoidal pattern. They demonstrate immunopositivity for ACTH, endorphins, and β-lipotrophin as well as varying degrees of PAS positivity. On electron microscopy, they possess some features similar to functioning corticotroph-cell adenomas. However, the cytoplasm is more electron–lucent and the secretory granules are smaller (up to 400 nm). Moreover, type I filaments, the ultrastructural marker of human corticotroph cells, are not detected in these tumors (102, 104, 106, 134).

Silent Gonadotroph-Cell Adenomas

It was mentioned in a previous section that, in many patients with gonadotroph cell adenomas, especially women, the serum gonadotropin levels are subnormal, or the hypersecretion of gonadotropic hormones is not accompanied by any obvious clinical syndrome. These tumors are diagnosed as silent gonadotroph-cell adenomas because of the presence of immunoreactive FSH/LH/α-subunit in the majority of the adenoma cells and their possession of ultrastructural features similar to those of gonadotroph adenoma cells (99, 134, 227, 279, 293). Tissue culture studies have indicated that the amount of hormone (FSH, LH, α-subunit) secreted by silent gonadotroph-cell adenomas is significantly lower than that secreted by functioning gonadotroph-cell adenomas that have given rise to a clinically detectable elevation of the serum gonadotropin levels (6). The reason for the silence of these tumors may be that the amount of hormone secretion is too small to raise the hormone level in vivo or to produce clinical changes (6). Alternatively, they may secrete altered hormones or hormone fragments that are immunochemically and biochemically inert once they reach the blood (6).

Silent Subtype-3 Adenomas

These tumors were originally classified as one of the histological subtypes of silent corticotroph-cell adenomas and were termed silent subtype-3 corticotroph-cell adenomas (93, 104, 134). Subsequent studies have indicated that these tumors show less consistent immunoreactivity for POMC-derived peptides and, ultrastructurally, have no resemblance to corticotroph-cell adenomas, so the term "corticotroph cell" was deleted (104). At this time, we have no conclusive evidence as to the cytogenesis of this type of tumor (104).

In women with silent subtype-3 adenomas, mild to moderate hyperprolactinemia is accompanied by galactorrhea or amenorrhea, often leading to a misdiagnosis of prolactinoma. Bromocriptine administration reduces serum Prl levels, but fails to reduce the tumor size. The tumors appear to be aggressive and are often invasive. In contrast, most such tumors in men behave like hormonally nonfunctioning adenomas and only become manifest due to local symptoms, although some of them are associated with elevated serum GH levels and acromegaly or mild to moderate hyperprolactinemia. These findings may suggest multidirectional differentiation of this type of tumor (104).

Histologically, subtype-3 adenomas are either chromophobic or show varying degrees of acidophilia and exhibit a diffuse or lobular pattern of growth. The fairly large adenoma cells often have moderately pleomorphic nuclei. Most such adenomas contain scattered cells showing immunopositivity for any of the known adenohypophyseal hormones, mainly GH, Prl, ACTH, endorphins, or the α-subunit of glycoprotein hormone (most commonly GH and POMC-derived peptides in females and GH in males). However, in some cases, the results of immunohistochemical studies are entirely negative. Electron microscopy is an indispensable tool for obtaining a definite diagnosis of this type of tumor. Such adenomas consist of medium-sized to large cells showing polarity. The nuclei are euchromatic and contain a large nucleolus and often spheridia as well. The ample cytoplasm is filled with well-developed, diffusely distributed RER, tubular SER, and prominent tortuous Golgi complexes. The secretory granules vary in number, are mostly spherical, measure between 50-250 nm in diameter, and often accumulate in the cytoplasmic processes (Fig. 15.15) (104, 106).

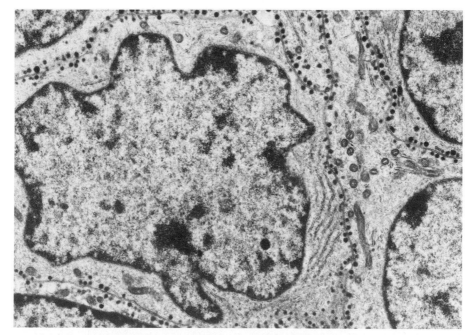

Figure 15.15. Electron micrograph of a silent subtype-3 adenoma. Medium-sized tumor cells with irregular nuclei have well-developed lamellar RER and many spherical secretory granules measuring 150-250 nm in diameter, $\times$ 13,200.

Null-Cell Adenomas

The term null-cell adenoma was introduced to designate pituitary adenomas that lacked histological, immunohistological, or ultrastructural markers that would allow the recognition of their cellular composition and cytogenesis (129). These adenomas were originally believed to be hormonally non-functioning, but have recently received considerable attention regarding their functional aspects (122). It has been found that many of them contain scattered cells or groups of cells that are immunoreactive for one or more of the adenohypophyseal hormones, (most commonly FSH and the α-subunit, less frequently LH, and very occasionally TSH, GH, Prl, or even more rarely ACTH) (29, 50, 122, 138, 246, 284). Interestingly, it seems likely that adenomas showing immunopositivity for either the α-subunit or β-subunit are more frequent than those exhibiting immunoreactivity for both the α- and β-subunits. Furthermore, in vitro studies (including cell culture (6, 138, 172, 311). RNA analysis (109, 248) and reverse hemolytic plaque assay (312)) have also suggested that many null-cell adenomas and oncocytomas can produce and secrete some hormones, most often gonadotropins. In fact, the amount of gonadotropin secreted into culture medium, or the percentage of tumor cells secreting gonadotropins, and the amount of gonadotropin secretion from individual tumor cells in the reverse hemolytic plaque assay are not significantly different between null-cell adenomas or oncocytomas and silent gonadotroph-cell adenomas (6, 312). It has been postulated that the subnormal serum levels of these hormones are due to hormone synthesis by only a small number of adenoma cells, to the production of very small quantities of hormone by a homogeneous tumor cell population, or to both factors (312). These in vitro studies support the suggestion that null-cell adenomas and gonadotroph-cell adenomas are closely related, and that there is a continuous spectrum from clinically detectable gonadotroph-cell adenomas to silent gonadotroph-cell adenomas and then on to null-cell adenomas or oncocytomas. Therefore, null-cell adenomas may have originated from progenitor cells that normally differentiate towards gonadotroph cells. Alternatively, these adenomas may be derived from multipotential precursor cells that can undergo multidirectional differentiation that is most often towards gonadotroph- or glycoprotein-hormone-producing cells.

Light microscopy shows null-cell adenomas to be chromophobic and to have either a diffuse or sinusoidal pattern of growth, often with pseudorosette formation (Fig. 15.16). Immunohistochemical studies either yield negative results or demonstrate small groups of cells or randomly scattered single cells that are positive for one or more of the pituitary hormones, as mentioned above (Fig. 15.17). Electron microscopy demonstrates that null-cell adenomas are composed of small, polyhedral cells with poorly-developed cytoplasm containing inconspicuous scattered RER, poorly or moderately developed Golgi complexes, numerous microtubules, and a modest number of small secretory granules measuring 100 to 250 nm in diameter (Fig. 15.18). These granules are spherical, vary in electron density, are often haloed, and frequently line up along the cell membrane. The majority of null-cell adenomas contain cells in which the number, size, and cytoplasmic volume density of the mitochondria are increased (oncocytic change) (102, 129, 134, 138).

Pituitary Oncocytomas

Oncocytomas are tumors composed of oncocytes, cells that are characterized by an abundance of cytoplasmic mitochondria (Fig. 15.18). Such tumors are usually benign and occur in various organs, including the salivary glands, thyroid, lungs, and kidneys. Pituitary oncocytomas were first described in 1973 (125, 145) and, subsequently, there have been a number of other reports on these tumors (17, 72, 115, 239, 241). Slight or moderate oncocytic transformation is also found in some functioning adenomas (72, 115) and some authors have suggested that a diagnosis of oncocytoma should be given when more than 50% of the observed adenoma cells show oncocytic transformation (150, 244), whereas others feel that nearly all the cells should be oncocytes (134). Recent morphometric studies have disclosed that the cytoplasmic volume density of organelles

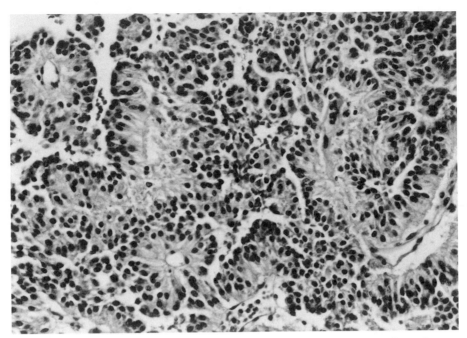

Figure 15.16.   Typical histologic feature of a null-cell adenoma. Tumor cells with elongated cytoplasm towards the blood vessels exhibit the characteristic pseudorosette arrangement, ×360.

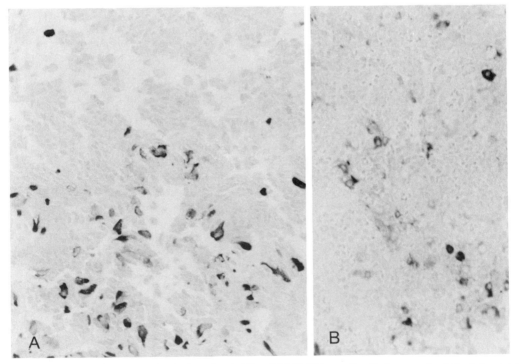

Figure 15.17.   Immunohistochemistry of α-subunit (A) and β-LH (B) in a null-cell adenoma. A relatively large number of α-subunit-immunoreactive cells are seen forming a cluster, while β-LH-immunoreactive cells are fewer and sparsely distributed, ×360.

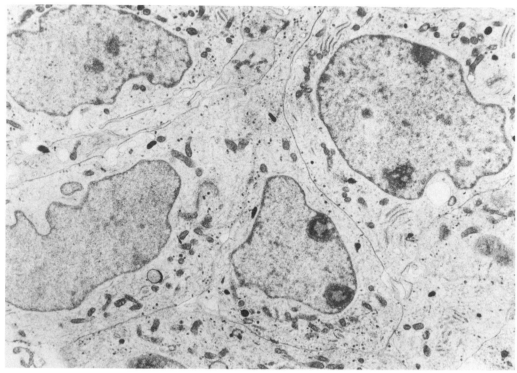

Figure 15.18. Electron micrograph of a null-cell adenoma. Polyhedral tumor cells have scanty cytoplasm with poorly developed RER and Golgi apparatus. Secretory granules are sparse and are located chiefly under the cell membrane, ×7900.

in oncocytomas is not significantly different from that in null-cell adenomas, except for the cellular enlargement and mitochondrial abundance noted in the former type of tumor (311). Moreover, taking into account their similarities with regard to epidemiological, clinical, and immunohistochemical characteristics, oncocytomas have been suggested to be variants of null-cell adenomas or to represent the end stage of the gradual oncocytic transformation of null-cell adenomas (102, 134, 260, 311).

Light microscopy shows oncocytomas to have varying degrees of acidophilia owing to uptake of the dye by the accumulated mitochondria rather than by secretory granules. These tumors usually show a diffuse growth pattern. Immunohistochemical and ultrastructural features are basically similar to those of null-cell adenomas, except for the mitochondrial abundance (102, 134, 138, 311). Electron microscopy is indispensable for the diagnosis of oncocytoma because the sole morphological marker of this tumor is

the presence of generalized oncocytic change (Fig. 15.19).

Plurihormonal Adenomas

As seen in many endocrine tumors arising in various other organs (48, 253), multiple hormones are often produced by a single pituitary adenoma. The application of sensitive immunohistochemical techniques has revealed that plurihormonality in pituitary tumors is not as rare as once considered (70, 136, 256). Recent in situ hybridization studies have shown that many adenomas express mRNA for more than one hormone simultaneously even if they may not undergo further processing to produce hormones (164). Therefore, it can perhaps be said that pituitary adenomas that produce exclusively one hormone, (i.e., monohormonal adenomas) may be in the minority. The term plurihormonal adenoma can be used as either a general term for all adenomas that express more than one hormone or as a strictly defined term for a special type of pituitary adenoma

(102, 103). In this chapter, we use the term in its broad sense to indicate all tumors that are not monohormonal adenomas, so that plurihormonal adenomas include various types of pituitary adenomas, as described below.

The hormones produced by pituitary adenomas are GH, Prl, ACTH, TSH, FSH, LH, and the free α-subunits of these glycoprotein hormones. Obviously, the combined expression of the α- and β-subunits of glycoprotein hormones is not regarded as evidence of plurihormonality. Adenomas containing either several POMC-related petides or both FSH and LH are also out of the category of plurihormonal adenomas, since such sets of hormones are normally produced in the same cells.

Plurihormonal adenomas are morphologically subclassified into two groups, monomorphous or polymorphous (102, 134). Monomorphous adenomas are composed of uniform tumor cells that are capable of the simultaneous production of more than one hormone. On the other hand, polymorphous adenomas are a mixture of structurally distinct cells that usually produce different hormones.

Plurihormonal adenomas include a wide range of adenoma types, with the largest group being adenomas associated with acromegaly. Many GH-cell adenomas can also produce other hormones, such as Prl, the α-subunit, and TSH (10, 21, 22, 94, 98). The coproduction of GH and Prl is a particularly common observation in these adenomas. Lloyd *et al.* (164) recently demonstrated by in situ hybridization that 87% of the adenomas causing acromegaly expressed both GH and Prl mRNA. Mixed GH and Prl cell adenomas consist of bimorphous cells: GH cells that are mostly of the densely granulated type, and Prl cells that are mostly of the sparsely granulated type (102, 134). Tumor cells containing both GH and Prl (mammosomatotroph cells) are sometimes intermingled in this type of adenoma. On the other hand, mammosomatotroph-cell adenomas are monomorphous and are almost exclusively composed of cells that share the ultrastructural features of densely-granulated GH cells as well as those of Prl cells and that produce GH and Prl concomitantly (60, 97, 134). Acidophil-stem-cell adenomas are also monomorphous and consist of cells showing

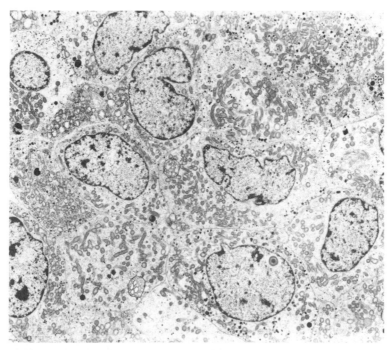

Figure 15.19. Electron micrograph of an oncocytoma. Note the marked, generalized abundance of mitochondria, ×3500.

the features of both Prl cells and sparsely granulated GH cells with fibrous bodies (94, 134). Usually, Prl is predominantly produced. Monomorphous densely granulated GH-cell adenomas also frequently contain a varying number of Prl-immunoreactive cells (136, 236), suggesting that some adenoma cells can produce both GH and Prl even though such cells display the ultrastructural profile of GH cells (236).

In addition to the bihormonal production of GH and Prl, the α-subunit is sometimes expressed by the adenomas that cause acromegaly, especially, in the densely granulated type of adenomas (10, 21, 70, 111, 136, 156, 214, 224, 256). In our study, more than 90% of densely-granulated GH-cell adenomas contained a varying number of the α-subunit-immunoreactive cells (Fig. 15.20). In contrast, sparsely granulated GH-cell adenomas exhibited no α-subunit immunoreactivity (254). Colocalization of GH and the α-subunit in the same tumor cells and in the same granules has been reported (21, 70, 214). Clinically elevated serum α-subunit

levels have been noted in some patients with acromegaly (10, 21, 224). In less frequent cases, GH-cell adenomas, usually of the densely granulated type, have been demonstrated by electron microscopy to contain many TSH cells or, by immunohistochemistry, to contain TSH-immunoreactive cells (10, 22, 70, 136, 168, 256) and to secrete TSH (10, 22, 168). Some patients with these adenomas show hyperthyroidism as well as acromegaly (22, 168). Among the adenomas associated with acromegaly, only sparsely granulated GH-cell adenomas produce only GH, although even a few of these adenomas contain a small number of Prl-immunoreactive cells.

The combination of TSH and gonadotropins (FSH and/or LH) has been demonstrated in some adenomas (215), but a careful evaluation of such immunoreactivity is required because of the frequent cross–reactions between antisera against glycoprotein hormones (294).

A rare but interesting combination is the free α-subunit and Prl or ACTH. Although

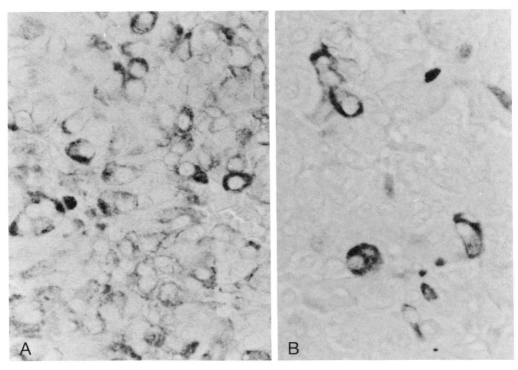

Figure 15.20. Plurihormonal adenoma. Many GH-immunoreactive cells (A) and a few α-subunit-immunoreactive cells (B) are demonstrated in this adenoma obtained from an acromegalic patient, $\times 720$.

both Prl-cell and corticotroph-cell adenomas are mostly monohormonal, the α-subunit has been immunohistochemically demonstrated in some of these adenomas (25, 111, 156, 179, 224). Elevated serum levels of the α-subunit have been reported in some patients (224), but there have been no clinical manifestations related to this.

A distinct adenoma type with frequent multihormonal expression is the silent subtype-3 adenoma (104). This rare type of adenoma is characterized by monomorphous cells with well developed organelles and immunoreactivity to various hormones, most commonly GH and ACTH (104).

There have been numerous, well-documented single case reports on the unusual coproduction of pituitary hormones in adenomas. They include ACTH and LH (252), ACTH and Prl (272, 318), TSH and Prl (110), and Prl and FSH/LH (281). However, most of the patients manifested symptoms due to only one of the hormones produced.

Several explanations can be applied to the mechanism of plurihormonal expression in pituitary adenomas. Before going into details, it should be noted that the recent observations on the monoclonal origin of pituitary adenomas shown by DNA analysis (84, 108) are not directly related to the mechanisms of the phenotypic expression of multiple hormones by these tumors. Firstly, tumors with plurihormonality may be derived from cells that are capable of producing more than one hormone but are inconspicuous under normal conditions. It has been reported that there are a few cells in the normal adenohypophysis that produce both GH and Prl (163) or GH and the α-subunit (214). In the neoplastic state, these tumor cells may undergo activation and then express their bihormonality. Secondly, tumors expressing two or more hormones may arise from multipotential progenitor cells that undergo multidirectional differentiation (136). Such cells may be either the mother cells from which the tumors have originated or cells that arise during tumor cell proliferation (dedifferentiation). Thirdly, microenvironmental factors, such as regulatory neuropeptides from the hypothalamus, growth factors, and disturbance of the blood supply may influence the phenotypic expression of individual tumor

cells (48, 305). Lastly, mutational changes in tumor cells may occur during adenoma growth and give rise to new clones, resulting in multiple-hormone secretion (136). Perhaps, none of these theories alone can fully explain the mechanism of plurihormonality (253) and a combination of these explanations may be more acceptable, because hormonal expression is believed to be regulated at several steps, including gene structure, translation, and transcription.

Ectopic Pituitary Adenomas

The ectopic pituitary adenoma was first described in 1909 (54). Subsequently, there have been a number of reports of these adenomas occurring in various (mainly extracranial) sites, such as the sphenoidal sinuses, nasal cavity, or cranial base (Fig. 15.21) (174). Intracranial ectopic pituitary adenomas have also occasionally been reported, including suprasellar (174, 238), parasellar (31), and temporal lobe (203), as well as those of the superior orbital fissure down to the clivus (213). As the most unusual ectopic adenoma, a corticotroph-cell adenoma occurring in pituitary tissue within an ovarian teratoma was reported (11).

The pharyngeal pituitary, remnants of the craniopharyngeal duct, or a suprasellar peri-infundibular ectopic adenohypophysis have each been thought to serve as the source of extracranial or intracranial ectopic pituitary adenomas (42, 88). They are usually nonfunctioning (including silent corticotroph-cell adenomas), but are sometimes associated with Cushing's disease, acromegaly, or hyperprolactinemia (174). Modern imaging techniques can help in the detection of small ectopic pituitary adenomas at an early stage. This type of adenoma also should be considered when a patient with Cushing's disease does not have a favorable result after pituitary exploration or hypophysectomy.

Invasive Adenomas

Invasive adenomas are those adenomas that infiltrate adjacent tissues, such as the remaining normal pituitary gland, dura, venous structures, cranial nerves, and nasal sinuses (Fig. 15.22) (257).

Taking into account their higher recurrence rates after surgery and the more com-

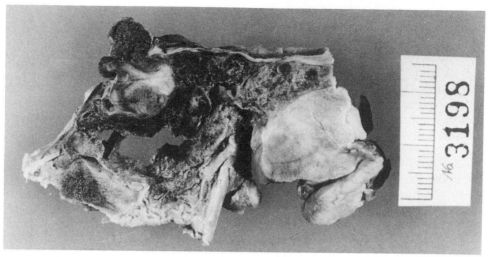

Figure 15.21.   Ectopic pituitary adenoma. This is a Prl-cell adenoma occurring in the sphenoidal sinus. It is demonstrated that the tumor occupies the sphenoidal sinus and surrounds the pituitary gland. (Reprinted with permission from Matsushita, H., Matsuya, S., Endo, Y., et al. A prolactin producing tumor originated in the sphenoid sinus. Acta. Pathol. Jpn., *34*:103–109, 1984)

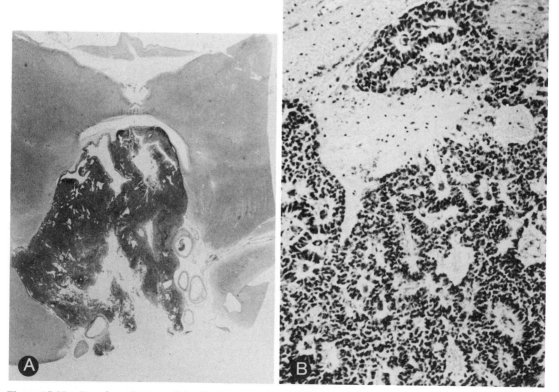

Figure 15.22.   Invasive adenoma. Prl-cell adenoma with striking suprasellar and third ventricular extension (A). Light microscopy shows finger-like invasion of the tumor to the hypothalamus (B) ×100.

mon occurrence of cellular pleomorphism and mitotic figures compared to noninvasive adenomas, invasive adenomas are still regarded as benign tumors, but they represent a biologically intermediate form between the sharply demarcated benign adenomas and metastasizing pituitary carcinomas (257). This intermediate biological behavior has been confirmed by recent studies using the Ki–67 monoclonal antibody. It has been reported that immunohistochemical demonstration of the Ki–67 antigen is useful in assessing the proliferative activity of tumors arising in various organs and that tumors with more Ki–67 immunoreactive cells show a more rapid growth rate and have a poorer prognosis than those with low cell counts (69, 209). Some authors have indicated that the number of Ki–67 immunopositive cells in invasive adenomas is significantly higher than that in noninvasive adenomas (124, 155).

Such an invasiveness can be identified by histological examination, by direct inspection during surgery, or (less frequently) by sophisticated neuroimaging techniques. It is generally assumed that the frequency of the histological demonstration of invasion is more than twice as common as that of its surgical identification (268). However, histological confirmation of invasiveness may be overlooked when the surgical specimen is small and does not include dura or bone.

Moreover, a positive correlation has been reported between the frequency of histological invasion and the tumor size or functional adenoma type; macroadenomas tend to invade more commonly than microadenomas (268). It has been mentioned by Scheithauer *et al.* that the estimated incidence of gross invasion is approximately 35% and that the most frequent invasive adenomas are silent corticotroph-cell adenomas followed by thyrotroph-cell adenomas and Prl-cell adenomas. In contrast, the less common invasive adenomas are corticotroph-cell adenomas or gonadotroph-cell adenomas (257).

Pituitary Carcinoma

Pituitary carcinoma is a rare condition that originates from the adenohypophyseal cells. The histological criteria for pituitary malignancy are still controversial (134, 257,

260). As with other endocrine tumors, cellular pleomorphism, nuclear atypia, and mitotic figures may indicate a rapid rate of growth, but they are not definitive indicators of malignancy in pituitary tumors (102, 257). Moreover, invasion of the surrounding tissues, despite being a reflection of an aggressive potential, is not in itself proof of malignancy (134, 257, 260).

Pituitary carcinoma can be diagnosed only when cerebrospinal or extracranial metastases are present (Fig. 15.23) (134, 257, 260). We cannot draw valid conclusions regarding the prevalence of various cell types giving rise to pituitary carcinoma, since endocrinological data and immunohistological or ultrastructural studies have been described in only a few of the reported cases (43, 66, 139, 171, 198, 262, 297). They may appear to be chromophobic nonfunctioning adenomas (167) or may produce GH (210), Prl (43, 171, 262, 297), or ACTH (57, 66, 225). Particularly important is the exclusion of metastatic carcinoma to the pituitary gland. In such instances, immunohistochemical analysis may be of considerable importance in establishing the proper diagnosis and exploring the cellular composition of a metastatic carcinoma whose primary site is unclear, since the presence of pituitary hormones in the tumor cells will indicate an adenohypophyseal origin for the lesion.

Pituitary Folliculo-Stellate-Cell Adenomas

Folliculo–stellate cells have been confirmed in the pituitary glands of various species and also in human pituitary adenomas (157, 195, 286). The term "folliculo–stellate cells" was proposed by Vila–Porcile, because these cells surround follicles and have a stellate form (299). The cytogenesis of these cells still remains controversial. Some authors have suggested a neuroectodermal origin because of their S-100 and/or GFAP immunostaining (157, 195, 286), whereas others have claimed that they are ectodermal and can differentiate towards glandular cells (89). This concept is supported by the presence of keratin–immunopositive folliculo–stellate cells (286). Moreover, the functions of these cells are also not well known, although several possibilities have been proposed, including that they are stem cells for adenohypophy-

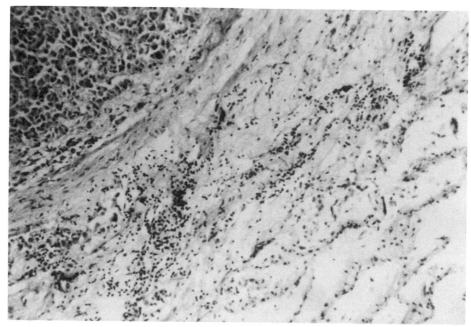

Figure 15.23. Pituitary carcinoma. Prl-cell adenoma (upper left) is metastasized to the lung, ×100.

seal cells (320), supporting cells (114), transport cells (62), or helper cells (273). These cells are estimated to comprise 3% to 4% of all the cells in a normal anterior pituitary gland (26).

A tumor that consisted of and arose from these folliculo–stellate cells, was first reported in 1984 (309). Light microscopy shows that these tumors consist of stellate, agranular cells, and appear to be chromophobic. Their most characteristic feature is the presence of numerous areas of a colloid-like substance which is PAS positive. By electron microscopy, these cells are stellate and are closely apposed with many desmosomes. The cytoplasm of the cells has few granules but contains large numbers of fine filaments. Colloid inclusions of varying sizes are found within intra- or intercellular lumens that are lined by many microvilli and occasional cilia (309).

These tumors appear to be extremely rare, but may be erroneously diagnosed as nonfunctioning adenomas. Vogel *et al.* claimed recently that these tumors may actually represent a secretory intrasellar meningioma on the basis of ultrastructural and immunohistochemical studies (300).

PITUITARY HYPERPLASIA

Hyperplasia of the adenohypophysis is a well–known entity, but its causes, pathogenesis, and histological definition are still obscure. Hypothalamic releasing factors may account for certain types of hyperplasia, whereas physiologic or compensatory states may cause hyperplasia under certain conditions, such as Prl-cell hyperplasia during pregnancy (65, 264) and thyrotroph-cell hyperplasia in prolonged hypothyroidism (219). Hyperplasia of unknown origin or primary hyperplasia of the pituitary includes corticotroph-cell hyperplasia in some cases of Cushing's disease (186, 266) and mammosomatotroph-cell hyperplasia in patients with or without McCane-Albright syndrome (132, 193).

A reversible process of pituitary hyperplasia has been well demonstrated by follow–up neuroimmaging studies in acromegalic patients with GHRH-producing tumors (250).

The enlarged sella turcica is markedly reduced and returns to its normal size after the removal of these tumors. On the other hand, Prl-cell hyperplasia associated with pregnancy may persist to some degree after delivery because the pituitary Prl-cell population is slightly greater in multiparous women than in nulliparous women (5, 264).

Microscopically, hyperplasia can be classified into two patterns: diffuse or nodular (105, 134). Diffuse hyperplasia is not associated with any circumscribed mass and the differential diagnosis between diffuse hyperplasia and adenoma causes few problems, but a careful investigation is required to distinguish hyperplasia from a normal pituitary gland. In contrast, it is very difficult to distinguish nodular hyperplasia from microadenoma with certainty (134). There are no established histological criteria for the differential diagnosis, but the following points would favor the diagnosis of adenoma: a) marked disruption or disappearance of the reticulin fiber network, b) compression of the adjacent tissue, and c) lack of interspersion with other cell types (103, 134, 186, 251). Nevertheless, as seen in other endocrine organs, such as the parathyroid, thyroid, and adrenal cortex, hyperplasia seems to represent part of a continuous spectrum leading eventually to neoplasia. In fact, thyrotroph-cell adenomas have been observed in pituitaries exhibiting thyrotroph-cell hyperplasia in patients with prolonged primary hypothyroidism (249, 261). Likewise, corticotroph-cell adenomas have been reported in patients with Addison's disease (85, 258). In animals, it seems likely that prolonged stimulation to certain pituitary cell types can cause, eventually, neoplasia on top of hyperplasia. Other than the well-known, estrogen-induced Prl-cell hyperplasia-adenoma (263), it has been recently demonstrated that excess GHRH secretion in GHRH transgenic mice evokes a massive mammosomatotroph-cell hyperplasia (282) and subsequent mammosomatotroph-cell adenoma (8).

GH-Cell Hyperplasia

GH-cell hyperplasia has been well known in cases with ectopic GHRH-producing tumors (250). The first case to be well documented was initially noticed by the histological observation of the pituitary resected from an acromegalic patient. This showed GH cell hyperplasia, but no adenoma (289). These extracranial GHRH-producing tumors include endocrine tumors arising in the pancreas, lung, and gastrointestinal tract (250). Hyperplastic GH cells are eosinophilic and strongly positive for GH over the cytoplasm. Prl-immunoreactive cells have also been observed in these hyperplastic areas (250). On electron microscopy, such hyperplastic cells are densely granulated and contain prominent Golgi complex and well developed RER. Mammosomatotroph-cell hyperplasia has been noted in McCane-Albright syndrome (132) and in GHRH transgenic mice (282). In the latter, a massive GH- or mammosomatotroph-cell hyperplasia was observed by eight months of age (282), and at the age of 16 to 24 months, mammosomatotroph-cell adenomas developed (8). More recently, mammosomatotroph-cell hyperplasia of unknown etiology was reported in the pituitary obtained from a girl with gigantism (193).

Prl-Cell Hyperplasia

Physiologic hyperplasia of Prl cells during pregnancy and lactation has been studied thoroughly (65, 264). Prl-cell hyperplasia develops in pregnant women as early as the second month of gestation (Fig. 15.24). At the time of delivery, the pituitary is significantly enlarged by massive Prl-cell hyperplasia, and this sometimes mimics an adenoma (264). It is unlikely that pregnancy affects the formation or growth of Prl-cell adenomas, since the incidence and the size of Prl-cell adenomas in pregnant or postpartum women is similar to that in age-matched, non-pregnant women (264). Prl-cell hyperplasia rarely develops in pituitary glands harboring various types of adenomas such as Prl-cell adenomas and corticotroph-cell adenomas (105), or in the glands of patients with long-standing hypothyroidism (261). Although estrogen-induced experimental Prl-cell hyperplasia and subsequent Prl-cell adenoma have been well known in rats, it has been reported that estrogen medication for patients with prostatic carcinoma may not cause Prl-cell hyperpla-

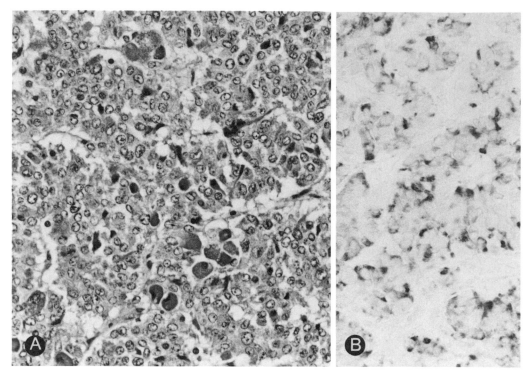

Figure 15.24. Prl-cell hyperplasia in the pituitary during pregnancy. Large, chromophobic cells are markedly increased to expand each acinus (A) and are intensively positive for Prl (B) ×360.

sia or adenoma (263). Idiopathic Prl-cell hyperplasia causing clinical symptoms is very rare. Hyperplastic Prl cells contain well-developed RER with Nebenkern formation and conspicuous Golgi complexes (101).

Corticotroph-Cell Hyperplasia

Corticotroph-cell hyperplasia may occur under several circumstances. Oversecretion of CRH from ectopic CRH–producing tumors leads to corticotroph-cell hyperplasia causing Cushing's disease (37). Such tumors include hypothalamic gangliocytomas and endocrine tumors arising in the lung, pancreas, and prostate (see Chapters 14 and 16). The untreated primary adrenocortical deficiency of Addison's syndrome is commonly accompanied by corticotroph-cell hyperplasia (258). In addition, there are a considerable number of cases of corticotroph-cell hyperplasia that are of unknown etiology (134, 186, 266). From the clinical point of view, the presence of such an idiopathic hyperplasia as a cause of Cushing's disease is the most difficult problem for both neurosurgeons and

surgical pathologists. In the pituitary of a patient with Cushing's disease, either corticotroph-cell adenoma or hyperplasia or both will be encountered. Although median wedge resection or total adenohypophysectomy is necessary for the curative treatment of corticotroph-cell hyperplasia, it is difficult to distinguish a microadenoma from hyperplasia or hyperplasia from a normal gland during surgery (103, 134, 186, 258). In hyperplastic corticotroph cells, well developed RER and Golgi complexes as well as varying amounts of type 1 filaments are observed, as are also found in corticotroph adenoma cells. Crook's hyaline change may be noticed within the corticotroph cells of a hyperplastic gland (37).

Thyrotroph-Cell Hyperplasia

Untreated prolonged hypothyroidism is known to cause thyrotroph-cell hyperplasia, resulting in the enlargement of the pituitary (103, 249, 261); adenoma formation has also been observed in such cases (249, 261). It is reported that about 50% of thyrotroph-cell adenomas occur in patients with preexisting hypothyroidism (260). Experimental thyroidectomy in rats can cause the pronounced hyperplasia, composed of large thyrotroph cells, named thyroidectomy cells (101, 103). Thyrotroph-cell hyperplasia may also be associated with Addison's disease (Schmidt's syndrome) (38). Histologically defined thyrotroph-cell hyperplasia has not been reported so far as an isolated cause of hyperthyroidism. Microscopically, hyperplastic or activated thyrotroph cells have abundant cytoplasm containing large amounts of RER with varying degrees of dilation and prominent, spherical Golgi complexes (Fig. 15.11) (101, 103).

Gonadotroph-Cell Hyperplasia

Although rare, enlargement of the pituitary and gonadotroph-cell hyperplasia may be observed in patients with insufficiently treated primary hypogonadism (280). Even gonadotroph-cell adenomas have been reported to arise in such patients (206, 308). However, it is unknown whether longstanding primary hypogonadism is responsible for the formation of gonadotroph-cell adenomas. Precocious puberty may result from excess GnRH release from hypothalamic gangliocytomas that contain GnRH–immunoreactive cells (313). Corticotroph-cell hyperplasia is the most common change in the pituitary, but the morphology of the pituitary has not yet become well known. The typical hyperplastic gonadotroph cells called gonadectomy cells, which are seen in experimental gonadectomized rats, exhibit a signet-ring-like appearance, because their cytoplasm is filled with markedly dilatated RER (101).

OTHER TUMORS AND TUMORLIKE CONDITIONS

Granular-Cell Tumors

Granular-cell tumors are benign tumors that are also called choristomas, or granular-cell myoblastomas. These tumors are most often encountered as incidental autopsy findings. They can also arise in other organs, such as the brain, tongue, and peripheral nervous system. In the pituitary, they are seen in up to 17% of unselected adult autopsy cases,

and are found most frequently in the infundibulum or the posterior lobe (166, 270). They are often multiple, usually very small, (less than 1 cm in diameter), and asymptomatic (102, 134). In some cases, however, they grow faster and enlarge to a considerable size that is detectable by imaging diagnosis (45) and subsequently cause visual disturbance; hypopituitarism, including diabetes insipidus; and even death (19, 285).

Histologically, granular-cell tumors in the pituitary are similar to those arising in other organs and consist of loosely apposed, large, spherical, oval, or polyhedral cells with an eccentrically located, moderately dense nucleus and abundant, strongly PAS-positive granules throughout the cytoplasm (Fig. 15.25-A). These granules are considered a marker for their histological diagnosis and are negative for adenohypophyseal hormones by immunostaining (19, 102, 134). Electron microscopy shows that these granules are membrane–bound and unevenly electron–dense lysosomal bodies (Fig. 15.25-B) (102, 134, 221).

The origin of these tumors is still controversial. Most granular-cell tumors arising in extracranial organs show immunopositivity for S–100 protein (51), NSE, and neural differentiation antigen PGP 9.5 (237), supporting a derivation from schwann cells. In contrast, immunopositivity for α-1 chymotrypsin (Fig. 15.25-A) and/or α-1 trypsin combined with immunonegativity for S–100 protein and NSE is seen in some granular-cell tumors arising in the posterior pituitary, brain, thyroid, and subcutaneous tissue; this pattern may suggest another origin (202). These differences in the expression of various immunohistochemical markers may suggest that granular-cell tumors, despite their uniform histological appearance on conventional microscopic examination, are actually heterogeneous (296). In the neurohypophysis, they may arise from pituicytes that are the glial cells of the stalk and the posterior pituitary gland (102, 134, 159). This theory is supported by the occasional finding of similar cells in astrocytomas (240).

Secondary Carcinoma

The pituitary gland is a relatively rare site of metastasis, but may be involved particu-

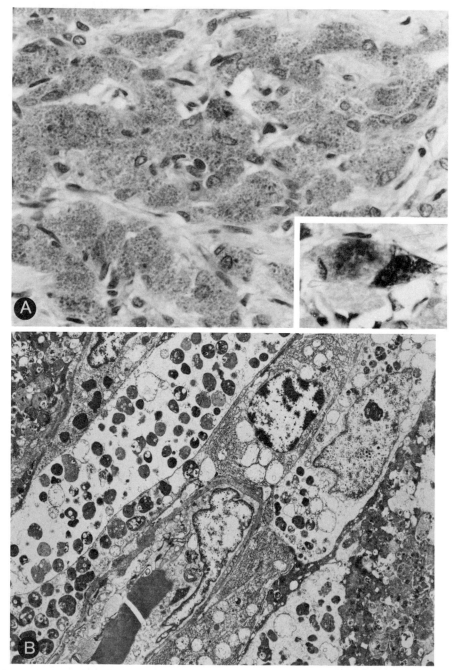

Figure 15.25. Granular-cell tumor in the posterior lobe. Abundant cytoplasm of the tumor cells is finely granular and strongly positive for PAS (A). Inset shows α1-antichymotripsine-immunoreactive cells. $\times$270 Electron micrograph shows the cells packed with heterolysosome (B) $\times$3600.

larly in patients with advanced and widely disseminated malignant tumors (77). In some instances, however, a metastasis to the pituitary may be the first and only manifestation of an otherwise occult carcinoma (34, 180). Moreover, there is no reliable clinical or radiological method to distinguish between pituitary metastasis and pituitary adenoma, although diabetes insipidus, extraocular palsy, and a prior history of malignancy may suggest a metastasis to the pituitary (34, 180, 204). Therefore, pituitary metastasis is often only diagnosed by histological examination after surgical intervention.

The incidence of carcinoma metastatic to the pituitary ranges from 1% to 1.8% in autopsies of patients with known malignancies (1, 34, 131, 176). Most pituitary metastases are asymptomatic and are an incidental autopsy finding, so such tumors are rare in neurosurgical practice (34, 180, 204). Various malignancies can give rise to metastases to the pituitary; the most common is breast carcinoma, followed by carcinoma of the lung, colon, prostate, and pancreas. Carcinoma of the thyroid, bladder, liver, and upper gastro-

intestinal tract as well as lymphoma, leukemia, and various sarcomas may also involve the pituitary (34). The pathological features depend on the primary tumor, but such lesions generally show a rich vascular network (Fig. 15.26). The posterior lobe is much more frequently involved than the anterior lobe and involvement of the anterior lobe is usually the result of contiguous spread of the tumor from the posterior lobe (180). The low incidence of anterior lobe involvement has been explained by the lack of a direct arterial blood supply to the anterior lobe of the pituitary (52, 77). Immunohistochemistry may be useful in making a differential diagnosis between pituitary metastasis and pituitary adenoma. However, it must be taken into account that pituitary adenomas themselves may rarely be a site of metastasis (223, 226, 323).

Rathke's Cleft Cysts

Rathke's cleft cysts are thought to be remnants of the apical portion of Rathke's pouch, which arises from the foregut and extends cranially to become the craniopharyngeal duct (271). Rathke's cleft cysts are usu-

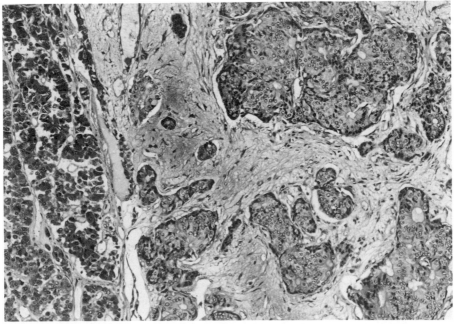

Figure 15.26. Metastatic deposits of a thyroid carcinoma are seen in the posterior lobe. In contrast, the anterior lobe (left) is spared such metastasis, ×180.

ally asymptomatic and are encountered in 13% to 33% of autopsy cases (18, 184, 271). Symptomatic Rathke's cleft cysts are quite uncommon and less than 100 such cases have been reported in the literature (306). They present with local compression symptoms, such as headache, visual disturbance, hypopituitarism, diabetes insipidus (169, 283, 306), or hyperprolactinemia (211, 303, 306). These cysts are mainly located in the sella turcica, but may extend into the suprasellar compartment. A purely suprasellar location, although extremely rare, has also been reported (12).

Small and asymptomatic Rathke's cleft cysts tend to be situated between the anterior and posterior lobes of the pituitary, and are generally lined with a single layer of columnar or cuboidal epithelium containing ciliated and goblet cells (107, 134). The lumens of these small cysts are filled with a slightly acidophilic homogenous colloid material (134) and the epithelium may show immunopositivity for some of the adenohypophyseal hormones. In contrast, large symptomatic Rathke's cleft cysts usually have pockets of stratified or squamous epithelium in addition to the cuboidal and columnar monolayer epithelium, and exhibit negative immunostaining for adenohypophyseal hormones (107). These histological data may support the hypothesis that large symptomatic Rathke's cysts do not arise simply from the enlargement of small cysts (107) but may actually represent a transitional form between the asymptomatic Rathke's cleft cyst and craniopharyngioma (175, 319), even though craniopharyngiomas exhibit a different histological differentiation and usually have a different biological behavior.

In rare instances, a Rathke's cleft cyst can be found in association with a pituitary adenoma (208). Adenohypophyseal cells are generally considered to derive from the cells in the anterior wall of Rathke's pouch. Kepes reported an unusual pituitary tumor consisting of a pituitary adenoma (nonfunctioning) and a Rathke's cleft cyst (120). He observed ultrastructurally the presence of intracytoplasmic tonofilaments and secretory granules in the tumor cells. Thus, this compound lesion was regarded as a Rathke's cleft cyst differentiating into a granulated pituitary ad-

enoma and these tumor cells were considered to be "transitional cells" (differentiating from Rathke's cleft cyst cells to adenohypophyseal cells). Accordingly, this type of tumor was termed a transitional cell tumor of the pituitary (120). However, some authors have claimed that the bundles interpreted as tonofilaments by Kepes are not actually tonofilaments but are the type 1 filaments usually found in Cushing's disease, and thus this tumor should be a silent subtype-1 adenoma because of the lack of Cushing's syndrome. Therefore, such compound lesions may represent the fortuitous association of a pituitary adenoma and a Rathke's cleft cyst (106).

Lymphocytic Adenohypophysitis

Lymphocytic adenohypophysitis is an uncommon pituitary disorder, although it is not as infrequent as was once considered. It occurs almost exclusively in women (one case has been reported in a man (76)), particularly during pregnancy and the puerperium. Patients present with headache and visual disturbance due to the expanding intrasellar mass and/or varying degrees of hypopituitarism (112, 182) (see Chapter 16). Hypopituitarism often occurs more rapidly in this disease than with pituitary adenomas, but subsequently resolves spontaneously in some cases (183). Hyperprolactinemia is also found in some instances (222). Imaging techniques delineate lymphocytic adenohypophysitis as a well–defined mass in the sella turcica with possible suprasellar extension that is often associated with optic compression, and it may thus be confused with a pituitary adenoma (13, 158). The pathogenesis is now assumed to be autoimmune (182) and this is probably one part of the polyglandular autoimmune syndrome (165), in view of the pituitary lymphocytic infiltration, the association with known autoimmune diseases (thyroiditis, pernicious anemia, adrenalitis, etc. (74, 141, 274)), and the common detection of antipituitary antibodies (177). However, it still remains to be determined whether the cause is cell–mediated, humoral autoimmune mechanisms, or both (112, 182).

The histological features are basically similar in all cases and resemble those found in

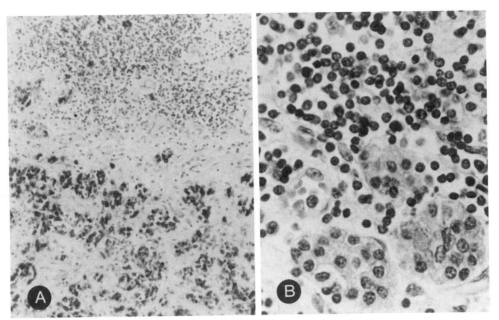

Figure 15.27. Lymphocytic adenohypophysitis. Massive lymphocytic infiltrations in the anterior lobe are depicted. Normal adenohypophyseal cells are found in the lower half in both figures, ×40 (A) ×250 (B).

many other autoimmune disorders; there are extensive infiltrates composed chiefly of lymphocytes and plasma cells that are associated with the destruction of adenohypophyseal cells; lymphoid follicles with germinal centers are also found (Fig. 15.27). No epithelioid cells or granulomatous features can be seen within the lesions. Immunohistochemical analysis is negative for the five known adenohypophyseal hormones within the involved areas, but shows varying degrees of immunopositivity within the surviving normal pituitary tissue. At the microscopic level, tuberculosis, syphilis, sarcoidosis, granulomatous hypophysitis, and postpartum hemorrhagic infarction must be considered in the differential diagnosis (182). Electron microscopy shows that all the different kinds of adenohypophyseal cells are either intact or suffering from varying degrees of damage. Interdigitated cells surrounded by infiltrating lymphocytes and oncocytic change associated with large lysosomal bodies fusing with secretory granules may also be found. The vessels show no pathological changes (4, 76, 158, 182, 274).

ACKNOWLEDGMENTS

The authors are grateful to Dr. Kalman Kovacs and Dr. Eva Horvath (St. Michael's Hospital, Toronto, Canada), for their continued encouragement and their generosity in offering some cases that are demonstrated as figures in this chapter.

REFERENCES

1. Abrams H.L., Spiro R., and Goldstein N. Metastases in carcinoma-analysis of 1000 autopsied cases. Cancer, *3:*74–85, 1950.
2. Afrasiabi A., Valenta L., and Gwinup G.A. A TSH-secreting pituitary tumour causing hyperthyroidism: presentation of a case review of the literature. Acta. Endocrinol. (Copen.), *92:*448–454, 1979.
3. Anniko M., and Wersall J. Morphological changes in bromocriptine-treated pituitary tumours. Acta. Otolaryngol. (Stockh.), *96:*337–353, 1983.
4. Asa, S.L., Bilbao, J.M., Kovacs, K., *et al.* Lymphocytic hypophysitis of pregnancy resulting in hypopituitarism: a distinct clinicopathological entity. Ann. Int. Med., *95:*166–171, 1981.
5. Asa S.L., Penz G., Kovacs K., *et al.* Prolactin cells in the human pituitary. A quantitative immunocytochemical analysis. Arch. Pathol. Lab. Med., *106:*360–363, 1982.

6. Asa S.L., Gerrie B.M., Singer W., *et al.* Gonadotropin secretion in vitro by human pituitary null cell adenomas and oncocytomas. J. Clin. Endocrinol. Metab., *62:*1011–1019, 1986.

7. Asa S.L., Gerrie B.M., Kovacs K., *et al.* Structure–function correlations of human pituitary gonadotroph adenomas in vitro. Lab. Invest., *58:*403–410, 1988.

8. Asa S.L., Kovacs K., Stefaneanu L., *et al.* Pituitary mammosomatotroph adenomas develop in old mice transgenic for growth hormone-releasing hormone. Proc. Soc. Exp. Biol. Med., *193:*232–235, 1990.

9. Asa S.L. In vitro culture techniques. In: *Functional Endocrine Pathology,* edited by K. Kovacs and S.L. Asar, pp. 109–123. Boston, Blackwell Scientific Publications, 1990.

10. Assadian H., Shimatsu A., Koshiyama H., *et al.* Secretion of alpha and TSH-beta subunits in patients with acromegaly: an in vivo study. Acta. Endocrinol. (Copenh.), *122:*729–734, 1990.

11. Axiotis C.A., Lippes H.A., Merino M.J., *et al.* Corticotroph cell pituitary adenoma within an ovarian teratoma. A new cause of Cushing's syndrome. Am. J. Surg. Pathol., *11:*218–224, 1987.

12. Barrow D.L., Spector R.H., Takei Y., *et al.* Symptomatic Rathke's cleft cysts located entirely in the suprasellar region: review of diagnosis, management, and pathogenesis. Neurosurgery, *16:*766–772, 1985.

13. Baskin D.S., Townsend J.J., and Wilson C.B. Lymphocytic adenohypophysitis of pregnancy simulating a pituitary adenoma: a distinct pathological entity. J. Neurosurg., *56:*148–153, 1982.

14. Bassetti M., Spada A., Pezzo G., *et al.* Bromocriptine treatment reduces the cell size in human macroprolactinomas: a morphometric study. J. Clin. Endocrinol. Metab., *58:*268–273, 1984.

15. Bassetti M., Arosio M., Spada A., *et al.* Growth hormone and prolactin secretion in acromegaly. Correlation between hormonal dynamics and immunocytochemical findings. J. Clin. Endocrinol. Metab., *67:*1195–1204, 1988.

16. Bassetti M., Brina M., Spada A., *et al.* Somatomammotrophic cells in GH-secreting and Prl-secreting human pituitary adenomas. J. Endocrinol. Invest., *12:*705–712, 1989.

17. Bauserman S.C., Hardman J.M., Schochet S.S., Jr., *et al.* Pituitary oncocytomas. Indispensable role of electron microscopy in its identification. Arch. Pathol. Lab. Med., *102:*456–459, 1978.

18. Bayoumi M.L. Rathke's cleft and its cysts. Edinburgh. Med. J., *55:*745–749, 1948.

19. Becker D.H. Parasellar granular cell tumors. In: *Neurosurgery,* Vol 1, edited by R.H. Wilkins and S.S. Rengachary, pp. 930–932, New York, McGraw-Hill, 1985.

20. Beckers A., Stevenaert A., Kovacs K., *et al.* The treatment of acromegaly with SMA 201–995. Advanc. Biosci., *69:*227–228, 1988.

21. Beck-Peccoz P., Bassettti M., Spada A., *et al.* Glycoprotein hormone α-subunit response to growth hormone (GH)-releasing hormone in patients with active acromegaly. Evidence for α-subunit and GH coexistence in the same tumoral cell. J. Clin. Endocrinol. Metab., *61:*541–546, 1985.

22. Beck-Peccoz P., Piscitelli G., Amr S., *et al.* Endocrine, biochemical, and morphological studies of a pituitary adenoma secreting growth hormone, thyrotropin (TSH), and α-subunit: evidence for secretion of TSH with increased bioactivity. J. Clin. Endocrinol. Metab., *62:*704–711, 1986.

23. Bendayan M., and Maestracci N.D. Pituitary adenomas: patterns of hPrl and hGH secretion as revealed by high resolution immunocytochemistry. Biol. Cell., *52:*129–138, 1984.

24. Bendayan M. Protein A-gold electron microscopic immunocytochemistry: methods, applications and limitations. J. Electron. Microsc. Tech., *1:*243–270, 1984.

25. Berg K.K., Scheithauer B.W., Felix I., *et al.* Pituitary adenomas that produce adrenocorticotropic hormone and alpha subunit: clinicopathological, immunohistochemical, ultrastructural and immunoelectron microscopic studies of nine cases. Neurosurgery, *26:*397–403, 1990.

26. Bergland R.M., and Torack R.M. An ultrastructural study of follicular cells in the human anterior pituitary. Am. J. Pathol., *57:*273–297, 1967.

27. Bevan J.S., Adams C.B.T., Burke C.W., *et al.* Factors in the outcome of transsphenoidal surgery for prolactinoma and nonfunctioning pituitary tumors, including pre-operative bromocriptine therapy. Clin. Endocrinol., (Oxf.), *26:*541–556, 1987.

28. Bilbao J.M., Horvath E., Hudson A.R., *et al.* Pituitary adenoma producing amyloid-like substance. Arch. Pathol., *99:*411–415, 1975.

29. Black P.M., Hsu D.W., Klibanski A., *et al.* Hormone production in clinically nonfunctioning pituitary adenomas. J. Neurosurg., *66:*244–250, 1987.

30. Boggan J.E., Tyrrell J.B., and Wilson C.B. Transsphenoidal microsurgical management of Cushing's disease. Report of 100 cases. J. Neurosurg., *59:*195–200, 1983.

31. Bonner R.A., Mukai K., and Oppenheimer J.H. Two unusual variants of Nelson's syndrome. J. Clin. Endocrinol. Metab., *49:*23–29, 1979.

32. Bonnyns M., Pasteels J.L., Herland M., *et al.* Comparison between thyrotropin concentration and cell morphology of anterior pituitary in asymptomatic atrophic thyroiditis. J. Clin. Endocrinol. Metab., *35:*722–728, 1972.

33. Borges J.L.C., Ridgway E.C., Kovacs K., *et al.* Follicle-stimulating hormone-secreting pituitary tumor with concomitant elevation of serum α-subunit levels. J. Clin. Endocrinol. Metab., *58:*937–941, 1984.

34. Branch C.L., and Laws E.R., Jr. Metastatic tumors of the sella turcica masquerading as primary pituitary tumors. J. Clin. Endocrinol. Metab., *65:*469–474, 1987.

35. Burrow G.N., Wortzman G., Rewcastle N.B., *et al.* Microadenomas of the pituitary and abnormal sellar tomograms in an unselected autopsy series. N. Engl. J. Med., *304:*156–158, 1981.

36. Cardell R.R., Jr., and Knighton R.S. The cytology

of a human pituitary tumor: an electron microscopic study. Trans. Am. Microsc. Soc., *85:*58–78, 1966.

37. Carey R.M., Varma S.K., and Drake C.R.Jr., *et al.* Ectopic secretion of corticotropin-releasing factor as a cause of Cushing's syndrome. N. Engl. J. Med., *311:*13–20, 1984.

38. Carpenter C.C.J., Solomon N., Silverberg S.G., *et al.* Schmidt's syndrome (thyroid and adrenal insufficiency): a review of the literature and a report of fifteen new cases including ten instances of coexistent diabetes mellitus. Medicine, *43:*153–180, 1964.

39. Chandler W.F., Schteingart D.E., Lloyd R.V., *et al.* Surgical treatment of Cushing's disease. J. Neurosurg., *66:*204–212, 1987.

40. Charpin C., Hassoun J., Oliver C., *et al.* Immunohistochemical and immunoelectron-microscopic study of pituitary adenomas associated with Cushing's disease. A report of 13 cases. Am. J. Pathol., *109:*1–7, 1982.

41. Chiodini P., Liuzzi A., Cozzi R., *et al.* Size reduction of macroprolactinomas by bromocriptine or lisuride treatment. J. Clin. Endocrinol. Metab., *53:*737–743, 1981.

42. Ciocca D.R., Puy L.A., and Stati A.O. Identification of seven hormone-producing cell types in the human pharyngeal hypophysis. J. Clin. Endocrinol. Metab., *60:*212–216, 1985.

43. Cohen D.L., Diengdoh J.V., Thomas D.G.T., *et al.* An intracranial metastasis from a Prl secreting pituitary tumour. Clin. Endocrinol. (Oxf.), *18:*259–264, 1983.

44. Comtois R., Bouchard J., and Robert F. Hypersecretion of gonadotropins by a pituitary adenoma: pituitary dynamic studies and treatment with bromocriptine in one patient. Fertil. Steril., *52:*569–573, 1989.

45. Cone L., Srinivasan M., and Romanul F.C.A. Granular cell tumor (choristoma) of the neurohypophysis: two cases and a review of the literature. A.J.N.R., *11:*403–406, 1990.

46. Corenblum B., Sirek A.M.T., Horvath E., *et al.* Human mixed somatotrophic and lactotrophic pituitary adenomas. J. Clin. Endocrinol. Metab., *42:*857–863, 1976.

47. Dakin A.C., and Marshall J.C. Medical therapy of hyperprolactinemia. In: *Medical Therapy of Endocrine Tumors,* vol. 18, edited by A.L. Barken, pp. 259–276, Endocrinol. Metab. Clin. North Am., Philadelphia, W.B. Saunders, 1989.

48. DeLellis R.A., Tischler A.S., and Wolfe H.J. Multidirectional differentiation in neuroendocrine neoplasms. J. Histochem. Cytochem., *32:*899–904, 1984.

49. Demura R., Jibiki K., Kubo O., *et al.* The significance of α-subunit as a tumor marker for gonadotropin-producing pituitary adenomas. J. Clin. Endocrinol. Metab., *63:*564–569, 1986.

50. Destephano D.B., Lloyd R.V., Pike A.M., *et al.* Pituitary adenomas: an immunohistochemical study of hormone production and chromogranin localization. Am. J. Pathol., *116:*464–472, 1984.

51. Dhillon A.P., Rode J. Immunohistochemical studies of S-100 protein and other neuronal characteristics expressed by granular cell tumors. Diagn. Histopathol., *6:*23–28, 1983.

52. Duchen L.W. Metastatic carcinoma in the pituitary gland and hypothalamus. J. Pathol. Bacteriol., *91:*247–355, 1966.

53. Duffy A.E., Asa S.L., and Kovacs K. Effect of bromocriptine on secretion and morphology of human prolactin cell adenomas in vitro. Horm. Res., *30:*32–38, 1988.

54. Erdheim J. Über einen hypophysentumor von ungewöhnlichem sitz. Beitr. Pathol. Anat., *46:*233–240, 1909.

55. Esiri M.M., Adams C.B.T., Burke C., *et al.* Pituitary adenomas: immunohistology and ultrastructural analysis of 118 tumors. Acta. Neuropathol. (Berl.), *62:*1–14, 1983.

56. Esiri M.M., Bevan J.S., Burke C.W., *et al.* Effect of bromocriptine treatment on the fibrous tissue component of prolactin-secreting and nonfunctioning macroadenomas of the pituitary gland. J. Clin. Endocrinol. Metab., *63:*383–388, 1986.

57. Fachnie J.D., Zafar M.S., Mellinger R.C., *et al.* Pituitary carcinoma mimics the ectopic adrenocorticotropin syndrome. J. Clin. Endocrinol. Metab., *50:*1062–1065, 1980.

58. Fatourechi V., Gharib H., Scheithauer B.W., *et al.* Pituitary thyrotropic adenoma associated with congenital hypothyroidism. Report of two cases. Am. J. Med., *76:*725–728, 1984.

59. Felix I.A., Horvath E., Kovaks K. Massive Crooke's hylinization in corticotroph cell adenomas of the human pituitary. A histological, immunocytological, and electron microscopic study of three cases. Acta. Neurochir. (Wien), *58:*235–243, 1982.

60. Felix I.A., Horvath E., Kovacs K., *et al.* Mammosomatotroph adenoma of the pituitary associated with gigantism and hyperprolactinemia. A morphological study including immunoelectron microscopy. Acta. Neuropathol. (Berl.), *71:*76–82, 1986.

61. Findling J.W., Aron D.C., and Tyrrell J.B. Cushing's disease. In: *The Pituitary Gland,* edited by H. Imura, pp. 441–466, New York, Raven Press, 1985.

62. Forbes M.S. Fine structure of the stellate cells in the pars distalis of the lizard Anolis carolinensis. J. Morphol., *136:*227–246, 1972.

63. Fossati P., Mazzuda M., Dwailly D., *et al.* Les adénomes gonadotropes hypophysaires. Presse. Med., *21:*937–939, 1988.

64. Friend J.N., Judge D.M., Sherman B.M., *et al.* FSH-secreting pituitary adenomas: stimulation and suppression studies in two patients. J. Clin. Endocrinol. Metab., *43:*650–657, 1976.

65. Friesen H.G., Fournier P., and Desjardins P. Pituitary prolactin in pregnancy and normal and abnormal lactation. Clin. Obstet Gynecol., *16:*25–45, 1973.

66. Gabrilove J.L., Anderson P.J., and Halmi N.S. Pituitary proopiomelanocortin-cell carcinoma occurring in conjunction with a glioblastoma in a patient with Cushing's disease and subsequent

Nelson's syndrome. Clin. Endocrinol. (Oxf.), *25:*117–126, 1986.

67. Gen M., Uozumi T., Ohta M., *et al.* Necrotic changes in prolactinomas after long term administration of bromocriptine. J. Clin. Endocrinol. Metab., *59:*463–470, 1984.

68. George S.R., Kovacs K., Asa S.L., *et al.* Effect of SMS 201–905, a long acting somatostatin analog on the secretion and morphology of a pituitary growth hormone cell adenoma. Clin. Endocrinol. (Oxf.), *26:*395–405, 1987.

69. Gerdes J., Lemke H., Baisch H., *et al.* Cell cycle analysis of a cell proliferation-associated human nuclear antigen defined by monoclonal antibody ki-67. J. Immunol., *133:*1710–1715, 1984.

70. Giannattasio G., and Bassetti M. Human pituitary adenomas. Recent advances in morphological studies. J. Endocrinol. Invest., *13:*435–454, 1990.

71. Girod C., Trouillas J., and Claustrat B. The human thyrotropic adenoma: pathologic diagnosis in five cases and critical review of the literature. Semin. Diagn. Pathol., *3:*58–68, 1986.

72. Gjerris A., Lindholm J., and Riishede J. Pituitary oncocytic tumor with Cushing's disease. Cancer, *42:*1818–1822, 1978.

73. Gold F.B. Epidemiology of pituitary adenomas. Epidemiol. Rev., *3:*163–183, 1981.

74. Goudie R.B., and Pinkerton P.H. Anterior hypophysitis and Hashimoto's disease in a young woman. J. Pathol., *83:*584–585, 1962.

75. Grisoli F., Leclerq T., Winteler J.P., *et al.* Thyroid-stimulating hormone pituitary adenomas and hyperthyroidism. Surg. Neurol., *25:*361–368, 1986.

76. Guay A.T., Agnello V., Tronic B.C., *et al.* Lymphocytic hypophysitis in a man. J. Clin. Endocrinol. Metab., *64:*631–634, 1987.

77. Hagerstrand I., and Schoneback J. Metastases to the pituitary gland. APMIS, *75:*64–70, 1969.

78. Halmi N.S., and Duello T. "Acidophilic" pituitary tumors. A reappraisal with differential staining and immunocytochemical techniques. Arch. Pathol. Lab. Med., *100:*346–351, 1976.

79. Halmi N.S. Immunostaining of growth hormone and prolactin in paraffin embedded and stored or previously stained materials. J. Histochem. Cytochem., *26:*486–495, 1978.

80. Halmi N.S. Occurrence of both growth hormone and prolactin-immunoreactive material in the cells of human somatotrophic pituitary adenomas containing mammotropic elements. Virchows. Arch. [A], *398:*19–31, 1982.

81. Hardy J. Cushing's disease: 50 years later. Can. J. Neurol. Sci., *9:*375–380, 1982.

82. Hassoun J., Charpin C., Jaquet P., *et al.* Cortico-lipotropin immunoreactivity in silent chromophobe adenomas. A light and electron microscopic study. Arch. Pathol. Lab. Med., *106:*25–30, 1982.

83. Hassoun J., Jacquel P., Devictor B., *et al.* Bromocriptine effects on cultured human prolactin-producing pituitary adenomas: in vitro, ultrastructural, morphometric and immunoelectron microscopic studies. J. Clin. Endocrinol. Metab., *61:*686–692, 1985.

84. Herman V., Fagin J., Gonsky R., *et al.* Clonal origin of pituitary adenomas. J. Clin. Endocrinol. Metab., *71:*1427–1433, 1990.

85. Himsworth R.L., Lewis J.G., and Rees L.H. A possible ACTH secreting tumour of the pituitary developing in a conventionally treated case of Addison's disease. Clin. Endocrinol. (Oxf.), *9:*131–139, 1978.

86. Ho K.Y., Weissberger A.J., Marbach P., *et al.* Therapeutic efficacy of the somatostatin analog SMA 201–995 (Octreotide) in acromegaly. Effects of dose and frequency and long-term safety. Ann. Intern. Med., *112:*173–181, 1990.

87. Holm R., Nesland J.M., Attramadal A., *et al.* Mixed growth hormone- and prolactin-cell adenomas of the pituitary gland. An immunoelectron microscopic study. J. Submicrosc. Cytol. Pathol., *21:*339–350, 1989.

88. Hori A. Suprasellar peri-infundibular ectopic adenohypophysis in fetal and adult brains. J. Neurosurg., *63:*113–115, 1985.

89. Horvath E., Kovacs K., Penz G., *et al.* Origin, possible function and the fate of follicular cells in the anterior lobe of the human pituitary. An electron microscopic study. Am. J. Pathol., *77:*199–206, 1974.

90. Horvath E., and Kovacs K. Ultrastructural classification of pituitary adenomas. Can. J. Neurol. Sci., *3:*9–21, 1976.

91. Horvath E., Kovacs K., Singer W., *et al.* Acidophil stem cell adenoma of the human pituitary. Arch. Pathol. Lab. Med., *101:*594–599, 1977.

92. Horvath E., and Kovacs K. Morphogenesis and significance of fibrous bodies in human pituitary adenomas. Virchows Arch. [B], *27:*69–78, 1978.

93. Horvath E., Kovacs K., Killinger D.W., *et al.* Silent corticotropic adenomas of the human pituitary gland. Am. J. Pathol., *98:*617–638, 1980.

94. Horvath E., Kovacs K., Singer W., *et al.* Acidophil stem cell adenoma of the human pituitary: clinicopathological analysis of 15 cases. Cancer, *47:*761–771, 1981.

95. Horvath E., and Kovacs K. Morphologic differentiation of sellar lesions associated with hyperprolactinemia. In: *Advances in Pathology (Anatomic and Clinical),* vol. 2, edited by E. Levy, pp. 363–366, Oxford, Pergamon Press, 1982.

96. Horvath E., Kovacs K., and Josse R. Pituitary corticotroph cell adenoma with marked abundance of microfilaments. Ultrastruct. Pathol., *5:*249–255, 1983.

97. Horvath E., Kovacs K., Killinger D.W., *et al.* Mammosomatotroph cell adenoma of the human pituitary: a morphologic entity. Virchows Arch. [A], *398:*277–289, 1983.

98. Horvath E., Kovacs K., Scheithauer B.W., *et al.* Pituitary adenomas producing growth hormone, prolactin, and one or more glycoprotein hormones: a histologic, immunohistochemical, and ultrastructural study of four surgically removed tumors. Ultrastruct. Pathol., *5:*171–183, 1983.

99. Horvath E., and Kovacs K. Gonadotroph adenomas of the human pituitary: sex related fine-structural dichotomy. A histologic, immunocytochem-

ical and electron microscopic study of 30 tumors. Am. J. Pathol., *117*:429–440, 1984.

100. Horvath E., and Kovacs K. Pathology of prolactin cell adenomas of the human pituitary. Semin. Diagn. Pathol., *3*:4–17, 1986.

101. Horvath E., and Kovacs K. Fine structural cytology of the adenohypophysis in rat and man. J. Electron. Microsc. Tech., *8*:401–432, 1988.

102. Horvath E., and Kovacs K. Pathology of the hypothalamus and pituitary gland. In: *Diagnosis and Pathology of Endocrine Diseases,* edited by G. Mendelsohn, pp. 379–412, Philadelphia, Lippincott, 1988.

103. Horvath E., and Kovacs K. Pituitary gland. Path. Res. Pract., *183*:129–142, 1988.

104. Horvath E., Kovacs K., Smyth H.S., *et al.* A novel type of pituitary adenomas: morphological features and clinical correlations. J. Clin. Endocrinol. Metab., *66*:1111–1118, 1988.

105. Horvath E. Pituitary hyperplasia. Path. Res. Pract., *183*:623–625, 1988.

106. Horvath E., and Kovacs K. The adenohypophysis. In: *Functional Endocrine Pathology,* edited by K. Kovacs, and S.L. Asa, pp. 245–281, Boston, Blackwell Scientific Publication, 1990.

107. Ikeda H., Yoshimoto T., and Suzuki J. Immunohistochemical study of Rathke's cleft cyst. Acta. Neuropathol. (Berl.), *77*:33–38, 1988.

108. Jacoby L.B., Hedley-Whyte E.T., Pulaski K., *et al.* Clonal origin of pituitary adenomas. J. Neurosurg., *73*:731–735, 1990.

109. Jameson J.L., Klibanski A., Black P.M., *et al.* Glycoprotein hormone genes are expressed in clinically nonfunctioning pituitary adenomas. J. Clin. Invest., *80*:1472–1478, 1987.

110. Jaquet P., Hassoun J., Delori P., *et al.* A human pituitary adenoma secreting thyrotropin and prolactin: immunohistochemical, biochemical, and cell culture studies. J. Clin. Endocrinol. Metab., *59*:817–824, 1984.

111. Jautzke G. Simultaneous production of the alpha-subunit of glycoprotein hormones and other hormones in pituitary adenomas. Path. Res. Pract., *183*:601–605, 1988.

112. Jensen M.D., Handwerger B.S., Scheithauer B.W., *et al.* Lymphocytic hypophysitis with isolated corticotroph deficiency. Ann. Int. Med., *105*:200–203, 1986.

113. Jordan R.M., and Köhler P.O. Recent advances in diagnosis and treatment of pituitary tumors. Adv. Intern. Med., *32*:299–324, 1987.

114. Kagayama M. The follicular cell in the pars distalis of the dog pituitary gland: an electron microscopic study. Endocrinology, *77*:1053–1060, 1965.

115. Kalyanaraman U.P., Halmi N.S., and Elwood P.W. Prolactin-secreting pituitary oncocytoma with galactorrhea-amenorrhea syndrome. Cancer, *46*:1584–1589, 1980.

116. Kameya T., Tsumuraya M., Adachi I., *et al.* Ultrastructure, immunohistochemistry and hormone release of pituitary adenomas in relation to prolactin production. Virchows Arch. [A], *387*:31–46, 1980.

117. Kanie N., Kageyama N., Kuwayama A., *et al.* Pi-

tuitary adenomas in acromegalic patients: an immunohistochemical and endocrinological study with special reference to prolactin-secreting adenoma. J. Clin. Endocrinol. Metab., *57*:1093–1101, 1983.

118. Katz M.S., Gregerman R.I., Horvath E., *et al.* Thyrotroph cell adenoma of the human pituitary gland associated with primary hypothyroidism: clinical and morphological features. Acta. Endocrinol. (Copenh.), *95*:41–48, 1980.

119. Kawakita S., Asa S.L., and Kovacs K. Effects of growth hormone-releasing hormone (GHRH) on densely granulated somatotroph adenomas and sparsely granulated somatotroph adenomas in vitro: a morphological and functional investigation. J. Endocrinol. Invest., *12*:443–448, 1989.

120. Kepes J.J. Transitional cell tumor of the pituitary gland developing from Rathke's cleft cyst. Cancer, *41*:337–343, 1978.

121. Klibanski A., Ridgway E.C., and Zervas N.T. Pure alpha subunit-secreting pituitary tumors. J. Neurosurg., *59*:585–589, 1983.

122. Klibanski A. Nonsecreting pituitary tumors. In: *Pituitary tumors: Diagnosis and Management.* Endocrinol. Metab. Clin. North Am. Vol 16, edited by M.E. Molitch, pp. 793–804. Philadelphia, W.B. Saunders, 1987.

123. Klibanski A., Zervas N.T., Kovacs K., *et al.* Clinically silent hypersecretion of growth hormone in patients with pituitary tumors. J. Neurosurg., *66*:806–811, 1987.

124. Knosp E., Kitz K., and Perneczky A. Proliferation activity in pituitary adenomas: measurement by monoclonal antibody Ki-67. Neurosurgery, *25*:927–930, 1989.

125. Kovacs K., and Horvath E. Pituitary "chromophobe" adenoma composed of oncocytes. Arch. Pathol., *95*:2351239, 1973.

126. Kovacs K., Horvath E., Bayley J.A., *et al.* Silent corticotroph cell adenoma with lysosomal accumulation and crinophagy. Am. J. Med., *64*:492–499, 1977.

127. Kovacs K., Horvath E., Van Look G.R., *et al.* Pituitary adenomas associated with elevated blood follicle-stimulating hormone levels: a histologic, immunocytologic, and electron microscopic study of two cases. Fertil. Steril., *29*:622–628, 1978.

128. Kovacs K., Horvath E., Rewcastle N.B., *et al.* Gonadotroph cell adenoma of the pituitary in a woman with long-standing hypogonadism. Arch. Gynecol., *229*:57–65, 1980.

129. Kovacs K., Horvath E., Ryan N., *et al.* Null cell adenoma of the human pituitary gland. Virchows Arch. [A], *387*:165–174, 1980.

130. Kovacs K., Horvath E., and Ryan N. Immunocytology of the human pituitary. In: *Diagnostic immunohistochemistry,* edited by R.A. Delellis, pp. 17–35, New York, Mason, 1981.

131. Kovacs K. Metastatic cancer of the pituitary gland. Oncology, *27*:533–542, 1983.

132. Kovacs K., Horvath E., Thorner M.O., *et al.* Mammosomatotroph hyperplasia associated with acromegaly and hyperprolactinemia in a patient with the McCune-Albright syndrome. A histologic, im-

munocytologic and ultrastructural study of the surgically-removed adenohypophysis. Virchows Arch. [A], *403:*77–86, 1984.

133. Kovacs K., and Horvath E. Pathology of growth hormone-producing tumors of the human pituitary. Semin. Diagn. Pathol., *3:*18–33, 1986.

134. Kovacs K., and Horvath E. Tumors of the pituitary gland. In: *Atlas of Tumor Pathology, Fascicle 21, 2nd series,* edited by W.H. Hartman, p. 1–269, Washington DC, Armed Forces Institute of Pathology, 1986.

135. Kovacs K. Pathology of growth hormone excess. Path. Res. Pract., *183:*565–568, 1988.

136. Kovacs K., Horvath E., Asa S.L., *et al.* Pituitary cells producing more than one hormone. Human pituitary adenomas. TEM 1989 Nov/Dec:104–107.

137. Kovacs K., Lloyd R.V., Horvath E., *et al.* Silent somatotroph adenomas of the human pituitary. A morphologic study of three cases including immunocytochemistry, electron microscopy, in vitro examination, and in situ hybridization. Am. J. Pathol., *134:*345–353, 1989.

138. Kovacs K., Asa S.L., Horvath E., *et al.* Null cell adenomas of the pituitary: attempts to resolve their cytogenesis. In: *Endocrine Pathology Update,* edited by J. Lechago, and T. Kameya, pp. 17–31, Philadelphia, Field and Wood Publishers, 1990.

139. Kuroki M., Tanaka R., Yokoyama M., *et al.* Subarachnoidal dissemination of a pituitary adenoma. Surg. Neurol., *28*71–76, 1987.

140. Kuwayama A., and Kageyama N. Current management of Cushing's disease. Part II. Contemp. Neurosurg., *7:*1–6, 1985.

141. Lack E.E. Lymphoid "hypophysitis" with end organ insufficiency. Arch. Pathol. Lab. Med., *99.*215–219, 1975.

142. Lambèrts S.W.V., deLange S.A., and Stefanko S.Z. Adrenocorticotropin-secreting pituitary adenomas originate from the anterior or the intermediate lobe in Cushing's disease: differences in the regulation of hormone secretion. J. Clin. Endocrinol. Metab., *54:*286–291, 1982.

143. Lambèrts S.W.J., Liuzzi A., Chiodini P.G., *et al.* The value of plasma prolactin levels in the prediction of the responsiveness of growth hormone secretion to bromocriptine and TRH in acromegaly. Eur. J. Clin. Invest., *12:*151–155, 1982.

144. Lambèrts S.W.J., Verleun T., Oosterom R., *et al.* The effects of bromocriptine, thyrotropin-releasing hormone, and gonadotropin-releasing hormone on hormone secretion by gonadotropin-secreting pituitary adenomas in vivo and in vitro. J. Clin. Endocrinol. Metab., *64:*524–530, 1987.

145. Landolt A.M., and Oswald U.W. Histology and ultrastructure of an oncocytic adenoma of the human pituitary. Cancer, *31:*1099–1105, 1973.

146. Landolt A.M. Ultrastructure of human sella tumors. Correlations of clinical findings and morphology. Acta. Neurochir. Suppl., (Wien), *27:*1–167, 1975.

147. Landolt A.M., Ryffel U., Hosbach H.U., *et al.* Ultrastructural tubular inclusions in endothelial cells of pituitary tumors associated with acromegaly. Virchows Arch. [A], *370:*129–140, 1976.

148. Landolt A.M., and Rothenbuhler V. Pituitary adenoma calcification. Arch. Pathol. Lab. Med., *101:*22–27, 1977.

149. Landolt A.M. Progress in pituitary adenoma biology: results of research and clinical applications. Adv. Tech. Stand. Neurosurg., *5:*3–49, 1978.

150. Landolt A.M., Rothenbühler V., and Kistler G.S. Morphology of the chromophobe adenoma. In: *Treatment of pituitary adenomas.,* edited by R. Fahlbusch, and K. von Werder, *et al.* 154–171, Stuttgart, 1st Eur. Workshop Rottach-Egern. Thieme, 1978.

151. Landolt A., Minder H., Osterwalder V., *et al.* Bromocriptine reduces the size of cells in prolactin-secreting pituitary adenomas. Experientia, *39:*625–626, 1983.

152. Landolt A.M., and Osterwalder V. Perivascular fibrosis in prolactinomas: is it increased by bromocriptine? J. Clin. Endocrinol. Metab., *58:*1179–1183, 1984.

153. Landolt A.M., Kleihues P., and Heitz P.U. Amyloid deposits in pituitary adenomas. Arch. Pathol. Lab. Med., *111:*453–458, 1987.

154. Landolt A.M., Osterwalder V., and Stuckmann G. Preoperative treatment of acromegaly with SMS 201–995: surgical and pathological observations. In: *Growth Hormone, Growth Factors, and Acromegaly,* edited by D.K. Lüdecke, and G. Tolis, pp. 229–244, New York, Raven Press, 1987.

155. Landolt A.M., Shibata T., and Kleihues P. Growth rate of human pituitary adenomas. J. Neurosurg., *67:*803–806, 1987.

156. Landolt A.M., Heitz P.U., and Zenklusen H.R. Production of the α-subunit of glycoprotein hormones by pituitary adenomas. Path. Res. Pract., *183:*610–612, 1988.

157. Lauriola L., Cocchia D., Sentinelli S., *et al.* Immunohistochemical detection of folliculo-stellate cells in human pituitary adenomas. Virchows Arch. [B], *47:*189–197, 1984.

158. Levine S.N., Benzel E.C., Fowler M.R., *et al.* Lymphocytic adenohypophysitis: clinical, radiological, and magnetic resonance imaging characterization. Neurosurgery, *22:*937–941, 1988.

159. Liss L., and Kahn E.A. Pituicytoma: tumor of the sella turcica: a clinicopathological study. J. Neurosurg., *15:*481–488, 1958.

160. Lloyd R.V., Gikes R.V., and Chandler W.F. Prolactin and growth hormone-producing pituitary adenomas. An immunohistochemical and ultrastructural study. Am. J. Surg. Pathol., *7:*251–260, 1983.

161. Lloyd R.V., Chandler W.F., McKeever P.E., *et al.* The spectrum of ACTH-producing pituitary lesions. Am. J. Surg. Pathol., *10:*618–626, 1986.

162. Lloyd R.V. Use of molecular probes in the study of endocrine disease. Hum. Pathol., *18:*1199–1211, 1987.

163. Lloyd R.V., Anagnostou D., Cano M., *et al.* Analysis of mammosomatotropic cells in normal and neoplastic human pituitary tissues by the reverse hemolytic plaque assay and immunocytochemistry. J. Clin. Endocrinol. Metab., *66:*1103–1110, 1988.

164. Lloyd R.V., Cano M., Chandler W.F., *et al.*

Human growth hormone and prolactin secreting pituitary adenomas analyzed by in situ hybridization. Am. J. Pathol., *134*:605–613, 1989.

165. Loriaux D.L. The polyendocrine deficiency sydromes (editorial). N. Engl. J. Med., *312*:1568–1569, 1985.

166. Luse S.A., and Kernohan J.W. Granular-cell tumors of the stalk and posterior lobe of the pituitary gland. Cancer, *8*:616–622, 1955.

167. Luzi P., Miracco C., Lio R., *et al.* Endocrine inactive pituitary carcinoma metastasizing to cervical lymph nodes: a case report. Hum. Pathol., *18*:90–92, 1987.

168. Malarkey W.B., Kovacs K., and O'Dorisio T.M. Response of a GH- and TSH-secreting pituitary adenoma to a somatostain analogue (SMS201–995): evidence that GH and TSH coexist in the same cell and secretory granules. Neuroendocrinology, *49*:267–274, 1989.

169. Martinez A.J. The pathology of nonfunctioning pituitary adenomas. Semin. Diagn. Pathol., *3*:83–94, 1986.

170. Martinez L.J., Osterholm J.L., Berry R.G., *et al.* Transsphenoidal removal of a Rathke's cleft cyst. Neurosurgery, *4*:63–65, 1979.

171. Martin N.A., Hales M., and Wilson C.B. Cerebellar metastasis during treatment with bromocriptine. J. Neurosurg., *55*:615–619, 1981.

172. Mashiter K., Adams E., and Van Noorden S. Secretion of LH, FSH and Prl shown by cell culture and immunocytochemistry of human functionless pituitary adenomas. Clin. Endocrinol. (Oxf.), *15*:103–112, 1981.

173. Mashiter K., Van Noorden S., Fahlbusch R., *et al.* Hyperthyroidism due to TSH secreting pituitary adenoma: case report, treatment and evidence for adenoma TSH by morphological and cell culture studies. Clin. Endocrinol. (Oxf.), *18*:473–483, 1983.

174. Matsumura A., Meguro K., Doi M., *et al.* Suprasellar ectopic pituitary adenoma. Case report and review of the literature. Neurosurgery, *26*:681–685, 1990.

175. Matsushima T., Fukui M., Ohta M., *et al.* Ciliated and goblet cells in craniopharyngioma: light and electron microscopic studies at surgery and autopsy. Acta. Neuropathol. (Berl.), *50*:199–205, 1980.

176. Max M.B., Deck M.D.F., and Rottenberg D.A. Pituitary metastasis: incidence in cancer patients and clinical differentiation from pituitary adenoma. Neurology, *31*:998–1003, 1981.

177. Mayfield R.K., Levine J.H., Gordon L., *et al.* Lymphoid adenohypophysitis presenting as a pituitary tumor. Am. J. Med., *69*:619–623, 1980.

178. McComb D.J., Kovacs K., Horvath E. Correlative ultrastructural morphometry of human prolactin-producing adenomas. Acta. Neurochir. (Wien), *53*:217–223, 1980.

179. McComb D.J., Bayley T.A., Horvath E., *et al.* Monomorphous plurihormonal adenoma of the human pituitary. A histologic, immunocytologic and ultrastructural study. Cancer, *53*:1538–1544, 1984.

180. McCormick P.C., Post K.D., Kandji A.D., *et al.* Metastatic carcinoma to the pituitary gland. Br. J. Neurosurg., *3*:71–80, 1989.

181. McCutcheon I.E., Weintraub B.D., OldField E.H. Surgical treatment of thyrotropin-secreting adenomas. J. Neurosurg., *73*:674–683, 1990.

182. McDermott M.W., Griesdale D.E., Berry K., *et al.* Lymphocytic adenohypophysitis. Can. J. Neurol. Sci., *15*:38–43, 1988.

183. McGrail K.M., Beyerl B.D., Black P.M., *et al.* Lymphocytic adenohypophysitis of pregnancy with complete recovery. Neurosurgery, *20*:791–793, 1987.

184. McGrath P. Cysts of sellar and pharyngeal hypophyses. Pathology, *3*:123–131, 1971.

185. McGregor A.M., Scanlon M.F.D., Hall R., *et al.* Effects of bromocriptine on pituitary tumour size. BMJ, *2*:700–703, 1979.

186. McKeever P.E., Koppelman M.C.S., Metcalf D., *et al.* Refractory Cushing's disease caused by multinodular ACTH-cell hyperplasia. J. Neuropathol. Exp. Neurol., *41*:490–499, 1982.

187. McNicol A.M. Current topics in neuropathology: Cushing's disease. Neuropathol. Appl. Neurobiol. II, 485–498, 1985.

188. McNicol A.M. A study of intermediate lobe differentiation in the human pituitary gland. J. Pathol., *150*:169–173, 1986.

189. McNicol A.M., Teasdale G.M., Beastall G.H. A study of corticotroph adenomas in Cushing's disease: no evidence of intermediate lobe origin. Clin. Endocrinol. (Oxf.), *24*:715–722, 1986.

190. McNicol A.M. Pituitary adenomas (invited review). Histopathology, *11*:995–1011, 1987.

191. Melmed S. Acromegaly. N. Engl. J. Med. *322*:966–977, 1990.

192. Miura M., Matsukado Y., Kodama T., *et al.* Clinical and histopathological characteristics of gonadotropin-producing pituitary adenomas. J. Neurosurg., *62*:376–382, 1985.

193. Moran A., Asa S.L., Kovacs K., *et al.* Gigantism due to pituitary mammosomatotroph hyperplasia. N. Engl. J. Med., *323*:322–327, 1990.

194. Mori H., Mori S., Saitoh Y., *et al.* Growth hormone-producing pituitary adenoma with crystal-like amyloid immunohistochemically positive for growth hormone. Cancer, *55*:96–102, 1985.

195. Morris C., Hitchock E. Immunocytochemistry of folliculo-stellate cells of normal and neoplastic human pituitary gland. J. Clin. Pathol., *38*:481–488, 1985.

196. Mukada K., Ohta M., Uozumi T., *et al.* Ossified prolactinoma: case report. Neurosurgery, *20*:473–475, 1987.

197. Mukai K. Pituitary adenomas: Immunocytochemical study of 150 tumors with clinicopathologic correlations. Cancer, *52*:648–653, 1983.

198. Myles S.T., Johns R.D., Curry C. Clinicopathological conference: carcinoma of the pituitary gland with metastases to bone. Can. J. Neurol. Sci., *11*:310–317, 1984.

199. Nagaya T., Doi T., Katsumata T., *et al.* Silent corticotroph cell adenoma with high levels of plasma ACTH. Case report. Neurol. Med. Chir. (Tokyo), *27*:795–798, 1987.

200. Nagaya T., Seo H., Kuwayama A., *et al.* Pro-opi-

omelanocortin gene expression in silent cortico-troph-cell adenoma and Cushing's disease. J. Neurosurg., *72:*262–267, 1990.

201. Nagaya T., Seo H., Kuwayama A., *et al.* Prolactin gene expression in human growth hormone-secreting adenomas. J. Neurosurg., *72:*879–882, 1990.

202. Nathrath W.B.J., Remberger K. Immunohistochemical study of granular cell tumors. Demonstration of neuron specific enolase, S 100 protein, laminin and α-1-antichymotrypsin. Virchows. Arch. [A], *408:*421–434, 1986.

203. Nelson K., de Chadarevian J.P. Ectopic anterior pituitary corticotropic tumour in a six-year-old boy. Histological ultrastructural and immunocytochemical study. Virchows. Arch. [A], *411:*267–273, 1987.

204. Nelson P.B., Robinson A.G., Martinez A.J. Metastatic tumor of the pituitary gland., *21:*941–944, 1987.

205. Neumann P.E., Goldman J.E., Horoupian D.S., *et al.* Fibrous bodies in growth hormone-secreting adenomas contain cytokeratin filaments. Arch. Pathol. Lab. Med., *109:*505–508, 1985.

206. Nicolis G.L., Modhi G., Gabrilove J.L. Gonadotropin-producing pituitary adenomas. A case report and review of the literature. Mt. Sinai J. Med., *49:*297–304, 1982.

207. Nicolis G., Shimshi M., Allen C., *et al.* Gonadotropin-producing pituitary adenoma in a man with long-standing primary hypogonadism. J. Clin. Endocrinol. Metab., *66:*237–241, 1988.

208. Nishio S., Mizuno J., Barrow D.L., *et al.* Pituitary tumors composed of adenohypophyseal adenoma and Rathke's cleft cyst element: a clinicopathological study. Neurosurgery, *2:*371–377, 1987.

209. Nishizaki T., Orita T., Furutani Y., *et al.* Flow-cytometric DNA analysis and immunohistochemical measurement of Ki-67 and BUdR labeling indices in human brain tumors. J. Neurosurg., *70:*379–384, 1989.

210. Ogilvy K.M., and Jakubowski J. Intracranial dissemination of pituitary adenomas. J. Neurol. Neurosurg. Psychiatry, *36:*199–205, 1973.

211. Okamoto S., Handa H., Ishikawa M., *et al.* Computed tomography in intra- and suprasellar epithelial cysts (symptomatic Rathke cleft cysts). A.J.N.R., *6:*515–519, 1985.

212. Oppizzi G., Liuzzi A., Chiodini P., *et al.* Dopaminergic treatment of acromegaly: different effects on hormone secretion and tumor size. J. Clin. Endocrinol. Metab., *58:*988–992, 1984.

213. Ortiz-Suarez H., Erickson D.L. Pituitary adenomas of adolescents. J. Neurosurg., *43:*437–439, 1975.

214. Osamura R.Y., Watanabe K. Immunohistochemical colocalization of growth hormone (GH) and subunit in human GH secreting pituitary adenomas. Virchows. Arch. [A], *411:*323–330, 1987.

215. Osamura R.Y., Watanabe K. Immunohistochemical studies of human FSH producing pituitary adenomas. Virchows. Arch. [A], *413:*61–68, 1988.

216. Parent A.D., Bebin J., Smith R.R. Incidental pituitary adenomas. J. Neurosurg., *54:*228–231, 1981.

217. Peterson R.E., Kourides I.A., Horwith M., *at al.* Luteinizing hormone and α-subunit-secreting pituitary tumor: positive feedback of estrogen. J. Clin. Endocrinol. Metab., *52:*692–698, 1981.

218. Phifer R.F., Spicer S.S., Orth D.H. Specific demonstration of the human hypophyseal cells which produce adrenocorticotropic hormone. J. Clin. Endocrinol. Metab., *31:*347–361, 1970.

219. Pioro E.P., Scheithauer B.W., Laws E.R., Jr., *et al.* Combined thyrotroph and lactotroph cell hyperplasia simulating prolactin-secreting pituitary adenoma in long-standing primary hypothyroidism. Surg. Neurol., *29:*218–226, 1988.

220. Popović V., Nešović M., Mićić D., *et al.* A comparison among the effectiveness of growth hormone suppression in active acromegaly of bromocriptine and long acting somatostatin analogue (SMS 201-995). Exp. Clin. Endocrinol., *95:*251–257, 1990.

221. Popovitch E.R., Sutton C.H., Becker N.H., *et al.* Fine structure and histochemical studies of choristomas of the neurohypophysis. J. Neuropathol. Exp. Neurol., *29:*155–156, 1970.

222. Portocarrero C.J., Robinson A.G., Taylor A.L., *et al.* Lymphoid hypophysitis: an unusual cause of hyperprolactinemia and enlarged sella turcica. J.A.M.A., *246:*1811–1812, 1981.

223. Post K.D., McCormick P.C., Hays A.P., *et al.* Metastatic carcinoma to pituitary adenoma. Surg. Neurol., *30:*286–292, 1988.

224. Preissner C.M., Klee G.G., Scheithauer B.W., *et al.* Free α subunit of the pituitary glycoprotein hormones. Measurement in serum and tissue of patients with pituitary tumors. Am. J. Clin. Pathol., *94:*417–421, 1990.

225. Queiroz L.S., Facure N.O., Facure J.J., *et al.* Pituitary carcinoma with liver metastases and Cushing syndrome. Arch. Pathol., *99:*32–35, 1975.

226. Ramsay J.A., Kovacs K., Scheithauer B.W., *et al.* Metastatic carcinoma to pituitary adenomas: a report of two cases. Exp. Clin. Endocrinol., *92:*69–76, 1988.

227. Randall R., Scheithauer B.W., Laws E.R., Jr. Hormone-containing, non-secreting pituitary tumors: clinically silent monohormonal pituitary adenomas. Trans. Am. Clin. Climatol. Assoc., *96:*98–103, 1984.

228. Rasmussen C., Larsson S.G., Bergh T. The occurrence of macroscopical pituitary calcifications in prolactinomas. Neuroradiology, *31:*507–511, 1990.

229. Reincke M., Allolio B., Saeger W., *et al.* A pituitary adenoma secreting high molecular weight adrenocorticotropin without evidence of Cushing's disease. J. Clin. Endocrinol. Metab., *65:*1296–1300, 1987.

230. Rengachary S.S., Tomita T., Jefferies B.F. *et al.* Structural changes in human pituitary tumor after bromocriptine therapy. Neurosurgery, *10:*242–252, 1982.

231. Riedel M., Saeger W., Lüdecke D.K. Grading of pituitary adenomas in acromegaly. Comparison of

light microscopical, immunocytochemical, and clinical data. Virchows. Arch. [A], *407*:83–95, 1985.

232. Riedel M., Noldus J., Saeger W., *et al.* Sellar lesions associated with isolated hyperprolactinemia: morphological, immunocytochemical, hormonal and clinical results. Acta. Endocrinol. (Copenh.), *113*:196–203, 1986.

233. Rilliet B., Mohr G., Robert F. Calcification in pituitary adenomas. Surg. Neurol., *15*:249–255, 1981.

234. Robert F. Electron microscopy of pituitary tumors. In: *Clinical Management of Pituitary Disorders,* edited by G.T. Tindall and W.F. Collins, pp. 113–131, New York, Raven Press, 1979.

235. Robert F., Hardy J. Human corticotroph cell adenomas. Semin. Diagn. Pathol., *3*:34–41, 1986.

236. Robert F., Pelletier G., Serri O., *et al.* Mixed growth hormone and prolactin-secreting human pituitary adenomas: a pathologic, immunocytochemical, ultrastructural, and immunoelectron microscopic study. Hum. Path., *19*:1327–1334, 1988.

237. Rode J., Dhillon A.P., Doran J.F., *et al.* PGP9.5, a new marker for human neuroendocrine tumors. Histopathology, *9*:147–158, 1985.

238. Rothman L.M., Sher J., Quencer R.M., *el al.* Intracranial ectopic adenoma. Case report. J. Neurosurg., *44*:96–99, 1976.

239. Roy S. Ultrastructure of oncocytic adenoma of the human pituitary gland. Acta. Neuropathol. (Berl.), *41*:169–171, 1978.

240. Russel D.S., Rubinstein L.J. Pathology of Tumours of the Nervous System, 4th ed., pp. 572–573, Baltimore, Williams & Wilkins, 1989.

241. Saeger W. Vergleichende licht- und elektronenmikroskopische Untersuchungen an oncocytären Hypophysenadenomen. Virchows. Arch. [A], *369*:29–44, 1975.

242. Saeger W. Morphology of ACTH-producing pituitary tumors. In: *Treatment of Pituitary Adenomas,* edited by R. Fahlbusch and K. von Werder, pp. 122–130, Stuttgart, Thieme, 1978.

243. Saeger W., Lüdecke D.K. Pituitary adenomas with hyperfunction of TSH. Frequency, histological classification, immunohistochemistry and ultrastructure. Virchows. Arch. [A], *394*:255–267, 1982.

244. Saeger W. Pathology of the pituitary gland. In: *Management of Pituitary Disease,* edited by P.E. Belchetz, pp. 253–289, London, Chapman and Hall, 1984.

245. Saeger W., Mohr K., Caselitz J., *et al.* Light and electron microscopical morphometry of pituitary adenomas in hyperprolactinemia. Path. Res. Pract., *181*:544–550, 1986.

246. Saeger W., Gunzl H., Meyer M., *et al.* Immunohistological studies on clinically silent pituitary adenomas. Endocr. Pathol., *1*:37–44, 1990.

247. Saitoh Y., Mori S., Arita N., *et al.* Cytosuppressive effect of bromocriptine on human prolactinomas: stereological analysis of ultrastructural alterations with special reference to secretory granules. Cancer Res., *46*:1507–1512, 1986.

248. Sakurai T., Seo H., Yamamoto N., *et al.* Detection of mRNA of prolactin and ACTH in clinically nonfunctioning pituitary adenomas. J. Neurosurg., *69*:653–659, 1988.

249. Samaan N.A., Osborne B.M., Mackay B., *et al.* Endocrine and morphologic studies of pituitary adenomas secondary to primary hypothyroidism. J. Clin. Endocrinol. Metab., *45*:903–911, 1977.

250. Sano T., Asa S.L., Kovacs K. Growth hormone-releasing hormone-producing tumors: clinical, biochemical, and morphological manifestations. Endocr. Rev., *9*:357–373, 1988.

251. Sano T., Kovacs K., Stefaneanu L., *et al.* Spontaneous pituitary gonadotroph nodules in aging male Lobund-Wistar rats. Lab. Invest., *61*:343–349, 1989.

252. Sano T., Kovacs K., Asa S.L., *et al.* Immunoreactive luteinizing hormone in functioning corticotroph adenomas of the pituitary. Immunohistochemical and tissue culture studies of two cases. Virchows. Arch. [A], *417*:361–367, 1990.

253. Sano T. Plurihormonality in neuroendocrine tumors [Editorial]. Endocr. Pathol., *1*:193–195, 1990.

254. Sano T., Ohshima T., Yamada S. Expression of glycoprotein hormones and intracytoplasmic distribution of cytokeratin in growth hormone-producing adenomas. Path. Res. Pract., *187*:530–533, 1991.

255. Scanlon M.F., Howells S., Peters J.R., *et al.* Hyperprolactinaemia, amenorrhoea and galactorrhoea due to pituitary thyrotroph adenoma. Clin. Endocrinol. (Oxf.), *23*:35–42, 1985.

256. Scheithauer B.W., Horvath E., Kovacs K., *et al.* Plurihormonal pituitary adenomas. Semin. Diag. Pathol., *3*:69–82, 1986.

257. Scheithauer B.W., Kovacs K., Laws E.R. Jr., *et al.* Pathology of invasive pituitary tumors with special reference to functional classification. J. Neurosurg., *65*:733–744, 1986.

258. Scheithauer B.W., Kovacs K., Randall R.V. The pituitary gland in untreated Addison's disease. Arch. Pathol. Lab. Med., *107*:484–487, 1983.

259. Scheithauer B.W. Surgical pathology of the pituitary: the adenomas. Pathol. Annu., 19 *(Part 1)*:313–374, 1984.

260. Scheithauer B.W. Surgical pathology of the pituitary: The adenomas. Pathol. Annu., 19 *(Part II)*:269–329, 1984.

261. Scheithauer B.W., Kovacs K., Randall R.V., *et al.* Pituitary gland in hypothyroidism: histologic and immunocytologic study. Arch. Pathol. Lab. Med., *109*:499–504, 1985.

262. Scheithauer B.W., Randall R.V., Laws E.R., Jr., *et al.* Prolactin cell carcinoma of the pituitary. Clinicopathologic, immunohistochemical, and ultrastructural study of a case with cranial and extracranial metastases. Cancer, *55*:598–604, 1985.

263. Scheithauer B.W., Kovacs K.T., Randall R.V., *et al.* Effects of estrogen on the human pituitary: a clinicopathologic study. Mayo. Clin. Proc., *64*:1077–1084, 1989.

264. Scheithauer B.W., Sano T., Kovacs K.T., *et al.* The pituitary gland in pregnancy: a clinicopathologic

and immunohistochemical study of 69 cases. Mayo Clin. Proc., *65*:461–474, 1990.

265. Schlechte J., Dolan K., Sherman B., *et al.* The natural history of untreated hyperprolactinemia: a prospective analysis. J. Clin. Endocrinol. Metab., *68*:412–418, 1989.

266. Schnall A.M., Kovacs K., Brodkey J.S., *et al.* Pituitary Cushing's disease without adenoma. Acta. Endocrinol. (Copenh.), *94*:297–303, 1980.

267. Schochet S.S. Jr., McCormick W.F., Halmi N.S. Acidophil adenomas with intracytoplasmic filamentous aggregates. Arch. Pathol., *94*:16–22, 1972.

268. Selman W.R., Laws E.R., Jr., Scheithauer B.W., *et al.* The occurrence of dural invasion in pituitary adenomas. J. Neurosurg., *64*:402–407, 1986.

269. Serri O., Comtois R., Jilwan N., *et al.* Distinctive features of prolactin secretion in acromegalic patients with hyperprolactinemia. Clin. Endocrinol. (Oxf.), *27*:429–436, 1987.

270. Shanklin W.M. On the origin of tumorlettes in the human neurohypophysis. Anat. Rec., *99*:297–327, 1947.

271. Shanklin W.M. The incidence and distribution of cilia in the human pituitary with a description of micro-follicular cysts derived from Rathke's cleft. Acta. Anat., (Basel), *11*:361–382, 1951.

272. Sherry S.H., Guay A.T., Lee A.K. *et al.* Concurrent production of adrenocorticotropin and prolactin from two distinct cell lines in a single pituitary adenoma: a detailed immunohistochemical analysis. J. Clin. Endocrinol. Metab., *55*:947–955, 1982.

273. Shiotani M.S. An electron microscopic study on stellate cells in the rabbit adenohypophysis under various endocrine conditions. Cell Tissue Res., *213*:237–246, 1980.

274. Simoes M.S., Brandao A., Paiva M.E., *et al.* Lymphoid hypophysitis in a patient with lymphoid thyroiditis, lymphoid adrenalitis, and idiopathic retroperitoneal fibrosis. Arch. Pathol. Lab. Med., *19*:230–233, 1985.

275. Smallman L.A., Dunn P.T.S., Curran R.C., *et al.* Pituitary adenomas producing growth hormone in acromegalic patients. J. Clin. Pathol., *37*:382–389, 1984.

276. Snyder P.J., Sterling F.H. Hypersecretion of LH and FSH by a pituitary adenoma. J. Clin. Endocrinol. Metab., *42*:544–549, 1976.

277. Snyder P.J., Johnson J., Muzyka R. Abnormal secretion of glycoprotein α-subunit and follicle-stimulating hormone (FSH) β-subunit in Men with pituitary adenomas and FSH hypersecretion. J. Clin. Endocrinol. Metab., *51*:579–584, 1980.

278. Snyder P.J., Muzyka P., Johnson J., *et al.* Thyrotropin-releasing hormone provokes abnormal follicle-stimulating hormone (FSH) and luteinizing hormone responses in men who have pituitary adenomas and FSH hypersecretion. J. Clin. Endocrinol. Metab., *51*:744–748, 1980.

279. Snyder P.J. Gonadotroph cell adenomas of the pituitary. Endocr. Rev., *6*:552–563, 1985.

280. Snyder P.J. Gonadotroph cell pituitary adenomas. In: *Pituitary tumors: Diagnosis and Management,*

edited by M.E. Molitch, Vol 16, pp. 755–764. Endocrinol Metab Clin North Am. Philadelphia, W.B. Saunders, 1987.

281. Spertini F., Deruaz J.-P., Perentes E., *et al.* Luteinizing hormone (LH) and prolactin-releasing pituitary tumor: possible malignant transformation of the LH cell line. J. Clin. Endocrinol. Metab., *62*:849–854, 1986.

282. Stefaneanu L., Kovacs K., Horvath E., *et al.* Adenohypophysial changes in mice transgenic for human growth hormone-releasing factor: a histological, immunocytochemical, and electron microscopic investigation. Endocrinology, *125*: 2710–2718, 1989.

283. Steinberg G.K., Koenig G.H., Golden J.B. Symptomatic Rathke's cleft cysts. J. Neurosurg., *56*:290–295, 1982.

284. Surmont D.W.A., Winslow C.L.J., Loizon M., *et al.* Gonadotropin and α subunit secretion by human "functionless" pituitary adenomas in cell culture: long term effects of luteinizing hormone releasing hormone and thyrotrophin releasing hormone. Clin. Endocrinol. (Oxf.), *19*:325–336, 1983.

285. Symon L., Granz J.C., Burston J. Granular cell myoblastoma of the neurohypophysis. Report of two cases. J. Neurosurg., *197*:82–89, 1971.

286. Tachibana O., Yamashima T. Immunohistochemical study of folliculo-stellate cells in human pituitary adenomas. Acta. Neuropathol. (Berl.), *76*:458–464, 1988.

287. Thorner M.O., Martin W.H., Rogol A.D., *et al.* Rapid regression of pituitary prolactinomas during bromocriptine treatment. J. Clin. Endocrinol. Metab., *51*:438–445, 1980.

288. Thorner M.O., Schran H.F., Evans W.S., *et al.* A broad spectrum of prolactin suppression by bromocriptine in hyperprolactinemic women: a study of serum prolactin and bromocriptine levels after acute and chronic administration of bromocriptine. J. Clin. Endocrinol. Metab., *50*:1026–1033, 1980.

289. Thorner M.O., Perryman R.L., Cronin M.J., *et al.* Somatotroph hyperplasia. J. Clin. Invest., *70*:965–977, 1982.

290. Tindall G.T., Kovacs K., Horvath E., *et al.* Human prolactin-producing adenoma and bromocriptine: a histological, immunocytochemical, ultrastructural and morphometric study. J. Clin. Endocrinol. Metab., *55*:1178–1183, 1982.

291. Tourniaire J., Trouillas J., Chalendar D., *et al.* Somatotropic adenoma manifested by galactorrhea without acromegaly. J. Clin. Endocrinol. Metab., *61*:451–453, 1985.

292. Trouillas J., Girod C., Lheritier M., *et al.* Morphological and biochemical relationships in 31 human pituitary adenomas with acromegaly. Virchows. Arch. [A], *389*:127–141, 1980.

293. Trouillas J., Girod C., Sassolas G., *et al.* Human pituitary gonadotropic adenoma: histological, immunocytochemical, and ultrastructural and hormonal studies in eight cases. J. Pathol., *135*:315–336, 1981.

294. Trouillas J., Girod C., Sassolas G., *et al.* The human gonadotropic adenoma: pathologic diag-

nosis and hormonal correlations in 26 tumors. Semin. Diagn. Pathol., *3:*42–57, 1986.

295. Trouillas J., Girod C., Loras B., *et al.* The TSH secretion in the human pituitary adenomas. Path. Res. Pract., *183:*596–600, 1988.

296. Ulrich J., Heitz PhU., Fisher T., *et al.* Granular cell tumors: evidence for heterogeneous tumor cell differentiation. Virchows. Arch. [B], *53:*52–57, 1987.

297. U S.H., Johnson C. Metastatic prolactin-secreting pituitary adenomas. Hum. Pathol., *15:*94–96, 1984.

298. Vanco M.L., Ridgway E.C., Thorner M.O. Follicle-stimulating hormone- and α-subunit-secreting pituitary tumor treated with bromocriptine. J. Clin. Endocrinol. Metab., *61:*580–584, 1985.

299. Vila-Porcile E. Le réseau des cellules folliculo-stellaires et les follicules de l'adénohypophyse du rat (pars distalis). Z. Zellforsch., *129:*328–369, 1972.

300. Vogel H., Horoupian D.S., Silverberg G. Do folliculo-stellate adenomas of the pituitary gland exist or are they intrasellar meningiomas? Acta. Neuropathol. (Berl.), *77:*219–223, 1988.

301. Von Westarp C., Weir B.K.A., Shnitka T.A. Characterization of pituitary stone. Am. J. Med., *68:*949–954, 1980.

302. Von Werder K. Recent advances in the diagnosis and treatment of hyperprolactinemia. In: *The Pituitary Gland,* edited by H. Imura, pp. 405–440, New York, Raven Press, 1985.

303. Wagle V.G., Nelson D., Rossi A., *et al.* Magnetic resonance imaging of symptomatic Rathke's cleft cyst: report of a case. Neurosurgery, *24:*276–278, 1989.

304. Wajchenberg B.L., Tsanaclis A.M.C., Marino R. Jr. TSH-containing pituitary adenoma associated with primary hypothyroidism manifested by amenorrhoea and galactorrhoea. Acta. Endocrinol. (Copenh.), *106:*61–66, 1984.

305. Webster J., Ham J., Bevan J.S., *et al.* Growth factors and pituitary tumors. TEM, 95–98, 1989; Nov/Dec.

306. Wenzel M., Salcman M., Kristt D.A., *et al.* Pituitary hyposecretion and hypersecretion produced by a Rathke's cleft cyst presenting as a noncystic hypothalamic mass. Neurosurgery, *24:*424–428, 1989.

307. Whitaker M.D., Prior J.C., Scheithauer B.W., *et al.* Gonadotropin-secreting pituitary tumour: report and review. Clin. Endocrinol. (Oxf.), *22:*43–48, 1985.

308. Woolf P.D., Schnenk E.A. A FSH-producing pituitary tumor in a patient with hypogonadism. J. Clin. Endocrinol. Metab., *38:*561–568, 1974.

309. Yagishita S., Itoh Y., Nakazima S., *et al.* Folliculostellate cell adenoma of the pituitary. A light- and electron-microscopic study. Acta. Neuropathol. (Copenh.), *62:*340–344, 1984.

310. Yalow R.S., Berson S.A. Characteristics of "big ACTH" in human plasma and pituitary extracts. J. Clin. Endocrinol. Metab., *36:*415–423, 1973.

311. Yamada S., Sylvia S.L., Kovacs K. Oncocytomas and null cell adenomas of the human pituitary: morphometric and in vitro functional comparison. Virchows. Archiv. [A]., *413:*333–339, 1988.

312. Yamada S., Sylvia S.L., Kovacs K., *et al.* Analysis of hormone secretion by clinically nonfunctioning human pituitary adenomas using the reverse hemolytic plaque assay. J. Clin. Endocrinol. Metab., *68:*73–79, 1989.

313. Yamada S., Stefaneanu L., Kovacs K., *et al.* Intrasellar gangliocytoma with multiple immunoreactivities. Endocr. Pathol., *1:*58–63, 1990.

314. Yamada S. The reverse hemolytic plaque assay in endocrine pathology [Editorial]. Endocr. Pathol., *1:*129–131, 1990.

315. Yamada S., Horvath E., Kovacs K., *et al.* Gonadotroph adenoma of the pituitary mimicking a prolactinoma. Neurosurgery, *28:*445–449, 1991.

316. Yamada S., Stefaneanu L., Kovacs K. Immunocytochemistry of pituitary tumors. Diagn. Oncol., *1:*218–230, 1991.

317. Yamada S., Horvath E., Kovacs K., *et al.* Morphological study of clinically non-secreting pituitary adenomas in patients under 40 years of age. J. Neurosurg., *75:*902–905, 1991.

318. Yamaji T., Ishibashi M., Teramoto A., *et al.* Prolactin secretion by mixed ACTH-prolactin pituitary adenoma cells in culture. Acta. Endocrinol. (Copenh.), *108:*456–463, 1985.

319. Yoshida J., Kobayashi T., Kageyama N., *et al.* Symptomatic Rathke's cleft cyst: morphological study with light and electron microscopy and tissue culture. J. Neurosurg., *47:*451–458, 1977.

320. Yoshimura F., Soji T., Sato S., *et al.* Development and differentiation of rat pituitary follicular cells under normal and some experimental conditions with special reference to an interpretation of renewal cell system. Endocrinol. Jpn., *24:*435–449, 1977.

321. Zárate A., Fonseca M.E., Mason M., *et al.* Gonadotropin-secreting pituitary adenoma with concomitant hypersecretion of testosterone and elevated sperm count. Treatment with LRH agonist. Acta. Endocrinol. (Copenh.), *113:*29–34, 1986.

322. Zülch K.J. Brain tumors. Their biology and pathology. Third (ed.), pp. 85–114, Berlin, Springer-Verlag, 1986.

323. Zwan A.V.D., Luyendijk W., Bots G.T.A.M. Metastasis of mammary carcinoma in a chromophobe adenoma of the hypophysis. J. Neurol. Neurosurg. Psychiatry, *74:*369–377, 1971.

CHAPTER 16

Neuropathology of the Effector Glands

TOSHIAKI SANO, M.D., Ph.D., SHOZO YAMADA, M.D., Ph.D.

Hypothalamic or pituitary lesions may produce the dysfunction of certain glands that are regulated by the central organs. Such secondary dysfunction of the effector glands, either hyperfunction or hypofunction, is designated as central dysfunction, in contrast to primary dysfunction, which is caused by diseases of the effector glands themselves. Central dysfunction is much less frequent than primary dysfunction, but it is essential to remember in the differential diagnosis of the endocrine disorders. Moreover, an understanding of the influence of hypothalamo-pituitary lesions on the various effector glands is important when assessing the clinical features of endocrine patients.

Central dysfunction is often associated with neurologic symptoms, such as headache, visual disturbance, papilledema, and mental changes, while primary dysfunction of the effector glands is not (32, 89). In addition, central dysfunction will often involve two or more pituitary hormones as well as antidiuretic hormone, depending on the extent of the disease.

This chapter will describe the etiology and pathogenesis of central dysfunction of the thyroid, adrenal cortex, and gonads. Histological features are only briefly referred to, since the features of the hypothalamic and pituitary lesions dealt with in this chapter are documented in detail in Chapters 14 and 15.

CENTRAL HYPERFUNCTION OF THE THYROID, ADRENAL CORTEX, AND GONADS

Hyperfunction of The Thyroid Gland

Thyroid hormone secretion is under the control of thyroid-stimulating hormone (TSH) released from adenohypophysial thyrotrophs, and TSH secretion is, in turn, regulated by hypothalamic thyrotropin releasing hormone (TRH). As shown in Table 16.1, the etiology of central hyperthyroidism (TSH–induced hyperthyroidism) can be classified into three categories: hypothalamic, pituitary, and idiopathic. Hypothalamic lesions (neoplastic, granulomatous, or inflammatory) may cause hypersecretion of TRH into the hypophysial portal vein, leading to TSH overproduction by the pituitary and, thus, to TSH-dependent hyperthyroidism (67, 85).

Far more frequent causes of central hyperthyroidism are lesions occurring in the pituitary. Thyrotroph-cell adenomas are the most common neoplastic process underlying TSH-induced hyperthyroidism (32, 38). Growth hormone- (GH) producing adenomas are also associated with hyperthyroidism, although much less frequently than thyrotroph-cell adenomas (8, 18, 116). Excessive autonomous TSH secretion by these adenomas usually causes hyperthyroidism

TABLE 16.1.
Etiology of Central Hyperthyroidism (TSH-induced Hyperthyroidism)

1. Hypothalamic hyperthyroidism
   neoplasia
   granuloma
   inflammation
2. Pituitary hyperthyroidism
   pituitary adenoma
   TSH-producing adenoma
   growth hormone-producing adenoma
   pituitary resistance hyperthyroidism
3. Idiopathic TSH-induced hyperthyroidism

and the plasma levels of T3, T4, and TSH are all elevated. However, since the biological activity of the TSH secreted differs from tumor to tumor, TSH-producing adenomas have been detected in patients with no evidence of hyperthyroidism or even with hypothyroidism (30, 38). On the other hand, normal plasma levels of TSH may be found in some patients with pituitary hyperthyroidism; this has been explained by the finding that the TSH produced in such cases is highly bioactive (8). Therefore, patients with TSH–producing adenomas may manifest one of three states of thyroid function: hyperthyroidism, euthyroidism, or hypothyroidism (38).

TSH secretion from the pituitary is further regulated by the negative feedback of thyroid hormones, which inhibit the TSH response of thyrotrophs to TRH. If the thyrotroph cells are resistant to the inhibitory effects of thyroid hormones, hyperthyroidism may occur. Patients with pituitary resistance hyperthyroidism are characterized by inappropriately high plasma TSH concentrations, no demonstrable pituitary tumor, and a supranormal TSH response to TRH (32, 36, 41, 87). There are a few case reports of idiopathic TSH-induced hyperthyroidism (31, 32). In such patients, the excessive plasma TSH level does not respond to TRH and there is no evidence of a hypothalamic or pituitary abnormality or of Graves' disease.

The clinical symptoms of central hyperthyroidism have shown little difference from those of Graves' disease, although no extrathyroidal manifestations (ophthalmopathy, pretibial myxedema, and finger clubbing) have been observed in central hyperthyroidism (32).

Goiter is present in more than 90% of patients with central hyperthyroidism, but most glands only show a slight increase above normal size. Microscopically, the thyroids in these patients show hyperplasia similar to that of Graves' disease (Fig. 16.1). The small and irregular follicles are lined by hyperplastic tall cuboidal epithelium with papillary infoldings, and contain pale staining colloid with a vacuolated appearance. In contrast to Graves' disease, however, lymphocytic infiltration is absent or minimal (17).

Hyperfunction of The Adrenal Cortex

Adrenocortical hyperfunction causing Cushing's syndrome may result from excessive secretion of ACTH by the pituitary or, rarely, by ectopic ACTH–producing tumors. In fact, about 75% of cases of Cushing's syndrome actually have a pituitary basis. The most common cause for primary overproduction of ACTH by the pituitary is a corticotroph-cell adenoma (75-90%) and the remaining 10-25% of cases are due to corticotroph-cell hyperplasia (25). Since approximately 80% of these adenomas are microadenomas (less than 10 mm in diameter) and more than half are smaller than 5 mm (25), it is often difficult to recognize them in patients with Cushing's syndrome either before or during surgery (75). In addition, the possible presence of corticotroph-cell hyperplasia often leads neurosurgeons to become confused when they cannot find any tumorous lesion in the pituitary (47, 48, 68, 73, 102). As described in Chapter 15, making a differential diagnosis between microadenoma and nodular hyperplasia is sometimes extremely difficult, or even impossible. Furthermore, the coexistence of adenoma and hyperplasia has actually been reported (47). Most cases of corticotroph-cell hyperplasia are of an unknown etiology, but certain hypothalamic disturbances have been considered to be responsible in some cases (25, 73, 89). The concomitant presence of corticotroph-cell hyperplasia and a CRH-producing gangliocytoma in a patient with Cushing's syndrome (4) suggests that hypothalamic CRH may play at least a partial role in the development of corticotroph-cell hyperplasia. Extrahypothalamic CRH-producing tumors

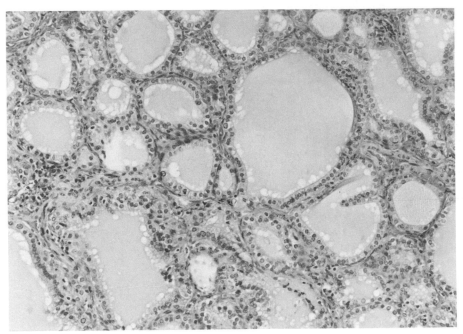

Figure 16.1. Hyperplasia of the thyroid. Follicles with varying sizes are lined by tall epithelium and contain colloid with a vacuolated appearance. Lymphoid infiltration is minimal. Hematoxylin-Eosin, X100.

are a very rare but important cause of corticotroph-cell hyperplasia. These tumors include pulmonary endocrine tumors, medullary carcinoma of the thyroid, pancreatic endocrine tumors, and small cell carcinoma of the prostate metastasizing to the hypothalamus and pituitary stalk (5, 9, 17, 103). Such tumors cause massive, diffuse, and multiple micronodular hyperplasia of corticotrophs (101).

Regardless of the type of central lesion, hypersecretion of ACTH leads to bilateral hyperplasia of the adrenal cortex. The total weight of both adrenal glands is 15 g in about one half and more than 24 g in a quarter of the patients, whereas the upper weight limit for both glands in the unstressed state is 12 g (12). Microscopically, the zona fasciculata and zona reticularis are most affected and enlargement of the cells in both zones is evident (Fig. 16.2). The thickened cortex is composed of an inner zone of compact cells and an outer zone of lipid-laden cells. The zona glomerulosa is usually compressed and is hard to recognize. It is claimed that the histological features of adrenocortical hyperpla-

sia due to an ectopic ACTH-producing tumor differ from those of hyperplasia of pituitary origin, and that this difference makes it possible to diagnose an ectopic ACTH-producing tumor simply by histological examination of the adrenal gland (12).

Nodular-cell nests mimicking microadenomas are often observed in the adrenal cortrx of patients with Cushing's disease and are especially common in young patients (12). In such cases, the nonadenomatous cortex, or the adrenal on the opposite side, exhibits hyperplasia, indicating that these adenomatous nodules are not truly autonomous adenomas. However, Hermus *et al.* (44) recently reported a case of hypercortisolism with a cortical adenoma and atrophy of the adjacent nonadenomatous cortex. After removal of the adenoma, the hypercortisolism persisted and, finally, hyperplasia of the other adrenal gland and a pituitary corticotroph-cell adenoma were detected and proved histologically. These cases suggest that there may be a hyperplasia-adenoma sequence of adrenocortical changes in patients with Cushing's disease, with the tissue chang-

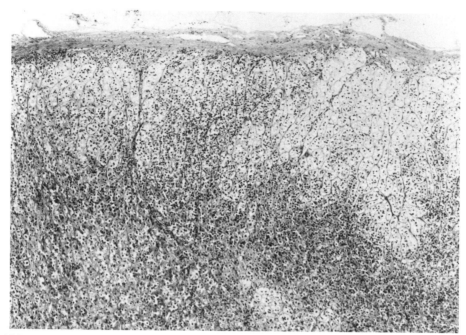

Figure 16.2. Hyperplasia of the adrenal cortex. The markedly thickened cortex is composed of an inner zone of compact cells and an outer zone of lipid-laden cells. Hematoxylin-eosin, X82.

ing from ACTH–dependent diffuse or nodular hyperplasia to become an autonomous adenoma (12, 44).

Hyperfunction of The Gonads

Hypergonadism is nearly always expressed as the earlier maturation of gonadal function and earlier manifestation of secondary sexual characteristics, i.e., precocious puberty (55, 91). In contrast to pseudoprecocious puberty due to primary adrenal or gonadal lesions, precocious puberty due to central lesions is acompanied by androgen secretion and spermatogenesis in boys or estrogen secretion and cyclic ovarian activity in girls (91). The diagnosis of precocious puberty can be made if it manifests itself before nine years of age in boys and 8 years in girls (55).

Although idiopathic precocious puberty is most frequent, demonstrable hypothalamic or suprasellar lesions are the second largest cause of precocious puberty (central precocious puberty, Table 16.2). Its incidence varies between the sexes, with about 42% to 45% of boy patients and 15% of girl patients having central precocious puberty. This condition is caused by tumorous and inflamma-

TABLE 16.2.
Etiology of Central Precocious Puberty

1. Tumorous lesion in the hypothalamus or suprasellar region
   hypothalamic neuronal hamartoma
   hypothalamic astrocytoma
   optic nerve glioma
   craniopharyngioma
   ependimoma
2. Tumorous lesion in the pineal gland
   choriocarcinoma
   germinoma
   teratoma
   pinealoma
3. Inflammatory lesion in the hypothalamus or suprasellar region
   tuberculosis
   encephalitis
   head injury
4. McCune-Albright syndrome
5. Carney's syndrome

tory lesions occurring in and around the hypothalamus (55). The tumors that can be responsible include hypothalamic neuronal hamartoma, hypothalamic astrocytoma, optic nerve glioma, and craniopharyngioma (55, 89, 101). Inflammatory lesions include tuberculosis, encephalitis, and head injury (55, 89, 101). Hypothalamic neuronal hamartomas are the most common underlying lesion (101) and about 70% to 90% of patients with such a hamartoma develop precocious puberty (66, 124). These patients often manifest precocious puberty prior to other signs of neuroendocrine dysfunction.

Two major mechanisms producing central precocious puberty have been proposed. One is that tumors may interfere with the inhibitory regulation of hypothalamic centers on the gonadotropin secretion or stimulate nuclei engaged in gonadotropin-releasing hormone (GnRH) production (70, 89, 101, 104). The other is that autonomous GnRH production by a hamartoma may lead to the development of precocious puberty (89). In this context, it should be noted that elevated GnRH levels have been detected in cerebrospinal fluid, and GnRH immunoreactivity has been observed in tumor cells (23, 52, 86).

The most common endocrinological symptom of McCune–Albright syndrome is precocious puberty. This syndrome is characterized by endocrine dysfunction, fibrous dysplasia of the bones, and cutaneous pigmentation, and is more common in girls than in boys (2, 54, 55, 65, 72, 91). Other endocrine abnormalities are only rarely noted, but they include acromegaly/gigantism, hyperthyroidism, and Cushing's syndrome (55, 59, 80). The etiology of such endocrine dysfunction is not known, but disturbed hypothalamo–pituitary function seems a likely candidate. An autopsy study failed to detect any demonstrable hypothalamic lesions (59, 65). In some cases of gigantism or acromegaly, pituitary hyperplasia or adenomas have been noted (59). A similar complex recently reported (Carey's syndrome) is characterized by myxoma, spotty cutaneous pigmentation, and endocrine dysfunctions, including Cushing's disease, acromegaly, and precocious puberty (19).

Tumors arising in the pineal region may cause precocious puberty with or without autonomous gonadotropin production (7, 55, 89, 106). Such tumors include choriocarcinoma, germinoma, teratoma, and pinealoma (27, 89, 101). Most of the patients affected are boys. The mechanism of the development of precocious puberty in these patients is obscure, but the possibility that the tumor has a mass effect on the adjacent hypothalamus and acts similarly to other destructive hypothalamic lesions must be considered (89). In addition, high levels of human chorionic gonadotropin production by the tumor may be responsible in some male cases (7, 61, 106).

It is of note that there has never been a case of precocious puberty caused by a demonstrable pituitary lesion (105). For example, detectable pituitary gonadotroph-cell adenomas are not associated with this form of gonadal dysfunction despite elevated plasma levels of gonadotropins. In contrast, prolonged hypogonadism may actually precede adenoma formation (82, 107).

Histopathological abnormalities in the gonads of precocious puberty patients are minimal. Development and maturation of the gonads is morphologically normal and only appears earlier than normal. Unfortunately, the early closure of the epiphyses due to high serum gonadotropin levels leads to permanent dwarfism.

CENTRAL HYPOFUNCTION OF THE THYROID, ADRENAL CORTEX, AND GONADS

Multiglandular Hypofunction

Hypothalamic and pituitary lesions often cause hypofunction of more than one effector gland, with the number of glands involved and the intensity of the changes depending on the size and location of the central lesion. The pituitary hormones most frequently affected are GH and gonadotropins, followed by ACTH and TSH (Fig. 16.3) (50). Such hypothalamopituitary lesions can be classified into several categories, as shown in Table 16.3.

Destructive hypothalamic lesions, either neoplastic, granulomatous, congenital, traumatic, or iatrogenic, may concurrently impair the synthesis or release of several hypothalamic-releasing factors, including GnRH, CRH, GHRH and TRH. Diabetes insipidus often occurs in patients with destructive lesions of the hypothalamus and the pituitary stalk, but is not seen, or is very rare, in other forms of hypothalamic dysfunction (89, 101). This is because the clinical signs of central diabetes insipidus only become manifest after the majority of the hypothalamic para-

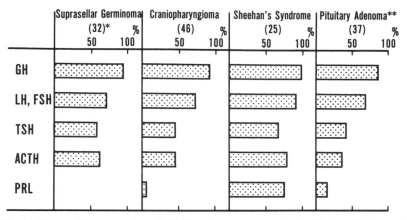

Figure 16.3. The incidence of hyposecretion of pituitary hormones associated with hypothalamo-pituitary lesions. *Parentheses indicate the number of cases studied; **clinically non-functioning adenoma. Modified from Imura, H., Kato, Y., and Nakai, Y. Hypopituitarism. Nihon Rinsho, (in Japanese), *44*:204–214, 1988.

ventricular and/or supraoptic neurons that secrete vasopressin have been destroyed or the pathways have been disrupted. Craniopharyngioma is an important cause of hypothalamic hypofunction, especially in childhood (101, 114). Combined deficits of several pituitary hormones often develop, with the most common being a GH deficit (114). Frolich's syndrome is the association of a space-occupying lesion in the hypothalamo-pituitary region (originally a craniopharyngioma), with growth retardation, obesity, and pubertal delay (88, 89).

Diencephalic syndrome or Russell's syndrome occurs in young children and is mostly caused by neoplastic lesions. It is characterized by marked emaciation, an alert appearance, and endocrine anomalies, such as high serum GH levels, varying degrees of hypopituitarism, and diabetes inspidus (10, 15, 93). Patients with this syndrome may also have types of hypothalamic dysfunction, such as low body temperature, abnormal sweating, euphoria, irritability, hypertension, tachycardia, mental retardation, involuntary movements, and nystagmus (15, 118). It has also been reported that a small number of these cases can develop obesity and/or precocious puberty after treatment (29, 34, 81). Most neoplastic lesions causing diencephalic syndrome are low–grade gliomas in the anterior hypothalamus (15) but, in rare cases, they may be malignant gliomas (118), ependymomas (1), or germinomas

(15). The underlying mechanism of this syndrome is still unknown (22, 81). However, taking into account that this syndrome seldom develops in children older than two years or in association with tumors other than benign gliomas, it is conceivable that it may be due to slowly progressive damage to an immature hypothalamus.

Rathke's cleft cysts are not a neoplasm, but are space–occupying lesions arising mainly in the sella turcica (112, 123) (Fig. 16.4). Usually these lesions are asymptomatic; they are a common incidental finding (13% to 33%) at autopsy (10, 101, 112). However, when they reach a size sufficient to compress the pituitary or suprasellar structures, i.e., approximately 1 cm in diameter, neuroendocrine symptoms may occur, including hypopituitarism (10, 112) with gonadal insufficiency or less commonly GH, TSH, or ACTH deficiency (101).

One of the congenital lesions affecting hypothalamo–pituitary function is septo–optic dysplasia, which was defined by de Morsier (111). This syndrome consists of midline structural abnormalities of the brain, hypoplasia of the optic nerves, and hypothalamo–pituitary dysfunction (101, 111). In spite of the name, the septum pellucidum is frequently present in this syndrome and the presence or absence of the septum is not related to the occurrence of endocrine dysfunction (111). Although the mid-brain lesion and visual defects are noted from birth, endocrine abnormalities, such as recurrent hypoglycemia and panhypopituitarism may appear considerably later (92, 111). Congenital hypopituitarism is similar to septo-optic dysplasia, in that both manifest with hypoglycemia and a spectrum of deficiencies of several pituitary hormones. However, septo-optic dysplasia is not present in congenital hypopituitarism (11, 13, 69, 78). Usually, in this disease, anterior pituitary and stalk are absent or only a remnant is present. A recent study using magnetic resonance imaging and hormonal assays showed that patients with this disease may exhibit a spectrum of hormonal responses, from a typical hypothalamic pattern to a primary pituitary one, and that the difference depends on the quantity of residual anterior pituitary tissue and may result from abnormal transport of hypothalamic hypophysial releasing hormones (13).

Cranial irradiation for the treatment of nasopharyngeal and brain tumors may damage the hypothalamo–pituitary region and produce central dysfunction after a variable latent period (63, 76, 95). The severity and extent of the neuroendocrine complications vary from subtle biochemical aberrations to dysfunction affecting the entire axis (76). The type of dysfunction depends on the time elapsed since irradiation and the age of the patients. Somnolence and anorexia develop frequently during or at early stage after radiation therapy, especially in children (35). However, such acute and early delayed reactions are transient and reversible, and resolve without any specific therapy. The late effects of radiation damage in young patients include endocrine dysfunction (growth retardation and impaired sexual development) and mental retardation (83). In adults, various kinds of hypothalamic disturbances such as hormonal, behavioral, and cognitive impairment are noted (76), and these usually antedate the onset of dementia, which appears in long-term survivors (26). Endocrine dysfunction seems to be caused by damage to the hypothalamus or hypothalamo–pituitary pathways, rather than by lesions of the pituitary (62), because the latter is more radioresistant than the former (56). It has been reported that endocrine deficits may be noted as early as one year after irradiation (63) and are progressive. By three to 20 years after irradiation, such deficits occur in approximately 80% of the patients given a dose of over 4000 cGy (96). Microscopic findings of

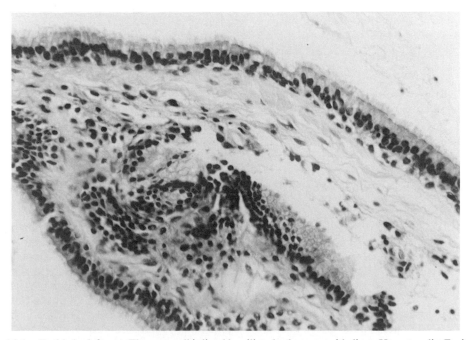

Figure 16.4.   Rathke's cleft cyst. The cyst wall is lined by ciliated columnar epithelium. Hematoxylin-Eosin, X420.

the irradiated brain in children include demyelination, focal necrosis, and cortical atrophy. Various vascular changes such as endothelial proliferation, vascular wall thickening and thrombosis are also observed at a later stage (83).

Tumorous or atrophic lesions (Table 16.3) within the pituitary may lead to deficits of multiple pituitary hormones and, thus, hypofunction of several effector glands. Large adenomas, generally prolactinomas and nonfunctioning adenomas, such as null-cell adenomas (60, 101), may cause hypopituitarism presumably due to the replacement and/or compression of adenohypophysial cells and the impaired delivery of hypothalamic releasing factors. Simultaneous deficiency of pituitary hormones is not infrequently observed (20, 50, 60, 107) (Fig. 16.3). The frequency of abnormal secretion of various hormones in 50 men with untreated pituitary adenomas was biochemically assessed by Snyder *et al.* (107). They found that 82% had GH deficiency, 74% had impaired gonadotropin secretion, 52% had TSH deficiency, 31% had Prl deficiency, and 30% had ACTH deficiency. Furthermore, hemorrhagic infarction of a preexisting pituitary adenoma may rarely occur and this causes clinical symptoms that include partial or complete hypopituitarism (3, 16, 48, 119) (Fig. 16.5). Hypopituitarism due to this rare condition of pituitary adenoma apoplexy is likely to be caused by compression of the portal circulation and pituitary stalk following the sudden increase in the intrasellar volume (3, 48). This process appears to be reversible and pituitary function is reported to be improved by surgical decompression (3). Lymphocytic hypophysitis has been known to cause deficiencies of multiple pituitary hormones (84, 101). This distinct autoimmune disease develops almost exclusively in females and in more than 80% of cases is pregnancy–associated (101). Heavy lymphocytic infiltration causes enlargement of the sella turcica and damages the adenohypophysial cells (46, 84). Panhypopituitarism is common, but a selective ACTH deficit has also been described (see below).

Postpartum pituitary necrosis, or Sheehan's syndrome, is still the major cause of panhypopituitarism in countries where perinatal care is inadequate (24, 25). Severe hemorrhage and subsequent prolonged circulatory collapse at the time of delivery is the etiology of this disease, but the mechanism of the pituitary damage is still obscure. It apparently includes thrombosis, Schwartzman reaction–induced vascular sensitization, vasospasm, and tissue anoxia (25, 105). It has been claimed that the increase in pituitary volume due to lactotroph hyperplasia during pregnancy may also be an important factor predisposing to adenohypophysial parenchymal damage (25). Pituitary edema caused by cellular damage could easily increase the intrasellar pressure in the presence of a hypertrophied gland and, thus, obstruct the pituitary circulation. The extent of adenohypophysial necrosis may reach 99% in the most severe cases. Since adenohypophysial cells cannot regenerate, the necrotic tissue is gradually replaced by fibrosis and reduced to a collagenous scar. Damage to the posterior

TABLE 16.3.
Hypothalamo-pituitary Lesion Causing "Central" Hypofunction of the Thyroid, Adrenal Cortex, and Gonads

1. Destructive hypothalamic lesion
   a. tumorous
      craniopharyngioma (Frölich's syndrome)
      diencephalic syndrome
      glioma, meningioma, ependymoma, germinoma
      Rathke's cleft cyst, aneurysm
   b. granulomatous
      sarcoidosis, histiocytosis X
   c. anomalous
      septo-optic dysplasia (de Morsier syndrome)
      basal encephalocele syndrome
   d. traumatic
   e. iatrogenic
      irradiation, pituitary stalk transection by surgery
   f. infectious
      tuberculosis, syphilis, encephalitis
2. Tumorous pituitary lesion
   a. neoplastic
      pituitary adenoma, metastatic carcinoma
   b. lymphocytic hypophysitis
3. Atrophic pituitary lesion
   Sheehan's syndrome (postpartum pituitary necrosis)
   lymphocytic hypophysitis, diabetic vascular damage
   hemochromatosis
4. Idiopathic
   Kallman's syndrome (isolated gonadotropin deficiency)
   familial (hereditary) cases of effector gland insufficiency
   congenital insufficiency of the effector gland
   isolated ACTH deficiency with autoantibody to corticotrophs

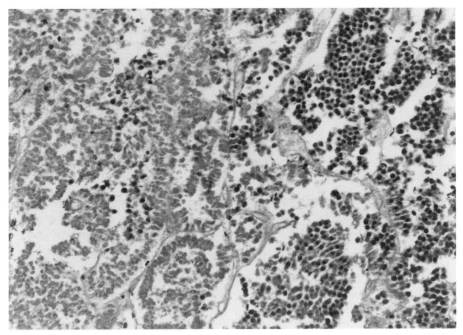

Figure 16.5. Pituitary apoplexy. Massive coagulation necrosis is seen in a clinically nonfunctioning ádenoma. Hematoxylin-Eosin, X360.

lobe and stalk also rarely occurs in the cases where at least 95% of anterior lobe becomes necrotic (105). Among a number of features of the endocrine dysfunction, failure of lactation and the failure to resume menstruation after delivery are the earliest manifestations (25). Deficiency of ACTH, gonadotropins, and TSH may develop later (32), but diabetes insipidus is an uncommon complication of this syndrome.

In some cases of endocrine hypofunction due to hypothalamo–pituitary disturbance, the underlying cause is not morphologically demonstrable. Such idiopathic dysfunction is likely to be caused by functional abnormalities, such as receptor malfunction or the presence of autoantibodies (89). Isolated deficiency of pituitary hormones may be noted, while multiple deficiencies may also occur (71, 89). Anorexia nervosa, in which amenorrhea is the most common and obvious manifestation, may be associated with various other endocrine abnormalities (28, 49, 100). These include low serum levels of gonadotropins and thyroid hormones, an absent or abnormal response to GnRH, and an abnormal response to the dexamethasone suppression test (6). Autopsy studies have not revealed any specific demonstrable changes in the hypothalamus or the pituitary in patients with anorexia nervosa (101). In addition, a recent immunohistochemical study by Scheithauer *et al.* (100) has disclosed that no specific or etiologic abnormalities are present in the pituitary and concluded that the altered secretion of pituitary hormones cannot be attributed to a primary pituitary disorder.

Central Hypothyroidism

Hypothalamo–pituitary lesions are a minor cause of hypothyroidism, but are important for both the differential diagnosis and treatment. Destructive hypothalamic lesions, such as neoplasms, granulomas, or injury result in a decrease in TRH, a subsequent decline in TSH and, ultimately, a reduction in thyroid hormones (51). TRH is known to be the hormone least affected among the hypothalamic-releasing hormones by lesions involving the hypothalamus. Thus, in most cases of central hypothyroidism of hypothalamic origin (i.e., tertiary hypothyroidism) the TRH deficit is associated with deficits of other hypothalamic releasing hormones (32, 51), and the causes mostly overlap with those for multihormone hypofunction described in the previous section (Table 16.3). The major cause of tertiary hypothyroidism is craniopharyngioma (114). Irradiation injury to the TRH–TSH system leads to a delayed TSH response to TRH, presumably due to the disturbance of TRH release (63). Such dysfunction may appear one year after irradiation (63). Irradiation can occasionally result in primary pituitary or thyroid failure (95). It is of note that a loss of the nocturnal increase in the TSH pulse amplitude has recently been observed in patients with hypothyroidism caused by destructive hypothalamic or pituitary lesions (97).

The term idiopathic hypothalamic hypothyroidism is applied to central hypothyroidism in patients who have no evidence of a space–occupying lesion as well as no evidence of a disease known to be associated with hypopituitarism, and can be made euthyroid by the administration of TRH (32, 37, 71). Several cases of this form of hypothyroidism have been reported and some of them are associated with deficiencies of other hormones (32, 71). Hormonally inactive TSH may play an important role in the mechanism of idiopathic central hypothyroidism (33). Since such abnormal TSH is immunologically active, these patients have significantly higher levels of serum TSH and TSH–β than those in normal subjects, whereas the α–subunit concentration does not differ (33). The cause of abnormal TSH and TSH–β secretion is not known, but TRH deficiency may be implicated, although it is not the sole cause (33). In addition, hormonally inactive TSH has also been reported to be produced by pituitary adenomas (30). In such cases, hypothyroidism occurs despite high serum levels of TSH. These patients must be distinguished from those with primary hypothyroidism who have high TSH levels and pituitary enlargement.

Pituitary hypothyroidism is caused by either tumorous or atrophic anterior pituitary lesions (Table 16.3), most of them again overlapping with those causing multi-hormonal hypofunction. Thus, isolated TSH deficiency is quite rare. Large Prl-cell adenomas and null-cell adenomas are the tumors causing pituitary hypothyroidism. In Sheehan's syndrome, which is a major cause of atrophic pituitary hypothyroidism, TSH deficiency usually develops concomitant with ACTH deficiency following Prl, gonadotropin, and GH deficiency (32).

In addition, pituitary hypothyroidism without any anatomical lesion, i.e., idiopathic pituitary hypothyroidism, has been reported (77, 94). This very rare form of central hypothyroidism is hereditary in some cases (43, 77) and defined as an intrinsic defect in the ability of the pituitary to synthesize or release TSH (32). TRH administration fails to increase serum TSH levels, but the disease is seldom associated with multiple pituitary hormone deficiencies, which distinguishes it from idiopathic hypothalamic hypothyroidism (32, 77). Recently a single-point mutation has been discovered by Hayashizaki *et al.* (43) in the gene coding TSH–β from patients with familial inhereted TSH deficiency including the cases of Miyai *et al.* (77). The mutant TSH–β subunit cannot associate with the α–subunit and thus becomes biologically inactive.

In some patients with central hypothyroidism, the thyroid has been shown to exhibit extensive fibrosis and lymphoplasmacytic infiltrates indistinguishable from primary hypothyroidism (79).

Adrenocortical Insufficiency Due To Hypothalamo–Pituitary Lesions

Adrenocortical insufficiency may result from destructive lesions occurring within the adrenal gland, such as Addison's disease, or from ACTH deficiency due to hypothalamo–pituitary lesions or iatrogenic causes. Among them, the most common cause is iatrogenic from the withdrawal of chronic high-dose glucocorticoid therapy (6). Hypothalamic or pituitary lesions producing adrenocortical hypofunction largely overlap with those described above that cause multiple hormone dysfunction and are classified as neoplastic, inflammatory, congenital, traumatic, or idiopathic. Therefore, this form of adrenocortical insufficiency usually occurs in association with deficiencies of other pituitary hormones as well as neurologic symptoms.

Isolated ACTH deficiency is a rare cause of secondary adrenocortical insufficiency (14, 109). Although there are several etiologies, including incomplete postpartum pituitary necrosis (40, 110), lymphocytic hypophysitis (90), and congenital defects (99), in most instances, no destructive lesion is demonstrated in the hypothalamus or pituitary gland. An autoimmune disorder of the pituitary gland seems to be the underlying etiology of these cases (90, 99), because a) other autoimmune diseases like Hashimoto's thyroiditis (45, 54) and type 1 diabetes mellitus (39) are often associated, b) selective loss of corticotrophs has been histologically proven in lymphocytic hypophysitis (90), and c) autoantibodies to pituitary tissue have been demonstrated in patients with isolated ACTH deficiency (113). Recently, an autoantibody to corticotroph antigen was detected in a patient with isolated ACTH deficiency (99). It is of interest that the antigen is located in the secretory granules of rat corticotrophs but is an unknown substance that differed from ACTH or proopiomelanocortin–derived peptides (99).

From the clinical point of view, ACTH deficiency may be the most serious endocrine disorder, since it is sometimes life–threatening when hypotension and shock develop under stress (6, 25, 32). However the symptoms are usually insidious and characterized by general fatigue, symptomatic hypoglycemia, and intolerance. It is of note that the clinical features of secondary adrenocortical insufficiency are in some ways different from those of primary deficiency. Loss of axillary and pubic hair is seen in women and presumably is due to combined ACTH and gonadotropin deficiencies (6, 25). In addition, the rare occurrence of hyperpigmentation of the skin, a greater tendency for hypoglycemia, and a lower frequency of hyperkalemia are characteristics of ACTH deficiency (6, 25). Hypocortisolism with undetectable serum levels of ACTH, normal adrenal responsiveness to ACTH administration, and an absent ACTH response to insulin–induced hypoglycemia and CRF are the laboratory findings that are essential for the diagnosis of ACTH deficiency (117).

The adrenal glands in patients with secondary adrenocortical insufficiency, due to either hypothalamo–pituitary lesions or iatrogenic causes, show marked atrophy of the cortex, especially of the zona fasciculata and zona reticularis, which are influenced by ACTH (25). By contrast, the zona glomerulosa is usually intact.

Central Hypogonadism

Central hypogonadism is a secondary form of hypogonadism caused by hypothalamo–pituitary lesions, which may or may not be demonstrable. Most of the anatomical lesions producing central hypogonadism are identical to those causing multiple hormone dysfunction; thus, central hypogonadism is usually associated with deficiencies of other pituitary hormones (6). Gonadotropins and GH are the hormones that are most frequently involved by the hypothalamo–pituitary lesions causing hypopituitarism. As far as the clinical manifestations are concerned, gonadotropins are the most commonly affected hormones.

Tumors, injuries, and anomalies occurring in the hypothalamo–pituitary region may cause hypogonadism as the major presenting symptom (6, 21). Such destructive lesions impair the synthesis or release of hypothalamic gonadotropin–releasing hormone (GnRH). Irradiation to this region can cause multiple hormone deficits, including hypogonadism. Either the hypothalamus or the pituitary is affected, but more commonly the former (62). It has been reported that the pulse frequency of LHRH is abnormal in patients with central hypogonadism due to irradiation (63).

Isolated hypogonadotropic hypogonadism is most probably caused by hypothalamic dysfunction and is best known as Kallmann's syndrome (64, 89, 101, 122). Although this disease was originally reported as a familial syndrome (53), sporadic cases are also not uncommon. The pattern of inheritance is reported to be autosomal recessive (64). The syndrome is characterized by the combination of anosmia or hyposmia due to agenesis of the olfactory lobe and sexual maldevelopment associated with low plasma levels of GnRH, FSH, and LH (64, 89). The secretion of other pituitary hormones is characteristically normal. Additional abnormalities have been observed, such as cryptorchidism and microphallus in some male patients and anomalies involving the midline facial and head structures in familial cases (Table 16.4) (64, 89, 122). On the other hand, a rare form of Kallmann's syndrome with isolated FSH or LH deficiency named the "fertile eunuch syndrome" has also been noted (122). The underlying defect producing hypogonadism in Kallmann's syndrome is most likely located in the part of the hypothalamus responsible for GnRH production and/or release. This hypothesis is supported by various clinical observations, e.g., that the administration of LHRH can increase plasma gonadotropin levels in patients with this disease (101, 122). Moreover, pathological studies have revealed marked hypoplasia of the lateral tuberal nuclei in the hypothalamus and a notable decrease in recognizable gonadotrophs in the adenohypophysis (58). Laurence–Moon–Bardet–Biedl syndrome (115, 121) is characterized by hypogonadism, obesity, and its occurrence in young children. Whether hypothalamic disorder or primary gonadal failure is the basis for the hypogonadism is obscure (121). Histological studies of patients with Laurence–Moon–Bardet–Biedl syndrome have revealed increased number of basophils and no demonstrable changes in the pituitary (121).

Central hypogonadism is also caused by destructive lesions in the pituitary, i.e., it is common in Sheehan's syndrome (24, 25). Almost all patients with this syndrome develop amenorrhea and the loss of axillary and pubic hair; a decrease in FSH and LH

TABLE 16.4.
Clinical Abnormalities of Kallmann's Syndrome

Anosmia or hyposmia
Hypogonadotropic hypogonadism
Cryptorchidism
Microphallus
Osteopenia
Color blindness
Neurosensory hearing loss
Obesity
Gynecomastia
Diabetes mellitus
Cleft lip and/or cleft palate
Renal agenesis
High-arched palate
Short fourth metacarpal

levels has been noted in more than one–third of such patients (24). Pituitary adenomas, either functional or not, may cause hypogonadism due to the replacement of gonadotrophs or the obstruction of GnRH release from the hypothalamus (6, 107). Infarction of a pituitary adenoma (pituitary apoplexy) may also lead to the hyposecretion of FSH and LH (3, 119). Gonadotroph-cell adenomas do not evoke any clinical signs and symptoms, even when high plasma levels of gonadotropins and testosterone are demonstrated. Instead, gonadotroph-cell adenomas tend to be observed in patients with hypogonadism and prolonged primary hypogonadism seems to have predated the development of such adenomas in most cases (82, 107). Hemochromatosis may also cause secondary hypogonadism in men, who present with loss of libido or impotence (57, 74, 120). Although iron–induced damage to the testicular Leydig cells cannot be excluded as an underlying cause, it seems most likely that the pituitary gonadotroph impairment by iron deposition is responsible for the hypogonadism (57).

Recently, an abnormal pulse secretion pattern for both FSH and LH has been noted in patients with central hypogonadism, both when the etiology is demonstrable and idiopathic (6, 97, 198). However, whether the hypothalamus or the pituitary is responsible for this abnormal pattern remains to be resolved (97).

Pathological changes in the gonads in the case of central hypogonadism include softening and atrophy of the testes and atrophies of the uterus and vagina. Microscopic findings of testicular biopsy from patients with Kallmann's syndrome are consistent with those of the normal infantile testis: The tissue contains immature seminiferous tubules with immature Sertoli cells and spermatogonia, and no definitive Leydig cells are recognized (42).

REFERENCES

1. Addy D.P., and Hudson F.P. Diencephalic syndrome of infantile emaciation. Analysis of literature and report of 3 cases. Arch. Dis. Child., 47:338–343, 1972.
2. Albright F., Butler A.M., Hampton A.O., *et al.* Syndrome characterized by ostetis fibrosa dissem-

inata, areas of pigmentation and endocrine dysfunction, with precocious puberty in females; report of 5 cases. N. Engl. J. Med., *216:*727–746, 1937.

3. Arafah B.M., Herrington J.F., Madhoun Z.T., *et al.* Improvement of pituitary function after surgical decompression for pituitary tumor apoplexy. J. Clin. Endocrinol. Metab., *71:*323–328, 1990.

4. Asa S.L., Kovacs K., Tindall G.T., *et al.* Cushing's disease associated with an intrasellar gangliocytoma producing corticotropin-releasing factor. Ann. Intern. Med., *101:*789–793, 1984.

5. Asa S.L., Kovacs K., Vale W., *et al.* Immunohistologic localization of corticotropin-releasing hormone in human tumors. Am. J. Clin. Pathol., *87:*327–333, 1987.

6. Asplin C.M., Carey R.M., Dunn J.T., *et al.* Biochemical tests. In: *Functional Endocrine Pathology,* edited by K. Kovacs and S.L. Asa, pp. 17–55. Boston, Blackwell Scientific Publications, 1991.

7. Axelrod L. Endocrine dysfunction in patients with tumors of the pineal region. In: *Pineal tumors,* edited by H.H. Schmidek, pp. 61–77. New York, Masson Publishers, 1977.

8. Beck-Peccoz P., Piscitelli G., Amr S., *et al.* Endocrine, biochemical, and morphological studies of a pituitary adenoma secreting growth hormone, thyrotropin (TSH), and α-subunit: evidence for secretion of TSH with increased bioactivity. J. Clin. Endocrinol. Metab. *62:*704–711, 1986.

9. Belsky J.L., Cuello B., Swanson L.W., *et al.* Cushing's syndrome due to ectopic production of corticotropin-releasing factor. J. Clin. Endocrinol. Metab. *60:*496–500, 1985.

10. Berry R.G., Schlezinger N.S. Rathke-cleft cysts. Arch. Neurol., *1:*48–58, 1959.

11. Blizzard R.M. Alberts M. Hypopituitarism, hypoadrenalism and hypogonadism in the newborn infant. J. Pediatr., *48:*782–792, 1956.

12. Bondy P.K. Disorders of the adrenal cortex. In: *Williams Textbook of endocrinology,* edited by D.J. Wilson and D.W. Foster, pp. 816–890. Philadelphia, W.B. Saunders Company, 1985.

13. Brown R.S., Bhatia V., Hayes E. An apparent cluster of congenital hypopituitarism in central Massachusetts: magnetic resonance imaging and hormone studies. J. Clin. Endocrinol. Metab., *72:*12–18, 1991.

14. Burke C.W. Adrenocortical insufficiency. J. Clin. Endocrinol. Metab. *14:*947–976, 1985.

15. Burr I.M., Slonim A.E., Danish R.K., *et al.* Dienchephalic syndrome revisited. J. Pediatr., *88:*439–444, 1976.

16. Cardoso E.R., Peterson E.W. Pituitary apoplexy: a review. Neurosurgery., *14:*363–372, 1984.

17. Carey R.M., Varma S.K., Drake C.R. Jr., *et al.* Ectopic secretion of corticotropin-releasing factor as a cause of Cushing's syndrome. A clinical, morphological, and biochemical study. N. Engl. J. Med., *311:*13–20, 1984.

18. Carlson H.E., Linfoot J.A., Braunstein G.D., *et al.* Hyperthyroidism and acromegaly due to a thyrotropin- and growth hormone-secreting pituitary tumor. Lack of hormonal response to bromocriptine. Am. J. Med., *74:*915–923, 1983.

19. Carney J.A., Gordon H., Carpenter P.C., *et al.* The complex of myxomas, spotty pigmentation, and endocrine overactivity. Medicine, *64:*270–283, 1985.

20. Christy N.P., Warren M.P. Other clinical syndromes of the hypothalamus and anterior pituitary, including tumor mass effects. In: *Endocrinology,* 2nd edition, edited by L.J. DeGroot, pp. 419–453, Philadelphia, W.B. Saunders Company, 1989.

21. Clark J.D.A., Raggatt P.R., Edwards O.M. Hypothalamic hypogonadism following major head injury. Clin. Endocrinol. (Oxf) *29:*153–165, 1988.

22. Connors M.H., Sheikholislam B.M. Hypothalamic symptomatology and its relationship to diencephalic tumor in childhood. Childs. Brain. *3:*31–36, 1977.

23. Culler F.L., James H.E., Simon M.L., *et al.* Identification of gonadotropin-releasing hormone in neurons of a hypothalamic hamartoma in a boy with precocious puberty. Neurosurgery, *17:*408–412, 1985.

24. Daughaday W.H. Sheehan's syndrome. In: *Endocrine causes of menstrual disorders,* edited by J.R. Givens, pp. 143–164, Chicago, Year Book Medical Publishers, 1978.

25. Daughaday W.H. The anterior pituitary. In: *Williams Textbook of endocrinology,* 7th edition. edited by D.J. Wilson, and D.W. Foster, pp. 568–613, Philadelphia, W.B. Saunders Company, 1985.

26. DeAngelis L.M., Delattre J.Y., Posner J.B. Radiation-induced dementia in patients cured of brain metastases. Neurology, *39:*789–796, 1989.

27. DeGirolami U., Schmidek H.H. Clinicopathological study of 53 tumors of the pineal region. J. Neurosurg., *39:*455–462, 1973.

28. DeRosa G., Corsello S.M., DeRosa E., *et al.* Endocrine study of anorexia nervosa. Exp. Clin. Endocrinol., *82:*160–172, 1983.

29. DeSousa A.L., Kalsbeck J.E., Mealey J. Jr., *et al.* Diencephalic syndrome and its relation to opticochiasmatic glioma: review of twelve cases. Neurosurgery, *4:*207–209, 1979.

30. Dickstein G., Barzilai D. Hypothyroidism secondary to biologically inactive thyroid-stimulating hormone secretion by a pituitary chromophobe adenoma. Arch. Intern. Med., *142:*1544–1545, 1982

31. Emerson C.H., Utiger R.D. Hyperthyroidism and excessive thyrotropin secretion. N. Engl. J. Med., *287:*328–333, 1972.

32. Emerson C.H. Central hypothyroidism and hyperthyroidism. Med. Clin. North. Amer., *69:*1019–1034, 1985.

33. Faglia G., Beck-Peccoz P., Ballabio M., *et al.* Excess of β-subunit of thyrotropin (TSH) in patients with idiopathic central hypothyroidism due to secretion of TSH with reduced biological activity. J. Clin. Endocrinol. Metab., *56:*908–914, 1983.

34. Fishman M.A., Peake G.T. Paradoxycal growth in a patient with the diencephalic syndrome. Pediatrics, *45:*973–982, 1970.

35. Freeman J.E., Johnston P.G.B., Voke J.M. Somnolence after prophylactic cranial irradiation in

children with acute lymphoblastic leukemia. Br. Med. (Bull.), *4:*523–525, 1973.

36. Gershengorn M., Weintraub B.D. Thyrotropin-induced hypothyroidism caused by selective pituitary resistance to thyroid hormone. J. Clin. Invest., *56:*633–642, 1975.

37. Gharib H., Abbound C.F. Primary idiopathic hypothalamic hypothyroidism. Am. J. Med. *83:*171–174, 1987.

38. Girod C., Trouillas J., Claustrat. The human thyrotropic adenoma: pathologic diagnosis in five cases and critical review of the literature. Semin. Diag. Pathol., *3:*58–68, 1986.

39. Guistina A., Candrina R., Cimino A., et al. Development of isolated ACTH deficiency in a man with type I diabetes mellitus. J. Endocrinol. Invest., *11:*375–377, 1988.

40. Haddock L., Vega L.A., Aguilo F., et al. Adrenocorticol, thyroidal, and human growth hormone reserve in Sheehan's syndrome. Johns Hopkins Med. J., *131:*80–86, 1972.

41. Hamon P., Bovier-LaPierre M, et al. Hyperthyroidism due to selective pituitary resistance to thyroid hormones in a 15-month-old boy. J. Clin. Endocrinol. Metab., *67:*1089–1093, 1988.

42. Hatakeyama S. The male reproductive system. In: *Functional endocrine pathology,* edited by K. Kovacs, and S.L. Asa, pp. 585–607, Boston, Blackwell Scientific Publications, 1991.

43. Hayashizaki Y., Hiraoka Y., Tatsumi K., et al. Deoxyribonucleic acid analyses of five families with familial inherited thyroid stimulating hormone deficiency. J. Clin. Endocrinol. Metab., *71:*792–796, 1990.

44. Hermus A.R., Pieters G.F., Smals A.G., et al. Transition from pituitary-dependent to adrenal-dependent Cushing's syndrome. N. Engl. J. Med., *318:*966–970, 1988.

45. Horii K., Adachi Y., Aoki N., et al. Isolated ACTH deficiency associated with Hashimoto's thyroiditis: report of a case. Jpn. J. Med., *23:*53–57, 1984.

46. Horvath E., Kovacs K. Pathology of the hypothalamus and pituitary gland. In: *Diagnosis and pathology of endocrine diseases,* edited by G. Medelsohn, pp. 379–412, Philadelphia, J.P. Lippincott Company, 1986.

47. Horvath E., Kovacs K. Pituitary gland. Path. Res. Pract., *183:*129–142, 1988.

48. Horvath E., Kovacs K. The adenohypophysis. In: *Functional endocrine pathology,* edited by K. Kovacs, and S.L. Asa, pp. 245–281, Boston, Blackwell Scientific Publications, 1991.

49. Hurd H.P. II, Palumbo P.J., Gharib H. Hypothalamic-endocrine dysfunction in anorexia nervosa. Mayo. Clin. Proc., *52:*711–716, 1977.

50. Imura H, Kato Y., Nakai Y. Hypopituitarism. Nihon Rinsho, (in Japanese), *44:*204–214, 1988.

51. Ingbar S.H. The thyroid gland. In: *Williams Textbook of endocrinology,* 7th ed., edited by D.J. Wilson, and D.W. Foster, pp. 682–815, Philadelphia, W.B. Saunders Company, 1985.

52. Judge D.M., Kulin H.E., Page R., et al. Hypothalamic hamartoma: a source of luteinizing hormone-releasing factor in precocious puberty. New. Engl. J. Med., *296:*7–10, 1977.

53. Kallmann F.J., Schoenfeld W.A., Barrera S.E. The genetic aspects of primary eunuchoidism. Am. J. Ment. Defic., *48:*203–236, 1944.

54. Kamijo K., Kato T., Saito A., et al. A case of isolated ACTH deficiency accompanying chronic thyroiditis. Endocrinol. Jpn. *29:*183–189, 1982.

55. Kaplan S.L., Grumbach M.M. Pathophysiology and treatment of sexual precocity. J. Clin. Endocrinol. Metab., *71:*785–789, 1990.

56. Kelly K.H., Feldsted E.T., Brown R.F., et al. Irradiation of the normal human hypophysis in malignancy: report of three cases receiving 8,000-10,000r tissue dose to the pituitary gland. J. Natl. Cancer. Inst., *11:*967–985, 1951.

57. Kelly T.M., Edwards C.Q., Meikle A.W., et al. Hypogonadism in hemochromatosis: reversal with iron depletion. Ann. Intern. Med., *101:*629–632, 1984.

58. Kovacs K., Sheehan H.L. Pituitary changes in Kallmann's syndrome: a histologic, immunocytologic, ultrastructural, and immunoelectron microscopic study. Fertil. Steril., *37:*83–89, 1982.

59. Kovacs K., Horvath E., Thorner M.O., et al. Mammosomatotroph hyperplasia associated with acromegaly and hyperprolactinemia in a patient with the McCune-Albright syndrome. A histologic, immunocytologic and ultrastructural study of the surgically-removed adenohypophysis. Virchows. Arch. [A] *403:*77–86, 1984.

60. Kovacs K., Horvath E. Tumors of the pituitary gland. Atlas of tumor pathology, 2nd series, fascicle 21. Washington, D.C.: Armed Forces Institute of Pathology, 1986.

61. Kubo O., Yamasaki N., Kamijo Y., et al. Human chorionic gonadotropin produced by ectopic pinealoma in a girl with precocious puberty. J. Neurosurg., *47:*101–105, 1977.

62. Lam R.T., Tse V.K., Wang C, et al. Hypothalamic hypopituitarism following cranial irradiation for nasopharyngeal carcinoma. Clin. Endocrinol. (Oxf) *24:*643–648, 1986.

63. Lam K.S.L., Tse V.K., Wang C., et al. Early effects of cranial irradiation on hypothalamic-pituitary function. J. Clin. Endocrinol. Metab., *64:*418–424, 1987.

64. Lieblich J.M., Rogol A.D., White B.J., et al. Syndrome of anosomia with hypogonadotropic hypogonadism (Kallmann syndrome): clinical and laboratory studies in 23 cases. Am. J. Med., *73:*506–519, 1982.

65. Lightner E.W., Penny R., Frasier S.D. Growth hormone excess and sexual precocity in polyostotic fibrous dysplasia (McCune-Albright syndrome): evidence for abnormal hypothalamic function. J. Pediatr., *87:*922–927, 1975.

66. Lin S.R., Bryson M.M., Gobien R.P., et al. Neuroradiologic study of hamartomas of the tuber cinereum and hypothalamus. Neuroradiology. *16:*17–19, 1978.

67. LiVolsi V.A. Surgical pathology of the thyroid. Philadelphia, W.B. Saunders Company, 1990.

68. Lloyd R.V., Chandler W.F., McKeever P.E., et al. The spectrum of ACTH-producing pituitary lesions. Am. J. Surg. Pathol., *10:*618–626, 1986.

69. Lovinger R.D., Kaplan S.L., Grumbach M.M.

Congenital hypopituitarism associated with neonatal hypoglycemia and microphallus: four cases secondary to hypothalamic hormone deficiencies. J. Pediatr., *87:*1171–1181, 1975.

70. Markin R.S., Leibrock L.G., Huseman C.A., *et al.* Hypothalamic hamartoma: a report of 2 cases. Pediatr. Neurosci., *13:*19–26, 1987.

71. Martin L.C., Martul P., Conner T.B., *et al.* Hypothalamic origin of idiopathic hypopituitarism. Metabolism. *21:*143–149, 1972.

72. McCune D.J. Ostetis fibrosa cystica: the case of a nine-year-old girl who also exhibits precocious puberty. Am. J. Dis. Child., *52:*743–744, 1936.

73. McKeever P.E., Koppelman M.C.S., Metcalf D. Refractory Cushing's disease caused by multinodular ACTH-cell hyperplasia. J. Neuropathol. Exp. Neurol., *41:*490–499, 1982.

74. McNeil L.W., McKee L.C. Jr., Lorber D., *et al.* The endocrine manifestations of hemochromatosis. Am. J. Med. Sci., *285:*7–13, 1983.

75. McNicol A.M. Current topics in neuropathology: Cushing's disease. Neuropathol. Appl. Neurobiol. II: 485–498, 1985.

76. Mechanick J.I., Hochberg F.H., LaRocque A.L. Hypothalamic dysfunction following whole-brain irradiation. J. Neurosurg., *65:*490–494, 1986.

77. Miyai K., Azukizawa M., Kumahara Y. Familial isolated thyrotropin deficiency with cretinism. N. Engl. J. Med., *285:*1043–1048, 1971.

78. Mosier H.D. Hypoplasia of the pituitary and adrenal cortex: report on occurrence in twin siblings and autopsy findings. J. Pediatr., *48:*633–639, 1956.

79. Murray D. The thyroid gland. In: *Functional endocrine pathology,* edited by K. Kovacs, and S.L. Asa, pp. 293–374, Boston, Blackwell Scientific Publications, 1991.

80. Nakagawa H., Nagasaka A., Sugiura T., *et al.* Gigantism associated with McCune-Albright's syndrome. Horm. Metab. Res., *17:*522–527, 1985.

81. Namba S., Nishimoto A., Yagyu Y. Diencephalic syndrome of emaciation (Russell's syndrome). Long-term survival. Surg. Neurol., *23:*581–588, 1985.

82. Nicolis G., Shimishi M., Allen C., *et al.* Gonadotropin-producing pituitary adenomas in a man with long-standing primary hypogonadism. J. Clin. Endocrinol. Metab. *66:*237–241, 1988.

83. Oi S., Kokunai T., Ijichi A., *et al.* Radiation-induced brain damage in children. Histological analysis of sequential tissue changes in 34 autopsy cases. Neurol. Med. Chir. (Tokyo) *30:*36–42, 1990.

84. Pestell R.G., Best J.D., Alford F.P. Lymphocytic hypophysitis. The clinical spectrum of the disorder and evidence for an autoimmune pathogenesis. Clin. Endocrinol. (Oxf) *33:*457–466, 1990.

85. Pittman J.A. Hypothalamic hyperthyroidism (?). N. Engl. J. Med., *287:* 356–357, 1972.

86. Price R.A., Lee P.A., Albright L., *et al.* Treatment of sexual precocity by removal a luteinizing hormone-releasing hormone secreting hamartoma. J.A.M.A., *251:*2247–2249, 1984.

87. Refetoff S., Salazar A., Smith T.J., *et al.* The consequences of inappropriate treatment because of failure to recognize the syndrome of pituitary and peripheral tissue resistance to thyroid hormone. Metabolism, *32:*822–834, 1983.

88. Reichlin S. Introduction. In: *The hypothalamus,* edited by S. Reichlin, and R.J. Baldessarini, pp. 1–14, New York, Raven Press, 1979.

89. Reichlin S. Neuroendocrinology. In: *Williams Textbook of endocrinology,* 7th ed., edited by J.D. Wilson, and D.W. Foster, pp. 492–567, 1985.

90. Richtsmeier A.J., Henry R.A., Bloodworth J.M.B. Jr., *et al.* Lymphoid hypophysis with selective adrenocorticotropic hormone deficiency. Arch. Intern. Med., *140:*1243–1245, 1980.

91. Ross G.T. Disorders of the ovary and female reproductive tract. In: *Williams Textbook of endocrinology,* 7th ed., edited by D.J. Wilson, and D.W. Foster, pp. 206–258, Philadelphia, W.B. Saunders Company, 1985.

92. Rush J.A., Bajandas F.J. Septo-optic dysplasia (de Morsier syndrome). Am. J. Ophthalmol., *86:*202–205, 1978.

93. Russell A. A diencephalic syndrome of emaciation in infancy and childhood. Arch. Dis. Child. *26:*274–280, 1951.

94. Sachson R., Rosen S.W., Cautrecasas P., *et al.* Prolactin stimulation by thyrotropin-releasing hormone in a patient with isolated thyrotropin deficiency. N. Engl. J. Med., *287:*972–973, 1972.

95. Samaan N.A., Bakdesh M.M., Caderao J.B., *et al.* Hypopituitarism after external irradiation: evidence for both hypothalamic and pituitary origin. Ann. Intern. Med., *83:*771–777, 1975.

96. Samaan N.A. Hypopituitarism after external irradiation of nasopharyngeal cancer. In: *Recent advances in the diagnosis and treatment of pituitary tumors,* edited by J.A. Linfoot, pp. 315–330, New York, Raven Press, 1979.

97. Samuels M.H., Lillehei K., Kleinschmidt-Demasters B.K., *et al.* Patterns of pulsatile pituitary glycoprotein secretion in central hypothyroidism and hypogonadism. J. Clin. Endocrinol. Metab., *70:*391–395, 1990.

98. Sasano N., Sasano H. The adrenal cortex. In: *Functional endocrine pathology,* edited by K. Kovacs, and S.L. Asa, pp. 546–583, Boston, Blackwell Scientific Publications, 1991.

99. Sauter N.P., Toni R., McLaughlin C.D., *et al.* Isolated adrenocorticotropin deficiency associated with an autoantibody to a corticotroph antigen that is not adrenocorticotropin or other proopiomelanocortin-derived peptides. J. Clin. Endocrinol. Metab., *70:*1391–1397, 1990.

100. Scheithauer B.W., Kovacs K.T., Jariwala L.K., *et al.* Anorexia nervosa: an immunohistochemical study of the pituitary gland. Mayo. Clin. Proc., *63:*23–28, 1988.

101. Scheithauer B.W. The hypothalamus and neurohypophysis. In: *Functional endocrine pathology,* edited by K. Kovacs, and S.L. Asa, pp. 170–244, Boston, Blackwell Scientific Publications, 1991.

102. Schnall A.M., Kovacs K., Brodkey J.S., *et al.* Pituitary Cushing's disease without adenoma. Acta. Endocrinol. (Copenh.), *94:*297–303, 1980.

103. Schteingart D.E., Lloyd R.V., Akil H., *et al.* Cushing's syndrome secondary to ectopic corticotropin-

releasing hormone-adrenocorticotropin secretion. J. Clin. Endocrinol. Metab., *63:*770–775, 1986.

104. Sharma R.R. Hamartoma of the hypothalamus and tuber cinereum: a brief review of the literature. J. Postgrad. Med., *33:*1–13, 1987.

105. Sheehan H.L., Kovacs K. Neurohypophysis and hypothalamus. In: *Endocrine pathology, general and surgical,* edited by J.M.B. Bloodworth Jr., pp. 45–99, Baltimore, Williams & Wilkins, 1982.

106. Sklar C.A., Conte F.A., Kaplan S.L., *et al.* Human chorionic gonadotropin-secreting pineal tumor: relation to pathogenesis and sex limitation of sexual precocity. J. Clin. Endocrinol. Metab., *53:*656–660, 1981.

107. Snyder P.J., Bigdeli H., Gardner D.F., *et al.* Gonadal function in fifty men with untreated pituitary adenomas. J. Clin. Endocrinol. Metab., *48:*309–314, 1979.

108. Spratt D.I., Carr D.B., Merriam G.R., *et al.* The spectrum of abnormal patterns of gonadotropin-releasing hormone secretion in men with idiopathic hypogonadotropic hypogonadism: clinical and laboratory correlations. J. Clin. Endocrinol. Metab., *64:*283–291, 1987.

109. Stacpoole P.W., Interlandi J.W., Nicholson W.E., *et al.* Isolated ACTH deficiency: a heterogeneous disorder. Critical review and report of four new cases. Medicine (Baltimore), *61:*13–24, 1982.

110. Stacpoole P.W., Kandell T.W., Fisher W.R. Primary empty sella, hyperprolactinemia, and isolated ACTH deficiency after postpartum hemorrhage. Am. J. Med., *74:*905–908, 1983.

111. Stanhope R., Preece M.A., Brook C.G.D. Hypoplastic optic nerves and pituitary dysfunction. A spectrum of anatomical and endocrine abnormalities. Arch. Dis. Child., *59:*111–114, 1984.

112. Steinberg G.K., Koenig G.H., Golden J.B. Symptomatic Rathke's cleft cysts: report of two cases. J. Neurosurg., *56:*290–295, 1982.

113. Sugiura M., Hashimoto A., Shizawa M., *et al.* Detection of antibodies to anterior pituitary cell surface membrane with insulin dependent diabetes mellitus and adrenocorticotropic hormone deficiency. Diabetes. Res., *4:*63–66, 1987.

114. Thomsett M.J., Conte F.A., Kaplan S.L., *et al.* Endocrine and neurologic outcome in childhood craniophryngioma: review of effect of treatment in 42 patients. J. Pediatr., *97:*728–735, 1980.

115. Toledo S.P.A., Medeiros-Neto G.A., Knobel M., *et al.* Evaluation of the hypothalamic-pituitary-gonadal function in the Bardet-Biedl syndrome. Metabolism, *26:*1277–1291, 1977.

116. Trouillas J., Girod C., Loras B., *et al.* The TSH secretion in the human pituitary adenomas. Path. Res. Pract., *183:*596–600, 1988.

117. Tsukada T., Nakai Y., Koh T., *et al.* Plasma adrenocorticotropin and cortisol responses to ovine corticotropin-releasing factor in patients with adrenocortical insufficiency due to hypothalamic and pituitary disorders. J. Clin. Endocrinol. Metab., *58:*758–760, 1984.

118. Waga S., Shimizu T., Sakakura M. Diencephalic syndrome of emaciation (Russell's syndrome). Surg. Neurol., *17:*141–146, 1982.

119. Wakai S., Fukushima T., Teratoma A., *et al.* Pituitary apoplexy: its incidence and clinical significance. J. Neurosurg., *55:*187–193, 1981.

120. Walsh C.H., Wright A.D., Williams J.W., *et al.* A study of pituitary function in patients with idiopathic hemochromatosis. J. Clin. Endocrinol. Metab., *43:*866–872, 1976.

121. Whitaker M.D., Scheithauer B.W., Kovacs K.T., *et al.* The pituitary gland in the Laurence-Moon syndrome. Mayo. Clin. Proc., *62:*216–222, 1987.

122. Whitcomb R.W., Crowley W.F. Jr. Clinical review 4: diagnosis and treatment of isolated gonadotropin-releasing hormone deficiency in men. J. Clin. Endocrinol. Metab., *70:*3–7, 1990.

123. Yoshida J., Kobayashi T., Kageyama N., *et al.* Symptomatic Rathke's cleft cyst. Morphological study with light and electron microscopy and tissue culture. J. Neurosurg., *47:*451–458, 1977.

124. Zuniga O.F., Tanner S.M., Wild W.O., *et al.* Hamartoma of CNS associated with precocious puberty. Am. J. Dis. Child., *13:*19–26, 1983.

CHAPTER 17

Diagnosis and Management of Hormone-Secreting Pituitary Adenomas[1]

ANNE KLIBANSKI, M.D., NICHOLAS T. ZERVAS, M.D.

Diagnostic, medical, and surgical advances over the past decade have greatly changed the management of secretory pituitary tumors. Improvements in magnetic resonance imaging have advanced the noninvasive visualization of smaller pituitary adenomas. Enhancement with gadolinium discloses the three-dimensional anatomy of most tumors and permits a precise assessment of their location and their volume, and the involvement of the carotid arteries, optic nerves, and chiasm. It is also possible to determine more confidently whether a tumor is fibrous or cystic and whether it has undergone necrosis or hemorrhage.

The advent of bilateral sampling of the petrosal sinus for corticotropin coupled with advances in microsurgery has had a major effect on the diagnosis and treatment of Cushing's disease. Microadenomas in Cushing's disease may be too small to identify with even the most contemporary imaging techniques. Sampling of the petrosal sinus, however, can verify the presence of disease in the pituitary. Advances in radioimmunoassays have made it possible to develop new tumor markers for the diagnosis and follow-up of adenomas that produce glycoprotein hormones. The radioimmunoassay for insulin-like growth factor I has become essential in the diagnosis and treatment of patients with acromegaly.

Microsurgery remains the treatment of choice for all pituitary adenomas except prolactinomas. In the past decade, technical advances have improved the outcome of surgery and decreased its risk. The removal of soft tissue has been enhanced by the use of intrasellar endoscopy to locate fragments of retained tissue, radiofrequency denaturation of residual tumor during surgery, and laser techniques. The success rate for the treatment of microadenomas has increased to more than 90% in the past decade in large referral centers with expertise in pituitary microsurgical techniques. Medical rather than surgical treatment has become the first choice for the vast majority of patients with prolactinomas. Finally, new treatments are beginning to change the adjunctive medical management of acromegaly and other hypersecretory states. In this short review, we consider selected aspects of current diagnostic and therapeutic approaches to the secretory adenomas of the pituitary.

CUSHING'S DISEASE

Diagnosis

Two excellent screening tests are widely used to identify patients with Cushing's syndrome: the overnight dexamethasone test and the measurement of 24-hr urinary excretion of cortisol. After hypercortisolism has been confirmed biochemically (a plasma cortisol concentration of more than 140 nmol per liter [5 μg per deciliter] in the morning, after oral administration of 1 mg of dexamethasone at midnight, or an increase in uri-

[1]This chapter is adopted with permission from N. Engl. J. Med. 1991: 822–831.

nary cortisol excretion) in a patient with clinical Cushing's syndrome, the site of hormone overproduction must be determined. Corticotropin-dependent sources, which are pituitary or ectopic, should be distinguished from corticotropin-independent sources, which are benign or malignant adrenal neoplasms. In the majority of patients with Cushing's syndrome, the disorder is pituitary-dependent (Cushing's disease). The diagnosis of Cushing's disease is based on dynamic cortisol and corticotropin testing, magnetic resonance imaging, and bilateral measurements of corticotropin in the inferior petrosal sinus. In patients with Cushing's disease, levels of urinary cortisol and 17-hydroxysteroids are increased in 24-hr measurements and, in contrast to its action in normal subjects, low-dose dexamethasone (0.5 mg orally every six hours for two days) fails to suppress urinary cortisol metabolites (60). However, high-dose dexamethasone (2 mg orally every six hours for two days) suppresses at least 50% of urinary steroid excretion in patients with Cushing's disease. In addition, an overnight suppression test for the diagnosis of Cushing's disease has been described that consists of a single high dose (8 mg) of oral dexamethasone (104). After such a dose, plasma cortisol concentrations are reduced to less than 50% of base-line values in 92% of patients with Cushing's disease. In contrast, plasma cortisol typically is not suppressed by dexamethasone in patients with adrenal tumors or ectopic overproduction of corticotropin due to malignant lung tumors.

Although suppression testing is critical for the diagnosis of Cushing's disease, both false-negative and false-positive results occur. In approximately 20% of patients with Cushing's disease, the two-day high-dose dexamethasone test does not suppress cortisol production as expected (29), and some patients may require up to 32 mg of dexamethasone for suppression to occur. Production of corticotropin by benign tumors, such as carcinoid tumors, may be suppressible in up to 40% of patients, and the tumor may not be apparent for many years (64). Because the dynamic test responses of such tumors may be similar to those of pituitary tumors, they are a major diagnostic problem. The failure to diagnose benign tumors producing ectopic corticotropin may explain the persistence of hypercortisolism after surgery in some patients (10). In addition, ectopic production of corticotropin–releasing hormone by benign tumors has also been reported, and such tumors may mimic Cushing's disease by demonstrating corticosteroid suppressibility on high–dose dexamethasone testing.

The secretion of corticotropin from the pituitary gland is regulated by hypothalamic corticotropin-releasing hormone. Testing with this hormone, which was isolated and purified in 1981 by Vale *et al.* (106), is useful in the differential diagnosis of Cushing's syndrome (13). Basal plasma levels of cortisol and corticotropin are typically higher in patients with Cushing's disease than in normal subjects and, in over 95% of cases, the levels of these hormones rise further after the intravenous administration of ovine corticotropin-releasing hormone (1 μg per kilogram of body weight) (13). In patients with Cushing's disease, a positive (exaggerated) response is defined as an increase in plasma corticotropin of 50% or more or an increase from the baseline cortisol level of 20% or more (40). Most patients with ectopic production of corticotropin have elevated basal plasma levels of cortisol and corticotropin and fail to respond to such stimulation; however, a small percentage of patients do respond, some of whom have tumors that produce ectopic corticotropin-releasing hormone (14). Nieman *et al.* (69) found that the ovine corticotropin-releasing hormone test was as effective as dexamethasone-suppression testing in distinguishing Cushing's disease from ectopic production of corticotropin and that the use of both tests increased the diagnostic accuracy to 98%. Corticotropin-releasing hormone testing may also be useful in separating patients with Cushing's disease from those with primary depression and associated hypercortisolism.

The majority of corticotroph adenomas (70%) are less than 10 mm in diameter and are difficult to discern by (computed tomography CT) or magnetic resonance imaging (MRI) (10, 62, 84, 103). CT scanning has a diagnostic accuracy of only 39% (85). The use of magnetic resonance imaging improves detection, especially when performed with gadolinium as a contrast agent (20, 22, 19). Magnetic resonance imaging with gadolinium enhancement has virtually supplanted

CT in the diagnosis of pituitary adenomas, especially for lesions that cause Cushing's disease (20, 22, 68). The use of gadolinium as a contrast agent facilitates the differentiation of normal tissue from adenomatous tissue because gadolinium rapidly enhances the image of normal pituitary tissue. In contrast, a microadenoma, which is usually avascular, is not enhanced on imaging for two to three minutes after the administration of the contrast agent. In one report, magnetic resonance imaging for the evaluation of suspected Cushing's disease had a sensitivity of 71% and a specificity of 87% (74). False-positives may occur because of coexisting incidental lesions; therefore, the identification of subtle abnormalities by magnetic resonance imaging does not eliminate the need for petrosal sampling.

A major advance in the diagnosis of Cushing's disease has been simultaneous bilateral sampling of corticotropin in the inferior petrosal sinuses. This radiologic technique is particularly important both in confirming a pituitary source of corticotropin secretion and in establishing the site of the adenoma (21, 70). In this technique, catheters are placed bilaterally into the femoral veins and are advanced into the right and left inferior petrosal sinuses. Placement is verified by the injection of contrast medium and timed samples are taken simultaneously from both catheters and from a peripheral vein for corticotropin determinations (70). If the ratio of central to peripheral corticotropin is greater than two to one, a pituitary source of corticotropin overproduction is confirmed. This is the single best test for distinguishing pituitary–based Cushing's disease from ectopic tumors secreting corticotropin. In a series of surgically cured patients with microadenomas (70), plasma corticotropin concentrations in the inferior petrosal sinus ipsilateral to the tumor were higher than in the contralateral sinus by a factor of more than 1.4 to 1. In patients in whom adenomas could not be located intraoperatively, a hemihypophysectomy of the side with higher corticotropin levels resulted in surgical cure. Simultaneous petrosal sampling with corticotropin-releasing hormone administration may assist in determining the site of the adenoma. We recommend bilateral catheterization of the inferior petrosal sinus before surgery in all patients for whom dynamic testing is consistent with pituitary tumor but pituitary imaging studies are inconclusive.

Therapy

The therapy of choice for patients with Cushing's disease is selective transsphenoidal adenomectomy performed at a large referral center by neurosurgeons experienced in pituitary surgery. The reported rates of surgical cure are as high as 90% in patients with microadenomas (10, 62, 84). If sellar exploration does not reveal a tumor, hemihypophysectomy can be performed with the use of the lateralization data obtained from preoperative bilateral measurement of corticotropin of the inferior petrosal sinuses. Hemihypophysectomy may induce a remission whether or not adenomatous tissue is found in the pathological specimen. Patients who are cured by surgery will require maintenance glucocorticoid therapy with periodic monitoring to determine when the pituitary-adrenal axis has recovered. The response of corticotropin to corticotropin-releasing hormone may become normal six months to one year after surgery in patients with Cushing's disease who are surgically cured (14); patients whose responses are normal rather than suppressed as early as one week after surgery are likely to be at high risk for recurrence. The effectiveness of surgery can be determined in the week after transsphenoidal surgery by assessment of both plasma cortisol and 24-hr urinary cortisol concentrations. At our institution, the patients are given small doses of dexamethasone during these assessments so that symptoms of severe adrenal insufficiency do not develop. If testing reveals persistent disease, the pituitary can be reexplored. In a series of 33 patients with recurrent or persistent Cushing's disease (26), surgery alleviated hypercortisolism in 73%. The cure rate increased to over 90% if a tumor was identified and a selective adenomectomy could be performed. The rate of remission of hypercortisolism was only 42% when a subtotal or total hypophysectomy was performed in the absence of an identifiable adenoma.

The role of radiation therapy is limited in Cushing's disease (39, 41) because of the delayed therapeutic effect. We recommend transsphenoidal surgery as the therapy of choice for children as well as adults. A remission rate of up to 85% has been reported one to 19 years after proton-beam therapy (41). However, the remission rate after two years was only 50% (41). Patients treated with radiation therapy typically require adjunctive medical therapy until the effect of radiation peaks. Another important disadvantage is the development of hypopituitarism in these patients.

Medical therapy of patients with Cushing's disease may be used to control severe hypercortisolism before curative surgery, as an adjunctive treatment in patients who have received radiotherapy, or to treat patients who are not surgical candidates. Agents that inhibit the production of cortisol are also useful in the treatment of patients with ectopic corticotropin syndrome. A number of pharmacologic agents block the adrenal system, including metyrapone, an inhibitor of 11β-hydroxylase; aminoglutethimide, which blocks the formation of pregnenolone from cholesterol; and mitotane, an adrenolytic drug. However, over the long term, these agents are limited by their lack of therapeutic efficacy and by side effects, including gastrointestinal symptoms (often severe) and, for aminoglutethimide and mitotane, somnolence. Cyproheptadine, a serotonin antagonist initially reported to be of some benefit in treating Cushing's syndrome, has limited effectiveness and is no longer recommended for medical management (11). Ketoconazole, an antimycotic agent that potently inhibits adrenal and gonadal steroidogenesis, rapidly suppresses cortisol (97) and is usually well tolerated. The most common side effects include gastrointestinal symptoms and elevations in liver-enzyme levels; severe clinical hepatitis has been reported. Ketoconazole should be considered the initial medical therapy of choice in the majority of patients with Cushing's syndrome who require adjunctive treatment. However, the effects of long-term use have not been established.

GLYCOPROTEIN HORMONE-SECRETING TUMORS

Diagnosis

The majority of tumors that produce glycoprotein hormones are slow-growing macroadenomas with extrasellar extension. Typically, such tumors do not have a characteristic clinical syndrome of excess hormone production and are manifested by symptoms of mass effect, including headache, insidious visual loss, and hypopituitarism. Advances in hormone radioimmunoassays and in techniques for investigating pituitary hormone production in vitro have increased the ability to detect such pituitary tumors (43). Elevations in the levels of follicle-stimulating hormone (FSH) and, less commonly, thyroid-stimulating hormone (TSH) or luteinizing hormone (LH) can be detected in the serum of some patients. In the majority of patients with such tumors, the production of glycoprotein hormone can be demonstrated only by in vitro studies of the tumor.

An important advance in our understanding of pituitary tumors that produce glycoprotein hormones has been the finding that free subunits of these hormones are often secreted. The pituitary glycoprotein hormones are composed of a common α subunit as well as β subunits specific to each hormone. An elevation of serum α-subunit concentrations may be independent of alterations in the levels of other pituitary hormones and may be the only tumor marker (78). Measurement of intact gonadotropins and free α subunit is useful in the diagnosis and follow-up of patients with pituitary tumors that produce glycoprotein hormones. Free serum α-subunit concentrations decrease after tumor resection or radiation therapy and may increase in parallel with tumor recurrence. The spectrum of glycoprotein hormone production ranges from elevated serum levels of intact glycoprotein hormones (most commonly FSH) or subunits (94, 95) to normal or low serum marker levels, but there is in vitro evidence of hormone production (38, 41). In addition, advances in immunocytochemical techniques and electron microscopy have been instrumental in our ability to characterize and identify these tumors (52). Recent studies using X-chromosome-inactivation analysis indicate a monoclonal cellular origin of these adenomas (1).

The secretion of α subunit by pituitary tumors may be accompanied by secretion of intact hormones (51), the β subunit of FSH

(FSHβ), or less often, the β subunit of LH (LHβ). At present, FSHβ and LHβ are only assayed in research laboratories: however, an α-subunit assay is commercially available. The prevalence of α-subunit hypersecretion in patients with clinically nonfunctioning tumors is 22%, according to a monoclonal assay (71). Serum FSHβ concentrations are significantly higher in men with hypersecretion of FSH than in men with primary hypogonadism (95). Patients with pituitary tumors and no clinical evidence of excess hormone production should have their serum levels of LH, FSH, and α subunit evaluated.

Hypersecretion of TSH by pituitary tumors, which occurs in less than 1% of cases, may result in clinical hyperthyroidism. A TSH-secreting pituitary tumor (thyrotroph adenoma) should be suspected in a patient with hyperthyroidism whose serum TSH levels are not suppressed in a sensitive radioimmunoassay. Although serum TSH levels are often markedly elevated in patients with pituitary tumors that produce TSH, in up to one-third of cases the levels are less than 10 mU per milliliter (92). Some adenomas, such as thyrotroph adenomas, that secrete growth hormone and α subunit have been reported to secrete TSH that has increased bioactivity and a lower molecular weight than normal (7). In over 80% of patients with thyrotroph adenomas, hypersecretion of free α subunit accompanies the production of TSH and is useful diagnostically.

Of the approximately 25% of pituitary tumors clinically classified as nonfunctional adenomas, the majority produce glycoprotein hormones, as determined by radioimmunoassay, immunocytochemical analysis, hormone secretion in cell culture, and the detection of messenger RNA specific to pituitary hormones (38, 45, 52, 72). In one series, 17% of patients with such tumors had evidence of a gonadotroph adenoma on the basis of the hypersecretion of FSH (93). Tumoral secretion of gonadotropins can also be confirmed by a finding of abnormal responses to hypothalamic releasing hormones. In contrast to its action in normal subjects, in whom thyrotropin-releasing hormone fails to stimulate the secretion of LH or FSH, thyrotropin-releasing hormone stimulates the secretion of LH and FSH in over 33% and 50%, respectively, of patients with tumors that secrete pituitary glycoprotein hormones. Thyrotropin-releasing hormone testing may be useful diagnostically in characterizing tumors that secrete glycoprotein hormones (93).

Therapy

The primary form of therapy for patients with pituitary tumors that produce glycoprotein hormones is transsphenoidal surgical decompression. Such surgery, which decompresses the optic chiasm, results in improved vision and decreased headaches. However, some patients with longstanding visual abnormalities and optic-nerve damage may have permanent visual loss despite decompressive surgery. At our institution, if a CT scan or magnetic resonance imaging done approximately four to six weeks after surgery shows no residual tumor, the patients are monitored with magnetic resonance imaging and assessments of visual fields at six-month intervals. In patients with elevated serum levels of FSH or α subunit before surgery, postoperative monitoring of the specific tumor marker may also be useful to detect recurrence (31). Surgery is rarely curative, and any residual tumor may grow (67). In 100 patients with clinically nonfunctioning pituitary tumors, tumors recurred after surgery in 16, despite radiation therapy in some (24). The current indications for postoperative radiation therapy remain controversial, and there are no large, controlled studies of its effectiveness.

Conventional radiation therapy should be considered for patients with substantial residual tumor as determined by radiographic studies immediately after surgery or for those with rapidly recurring tumors. In our institution, if a tumor recurs after four to five years, a second operation may be advised. We carefully follow all patients in whom postoperative scanning reveals little residual tumor. If a mass appears to be growing rapidly, radiotherapy is instituted promptly. Conventional radiotherapy administered through a wide beam to the tumor area through multiple ports to deliver 45 Gy (4500 rad) at 1.8 Gy (180 rad) per day is the accepted norm.

In patients with TSH-producing adenomas, the therapeutic goals include cure of hyperthyroidism and reduction of tumor mass. Because of the large size of the majority of such tumors, the surgical cure rates are relatively low. Pituitary surgery alone has a reported cure rate of 38% for hyperthyroidism; the combination of radiation and surgery has a 46% rate of cure (91). Although effective adjunctive medical therapy for this group of pituitary tumors is needed, there are no reports of large series. A recent development in the treatment of thyrotroph adenomas is the use of a somatostatin analogue. In one study (17), four of five patients with thyrotroph adenomas who were treated with 50 to 100 μg of this analogue every 8 to 12 hours had a decrease of 38% to 90% in serum TSH levels, and α-subunit secretion decreased in all five patients. Despite the reduction in serum hormone concentrations, there was no parallel decrease in tumor mass. In addition, in one long-term study, TSH-induced hyperthyroidism progressed despite an initial response to therapy with a somatostatin analogue (112). The long-term efficacy of somatostatin analogue in patients with TSH-secreting tumors remains to be determined.

Adjunctive medical therapy of tumors that produce glycoprotein pituitary hormones has also been investigated. Somatostatin can inhibit the release of α subunit from bovine pituitary cells in vitro (79). Receptors for somatostatin have been identified on clinically nonfunctioning human pituitary adenomas (35). Somatostatin analogue has been reported to decrease levels of tumor-produced α subunit (86): however, further studies are needed to determine the effects of this analogue on tumor size.

Because dopamine suppresses intact gonadotropin levels in normal subjects, dopamine and dopamine agonists have been tested as suppressors of hormone secretion by pituitary tumors. Dopamine may decrease concentrations of free α subunit in patients with tumors that secrete glycoprotein pituitary hormones. Several investigators have used the dopamine agonist bromocriptine to treat such patients (48). Short-term administration of bromocriptine decreases hormone levels in vivo and in vitro (54) and can decrease levels of α-subunit messenger RNA in cultured human pituitary tumor cells (48). Long-term treatment with bromocriptine suppresses the production of gonadotropins in patients with pituitary tumors and has also been reported to suppress subunit secretion in a subgroup of patients with pituitary tumors associated with the hypersecretion of this subunit (48, 109). In a limited number of these patients, the suppression of hormone production was accompanied by small decreases in the size of the pituitary tumor on CT scanning or improvement in visual fields. The use of dopamine agonists as adjunctive therapy in this heterogeneous group of patients awaits further study.

In normal subjects, long-term administration of gonadotropin-releasing hormone initially stimulates the secretion of gonadotropins and subsequently causes desensitization of gonadotrophs and suppression of gonadotropin production. A few patients with hypersecretion of gonadotropins have therefore received analogues of gonadotropin-releasing hormone agonists in an attempt to desensitize the gonadotrophs and suppress hormone production. In the majority of these patients, gonadotropin-releasing hormone has a persistent agonist effect on the production of pituitary glycoprotein hormones (47, 81, 114), but in approximately 5%, hormone secretion decreases. A new approach is the use of a gonadotropin-releasing hormone antagonist to treat hypersecretion of gonadotropins by these tumors. The administration of a gonadotropin-releasing hormone antagonist for seven days was reported to decrease FSH secretion significantly in four of five patients with gonadotroph adenomas (18). Although these findings are useful in our understanding of the secretion of pituitary glycoprotein hormones by tumors, the long-term therapeutic efficacy of gonadotropin-releasing hormone antagonists has not yet been established. Large, controlled studies are needed to clarify the role of these potential adjunctive therapies in the management of tumors that secrete pituitary glycoprotein hormones.

ACROMEGALY

Diagnosis

The pathophysiologic features and therapy of acromegaly have been the subject of a recent review in the *New England Journal of Medicine* (65), but we will comment on several current controversies in the management of acromegaly. The two most sensitive tests for biochemical confirmation of the hypersecretion of growth hormone are measurements of plasma insulin-like growth factor I and an oral glucose test. Hypersecretion is confirmed by elevated plasma insulin-like growth factor I levels and the nonsuppressibility of growth hormone levels to less than 2 ng per milliliter after the oral administration of 100 g of glucose. Random determinations of growth hormone levels are rarely useful in the diagnosis of acromegaly. Insulin-like growth factor I levels are specific in the diagnosis of grwoth hormone excess (16) and correlate well with mean 24-hr plasma measurements of hormone (4). The production of growth hormone by a tumor may be accompanied by hypersecretion of prolactin in 20% to 40% of cases, and immunocytochemical staining for prolactin is observed in a majority of somatotroph adenomas. Hypersecretion of α subunit or TSH may also occur. Immunohistochemical colocalization of growth hormone and α subunit in the same cell has been reported in human somatotroph adenomas (73). Serum levels of α subunit are increased in a subgroup of patients with acromegaly (36); such increases may affect up to 37% of patients, according to monoclonal-assay results (71).

After the biochemical documentation of acromegaly, pituitary magnetic resonance imaging with gadolinium as a contrast agent should be performed; many patients with acromegaly have macroadenomas at the time of presentation. Infrequently, acromegaly may result from the ectopic production of growth hormone–releasing hormone. In 1982 Thorner *et al.* described ectopic production of growth hormone–releasing hormone from a pancreatic islet–cell tumor that caused somatotroph hyperplasia and clinical acromegaly (101). Three of 177 patients with acromegaly studied by Thorner *et al.* were found to have elevated plasma growth hormone–releasing hormone levels (98). Gangliocytomas in the hypothalamus associated with the production of growth hormone–releasing hormone are also rare causes of acromegaly (2). Plasma growth hormone–releasing hormone concentrations should be measured in patients with clinical acromegaly who do not have a demonstrable tumor. In patients in whom ectopic production of hormone is suspected, abdominal and chest imaging studies should be done.

Therapy

Surgical, medical, and radiation therapy are all important in the treatment of acromegaly. Neurosurgical intervention, typically transsphenoidal, is the primary therapeutic choice for almost all patients. Decreases in growth hormone concentrations can cause rapid clinical improvement, particularly in patients with soft-tissue involvement, diabetes, hyperhidrosis, or arthralgias. A reduction in tumor mass and chiasmal decompression are realistic goals of therapy for patients with larger tumors that have widespread extrasellar extension. Surgical success rates in the literature are often difficult to compare because insulin-like growth factor I levels in the patients studied are often unavailable. Basal plasma levels of growth hormone in patients after successful surgery are less than 5 ng per milliliter and should decrease to 2 ng per milliliter or less after the administration of glucose. Insulin-like growth factor I levels should become normal, since a persistent elevation indicates residual disease; however, normalization of the levels may require two or more weeks. In a series of 214 patients with acromegaly, 59% of the patients with microadenomas or intrasellar macroadenomas were cured by surgery (83). In another study, approximately 78% of patients with intrasellar lesions were cured (28). In one series, the tumors recurred one to six years after surgery in 14% of the patients (89), almost all of whom had macroadenomas. Hypopituitarism occurs in a minority of patients after surgery, depending on both the degree of expertise of the surgeon and the preoperative degree of pituitary reserve function (81, 83).

Radiation therapy is a primary treatment option for the few patients with acromegaly who are not surgical candidates. It has also been used for patients with persistent excess of growth hormone after surgery. External conventional (45 Gy [4500 rad]) as well as proton-beam (150 Gy [15,000 rad]) radiation reduces growth hormone levels in the majority of patients to less than 5 ng per milliliter after 10 and 5 years, respectively (23, 49), although the long-term rates of cure are comparable. A major problem with radiotherapy is the likelihood of panhypopituitarism, an effect that is uncommon after transsphenoidal adenomectomy. Acquired hypogonadism due to the loss of gonadotropin-releasing hormone, gonadotropin, or both is a common deficiency with a frequency that approaches 50% (96). As more effective pharmacologic agents become available for the treatment of acromegaly, the role of radiotherapy will become more limited.

A major advance in the adjunctive treatment of acromegaly has been the use of octreotide, a cyclic octapeptide analogue of somatostatin, to decrease growth hormone concentrations (6, 53, 55). Although approval of this agent by the Food and Drug Administration extends only to secretory gastrointestinal tumors, octreotide has been used extensively both in this country and abroad to treat acromegaly. The response of growth hormone to octreotide therapy may vary depending on the number of somatostatin receptors on adenomatous somatotrophs (77). In 19 patients who received 100 μg of octreotide subcutaneously two or three times daily, the concentrations of growth hormone and insulin-like growth factor I were significantly reduced, with growth hormone levels becoming normal in 40% of the patients. It is unclear whether continued escalations in the dose increase the rate of remission (33, 75). Continuous subcutaneous infusion of octreotide (15) or frequent subcutaneous injections (107) may be more effective than intermittent doses in decreasing the secretion of growth hormone. Although octreotide therapy is usually well tolerated, somatostatin inhibits gallbladder contraction (76) and octreotide has been reported to inhibit postprandial gallbladder contractility (105). In one study (33), new gallstones developed in four of nine patients after 12 months of therapy. More data on the clinical importance of cholelithiasis in treated patients are needed. Insulin-like growth factor I concentrations returned to normal in 37% to 81% of the patients in several large series (3, 32, 55, 76). Although some degree of tumor shrinkage has also been reported in patients undergoing long-term treatment, the long-

term efficacy of this analogue in reducing tumor mass awaits further study (5, 55). Pretreatment with octreotide has been proposed as a method of increasing surgical cure rates, and data from one study support this (5); however, a large prospective randomized study is needed to clarify this point.

Bromocriptine has been widely used in treating acromegaly since 1974 (61) and is a useful adjunctive therapy, particularly in patients with mild disease. Data on insulin-like growth factor I levels are not available in most large clinical series of patients with acromegaly who are treated with bromcriptine. Growth hormone levels are suppressed to less than 5 ng per milliliter in 5% to 41% of such patients (8, 60, 111). Growth hormone levels normalize in a minority of patients treated with bromocriptine (8), and side effects, primarily gastrointestinal, are common. In three reports, the administration of a somatostatin analogue suppressed the secretion of growth hormone more effectively than bromocriptine in most patients (12, 30, 56). Concomitant use of both agents is suggested for patients who do not respond to therapy with either agent alone. Both the somatostatin analogue and bromocriptine are potential treatment options for patients with acromegaly in whom hypersecretion of growth hormone persists after surgery.

PROLACTINOMAS

Diagnosis

Prolactinomas represent approximately 40% of pituitary adenomas. Confirmed elevation of serum prolactin concentrations in the absence of pregnancy, renal failure, hypothyroidism, or the use of medication known to induce hyperprolactinemia warrants neuroradiologic investigation of the pituitary gland. Although a sellar abnormality in a patient with hyperprolactinemia may be due to a prolactinoma, the differential diagnosis should also include nonfunctioning tumors, mixed pituitary adenomas, and other sellar or hypothalamic disorders. In patients with prolactinomas, the size of the sellar mass typically correlates well with the serum prolactin level. A mild degree of hyperprolactinemia (less than 200 ng per milliliter) in association with a macroadenoma, particularly with extrasellar extension, is usually not consistent with a prolactinoma. In this setting, the elevation in prolactin levels is most likely due to compression of the pituitary stalk. Further testing is needed to look for excess production of growth hormone, corticotropin, or pituitary glycoprotein hormone. In addition, transsphenoidal exploration needs to be considered for diagnostic and therapeutic purposes. As with other pituitary lesions, magnetic resonance imaging is the preferred initial radiologic tool in the evaluation of prolactinomas.

Therapy

Therapeutic considerations depend on the associated symptoms and the size of the lesion on pituitary scanning. An important consideration in the treatment of microprolactinomas is the natural history of untreated hyperprolactinemia. A number of reports (50, 63, 87, 90) indicate that neither tumor size nor prolactin levels change over a number of years in the majority of women with microprolactinomas. In a prospective series of 43 women with microprolactinomas followed for a period of 3 to 20 years, radiologic findings did not change significantly in 41 of the women. CT scans were unchanged in all 38 untreated women in a confirmatory prospective study (90). In a retrospective assessment of 25 women (50), the mean serum prolactin levels decreased significantly over time, and menses resumed spontaneously in seven patients. In a recent prospective report, 30 untreated women with hyperprolactinemia were followed for three to seven years (87). Serum prolactin levels increased in six women, decreased in 10, and did not change in 14. Decreases in serum prolactin levels and normalization of menstrual status were more likely to occur in women who presented with oligomenorrhea or normal menses, rather than amenorrhea. In 22% of the patients, however, radiographic changes were consistent with the appearance of the tumor or its pattern of growth, and no correlation was found between serum prolactin levels and radiographic changes. Therefore, in patients with untreated microadenomas, clinical symptoms, serum prolactin levels, and the appearance of the pituitary gland must be carefully monitored.

Despite the relative stability in tumor size, therapy may be necessary because of reproductive dysfunction, including infertility, menstrual abnormalities, and extreme galactorrhea in women and sexual dysfunction in men. Presumed abnormalities in pulsatile secretion of gonadotropin-releasing hormone (58) and gonadotropins lead to a relative or absolute estrogen deficiency in many women with prolactinomas (37). This hypogonadal state is associated with osteoporosis (46). The decrease in bone mass appears to be related to the degree and duration of estrogen deficiency rather than to a direct effect of prolactin (44). Cortical bone mass increases, but does not return to normal after treatment in the majority of women with hyperprolactinemia. A significant number of both treated and untreated women may enter menopause with an already substantial decrease in bone density. In men, hyperprolactinemic hypogonadism is also associated with both cortical and trabecular osteopenia (27).

Treatment of microadenomas primarily consists of the dopamine agonist bromocriptine. Neurosurgery is not always curative, and recurrences are possible (80, 88). A 16% rate of biochemical recurrence has been reported in the absence of radiographic evidence of tumor recurrence (88). Radiation therapy has now been abandoned for microprolactinomas because of the associated hypopituitarism and the proved efficacy of drug therapy. Bromocriptine rapidly lowers serum prolactin levels, restores normal gonadal function, and decreases the size of the tumor (97, 108). Discontinuation of bromocriptine therapy leads to the reemergence of hyperprolactinemia in most patients (113). However, hyperprolactinemia can resolve spontaneously, and prolactin levels remain normal in a small subgroup of patients after therapy is discontinued. Therefore, bromocriptine can be discontinued every two years on a trial basis to determine the need for continued therapy.

Bromocriptine is also the initial therapy for the majority of patients with macroprolactinomas, including those with visual loss, because surgical cure is unlikely and the risk of tumor recurrence is high (88). In a prospective multicenter trial of 27 patients with macroprolactinomas who were receiving bromocriptine alone (66), serum prolactin levels decreased to normal in 18 (67%), and tumor size was reduced 50% or more in 13 (48%). It is important to emphasize that patients with large tumors and those with severe compression of the optic chiasm and visual loss often have objective decreases in tumor mass and visual improvement within days to weeks of the initiation of therapy (99). Most patients require bromocriptine indefinitely because discontinuation of therapy may be associated with rapid expansion of the tumor (102). A very rare complication in patients with large adenomas is the development of a leak of cerebrospinal fluid during treatment. Other ergot derivatives, including lisuride and the longer-acting pergolide (42), are also effective in lowering prolactin levels; however, side effects have limited the therapeutic usefulness of these medications. A nonergot dopamine agonist, CV 205-502, with specific D_2 activity, also effectively suppresses prolactin levels when administered once daily and has been found to be well tolerated (107). At present, however, only bromocriptine is approved for the treatment of hyperprolactinemia in the U.S.

Neurosurgical therapy may be required in several groups of patients: patients whose tumors are unresponsive to bromocriptine treatment (particularly cystic prolactinomas), patients with rapidly progressive visual loss, patients who are unable to tolerate dopamine agonists, and patients whose tumors grow during bromocriptine treatment. Because the surgical rates of cure are higher for microadenomas than for macroadenomas, attempts have been made to treat patients with bromocriptine before surgery, to decrease tumor size. No study has yet reported higher surgical cure rates after such preoperative treatment with bromocriptine (25, 34). In addition, long-term administration of bromocriptine may cause pituitary fibrosis (57) with consequent surgical difficulties (9). Because of this possibility, surgery for prolactinomas is best performed within the first 12 months of bromocriptine therapy. Radiation therapy should be considered primarily in patients with macroprolactinomas who require additional treatment and cannot tolerate medication.

REFERENCES

1. Alexander J.M., Biller B.M.K., Bikkal H., *et al.* Clinically nonfunctioning pituitary tumors are monoclonal in origin. J. Clin. Invest., *86:*336–340, 1990.
2. Asa S.L., Scheithauer B.W., Bilbao J.M., *et al.* A case for hypothalamic acromegaly: a clinicopathological study of six patients with hypothalamic gangliocytomas producing growth hormone-releasing factor. J. Clin. Endocrinol. Metab., *58:*796–803, 1984.
3. Barkan A., Lloyd R.V., Chandler W.F., *et al.* Treatment of acromegaly with SMS 201-995 (sandostatin): clinical, biochemical and morphologic study. In: *Sandostatin in the treatment of acromegaly,* edited by S.W.J. Lamberts, pp. 103–8, New York, Springer, 1988.
4. Barkan A.L., Beitins I.Z., Kelch R.P. Plasma insulin-like growth factor-I/somatomedin-C in acromegaly: correlation with the degree of growth hormone hypersecretion. J. Clin. Endocrinol. Metab., *67:*69-73, 1988.
5. Barkan A.L., Lloyd R.V., Chandler W.F., *et al.* Preoperative treatment of acromegaly with long-acting somatostatin analog SMS 201-995; shrinkage of invasive pituitary macroadenomas and improved surgical remission rate. J. Clin. Endocrinol. Metab., *67:*1040–8, 1988.
6. Bauer W., Briner U., Doepfner W., *et al.* SMS 201-995: a very potent and selective octapeptide analogue of somatostatin with prolonged action. Life. Sci., *31:*1133–40, 1982.
7. Beck-Peccoz P., Piscitelli G., Amr S., *et al.* Endocrine, biochemical, and morphological studies of a pituitary adenoma secreting growth hormone, thyrotropin (TSH), and α-subunit: evidence for secretion of TSH with increased bioactivity. J. Clin. Endocrinol. Metab., *62:*704–11, 1986.
8. Bell P., Atkinson A.B., Hadden D.R., *et al.* Bromocriptine reduces growth hormone in acromegaly. Arch. Intern. Med., *146:*1145–9, 1986.
9. Bevan J.S., Adams C.B.T., Burke C.W., *et al.* Factors in the outcome of transsphenoidal surgery for prolactinoma and non-functioning pituitary tumor, including pre-operative bromocriptine therapy. Clin. Endocrinol. (Oxf.), *26:*541–56, 1987.
10. Boggan J.E., Tyrrell J.B., Wilson C.B. Transsphenoidal microsurgical management of Cushing's disease: report of 100 cases. J. Neurosurg., *59:*195–200, 1983.
11. Carpenter P.C. Cushing's syndrome: update of diagnosis and management. Mayo. Clin. Proc., *61:*49–58, 1986.
12. Chiodini P.G., Cozzi R., Dallabonzana D., *et al.* Medical treatment of acromegaly with SMS 201-995, a somatostatin analog: a comparison with bromocriptine. J. Clin. Endocrinol. Metab., *64:*447–53, 1987.
13. Chrousos G.P., Schuermeyer T.H., Doppman T., *et al.* Clinical applications of corticotropin-releasing factor. Ann. Intern. Med., *102:*344–58, 1985.
14. Chrousos G.P., Schulte H.M., Oldfield E.H., *et al.*

The corticotropin-releasing factor stimulation test: an aid in the evaluation of patients with Cushing's syndrome. N. Engl. J. Med., *310:*622–6, 1984.

15. Christensen S.E., Weeke J., Orskov H., *et al.* Continuous subcutaneous pump infusion of somatostatin analogue SMS 201-995 versus subcutaneous injection schedule in acromegalic patients. Clin. Endocrinol. (Oxf) *27:*297–306, 1987.

16. Clemmons D.R., Van Wyk J.J., Ridgway E.C., *et al.* Evaluation of acromegaly by radioimmunoassay of somatomedin-C. N. Engl. J. Med., *301:*1138–42, 1979.

17. Comi R.J., Gesundheit N., Murray L., *et al.* Response of thyrotropin-secreting pituitary adenomas to a long-acting somatostatin analogue. N. Engl. J. Med., *317:*12–7, 1987.

18. Daneshdoost L., Molitch M.E., Snyder P.J. Inhibition of follicle-stimulating hormone secretion from gonadotroph adenomas by repetitive administration of a GnRH antagonist. In: *Program and abstracts of the 72nd annual meeting of the Endocrine Society,* Bethesda, Md, Endocrine Society, abstract, 1990.

19. Davis P.G., Hoffman J.C. Jr., Malko J.A., *et al.* Gadolinium-DTPA and MR imaging of pituitary adenomas: a preliminary report. A.J.N.R., *8:*817–23, 1987.

20. Doppman J.L., Frank J.A., Dwyer A.J., *et al.* Gadolinium DTPA enhanced MR imaging of ACTH-secreting microadenomas of the pituitary gland. J. Comput. Assist. Tomogr., *12:*728–35, 1988.

21. Doppman J.L., Oldfield E., Krudy A.G., *et al.* Petrosal sinus sampling for Cushing syndrome: anatomical and technical considerations: work in progress. Radiology., *150:*99–103, 1984.

22. Dwyer A.J., Frank J.A., Doppman J.L., *et al.* Pituitary adenomas in patients with Cushing's disease: initial experience with Gd-DTPA-enhanced MR imaging. Radiology., *163:*421–6, 1987.

23. Eastman R.C., Gorden P., Roth J. Conventional supervoltage irradiation is an effective treatment for acromegaly. J. Clin. Endocrinol. Metab., *48:*931–40, 1979.

24. Ebersold M.J., Quast L.M., Laws E.R. Jr., *et al.* Long-term results in transsphenoidal removal of nonfunctioning pituitary adenomas. J. Neurosurg., *64:*713–9, 1986.

25. Fahlbusch R., Buchfelder M., Schrell U. Short-term preoperative treatment of macroprolactinomas by dopamine agonists. J. Neurosurg., *67:*807–15, 1987.

26. Friedman R.B., Oldfield E.H., Nieman L.K., *et al.* Repeat transsphenoidal surgery for Cushing's disease. J. Neurosurg., *71:*520–7, 1989.

27. Greenspan S.L., Oppenheim D.O., Klibanski A. Importance of gonadal steroids to bone mass in men with hyperprolactinemic hypogonadism. Ann. Intern. Med., *110:*526–31, 1989.

28. Grisoli F., Leclercq T., Jaquet P., *et al.* Transsphenoidal surgery for acromegaly—long-term results in 100 patients. Surg. Neurol., *25:*513–9, 1985.

29. Grossman A.B., Howlett T.A., Perry L., *et al.* CRF in the differential diagnosis of Cushing's syndrome: a comparison with the dexamethasone suppression test. Clin. Endocrinol. (Oxf.), *29:*167–78, 1988.

30. Halse J., Harris A.G., Kvistborg A., *et al.* A randomized study of SMS 201-995 versus bromocriptine treatment in acromegaly: clinical and biochemical effects. J. Clin. Endocrinol. Metab., *70:*1254–61, 1990.

31. Harris R.I., Schatz N.J., Gennarelli T., *et al.* Follicle-stimulating hormone-secreting pituitary adenomas: correlation of reduction of adenoma size with reduction of hormonal hypersecretion after transsphenoidal surgery. J. Clin. Endocrinol. Metab., *56:*1288–93, 1983.

32. Harris A.G., Prestele H., Herold K., *et al.* Long-term efficacy of sandostatin (SMS 201-995, octreotide) in 178 acromegalic patients: results from the International Multicentre Acromegaly Study Group. In: *Sandostatin in the treatment of acromegaly,* edited by S.W.J. Lamberts, pp. 117–25, New York, Springer, 1988.

33. Ho K.Y., Weissberger A.J., Marbach P., *et al.* Therapeutic efficacy of the somatostatin analog SMS 201-995 (octreotide) in acromegaly: effects of dose and frequency and long-term safety. Ann. Intern. Med., *112:*173–81, 1990.

34. Hubbard J.L., Scheithauer B.W., Abboud C.F., *et al.* Prolactin-secreting adenomas: the preoperative response to bromocriptine treatment and surgical outcome. J. Neurosurg., *67:*816–21, 1987.

35. Ikuyama S., Nawata H., Kato K., *et al.* Specific somatostatin receptors on human pituitary adenoma cell membranes. J. Clin. Endocrinol. Metab., *61:*666–71, 1985.

36. Ishibashi M., Yamaji T., Takaku F., *et al.* Secretion of glycoprotein hormone α-subunit by pituitary tumors. J. Clin. Endocrinol. Metab., *64:*1187–93, 1987.

37. Jacobs H.S., Franks S., Murray M.A.F., *et al.* Clinical and endocrine features of hyperprolactinaemic amenorrhoea. Clin. Endocrinol. (Oxf) *5:*439–54, 1976.

38. Jameson J.L., Klibanski A., Black P., *et al.* Glycoprotein hormone genes are expressed in clinically nonfunctioning pituitary adenomas. J. Clin. Invest., *80:*1472–8, 1987.

39. Jennings A.S., Liddle G.W., Orth D.N. Results of treating childhood Cushing's disease with pituitary irradiation. N. Engl. J. Med., *297:*957–62, 1977.

40. Kaye T.B., Crapo L. The Cushing syndrome: an update on diagnostic tests. Ann. Intern. Med., *112:*434–44, 1990.

41. Kjellberg R.N., Kliman B., Swisher B., *et al.* Proton beam therapy of Cushing's disease and Nelson's syndrome. In: *Secretory tumors of the pituitary gland,* edited by P.M. Black, N.T. Zervas, E.C. Ridgway, and J.B. Martin, pp. 295–307, New York, Raven Press, 1984.

42. Kleinberg D.L., Boyd A.E. III, Wardlaw S., *et al.* Pergolide for the treatment of pituitary tumors secreting prolactin or growth hormone. N. Engl. J. Med., *309:*704–9, 1983.

43. Klibanski A. Nonsecreting pituitary tumors. Endocrinol. Metab. Clin. North. Am., *16:*793–804, 1987.

44. Klibanski A., Biller B.M.K., Rosenthal D.I., *et al.* Effects of prolactin and estrogen deficiency in amenorrheic bone loss. J. Clin. Endocrinol. Metab., *67:*124–30, 1988.

45. Klibanski A., Deutsch P.J., Jameson J.L., *et al.* Luteinizing hormone-secreting pituitary tumor: biosynthetic characterization and clinical studies. J. Clin. Endocrinol. Metab., *64:*536–42, 1987.

46. Klibanski A., Greenspan S.L. Increase in bone mass after treatment of hyperprolactinemic amenorrhea. N. Engl. J. Med., *315:*542–6, 1986.

47. Klibanski A., Jameson J.L., Biller B.M.K., *et al.* Gonadotropin and α-subunit responses to chronic gonadotropin-releasing hormone analog administration in patients with glycoprotein hormone-secreting pituitary tumors. J. Clin. Endocrinol. Metab., *68:*81–6, 1989.

48. Klibanski A., Shupnik M.A., Bikkal H.A., *et al.* Dopaminergic regulation of α-subunit secretion and messenger ribonucleic acid levels in α-secreting pituitary tumors. J. Clin. Endocrinol. Metab., *66:*96–102, 1988.

49. Kliman B., Kjellberg R.N., Swisher B., *et al.* Long-term effects of proton beam therapy for acromegaly. In: *Acromegaly: A Century of Scientific and Clinical Progress,* edited by R.J. Robbins, and S. Melmed, pp. 221–8, New York, Plenum Press, 1987.

50. Koppelman M.C.S., Jaffe M.J., Rieth K.G., *et al.* Hyperprolactinemia, amenorrhea, and galactorrhea: a retrospective assessment of 25 cases. Ann. Intern. Med., *100:*115–21, 1984.

51. Kourides I.A., Weintraub B.D., Rosen S.W., *et al.* Secretion of α subunit of glycoprotein hormones by pituitary adenomas. J. Clin. Endocrinol. Metab., *43:*97–106, 1976.

52. Kovacs K., Horvath E. Pathology of pituitary tumors. Endocrinol. Metab. Clin. North. Am., *16:*529–51, 1987.

53. Lamberts S.W.J. The role of somatostatin in the regulation of anterior pituitary hormone secretion and the use of its analogs in the treatment of human pituitary tumors. Endocr. Rev., *9:*417–36, 1988.

54. Lamberts S.W.J., Verleun T., Oosterom R., *et al.* The effects of bromocriptine, thyrotropin-releasing hormone, and gonadotropin-releasing hormone on hormone secretion by gonadotropin-secreting pituitary adenomas in vivo and in vitro. J. Clin. Endocrinol. Metab., *64:*524–30, 1987.

55. Lamberts S.W.J., Uitterlinden P., Verschoor L., *et al.* Long-term treatment of acromegaly with the somatostatin analogue SMS 201-995. N. Engl. J. Med., *313:*576–80. 1985.

56. Lamberts S.W.J., Zweens M., Verschoor L., *et al.* A comparison among the growth hormone-lowering effects in acromegaly of the somatostatin analog SMS 201-995, bromocriptine, and the combination of both drugs. J. Clin. Endocrinol. Metab., *63:*16–9, 1986.

57. Landolt A.M., Osterwalder V. Perivascular fibrosis in prolactinomas: is it increased by bromocriptine? J. Clin. Endocrinol. Metab., *58:*1179–83, 1984.

58. Leyendecker G., Struve T., Plotz E.J. Induction of ovulation in chronic intermittent (pulsatile) administration of LH-RH in women with hypothalamic and hyperprolactinemic amenorrhea. Arch. Gynecol., *229:*177–90, 1980.

59. Liddle G.W. Tests of pituitary-adrenal suppressibility in the diagnosis of Cushing's syndrome. J. Clin. Endocrinol. Metab., *20:*1539–60, 1960.

60. Lindholm J., Riishede J., Verstergaard S., *et al.* No effect of bromocriptine in acromegaly: a controlled trial. N. Engl. J. Med., *304:*1450–4, 1981.

61. Liuzzi A., Chiodini P.G., Botalla A., *et al.* Decreased plasma growth hormone (GH) levels in acromegalics following CB 154(2-Br-α-ergocriptine) administration. J. Clin. Endocrinol. Metab., *38:*910–2, 1974.

62. Mampalam T.J., Tyrrell J.B., Wilson C.B. Transsphenoidal microsurgery for Cushing disease: a report of 216 cases. Ann. Intern. Med. *109:*487–93, 1988.

63. March C.M., Kletzky O.A., Davajan V., *et al.* Longitudinal evaluation of patients with untreated prolactin-secreting pituitary adenomas. Am. J. Obstet. Gynecol., *139:*835–44, 1981.

64. Mason A.M.S., Ratcliffe J.G., Buckle R.M., *et al.* ACTH secretion by bronchial carcinoid tumours. Clin. Endocrinol. (Oxf) *1:*3–25, 1972.

65. Melmed S. Acromegaly. N. Engl. J. Med., *322:*966–77, 1990.

66. Molitch M.E., Elton R.L., Blackwell R.E., *et al.* Bromocriptine as primary therapy for prolactin-secreting macroadenomas: results of a prospective multicenter study. J. Clin. Endocrinol. Metab., *60:*698–705, 1985.

67. Nelson A.T. Jr., Tucker H.S. Jr., Becker D.P. Residual anterior pituitary function following transsphenoidal resection of pituitary macroadenomas. J. Neurosurg., *61:*577–80, 1984.

68. Newton D.R., Dillon W.P., Norman D., *et al.* Gd-DTPA-enhanced MR imaging of pituitary adenomas. A.J.N.R., *10:*949–54, 1989.

69. Nieman L.K., Chrousos G.P., Oldfield E.H., *et al.* The ovine corticotropin-releasing hormone stimulation test and the dexamethasone suppression test in the differential diagnosis of Cushing's syndrome. Ann. Inter. Med., *105:*862–66, 1986.

70. Oldfield E.H., Chrousos G.P., Schulte H.M., *et al.* Preoperative lateralization of ACTH-secreting pituitary microadenomas by bilateral and simultaneous inferior petrosal venous sinus sampling. N. Engl. J. Med., *312:*100–3, 1985.

71. Oppenheim D.S., Kana A.R., Sangha J.S., *et al.* Prevalence of α-subunit hypersecretion in patients with pituitary tumors: clinically nonfunctioning and somatotroph adenomas. J. Clin. Endocrinol. Metab., *70:*859–64, 1990.

72. Oppenheim D.S., Klibanski A. Medical therapy of glycoprotein hormone-secreting pituitary tumors. Endocrinol. Metab. Clin. North. Am., *18:*339–58, 1989.

73. Osamura R.Y., Watanabe K. Immunohistochemical colocalization of growth hormone (GH) and α subunit in human GH secreting pituitary adenomas. Virchows. Arch. [A] *411:*323–30, 1987.

74. Peck W.W., Dillon W.P., Norman D., *et al.* High-

resolution MR imaging of pituitary microadenomas at 1.5 T: experience with Cushing disease. A.J.R., *152*:145–51, 1989.

75. Quabbe H.J., Plockinger U. Dose-response study and long term effect of the somatostatin analog octreotide in patients with therapy-resistant acromegaly. J. Clin. Endocrinol. Metab., *68*:873–81, 1989.

76. Reichlin S. Somatostatin. N. Engl. J. Med., *309*:1556–63, 1983.

77. Reubi J.C., Landolt A.M. The growth hormone responses to octreotide in acromegaly correlate with adenoma somatostatin receptor status. J. Clin. Endocrinol. Metab., *68*:844–50, 1989.

78. Ridgway E.C., Klibanski A., Ladenson P.W., *et al.* Pure α-secreting pituitary adenomas. N. Engl. J. Med., *304*:1254–9, 1981.

79. Ridgway E.C., Klibanski A., Martorana M.A., *et al.* The effect of somatostatin on the release of thyrotropin and its subunits from bovine anterior pituitary cells in vitro. Endocrinology. *112*:1937–42, 1983.

80. Rodman E.F., Molitch M.E., Post K.E., *et al.* Long-term follow-up of transsphenoidal selective adenomectomy for prolactinoma. J.A.M.A., *252*:921–24, 1984.

81. Roelfsema F., van Dulken H., Frolich M. Long-term results of transsphenoidal pituitary microsurgery in 60 acromegalic patients. Clin. Endocrinol. (Oxf), *23*:555–65, 1985.

82. Roman S.H., Goldstein M., Kourides I.A., *et al.* The luteinizing hormone-releasing hormone (LHRH) agonist [D-Trp^6-Pro^9-NEt] LHRH increased rather than lowered LH and α-subunit levels in a patient with an LH-secreting pituitary tumor. J. Clin. Endocrinol. Metab., *58*:313–9, 1984.

83. Ross D.A., Wilson C.B. Results of transsphenoidal microsurgery for growth hormone-secreting pituitary adenomas in a series of 214 patients. J. Neurosurg. *68*:854–67, 1988.

84. Salassa R.M., Laws E.R. Jr., Carpenter P.C., *et al.* Transsphenoidal removal of microadenoma in Cushing's disease. Mayo. Clin. Proc., *53*:24–8, 1978.

85. Saris S.C., Patronas N.J., Doppman J.L., *et al.* Cushing syndrome: pituitary CT scanning. Radiology., *162*:775–7, 1987.

86. Sassolas G., Serusclat P., Claustrat B., *et al.* Plasma α-subunit levels during the treatment of pituitary adenomas with the somatostatin analog (SMS 201-995). Horm. Res., *29*:124–8, 1988.

87. Schlechte J., Dolan K., Sherman B., *et al.* The natural history of untreated hyperprolactinemia: a prospective analysis. J. Clin. Endocrinol. Metab., *68*:412–8, 1989.

88. Serri O., Rasio E., Beauregard H., Hardy J., *et al.* Recurrence of hyperprolactinemia after selective transsphenoidal adenomectomy in women with prolactinoma. N. Engl. J. Med., *309*:280–2, 1983.

89. Serri O., Somma M., Comtois R., *et al.* Acromegaly: biochemical assessment of cure after long term follow-up of transsphenoidal selective adenomec-

tomy. J. Clin. Endocrinol. Metab., *61*:1185–1, 1985.

90. Sisam D.A., Sheehan J.P., Sheeler L.R. The natural history of untreated micropoolactinomas. Fertil. Steril., *48*:67–71, 1987.

91. Smallridge R.C. Thyrotropin-secreting pituitary tumors. Endocrinol. Metab. Clin. North. Am., *16*:765–92, 1987.

92. Smallridge R.C., Smith C.E. Hyperthyroidism due to thyrotropin-secreting pituitary tumors: diagnostic and therapeutic consideration. Arch. Intern. Med., *143*:503–5, 1983.

93. Snyder P.J. Gonadotroph cell adenomas of the pituitary. Endocr. Rev. 6:552–63, 1985.

94. Snyder P.J., Bashey H.M., Kim S.U., *et al.* Secretion of uncombined subunits of luteinizing hormone by gonadotroph cell adenomas. J. Clin. Endocrinol. Metab., *59*:1169–75, 1984.

95. Snyder P.J., Johnson J., Muzyka R. Abnormal secretion of glycoprotein α-subunit and follicle stimulating hormone (FSH) β-subunit in men with pituitary adenomas and FSH hypersecretion. J. Clin. Endocrinol. Metab., *51*:579–84, 1980.

96. Snyder P.J., Fowble B.F., Schatz N.J., *et al.* Hypopituitarism following radiation therapy of pituitary adenomas. Am. J. Med., *81*:457–62, 1986.

97. Sonino N., Boscaro M., Merola G., *et al.* Prolonged treatment of Cushing's disease by ketoconazole. J. Clin. Endocrinol. Metab., *61*:718–22, 1985.

97. Thorner M.O., McNeilly A.S., Hagan C., *et al.* Long-term treatment of galactorrhea and hypogonadism with bromocriptine. B.M.J., *2*:419–22, 1974.

98. Thorner M.O., Frohman L.A., Leong D.A., *et al.* Extrahypothalamic growth-hormone-releasing factor (GRF) secretion is a rare cause of acromegaly: plasma GRF levels in 177 acromegalic patients. J. Clin. Endocrinol. Metab., *59*: 846–9, 1984.

99. Thorner M.O., Martin W.H., Rogol A.D., *et al.* Rapid regression of pituitary prolactinomas during bromocriptine treatment. J. Clin. Endocrinol. Metab., *51*:438–45, 1980.

101. Thorner M.O., Perryman R.L., Cronin M.J., *et al.* Somatotroph hyperplasia: successful treatment of acromegaly by removal of a pancreatic islet cell tumor secreting a growth hormone-releasing factor. J. Clin. Invest., *70*:965–77, 1082.

102. Thorner M.O., Perryman R.L., Rogol A.D., *et al.* Rapid changes of prolactinoma volume after withdrawal and reinstitution of bromocriptine. J. Clin. Endocrinol. Metab., *53*:480–83, 1981.

103. Tyrrell J.B., Brooks R.M., Fitzgerald P.A., *et al.* Cushing's disease: selective trans-sphenoidal resection of pituitary microadenomas. N. Engl. J. Med., *298*:753–7, 1978.

104. Tyrrell J.B., Findling J.W., Aron D.C., *et al.* An overnight high-dose dexamethasone suppression test for rapid differential diagnosis of Cushing's syndromes. Ann. Intern. Med., *104*:180–6, 1986.

105. van Liessum P.A., Hopman W.P.M., Pieters G.F.F.M., *et al.* Postprandial gallbladder motility during long term treatment with the long-acting

somatostatin analog SMS 201-995 in acromegaly. J. Clin. Endocrinol. Metab., *69:*557–62, 1989.

106. Vale W., Spiess J., Rivier C., Rivier J. Characterization of a 41-residue ovine hypothalamic peptide that stimulates secretion of corticotropin and β-endorphin. Science., *213:*1394–397, 1981.

107. Vance M.L., Cragun J.R., Reimnitz C., *et al.* CV 205-502 treatment of hyperprolactinemia. J. Clin. Endocrinol. Metab., *68:*336–69, 1989.

108. Vance M.L., Evans W.S., Thorner M.O. Bromocriptine. Ann. Intern. Med., *100:*78–91, 1984.

109. Vance M.L., Ridgway E.C., Thorner M.O. Follicle-stimulating hormone- and α-subunit-secreting pituitary tumor treated with bromocriptine. J. Clin. Endocrinol. Metab., *61:*580–4, 1985.

110. Wang C., Lam K.S.L., Arceo E., Chan F.L., Comparison of the effectiveness of 2-hourly versus 8-hourly subcutaneous injections of a somatostatin analog (SMS 201-995) in the treatment of acromegaly. J. Clin. Endocrinol. Metab., *69:*670–7, 1989.

111. Wass J.A.H., Thorner M.O., Morris D.V., *et al.* Long-term treatment of acromegaly with bromocriptine. B.M.J., *1:*875–8, 1977.

112. Wemeau J.L., Dewailly D., Leroy R., *et al.* Long term treatment with a somatostatin analog SMS 201-995 in a patient with a thyrotropin- and growth hormone-secreting pituitary adenoma. J. Clin. Endocrinol. Metab., *66:*636–9, 1988.

113. Zarate A., Canales E.S., Cano C., *et al.* Follow-up of patients with prolactinomas after discontinuation of long-term therapy with bromocriptine. Acta. Endocrinol. (Copenh) *104:*139–42, 1983.

114. Zarate A., Fonseca M.E., Mason M., *et al.* Gonadotropin-secreting pituitary adenoma with concomitant hypersecretion of testosterone and elevated sperm count: treatment with LRH agonist. Acta. Endocrinol. (Copenh) *113:*29–34, 1986.

CHAPTER 18

Radiation Therapy of Pituitary Tumors[1]

JACOB I. FABRIKANT, M.D., Ph.D., RICHARD P. LEVY, M.D., PhD.

INTRODUCTION

Almost all pituitary tumors are benign adenomas, but depending on type, may grow aggressively, extend beyond the sella turcica, and invade adjacent neural and vascular structures (9). About 70% to 75% of pituitary tumors secrete excess hormones and the remainder are hormonally silent and nonfunctioning. About 12% of all intracranial tumors arise in the pituitary gland (34); of the hormonally-active pituitary tumors, Prl-secreting adenomas (hyperprolactinemia) are the most common, followed by growth-hormone–secreting adenomas (acromegaly) (2). The effects of excess hormones produced by the tumor are responsible for the characteristic signs and symptoms of the class of neoplasm; the increasing mass may produce signs and symptoms of hypopituitarism by compression of the normal pituitary tissue or stalk, or it may extend outside the sella into adjacent neural structures, leading to impairment of vision (visual field defects and extraocular motor palsies) and headaches.

Evaluation of the biochemical and metabolic alterations and the neuroradiologic features of the hypothalamopituitary region are necessary for accurate diagnosis of pituitary tumors. Pituitary function testing is essential; the integrity of the hypothalamopituitary system is assessed by stimulation or suppression tests for each of the pituitary hormones, involving hormone–specific factors regulating the anterior pituitary cells re-

sponsible for excess secretion. Radiologic studies for suspected disease include computed tomography (CT) scans and magnetic resonance imaging (MRI). For large tumors, MRI demonstrates mass effects resulting from extrasellar extension and, particularly, the integrity of the optic chiasm. Both CT and MRI can detect microadenomas of 3 to 4 mm; however, a normal scan does not exclude the presence of a small tumor, and false-positive results can arise from normal variants (1,2).

Pituitary adenomas are currently managed therapeutically according to their anatomic staging and endocrine dysfunction; thus, the neuroradiologic characteristics and biochemical and metabolic assays are important for guiding immediate and long-term management of each patient. The neurosurgical classification proposed by Hardy (27) is based on radiologic characteristics and includes Grade I and II (pituitary adenomas confined to an intact sella) and Grade III and IV (invasive adenomas), and Types A through D, which are secondary designations for suprasellar and inferior extensions. Invasion of the brain, cavernous sinus, optic chiasm, and other intracranial structures are important determinants for guiding therapeutic management—medical, radiotherapeutic, and surgical therapies alone or in combination.

The human anterior pituitary gland contains five major secretory cell types, which can be distinguished by immunohistochemical staining for specific hormones and morphologic characteristics on electron microscopy (2, 66). The cells responsible for production and release of anterior pituitary hormones include: (1) somatotrophs, which

[1]Portions of this chapter are adopted with permission from the following: Levy, R.P., Fabrikant, J.I., Frankel, K.A., *et al*. Charged particle radiosurgery of the brain. Neurosurg. Clin. North Am., *4:* 955–990, 1990.

secrete growth hormone (GH, somatotropin); (2) lactotrophs, which secrete prolactin (Prl); (3) thyrotrophs, which produce thyroid-stimulating hormone (TSH, thyrotropin); (4) corticotrophs, which produce adrenocorticotrophic hormone (ACTH, corticotropin) and β-lipotropin; and (5) gonadotrophs, which secrete luteinizing hormone (LH) and follicle-stimulating hormone (FSH) (39). Thus, GH, ACTH, TSH, and Prl are secreted by specific pituitary cells; GH and Prl arise from subtypes of acidophilic cells and ACTH, TSH, LH, and FSH are secreted by different basophilic cells. TSH, GH, ACTH, and Prl-secreting adenomas, and the nonfunctional adenomas differ in clinical presentation and evaluation, disease progression and complications, and treatment and prognosis.

The pathologic and metabolic determinants of the complex of clinical diseases resulting from functioning and nonfunctioning pituitary adenomas characterize the selection of therapeutic modalities and assessment of long-term results. Three measures are important: (1) the extent and degree of anatomic and metabolic abnormality; (2) the reversibility of the endocrine dysfunction to normal or near-normal levels, and of the extension of the neoplasm causing distortion and destruction of adjacent neural and vascular structures; and (3) the temporal pattern of therapeutic response and the duration of remission. The diagnostic and therapeutic goals, whether medical, radiotherapeutic or surgical, are directed to define the limits of the neoplasm and the extent of the endocrinopathies, remove or destroy the tumor, preserve adjacent neural and vascular structures, and control and correct endocrine dysfunctions without producing hypopituitarism. All measures of health outcomes of the various clinical series of the management of patients with pituitary tumors must consider how well these goals are accomplished to assess and compare the efficacy of treatment and therapeutic strategies.

GENERAL CONSIDERATIONS OF MEDICAL AND SURGICAL MANAGEMENT

The management of complex endocrine disorders arising from the different pituitary

tumors has undergone considerable change in recent decades, and multistage medical, surgical, and radiotherapeutic procedures now have clearly defined indications. Medical management as primary therapy attempts to suppress pituitary hyperfunction, primarily by the use of dopamine agonists (e.g., bromocriptine), but this approach is not universally successful. These drugs usually have undesirable side effects which may lead to the discontinuation of therapy and the inevitable relapse of the disease. Medical therapy also is used to control or maintain remission following radiotherapy to augment the delayed induction of permanent hormone suppression (2).

Over the past decade, improved diagnostic reliability of biochemical and radiologic determinants of pituitary disease during its earliest stages, combined with transsphenoidal microsurgery, have changed the role of surgery in the management of patients with pituitary tumors. In major neurosurgical centers, more than 95% of surgery in the management of pituitary tumors is transsphenoidal microsurgery, both for the selective removal of intrasellar microadenomas and for macroadenomas with extension beyond the sella. The indications for transsphenoidal surgery are now well defined, and particularly when considering the neurosurgical classification of pituitary tumors by Hardy (27), so that comparisons of efficacy and advances as regards combined pituitary tumor therapies may be evaluated.

Acromegaly

The treatment of acromegaly involves ablation of the pituitary adenoma; transsphenoidal hypophysectomy is usually preferred and results in successful long-term control, with permanent remission associated with very low morbidity and prompt biochemical response (9, 19). Successful surgery lowers serum GH to normal (less than 4 ng/mL) and with normal circulating insulin-like growth factor I (somatomedin–C). Conventional radiotherapy of the pituitary tumor is also effective and has similar cure rates, but biochemical response is slow, requiring two to 10 years for complete and sustained remission. Radiotherapy carries a substantial risk of hypopituitarism (approaching 30% or more in some clinical series) occurring by 10 years; this is less common following surgery, unless the normal pituitary is injured. Medical treatment may be offered if ablative therapy does not result in cure. Bromocriptine frequently induces a fall in serum GH when given in large doses, but only infrequently is the response sufficient to lower serum GH or serum somatomedin–C to normal or near-normal levels (2, 9). Octreotide is a more effective pharmacologic treatment; it suppresses serum GH in nearly all patients and is frequently associated with mild to moderate tumor shrinkage (2).

Prolactin-Secreting Adenomas

Serum Prl levels over 100 ng/mL may be due to a wide variety of medical conditions and medications; in the absence of an obvious cause, pituitary adenoma should be considered. A negative CT or MRI scan does not exclude a microadenoma, but such a radiologic finding indicates that surgical intervention is not required (2). Most patients with idiopathic hyperprolactinemia have pituitary microadenomas and they are generally treated with bromocriptine to lower serum Prl levels and restore gonadal function; those patients with large Prl-secreting microadenomas (less than 10 mm diameter) are also treated with bromocriptine. Patients with macroadenomas (greater than 10 mm diameter) are frequently given bromocriptine initially; those with massive elevations of serum Prl (e.g., greater than 1,000 ng/mL) may never achieve normal levels, and about 10% to 15% of prolactinomas fail to respond to bromocriptine therapy. While bromocriptine will reduce the size of the tumor in about 60% to 80% of the patients, shrinkage is frequently incomplete, with failure to relieve neurologic compressive symptoms in many patients (2, 9).

Transsphenoidal microsurgery may be used in patients who respond poorly to bromocriptine. Surgery or conventional radiotherapy are usually not given as primary therapeutic management for prolactinomas. Following surgical therapy, the recurrence rate is 10% to 50% at five years, and the initial cure rate with surgery is low, only 10% to 30% for macroadenomas (2, 19, 28). Radiotherapy may also be used for the treatment of prolactinomas. However, while control and shrinkage are achieved in most cases, serum Prl levels fall quite slowly over a two- to 15-year period, during which time bromocriptine therapy is required. Radiotherapy is a useful adjunct to surgery in patients who respond poorly to bromocriptine therapy.

Cushing's disease

Cushing's disease is pituitary–dependent hypocortisolism; the characteristic clinical manifestations of Cushing's syndrome in 60% to 70% of patients are due to ACTH–secreting pituitary microadenomas (9). Precise localization of the tumor on high–resolution CT scans of the pituitary region may be made in only 50% of cases; however, MRI of the pituitary appears to be more reliable (9). Transsphenoidal microsurgery is usually the preferred treatment. Elevated ACTH levels can be determined by petrosal vein sampling to guide the surgical ablation of an identifiable microadenoma or a hemihypophysectomy, as is required on the side with elevated ACTH levels.

Glycoprotein-Hormone–Secreting Adenomas

True tumors of thyrotroph and gonadotroph cells are not uncommon, but hypersecretion of TSH, LH, or FSH is rare (2, 9). Tumors producing TSH lead to hyperthyroidism. Gonadotropin-containing pituitary adenomas are relatively common but, frequently, behave as nonfunctioning tumors and possess no biological effects. Some rapidly growing tumors of pituitary thyrotrophs and gonadotrophs may cause enlargement of the pituitary gland and sella turcica, with concomitant selective elevation of serum hormone levels. Glycoprotein-hormone–secreting tumors are usually treated with surgery primarily, with or without radiotherapy; radiotherapy is given when extirpation is incomplete and some tumor persists following surgery.

CONVENTIONAL RADIATION THERAPY OF PITUITARY TUMORS

Conventional radiotherapy, that is, external irradiation with photon energies of 1 MV to 20 MV, was a primary therapy for most pituitary tumors until the emergence of pharmacologic treatment (e.g., bromocriptine), and the development and widespread application of transsphenoidal microsurgery. Irradiation has proven effective for suppression of hypersecretion and reduction of large tumor masses with relief of signs and symptoms of neurologic compression. Control of hypersecretion can be achieved in about 80% of patients with acromegaly and in about 50% to 80% of patients with Cushing's disease (19). Rarely, primary radiotherapy may be effective in shrinking large tumors; biopsy, decompression of the optic chiasm, surgical ablation of the neoplasm, and postoperative irradiation are preferable combined therapeutic strategies for these neoplasms. In acromegaly and in Cushing's disease, therapeutic outcomes may be related to three distinct goals, viz., the effects on the tumor itself, the metabolic effects, and the cosmetic effects. In acromegaly, a successful metabolic response to therapy involves a reduction of serum GH to values of less than 4 ng/mL, with long-term maintenance of normal levels. For Cushing's disease, the therapeutic strategy is to lower plasma and urine steroids and plasma ACTH levels to the normal range. Similarly, the therapeutic goal in patients with Prl-secreting tumors is suppression of elevated serum Prl to normal levels. Complete endocrine profiles, including thyroid, gonadal and adrenal function, are necessary for follow-up of patients treated for all classes of pituitary tumors, since hypopituitarism is a frequent complication of radiotherapeutic and surgical ablation; following radiotherapy, signs and symptoms of pituitary hyposecretion may develop only after a number of years (9).

Clinical experience in thousands of pituitary tumor patients indicates that for photon radiation therapy, at the 95% isodose contour, a daily dose of 1.8 Gy to 2.0 Gy, and a total dose of 45 Gy to 50 Gy delivered over a period of four to five weeks is adequate to obtain a satisfactory tumor response for most pituitary microadenomas, with virtually no adverse sequelae or complications and with no mortality (19). Grigsby (19) has provided an effective dose treatment schedule for the radiotherapeutic management of pituitary adenomas. When radiation alone is given as the primary method of treatment for Cushing's disease, a total dose of 45 Gy to 50 Gy

delivered in daily fractions of 1.8 Gy over a period of four to five weeks is used. For other pituitary microadenomas, 50 Gy at 1.8 Gy per day for five to six weeks is delivered. For inoperable macroadenomas, where conventional medical management is not indicated, a radiotherapeutic does of 50 to 54 Gy at 1.8 Gy per day for five to six weeks is prescribed. For invasive pituitary tumors or incomplete microsurgical resection, postoperative radiotherapy is given. In the former case, a dose of 50 Gy at 1.8 Gy per day for five to six weeks is delivered; in the latter situation, a dose of 54 Gy at 1.8 Gy per day for six weeks is given.

Radiotherapeutic Treatment Procedures

A number of reliable conventional radiotherapeutic techniques for photon irradiation have been developed and have proven to be clinically effective (19, 61, 69, 71, 74, 76, 80). Fixed fields (including bilateral/coaxial wedge fields augmented with a coronal field), moving arc rotation with wedge fields, and 360° rotating fields may be used, with the goal of delivering an effective tumor dose uniformly to a defined target volume, i.e., to restrict the high–dose region to the treatment volume while protecting the adjacent neural tissues (optic nerves and chiasm, temporal lobes, hypothalamus, cranial nerves, and the structures of the eye) (19, 61, 64, 69, 71, 74, 76, 80). The treatment volume is usually confined to portals or shaped fields of 5 cm × 5 cm to 6 cm × 6 cm; wedges are used to produce a reliably homogeneous dose distribution while minimizing the dose to critical adjacent structures, particularly the optic chiasm (Fig. 18.1). The target volume is usually confined to the 95% isodose contour and, with a satisfactory isodose distribution, the dose fall-off is rapid, within millimeters outside the target volume. The isodose contours and homogeneity of the dose distribution are altered as required, depending on the size and location of the tumor and adjacent normal structures; this is accomplished by altering the axis of rotation, size of fields, length of arcs, and thickness of wedges.

Clinical Results

Acromegaly

Earlier clinical data, prior to reliable biochemical assay of serum GH, demonstrated

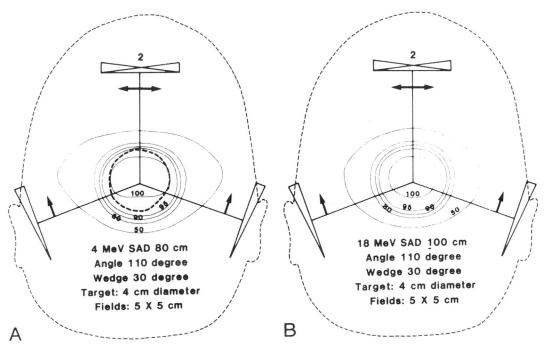

Figure 18.1.   Isodose curves and dose distributions for conventional external radiation therapy of pituitary adenomas. (A) Isodose curves and dose distribution for a 4-cm diameter target volume (dotted circle) centered in the sella turcica, using a 4 MV linear accelerator, bilateral coronal arc (110-degree) 5 cm × 5 cm fields with moving wedge (30°) filters. (B) Isodose curves and dose distribution for similar beam arrangement using an 18 MV linear accelerator, coronal arc (110 degree) and moving wedge (30°) filters for treatment of a centrally–located pituitary tumor. Isodose contours are shown for 50%, 80%, 90%, 95%, and 100% of the maximum central dose. (Reprinted with permission from Grigsby P.W., and Sheline G.E. In: *Principles and Practice of Radiation Oncology,* edited by C.A. Perez and L.A. Brady, p. 573. Philadelphia, J.B. Lippincott Company, 1990.)

TABLE 18.1.
Clinical Results of Radiotherapy for Acromegaly[a]

Study [Ref. No.]	No. Patients	Visual Field Defects (%)	Dose (Gy)	No. Treated Patients Controlled (%)	Hypopituitarism
Sheline et al. (1961) [72]	37	15/37 (41%)	≤35	5/19 (26%)	0
			>35	14/18 (78%)	0
Pistenma et al (1976) [63]	19	6/19 (32%)	58[b]	17/19 (90%)	1/11
Kramer (1973) [40]	29	—	44–50	25/29 (86%)	—
Grigsby et al (1988) [23]	22	—	40–56	17/22 (77%)	0

[a]Modified from Grigsby and Sheline [19]
[b]Average dose

five-year tumor-control rates ranging from a high of 90% down to 25% using doses of 45 to 55 Gy. A number of clinical radiotherapy studies (Table 18.1) (22, 23, 40, 63, 72) indicated that satisfactory control of acromegaly was achieved in about 80% to 90% of patients, but was often associated with some visual field defects; hypopituitarism was rarely induced. Eastman *et al.* (12) treated 47 patients with acromegaly with total doses of 40 Gy to 50 Gy (daily dose of 2 Gy or less); in 16 patients followed for more than 10 years, the mean decrease in plasma growth hormone five years after therapy was 77%.

Plasma growth hormone levels of < 10 ng/mL were present in 13% of patients prior to therapy, 73% at five years, and 81% at 10 years after therapy. There was a slight increase in the incidence of hypothyroidism and hypoadrenalism, and there were no nonendocrine complications.

Ross et al. (68) described their results of transsphenoidal microsurgery alone in a series of 214 acromegalic patients; 54% of patients had plasma GH levels of less than 5 ng/mL and 74% had levels below 10 ng/mL immediately after surgery. About 11% of surgical patients in the former group required additional therapy, whereas 21% with levels between 5 and 10 ng/mL required additional treatment. Complications of the surgical procedure were low; about 2% experienced meningitis and 2%, cerebrospinal fluid leakage requiring surgical repair. Hardy et al. (29) reported a cure rate of 80% to 90% (plasma GH < 5 ng/mL) following transsphenoidal resection of tumors in 57 acromegalic patients; about 12% of the patients experienced hypopituitarism.

Grigsby et al. (20, 21) reported on a number of acromegalic patients treated with radiation postoperatively when surgical resection failed to control plasma GH levels; a 76% control rate 10 years following treatment was achieved. Similar results of postoperative radiotherapy, exceeding 80% control (i.e., patients with normal plasma-GH) within a few years of radiotherapy, have been reported by a number of other investigators (12, 71, 81, 82).

Prolactin–Secreting Adenomas

The diagnosis and treatment of patients with Prl–secreting adenomas is largely dependent on biochemical assay of serum Prl; since the assay has been recently introduced, reliable long-term radiotherapeutic results are presently lacking. Combined treatment series indicate that, whether therapy was by irradiation alone or combined with surgery, mean Prl levels after irradiation ranged from 50% down to 25% of pretreatment levels; however, cessation of galactorrhea and return of menses failed to occur in the majority of patients and few patients reached normal or near–normal levels of plasma Prl (2, 9, 17, 19).

The long-term clinical data for the results of primary irradiation are limited, since outcomes reported are not necessarily subsequent to initial pharmacologic treatment with dopamine agonists. Moreover, transsphenoidal microsurgery has been used frequently and patient selection protocols are not available. Thus, comparison of clinical trials to assess optimal multistage, multimodality therapy is not possible. Grossman et al. (25) treated 36 women with small Prl-secreting adenomas; after irradiation, a dopamine agonist was given. A progressive decrease in serum Prl levels occurred in 26 of 27 patients, and four years after irradiation, Prl levels returned to normal levels in one–third of patients. Rush and Newall (69) treated 10 patients with prolactinomas; seven reverted to normal serum Prl levels within three to eight years. Antunes et al. (3) examined the clinical results of 30 patients treated with radiation alone, surgery alone, or combined; similar clinical responses of decrease in serum Prl levels, cessation of galactorrhea, and return of menses were observed for the three treatment groups. Whereas normal Prl levels occurred more frequently (seven of 16) inpatients after transsphenoidal microsurgery only, Sheline et al. (73) found combined transsphenoidal resection and postoperative radiotherapy to be most effective for large, invasive tumors. In summary, pituitary irradiation for prolactinomas appears to be of value following incomplete surgical ablation, particularly in patients contemplating pregnancy. As primary therapy for Prl-secreting adenomas, the results appear to be less certain than with initial medical therapy and with surgical ablation.

Cushing's Disease

The number of Cushing's disease patients treated with primary radiotherapy has been limited since the introduction of transsphenoidal microsurgery. In general, the metabolic effects are usually reversible, as are the cosmetic effects. Increasing clinical data available suggest that most (perhaps 80%) or all patients with Cushing's disease harbor a small pituitary ACTH-secreting adenoma warranting microsurgical removal (2, 9, 19). Since about 90% of these tumors produce no direct neurologic compression symptoms, treatment of all Cushing's disease patients by ablative procedures must be performed with very low risk. Transsphenoidal microsurgery fulfills these requirements and appears to be the preferred therapeutic strategy for Cushing's disease patients.

Aristizabal *et al.* (4) found doses of 45 Gy to 50 Gy delivered over four to five weeks with daily fractions no greater than 2 Gy, cured about 25% of Cushing's disease patients and produced partial benefit in about another 25%. A summary of recent clinical reports (Table 18.2) since the introduction of microsurgery for Cushing's disease indicates that with doses of 35 Gy to 50 Gy delivered at less than 2 Gy per fraction, five times per week, control rates ranged from 50% (62) to 100% (22, 23) depending on the follow–up criteria chosen (Table 18.2). Each series is relatively small, but, together, they provide a reliable trend of the results of radiation therapy for Cushing's disease.

Transsphenoidal resection has emerged as the primary treatment of Cushing's disease in adults; radiation therapy may be used if a tumor cannot be identified or surgical ablation fails to correct the hypercortisolism. The main limitation of pituitary irradiation is the prolonged delay in endocrine response. In Hardy's (26) clinical series of 25 patients with transsphenoidal microsurgery, selective removal was completed in 19; 17 (68%) patients were cured, and three required cortisone replacement. Boggan *et al.* (7) reported

a series of 100 Cushing's disease patients who underwent transsphenoidal resection; hypercortisolism was controlled in 74%, 67% by selective removal and 7% by total hypophysectomy.

Pituitary Adenomas in Children

Cushing's disease is the most common pituitary adenoma in children (23, 31). Radiation therapy has been used (see Jennings *et al.* (32), Table 18.2) with considerable success; control rates of 80% to 100% have been reported in small series. Styne (75) reported control in 14 of 15 pediatric patients (93%) following transsphenoidal microsurgery only; others have reported excellent results in children treated for prolactinomas, acromegaly (gigantism), and nonfunctioning adenomas.

Nonfunctioning Pituitary Adenomas

Endocrine–inactive pituitary adenomas may grow to a large size before clinical signs and symptoms associated with pressure effects become manifest (9). Growth of such nonfunctioning pituitary tumors beyond the sella, when sufficiently large, can result in pressure effects, particularly compression of adjacent cranial nerves, temporal lobe, optic nerves and chiasm, and extension into the cavernous sinus. In such cases, the clinical presentation may be associated with decreased visual acuity and visual field defects, papilledema, ophthalmoplegia, and ocular

TABLE 18.2.
Clinical Results of Radiation Therapy for Cushing's Disease[a]

Study [Ref. No.]	No. Patients	Radiation Dose (Gy)	Duration (wk)	No. Pts. Cured	Time to Remission (mo)	Complications	Recurrences	Follow-up (y) Range	(Mean)
Dohan *et al.* (1957 [11]	6	38–52	5–7	5/6	3–6	0	0	5–7.5	(6)
Heuschele, Lampe (1967) [30]	16	40	4–5	10/16	5–7	—	—	3–7	—
Orth, Liddle (1971) [62]	44	40–50	1 mo	23/44	—	0	0	1–14	(9)
Edmonds *et al.* (1972) [13]	15	35–50	3–5	9/15	1–6	0	0	0.25–10	(2.5)
Jennings *et al.* (1977) [32]	15[b]	40–50	—	12/15	<18	0	0	1–19	(8)
Grigsby *et al.* (1988) [23]	6	45–50	5.6	6/6	—	0	0	6–29	(16)

[a]Modified from Grigsby and Sheline [19]
[b]Children

motor abnormalities. Pressure-induced pituitary gland atrophy may give rise to hypopituitarism. Two large clinical series of treatment of patients with nonfunctioning pituitary adenomas (15, 16, 20, 21) demonstrate that, when large nonfunctioning tumors without invasion present with mass effect, particularly with advanced visual field deficits, surgical resection with postoperative radiation therapy provides better results than do surgery or radiation alone (Table 18.3). With very large invasive tumors, however, radiation therapy alone is preferred; surgical resection and decompression is frequently unsuccessful, and associated with high mortality and morbidity rates.

Grigsby *et al.* (20, 21) reported on 124 patients with pituitary adenomas treated with surgery and radiation therapy (Table 18.3); 82 patients with nonfunctioning adenomas received postoperative irradiation. Approximately 95% of all patients treated with radiation alone experienced improvement in visual field deficits. A significant dose response was observed for those with nonfunctioning adenomas, prolactinomas, and acromegaly; local recurrence of the pituitary tumor decreased significantly with higher doses.

Interstitial Radiation Therapy for Pituitary Adenomas

Joplin and his colleagues (18, 33) implanted radioactive yttrium-90 and gold-198 seeds for treatment of pituitary adenomas; this approach succeeded in suppressing hormone output from hypersecreting tumors, prevented further tumor growth, and produced tumor shrinkage. Yttrium-90 was used in doses of 200 Gy to 1500 Gy at the tumor surface for all pituitary tumors except for certain cases of Cushing's disease, where gold-198 was used with a surface dose of 100 Gy. In almost 200 patients treated, and based on specific patient selection criteria, the majority of cases of prolactinoma, Cushing's disease, Nelson's syndrome, and acromegaly treated by implantation of radioactive seeds had clinical results that were very similar to most surgical series, and with much more rapid responses than occurred following conventional radiotherapy. In over 80 consecutive implants, there was minimal early morbidity; there are no reports on delayed late effects, including hypopituitarism or injury to adjacent neural structures.

Complications and Sequelae of Radiation Therapy

Three potential late, delayed complications of pituitary irradiation with conventional methods include hypopituitarism, optic or other cranial nerve injury, and brain necrosis (70, 73). The incidence of late hypopituitarism is a function of radiation dose; repeated courses of radiation therapy for tumor recurrence carries an increased risk of pituitary hypofunction. Samaan *et al.* (70) reported on 65 patients with hypopituitarism after therapeutic irradiation for extracranial neoplasms, in whom the hypothalamic-pituitary axis received doses from 30 Gy to 85 Gy and with 92% of doses greater than 45 Gy; three to 20 years following treatment, 54 had evidence of hypothalamic-pituitary impairment, 25 had primary hypopituitarism, and 13 had growth failure with delayed bone age. In 36 women with prolactinomas treated by radiation and dopamine agonists and fol-

TABLE 18.3.
Dose Response and Clinical Outcomes in 124 Patients with Pituitary Adenomas Treated with Surgery and Postoperative Radiation Therapy[a]

| Clinical Syndrome | No. Pts. | Failures and Dose Levels (Gy) | | | | | Total Failures |
		<30	30–40	40–50	50–54	>54	
Nonfunctioning adenoma	82	3/4	3/13	1/13	2/49	0/3	9/82
Amenorrhea/ galactorrhea	30	2/3	2/8	0/3	1/14	0/2	5/30
Acromegaly	12	0	1/3	2/4	1/5	0	4/12
Total	124	5/7	6/24	3/20	4/68	0/5	18/124
Failures (%)		71	25	15	6	0	15

[a]Modified from Grigsby et al [20].

lowed for two to 10 years, Sheline *et al.* (73) found 21 patients with growth hormone deficiency. In patients treated with radiation for acromegaly, an increased incidence of hypopituitarism has been found, although reported series are small. Delayed hypopituitarism following pituitary irradiation can occur after many years and can readily be corrected by appropriate endocrine replacement therapy (9).

Radiation injury to the optic nerves or optic chiasm following pituitary irradiation is uncommon; in almost 1,000 pituitary tumor patients in different clinical series treated with conventional radiotherapy, the incidence of injury was less than 2%, and only two cases of brain necrosis have been reported (19). Except for cases of acromegaly, most cases of patients with damage to the optic apparatus have received radiation doses in excess of 50 Gy or daily fractions greater than 2 Gy, or both. Radiation-induced fibrosarcomas and osteosarcomas have been reported following orthovoltage therapy with multiple courses of radiation to very high total doses, although the incidence is extremely rare.

STEREOTACTIC RADIOSURGERY[1]

Stereotactic radiosurgery can be defined as an external beam radiation treatment procedure applied to a relatively small volume of intracranial tissue in which the total dose is delivered in a single or limited number of fractions, with the intent to alter structure and/or function of a designated population of cells within the target volume. This procedure is contrasted with external radiotherapy, which generally involves a larger tissue volume with the total dose delivered by a large number (typically, 12 to 35 fractions) of daily treatments over a longer period of time (three to seven weeks) with the intent to destroy the clonogenic capacity of tumor cells. "Stereotactic" refers to the system in which the coordinates and spatial relationships of

the intracranial target volume are determined in three dimensions from high-resolution neuroradiologic images. The coordinates are related to an externally applied device (a stereotactic frame) which is attached to the head and is used to effect reliable patient immobilization.

Ionizing radiations used for stereotactic pituitary irradiation may be classified as high–energy photons (e.g., X-rays or gamma rays) or accelerated charged particles (e.g., protons or helium ions). The physical characteristics of both classes have been adapted for application to pituitary irradiation, but in very different ways. Photons are attenuated as they traverse tissues; as they interact with matter, the ionization events occurring in tissue decrease exponentially with depth in tissue and, therefore, treatment planning must take into account the absorption of relatively high-dose radiation in the overlying normal tissues through which the radiation beams must traverse (Fig. 18.2).

Protons and helium ions manifest very different physical properties from those of high energy photons (8). Beams of these charged particles have several physical properties that can be exploited in stereotactic radiosurgery procedures to place a high dose of radiation preferentially within the boundaries of the pituitary gland (Table 18.4). These include: (1) an initial region of low dose (the "plateau") as the beam penetrates through matter, followed by a region of high dose (the "Bragg ionization peak") at the end of the range of the beam and deep within the tissue, which can be adjusted to conform to the length of the target, so that the entrance dose can be kept to a minimum; (2) a well–defined range that can be modulated so that the beam stops at the distal edge of the target, resulting in little or no exit dose beyond the Bragg peak; and (3) very sharp lateral edges that can readily be made to conform to the projected cross-sectional contour of the target, so that little or no dose is absorbed by the adjacent normal tissues (Fig. 18.2).

When charged-particle beams of sufficiently high energy, and hence greater depth of penetration, are available, radiosurgery can also be performed with the plateau portions of the narrow beams, using several intersecting arcs or multiple discrete, stereotac-

[1]Portions of this section are adapted with permission from: Levy, R.P., Fabrikant, J.I., Frankel, K.A., Phillips, M.H., and Lyman, J.T.: Charged-particle radiosurgery of the brain. Neurosurg. Clin. North. Am., *1*:955–990, 1990.

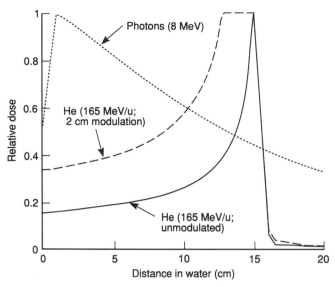

Figure 18.2. Relative dose as a function of depth measured in water is shown for 8 MeV photons (dotted line), an *unmodulated* helium-ion (165 MeV/u) plateau and Bragg ionization peak curve (solid line) and a *spread-out* helium-ion Bragg peak (SOBP) *modulated* to 2 cm width (dashed line) using beam filters; the increased dose with depth is demonstrated for the charged-particle beams. The unmodulated Bragg peak produces a narrow beam with high intensity at the end of the range, and is suitable for stereotactic irradiation of small intracranial targets. For uniform irradiation of larger intracranial target volumes it is often necessary to spread out the width of the Bragg peak to the precise target volume to insure optimum dose-localization and dose-distribution throughout the lesion. This is done by interposing variable-thickness absorbers in the beam path and tissue compensators at appropriate sites. (Reprinted with permission from Levy R.P., Fabrikant J.I., Frankel K.A., *et al.* Charged-particle radiosurgery of the brain. Neurosurg. Clin. North Am., *1*:958, 1990.)

TABLE 18.4.
Physical Properties of Charged-Particle Beams

- Well-defined range
- Low entry dose ("plateau")
- Increased dose at depth ("Bragg peak")
- Adjustable width of Bragg peak
- Very sharp lateral edges
- Little or no exit dose

tically directed, intersecting beams. In this procedure, through–and–through irradiation techniques are employed, so that the plateau ionization regions pass through the entire brain; the Bragg peak regions of the individual beams occur outside the patient and their radiant energy is dissipated harmlessly in the air.

Charged–Particle Irradiation of the Pituitary Gland

A beam delivery system was developed by Lawrence and his colleagues (43, 46, 77, 78, 79) for irradiation with plateau beams of ac-celerated charged particles, protons, and helium ions, to ensure precise dose–localization and dose–distribution within the target volume of the pituitary gland. A stereotactic positioning table and integrated stereotactic head frame were constructed and individually-fabricated plastic head masks were used to immobilize the patient's head relative to the stereotactic frame (Fig. 18.3). Until the introduction of high-resolution CT and MRI scanning, it was necessary to define the precise location of the pituitary gland and adnexal structures with pneumoencephalography and polytomography. Following delineation of the isocenter within the pituitary gland, the charged-particle beams are centered on the sella turcica by means of orthogonal diagnostic X–ray projections and beam-localizing charged-particle autoradiographs, and the beam contour is shaped by brass apertures (Figs. 18.3, 18.4, 18.5). During irradiation, the immobilized head is turned in pendulum motion around a horizontal axis while the patient is positioned at 12 discrete angles around a vertical axis (Fig. 18.3). The dose fall-off is very rapid in the anteroposterior direction and toward the optic chiasm, and decreases more slowly in the lateral direction toward the temporal lobe (Fig. 18.5). The isodose curves achieved are much better than the isodose curves obtained with conventional photon irradiation, which usually cannot avoid sensitive neural structures adjacent to the pituitary. With this method, the optic chiasm, hypothalamus, and outer portions of the sphenoid sinus receive less than 10% of the central–axis pituitary dose (41). Doses used ranged considerably, depending on the disease and the size of the target volume. Although necrotizing doses were used, they were selected so that the cortex of the temporal lobes received no more than 15 Gy.

The high–dose regions attained with the plateau irradiation technique are usually as sharply-delineated as those attained with the Bragg peak technique; differences tend to be relatively minor for small target volumes (i.e., pituitary gland). With the plateau irradiation technique, consideration of the tissue inhomogeneity normally encountered in the head is not important, but accurate stereotactic localization of the intracranial target volume and precise isocentric technique are essential (47).

In 1954, the first stereotactic irradiation procedures utilizing charged particles in clinical patients were performed at the University of California at Berkeley-Lawrence Berkeley Laboratory for pituitary hormone suppression in the treatment of metastatic breast carcinoma (46, 78, 79). Since that

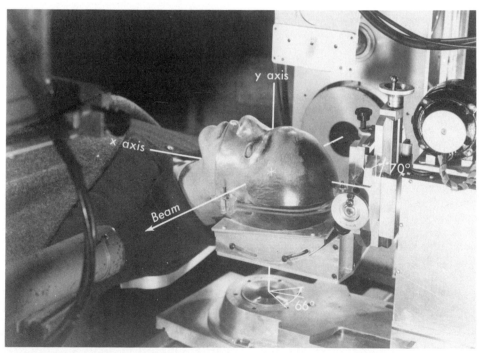

Figure 18.3. Stereotactic frame and mask immobilization technique as part of the irradiation stereotactic apparatus for humans (ISAH) system for stereotactic multiport helium-ion irradiation developed for pituitary irradiation at the University of California at Berkeley-Lawrence Berkeley Laboratory 184-inch Synchrocyclotron. The ISAH immobilization system is designed to place the unmodulated Bragg peak within 0.1 mm in water medium in coplanar and noncoplanar entry angles relative to three planar *(x, y, z)* coordinates. The mask is a rigid transparent polystyrene heat-vacuum molded unit that has been tailored to each individual patient; the system is an integral part of the overall immobilization facility and is designed in coordination with the charged-particle beam delivery system. The immobilization technique has provided satisfactory immobilization for stereotactic charged-particle radiosurgery in over 1,000 patients. (Reprinted with permission from Levy R.P., Fabrikant J.I., Frankel K.A., *et al.* Charged-particle radiosurgery of the brain. Neurosurg. Clin. North Am., *1*:971, 1990.)

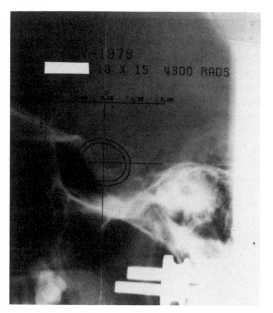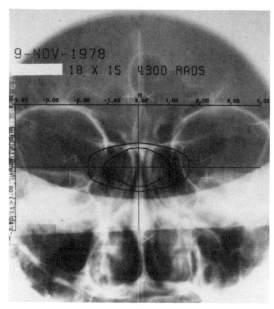

Figure 18.4. Localization radiographs obtained during the pituitary tumor treatment procedure with stereotactic helium-ion plateau radiosurgery at the University of California at Berkeley - Lawrence Berkeley Laboratory 184-inch Synchrocyclotron. The isodose contours are superimposed on lateral (left) and anteroposterior (right) X-ray radiographs of the sella turcica and parasellar structures. The dose selected for treatment resulted in no more than 15 GyE to the cortex of the adjacent mesial temporal lobes, to protect against temporal lobe injury. (Reprinted with permission from Levy R.P., Fabrikant J.I., Frankel K.A., *et al.* Charged-particle radiosurgery of the brain. Neurosurg. Clin. North. Am., *1:*965, 1990.)

time, more than 3,500 patients worldwide have been treated with stereotactic charged–particle irradiation of the pituitary gland for various localized and systemic, malignant and benign disorders (Table 18.5). Nearly all of these patients have been treated at the University of California at Berkeley - Lawrence Berkeley Laboratory (41, 44, 45, 46, 48, 50, 51), the Harvard Cyclotron Laboratory-Massachusetts General Hospital (35, 37), the Burdenko Neurosurgical Institute in Moscow (ITEP) (57, 59), or the Institute of Nuclear Physics in St. Petersburg (38). Charged-particle radiosurgery of the pituitary gland has proven to be a highly effective method for treatment, alone or in combination with surgical hypophysectomy and/or medical therapy. Disorders treated include primarily: (1) pituitary adenomas (35, 38, 44, 48, 49, 55, 58); and (2) conditions responsive to pituitary suppression, such as hormone-responsive metastatic carcinomas (i.e., breast and prostate cancer) (38, 52, 57, 59, 60, 77),

and proliferative diabetic retinopathy (36, 38, 57, 59, 60).

The emphasis in this section on helium-ion radiosurgery reflects the authors' experience at the University of California at Berkeley - Lawrence Berkeley Laboratory; these developments have been paralleled by extensive experience with proton beam therapy at the Harvard Cyclotron Laboratory, in Russia, and elsewhere (47). At Lawrence Berkeley Laboratory, stereotactically-directed focal charged-particle irradiation was used to treat 840 patients to destroy tumor growth and/or suppress pituitary function; this includes patients with acromegaly, Cushing's disease, Nelson's syndrome, and Prl-secreting adenomas, and patients with metastatic breast carcinoma and diabetic retinopathy (Table 18.5). The initial 30 patients were treated with plateau proton beams. Subsequently, almost all of these patients were treated with plateau helium-ion irradiation, although selected patients with larger tumor volumes received Bragg-peak helium-ion ir-radiation. Stereotactic plateau–beam radio-surgery has also been employed at the proton irradiation centers in Russia for the treatment of small intracranial targets for various disorders (38, 57, 59).

Pituitary Adenomas

Charged-particle radiosurgery has been used as a primary noninvasive treatment for pituitary adenomas, as adjunctive radiation therapy for incomplete operative resection,

and as treatment for late recurrences after surgery. At the University of California at Berkeley - Lawrence Berkeley Laboratory, helium–ion radiosurgery has resulted in the reliable control of tumor growth and suppression of hypersecretion in a great majority of the 475 patients treated for pituitary adenomas (primarily acromegaly, Cushing's disease, Nelson's syndrome, and Prl–secreting tumors). The objective has been to destroy the tumor or the central core of the pituitary gland, while generally preserving a narrow

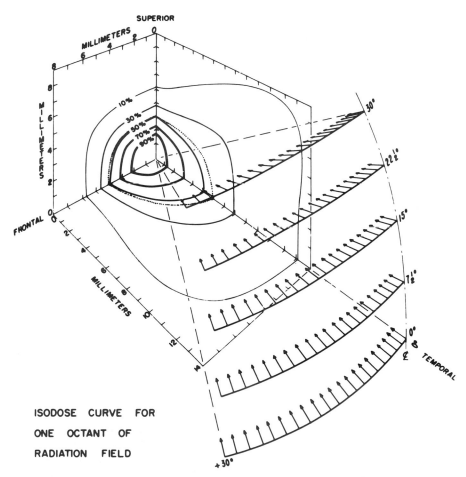

Figure 18.5. Stereotactic irradiation with the plateau portion of a charged-particle beam (helium ions, 230 MeV/u) designed for pituitary irradiation at the University of California at Berkeley-Lawrence Berkeley Laboratory 184-inch Synchrocyclotron; the three-dimensional isodose contours (90% to 10% isodose curves) for one octant of the radiation field used to treat pituitary adenomas are illustrated. The dose fall-off from 90% to 10% occurs in less than 4 mm in the frontal plane. The technique produces very favorable dose distributions for the treatment of small intracranial lesions. (Reprinted with permission from Tobias C.A. Pituitary radiation: Radiation physics and biology. In: *Recent Advances in the Diagnosis and Treatment of Pituitary Tumors,* edited by J.A. Linfoot, p. 234. New York, Raven Press, 1979.)

TABLE 18.5.
Charged-Particle Radiosurgery of the Pituitary Gland[a]

Disorder	UCB-LBL[b] 1954-Mar.	1990	HCL-MGH[c] 1965-Oct.	1989	ITEP[d] 1972-Feb.	1990	INPh[e] 1975-Feb.	1990
Pituitary tumors (total)	**475**		**1083**		**366**		**312**	
Acromegaly		318		580		93		158
Cushing's disease		83		177		224		51
Nelson's syndrome		17		36		1		3
Prolactin-secreting		23		132		34		75
Nonfunctioning adenomas		34		157		4		25
TSH-secreting [f]		—		1		1		—
Mixed		—		—		9		—
Pituitary suppression (total)	**365**		**220**		**583**		**146**	
Diabetic retinopathy		169		183		2		25
Breast cancer		183		31		489		93
Prostate cancer		3		5		92		1
Ophthalmopathy		3		—		—		27
Other		7		1		—		—
Total	**840**		**1303**		**949**		**458**	

[a]Modified from Levy *et al.* [47].
[b]UCB-LBL: University of California at Berkeley - Lawrence Berkeley Laboratory
[c]HCL-MGH: Harvard Cyclotron Laboratory - Massachusetts General Hospital (personal communication, R. N. Kjellberg)
[d]ITEP: Institute for Theoretical and Experimental Physics - Burdenko Neurosurgical Institute (personal communication, Ye. I. Minakova)
[e]INPh: Institute of Nuclear Physics, St. Petersburg (personal communication, B. A. Konnov)
[f]TSH: thyroid-stimulating hormone

rim of functional pituitary tissue. Variable degrees of hypopituitarism resulted in a number of cases, but endocrine deficiencies were readily corrected with appropriate hormone supplemental therapy. Excellent clinical results have also been achieved with proton-beam Bragg-peak radiosurgery in nearly 1,100 patients at the Harvard Cyclotron Laboratory-Massachusetts General Hospital (35, 37), and with plateau proton-beam radiosurgery in over 360 patients at the Burdenko Neurosurgical Institute in Moscow (55, 58) and in over 300 patients at the Institute of Nuclear Physics in St. Petersburg (38).

Acromegaly

At the University of California at Berkeley-Lawrence Berkeley Laboratory, stereotactic helium–ion plateau-beam radiosurgery has proven to be very effective for the treatment of acromegaly in 318 patients (42, 44, 49). The maximum dose to the pituitary tumor ranged from 30 to 50 Gy, most often delivered in four fractions over five days. Clinical and metabolic improvement (i.e., improved glucose tolerance, normalization of serum phosphorus levels) was observed in most patients within the first year, even before a significant fall in serum–GH level was noted. A

sustained decrease in serum-GH secretion was observed in most patients; the mean serum-GH level in a cohort of 234 of these patients decreased nearly 70% within one year, and continued to decrease thereafter (Fig. 18.6). Normal levels were sustained during more than 10 years of follow-up. Comparable long-term results were observed in a cohort of 65 patients who were irradiated with helium ions because of residual or recurrent metabolic abnormalities persisting after surgical hypophysectomy. Treatment failures following helium-ion irradiation generally resulted from failure to assess the degree of extrasellar tumor extension (42, 44, 49). The clinical results and long-term metabolic assays indicate that focal charged-particle irradiation treatment is as effective as transsphenoidal microsurgery.

A direct correlation was found between sellar volume and fasting plasma GH level. Serial GH levels were examined before and after helium-ion irradiation as a function of neurosurgical grade. Statistically significant differences ($p < 0.01$) in fasting GH existed only between the microadenoma patients with normal sellar volumes (Hardy's Grade I (26)) and patients with macroadenomas (Grades II through IV) (49). Grade I patients responded very well and have a good prognosis for cure; a lower incidence of post-treatment hypopituitarism was also observed in these patients. The more invasive tumors were slower to respond, but by four years after irradiation were associated with GH levels not statistically different than levels found in patients with grade I tumors (Fig. 18.7).

Kjellberg *et al.* (35, 36, 37) have now treated over 580 patients with acromegaly with Bragg-peak proton irradiation at the Harvard Cyclotron Laboratory-Massachusetts General Hospital. Therapy has resulted in objective clinical improvement in about 90% of a cohort of 145 patients 24 months after irradiation. By this time, 60% of patients were in remission (GH level $\leq$ 10 ng/mL); after 48 months, 80% were in remission. About 10% of patients failed to enter remission or to improve and they required additional treatment (usually transsphenoidal hypophysectomy).

In the Russian experience, plateau proton-beam radiosurgery has also proven successful for treatment of acromegalic tumors. Minakova *et al.* (58) reported excellent results in 93 patients with acromegaly treated at the Burdenko Neurosurgical Institute in Moscow. Konnov *et al.* (38) observed partial or total remission in 89% of 145 patients treated with doses of 100 to 120 Gy at the Institute of Nuclear Physics in St. Petersburg.

Cushing's Disease

Cushing's disease has been treated successfully at the University of California at Berkeley-Lawrence Berkeley Laboratory, using stereotactic helium–ion plateau–beam irradiation (42, 44). In 83 patients (aged 17–78 years) thus far treated, mean basal cortisol levels in a cohort of 44 patients and dexamethasone-suppression testing in a cohort of 35 patients returned to normal values within one year after treatment and remained normal during more than 10 years of follow–up

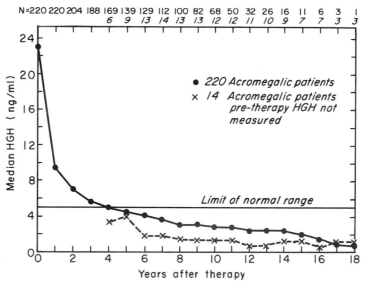

Figure 18.6. Changes in plasma human growth hormone (GH) levels in 234 patients with acromegaly one or more years after stereotactic helium-ion (230 MeV/u) plateau radiosurgery at the University of California at Berkeley-Lawrence Berkeley Laboratory 184-inch Synchrocyclotron. At the top of the graph are the numbers of patients used to calculate the median plasma levels for each time interval following radiosurgery. Fourteen patients did not have pretreatment GH measurements, but their GH levels determined four to 18 years after radiosurgery are comparable with those of the other 220 patients. Excluded from this series were 63 patients who had undergone prior pituitary surgery and five patients whose preradiosurgery growth hormone levels were less than 5 ng/ml. The 20 patients in the series who subsequently underwent pituitary surgery or additional pituitary irradiation were included until the time of the second procedure. (Reprinted with permission from Lawrence J.H. Heavy particle irradiation of intracranial lesions. In: *Neurosurgery,* edited by R.H. Wilkins and S.S. Rengachary, p. 1121. New York, McGraw-Hill, 1985.)

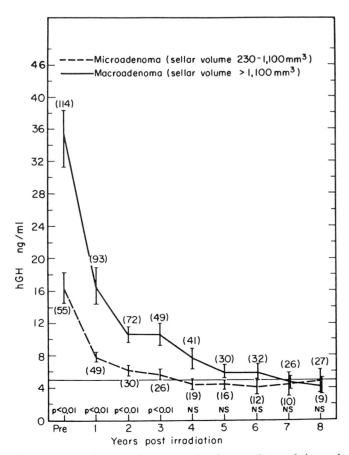

Figure 18.7. Results of helium-ion radiosurgery in acromegaly prior to and at yearly intervals after treatment. Serial fasting plasma growth hormone (GH) levels are shown for grade I microadenoma patients and for patients with Grade II through IV macroadenomas. Microadenoma patients have lower initial GH levels and respond more rapidly to treatment. However, by four years after treatment, macroadenoma response is no longer statistically different than microadenoma response. Results are shown as mean ± SEM. (Reprinted with permission from Linfoot J.A. Heavy ion therapy: alpha particle therapy of pituitary tumors. In: *Recent Advances in the Diagnosis and Treatment of Pituitary Tumors,* edited by J.A. Linfoot, p. 258. New York, Raven Press, 1979.)

(49). Doses to the pituitary gland ranged from 50 to 150 Gy, most often delivered in three or four daily fractions. All five teenage patients were cured by doses of 60 to 120 Gy without inducing hypopituitarism or neurologic sequelae; however, nine of 59 older patients subsequently underwent bilateral adrenalectomy or surgical hypophysectomy due to relapse or failure to respond to treatment. Of the nine treatment failures, seven occurred in the earlier group of 22 patients treated with 60 to 150 Gy in six alternate–day fractions; when the same doses were given in three or four daily fractions, 40 of 42 patients were successfully treated (49). The

marked improvement in response to reduced fractionation in the Cushing's disease group of patients has provided the clinical rationale for single-fraction treatment of pituitary disorders with stereotactically directed beams of charged particles (vide infra).

Figure 18.8 illustrates the biochemical results of helium-ion radiosurgery in our Cushing's disease series (47, 49). In a cohort of 37 Cushing's disease patients, the mean urinary fluorogenic cortisol was 1,350 μg/24 hours prior to treatment. Following radiosurgery, this mean value fell to a normal level of 200 μg/24 hours, and normal levels were maintained in patients followed-up at least 10 years. Mean plasma cortisol levels decreased from 30 μg/dL before treatement to 16 μg/dL following treatment and also remained in the normal range for at least 10 years. These changes in urinary and plasma cortisol levels were highly significant (p, 0.001) at one year following treatment. Response time varied from a few weeks to 24 months, but most patients responded within six to 12 months.

Plasma ACTH (14 patients), cortisol (30 patients), and urinary fluorogenic cortisol (21 patients) levels were measured pre- and one-year post–treatment (49). Results are statistically significant ($p < 0.01$) for plasma and urinary cortisol measurements but not for ACTH levels ($p > 0.1$). The mean ACTH level decreased from 90 pg/ml pretreatment to 58 pg/ml one year after treatment. Plasma cortisol suppression by dexamethasone and plasma 11-deoxycortisol response to metyrapone normalized at one year after treatment and remained normal for at least 10 years of follow–up (49). Relapse has been rare and normal ACTH reserve has been maintained in most patients. Prior to helium-ion treatment, mean plasma cortisol was elevated to 30 μg/dL and this baseline level was incompletely suppressed to 19 μg/dL by dexamethasone. Following treatment, the baseline cortisol levels became normal and suppression to values < 5 μg/dL occurred. Response to metyrapone stimulation was highly variable

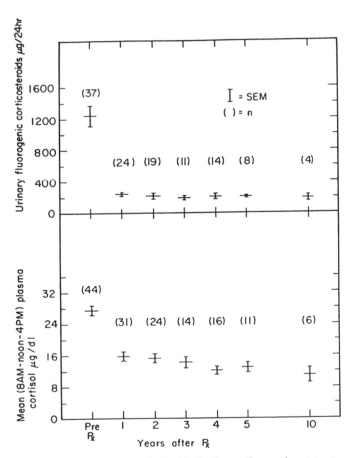

Figure 18.8. Results of helium-ion radiosurgery in Cushing's disease. Pre- and post-treatment levels in mean ($\pm$ SEM) urinary fluorogenic corticosteroids (upper) and plasma cortisol (lower) are shown. Normal plasma and urinary cortisol levels were found at one year and maintained for at least 10 years follow-up. The number of patients studied is shown in parentheses. (Reprinted with permission from Linfoot J.A. Heavy ion therapy: alpha particle therapy of pituitary tumors. In: *Recent Advances in the Diagnosis and Treatment of Pituitary Tumors,* edited by J.A. Linfoot, p. 250. New York, Raven Press, 1979.)

prior to treatment; many patients showed hyper–responsiveness but others had normal responses. One year after treatment, metyrapone responses became normal and normal ACTH reserve was maintained in most patients. Relapse has not been seen in patients whose metyrapone response has returned to normal (49). The clinical results indicate that focal charged-particle irradiation is as effective as transsphenoidal resection.

Kjellberg et al. (35) have treated more than 175 Cushing's disease patients with Bragg-peak proton–beam irradiation at the Harvard Cyclotron Laboratory–Massachusetts General Hospital; complete remission with restoration of normal clinical and laboratory findings has occurred in about 65% of a cohort of 36 patients; another 20% were improved to the extent that no further treatment was considered necessary.

Minakova et al. (57, 58) have reported excellent results in 224 patients treated with plateau proton–beam radiosurgery at the Burdenko Neurosurgical Institute. Konnov et al. (38) reported that plateau proton-beam radiosurgery (doses, 100 to 120 Gy) in 51 patients with Cushing's disease induced partial or total remission in 34 of 37 patients who were followed six to 15 months after treatment at the Institute of Nuclear Physics in St. Petersburg.

Nelson's Syndrome

Helium-ion beam radiosurgery has been used at the University of California at Berkeley–Lawrence Berkeley Laboratory in 17 patients with Nelson's Syndrome (49). Treatment doses and fractionation schedules were comparable to those for the Cushing's disease group, i.e., 50 to 150 Gy in four fractions. Six patients had prior pituitary surgery, but persistent tumor or elevated serum adrenocorticotrophic hormone (ACTH) levels warranted radiosurgery. All patients exhibited marked decrease in ACTH levels, but rarely to normal levels. However, all but one patient had neuroradiologic evidence of local tumor control (42, 44).

Kjellberg and Kliman (35) reported similar findings in 36 patients thus far treated with Bragg peak proton irradiation. Of a cohort of 19 patients treated, 12 of 14 patients experienced some degree of depigmentation

following treatment, and headache was reduced or eliminated in eight of 11 patients. ACTH levels were decreased in all four patients on whom data were available, but became normal in only one patient.

Prolactin–Secreting Adenomas

At the University of California at Berkeley–Lawrence Berkeley Laboratory, serum Prl levels were successfully reduced in most of 29 patients with Prl-secreting pituitary tumors following stereotactic helium–ion plateau radiosurgery. Of 20 patients followed one year after irradiation, 19 had a marked fall in Prl level (12 to normal levels) (Fig. 18.9) (42, 49). Treatment dose and fractionation were comparable to that in the Cushing's disease and Nelson's syndrome groups, i.e., 50 to 150 Gy in four fractions. Helium-ion irradiation was the sole treatment in 17 patients; the remaining patients were irradiated after surgical hypophysectomy had failed to provide complete or permanent improvement. Amenorrhea and galactorrhea frequently resolved before Prl levels returned to normal (49). Resumption of menses usually preceded resolution of galactorrhea. Two patients became pregnant after sucessful radiosurgery. In this clinical series, stereotactic charged–particle radiosurgery has proven to be more effective than medical management alone or transsphenoidal microsurgery for prolactin–secreting adenomas.

Konnov et al. (38) have reported partial or total remission in about 85% of patients with Prl-secreting tumors treated with plateau-proton radiosurgery (doses, 100 to 120 Gy) at the Institute of Nuclear Physics in St. Petersburg. Excellent results have also been obtained in 75 patients treated with plateau-proton radiosurgery at the Burdenko Neurosurgical Institute (Ye. I. Minakova, personal communication), and in 132 patients treated with Bragg-peak-proton therapy at the Harvard Cyclotron Laboratory–Massachusetts General Hospital (R.N. Kjellberg, personal communication).

Complications

Following stereotactic helium-ion plateau-beam radiosurgery, variable degrees of hypopituitarism developed as sequelae of attempts at subtotal destruction of pituitary

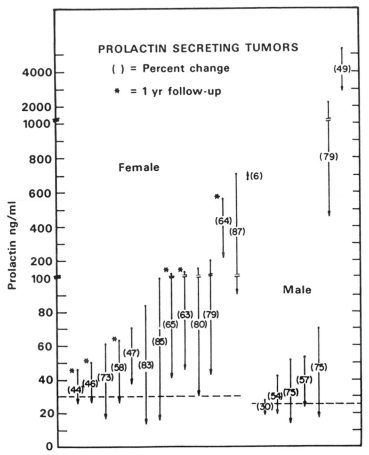

Figure 18.9. Results of helium-ion radiosurgery in prolactin-secreting tumors. Fasting plasma prolactin levels are shown pre- and post-treatment for females (left) and males (right). Arrows indicate the direction of change in prolactin levels after treatment. A marked decrease in prolactin, usually to normal levels (dashed line), was observed in many patients at 1 year (*) post-treatment. Percent change is shown in parentheses. (Reprinted with permission from Linfoot J.A. Heavy ion therapy: Alpha particle therapy of pituitary tumors. In: *Recent Advances in the Diagnosis and Treatment of Pituitary Tumors,* edited by J.A. Linfoot, p. 264. New York, Raven Press, 1979.)

function in about one-third of the patients, although endocrine deficiencies were rapidly corrected in most patients with appropriate hormonal replacement therapy (49, 67). Diabetes insipidus has not been observed in any pituitary patients treated with helium–ion irradiation (49). Other than hormonal insufficiency, complications in the pituitary tumor patients treated with helium-ion plateau radiosurgery were relatively few and limited, most frequently, to patients who had received prior photon treatment. These included seizures due to limited temporal lobe injury, mild or transient extraocular nerve palsies, and partial visual field deficits (49).

There were few significant complications after the initial high-dose group of patients. After appropriate adjustments of dose and fractionation schedules based on this early experience, focal temporal lobe necrosis and transient cranial nerve injury have been rare sequelae, in the range of 1% or less, and no other permanent therapeutic sequelae have occurred (49, 56, 67). A very low incidence of significant adverse sequelae has also been reported in patients treated with Bragg-peak-proton irradiation in the Harvard and Moscow experience and with plateau-proton irradiation in the St. Petersburg series (35,38).

Pituitary Hormonal Suppression

Hormone-Dependent Metastatic Carcinoma

Between 1954-1972, at the University of California at Berkeley - Lawrence Berkeley Laboratory, stereotactically-directed proton (initial 26 cases) or helium-ion beams (157 cases) were used for pituitary ablation in 183 patients with metastatic breast carcinoma. Patients received 180 to 220 Gy stereotactic plateau helium-ion beam irradiation to the pituitary gland, in order to control the malignant spread of carcinoma by effecting hormonal suppression through induction of hypopituitarism (45). Radiation was delivered in six to eight fractions over two to three weeks in the early years of the clinical program, and in three or four fractions over five days in later years. Many patients experienced long-term remissions. Eight cases of focal radiation necrosis limited to the adjacent portion of the temporal lobe occurred; all were from an earlier treatment group of patients entered in a dose-searching protocol who had received higher doses to suppress pituitary function as rapidly as possible (56). Clinical manifestations of temporal lobe injury and transient third, fourth, and sixth cranial nerve involvement occurred in only four of these patients.

Minakova *et al.* (52, 60) have reported excellent results following stereotactic plateau-beam proton radiosurgery in Moscow in a series of 489 patients with metastatic breast carcinoma and a series of 92 patients with metastatic prostate carcinoma (Ye. I. Minakova, personal communication). Konnov *et al.* (38) have also reported excellent clinical results in patients treated with 120 to 180 Gy plateau proton beam radiosurgery in St. Petersburg. In a series of 91 patients with bone metastases, 93% had relief of pain following treatment. Of 45 patients treated for metastatic disease with combined medical therapy and proton beam hypophysectomy, 20 had no signs of recurrence or metastases after a follow-up period of two to six years. Kjellberg *et al.* have used Bragg peak proton beam therapy of the pituitary to treat 31 patients with metastatic breast cancer at the Harvard Cyclotron Laboratory–Massachusetts General Hospital (R.N. Kjellberg, personal communication, 1989).

Diabetic Retinopathy

Between 1958 and 1969 at the University of California at Berkeley - Lawrence Berkeley Laboratory, 169 patients with proliferative diabetic retinopathy received plateau-beam helium–ion focal pituitary irradiation. This was done to follow the effects of pituitary hormonal suppression on diabetic retinopathy and to control the effects of insulin- and growth hormone–dependent retinal proliferative angiogenesis, which could result in progressive blindness. Previous clinical studies had suggested that surgical hypophysectomy resulted in regression of proliferative retinopathy in many diabetic patients, presumably as a result of decreased insulin requirements and lowered growth hormone levels (53, 54, 65). The first 30 patients were treated with 160 to 320 Gy delivered over 11 days to effect total pituitary ablation; the subsequent 139 patients underwent subtotal pituitary ablation with 80 to 150 Gy delivered over 11 days. Most patients had a 15% to 50% decrease in insulin requirements; this result occurred sooner in patients receiving higher doses but, ultimately, both patient groups had comparable insulin requirements. Fasting growth hormone levels and reserves were lowered within several months after irradiation. Moderate to good vision was preserved in at least one eye in 59 of 114 patients at five years after pituitary irradiation (J.H. Lawrence, unpublished). Of 169 patients treated, 69 patients (41%) ultimately required thyroid replacement and 46 patients (27%) required adrenal hormone replacement. There were four deaths from complications of hypopituitarism. Focal temporal lobe injury was limited to an early group of patients that had received at least 230 Gy in order to effect rapid pituitary ablation in advanced disease; four patients in this high-dose group developed extraocular palsies. Neurologic injury was rare in those patients received doses less than 230 Gy (J.H. Lawrence, unpublished).

In a series of 25 patients treated with 100 to 120 Gy plateau-proton radiosurgery in Russia, Konnov *et al.* (38) found that those with higher visual acuity and without proliferative changes in the fundus demonstrated stabilization and regression of retinopathy; microaneurysms decreased and visual acuity stabilized or improved. Patients with poor visual acuity and progressive proliferative retinopathy responded less favorably. A reduction in insulin requirements was observed in all patients. Kjellberg *et al.* (36) reported comparable results following stereotactic Bragg-peak-proton radiosurgery in 183 patients.

Histopathological Studies

Histopathological observations on autopsies from early patients, who received pituitary helium-ion therapy for hormonal suppression of metastatic breast carcinoma, confirmed that more than 95% of pituitary cells can be eradicated and replaced with connective tissue in a period of several months with nominal doses of 180 to 220 Gy delivered in two or three weeks total time (Fig. 18.10) (56, 83). At lesser doses, it appears that the magnitude of the histological effects depended on the dose at the periphery of the pituitary gland (47, 77). Viable hormone–secreting cells are usually found at the periphery. Surviving cells from the center of the pituitary gland tend to migrate to the periphery where blood supply is better.

Woodruff *et al.* (83) performed autopsies on 15 patients who had been treated with stereotactic plateau-beam helium–ion irradiation of the pituitary gland at the University of California at Berkeley–Lawrence Berkeley Laboratory. Ten of these patients had been treated for progressive diabetic retinopathy with average doses of 116 Gy delivered in six fractions. All patients demonstrated progressive pituitary fibrosis. Five patients had been treated for acidophilic adenomas with average doses of 56 Gy in six fractions; these adenomas developed cystic cavitation, suggesting greater radiosensitivity of the tumor than the surrounding normal anterior pituitary gland (Fig. 18.10). The anterior pituitary gland proved to be more radiosensitive than the posterior pituitary gland. However, no radiation changes were found in the surrounding brain or cranial nerves, demonstrating that charged–particle beams applied

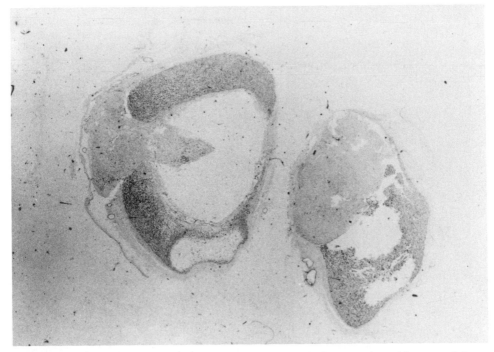

Figure 18.10. Pathologic autopsy specimen of the pituitary gland of a female patient with metastatic breast carcinoma 14 years after stereotactic helium-ion radiosurgery for hormonal suppression. The precise demarcation of normal tissue, the central coagulative necrosis, and the peripheral rim of preserved functioning pituitary gland epithelium are readily identified. (Reprinted with permission from Fabrikant J.I., Levy R.P., Phillips M.H., Frankel K.A., Lyman J.T.: Neurosurgical applications of ion beams. Nucl. Instrum. Methods Phys. Res., *B40/41:*1378, 1989.)

with relatively high doses create a sharply de-lineated focal lesion in the pituitary gland, without injury to the adjacent critical brain structures.

Future Directions

Improved anatomic resolution now possi-ble with MRI and CT scanning has made possible the better localization of pituitary microadenomas and adjacent neural struc-tures, and the more accurate assessment of extrasellar tumor extension (Fig. 18.11). These recent neuroradiologic advances should result in improved cure and control rates, decreased treatment sequelae, and a decrease in the number of treatment failures

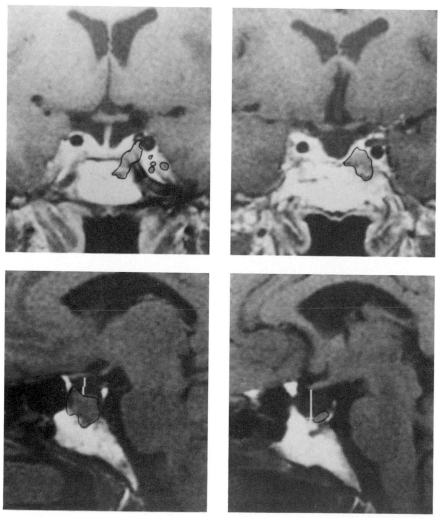

Figure 18.11. MRI scans of the pituitary region of a 49-year-old woman 14 years after transsphenoidal hypophysec-tomy for acromegaly. Recurrent tumor has resulted in endocrinologic changes associated with increased levels of growth hormone. The acromegalic tumor is identified and there is extension into the left cavernous sinus, lying directly on the left internal carotid artery. Upper scan: Coronal views demonstrate the recurrent tumor and its relationship to the optic nerves, chiasm, and tracts, and the left carotid artery and adjacent cranial nerves. The tumor and cranial nerves are outlined for radiosurgical treatment planning. Lower scan: Sagittal views demonstrate the precise distance between the upper edge of the recurrent tumor (outlined) and the optic chiasm (see Fig. 18.12). The MRI technique is part of the treatment planning procedure for stereotactic charged-particle radiosurgery. (Reprinted with permission from Levy R.P., Fabrikant J.I., Frankel K.A., *et al.* Charged-particle radiosurgery of the brain. Neurosurg. Clin. North Am., *1:*972, 1990.)

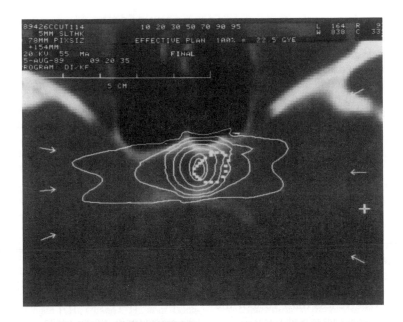

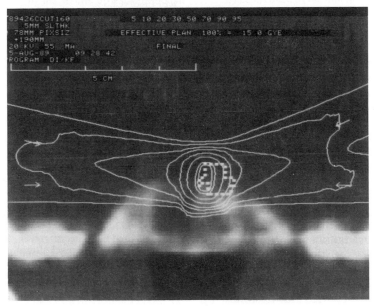

Figure 18.12. Stereotactic helium-ion Bragg-peak radiosurgery treatment plan for the recurrent acromegalic tumor in the patient illustrated in Figure 18.11. The radiosurgical target is defined by the inner ring of white dots. The helium-ion beam was modulated 0.50 cm and collimated by a 15 × 13 mm individually-shaped brass and cerrobend aperture. A dose of 30 GyE† was delivered to a volume of 800 mm³ through eight ports in one day at the University of California at Berkeley - Lawrence Berkeley Laboratory Bevatron. Isodose contours are calculated for 95, 90, 70, 50, 30, 20 and 10% of the maximum central dose in the axial (upper) and coronal (lower) planes. The 5% isodose contour is also calculated in the coronal plane and demonstrates the rapid fall-off of the radiation dose within a few millimeters of the irradiated target volume. The treatment plan was designed with an eccentric isocenter in order to place higher dose in the tumor mass lying within the sella and lower dose in the tumor lying against the internal carotid artery in the cavernous sinus; the optic chiasm, nerves, and tracts received less than 10% of the central dose, i.e., less than 3 GyE† , and the parasellar cranial nerves only a fraction of this dose. (From Levy R.P., Fabrikant J.I., Frankel K.A., *et al.* Charged-particle radiosurgery of the brain. Neurosurg. Clin. North Am. *1*:973, 1990.) [XBB 898-6680]

†GyE = gray-equivalent; represents the absorbed dose in Gy multiplied by a factor to account for the increased biological effectiveness of the Bragg ionization peak [47]

389

of pituitary tumors by external radiation. In: *Diagnosis and Treatment of Pituitary Tumors,* edited by P.O. Kohler, and G.T. Ross, pp. 217–229, New York, Excerpta Medica, 1973.

41. Lawrence J.H. Proton irradiation of the pituitary. Cancer, *10:*795–798, 1957.

42. Lawrence J.H. Heavy particle irradiation of intracranial lesions. In: *Neurosurgery,* edited by R.H. Wilkens, and S.S. Rengachary, pp. 1113–1132, New York, McGraw-Hill, 1985.

43. Lawrence J.H., Born J.L., Tobias C.A., *et al.* Clinical and metabolic studies in patients after alpha particle subtotal or total hypophysectomy. In: *Medicine in Japan in 1959. Proceedings of the 15th General Assembly of the Japan Medical Congress,* pp. 859–862, Tokyo, 1959.

44. Lawrence J.H., and Linfoot J.A. Treatment of acromegaly, Cushing disease and Nelson syndrome. West. J. Med., *133:*197–202, 1980.

45. Lawrence J.H., Tobias C.A., Born J.L., *et al.* Heavy-particle irradiation in neoplastic and neurologic disease. J. Neurosurg., *19:*717–722, 1962.

46. Lawrence J.H., Tobias C.A., Linfoot J.A., *et al.* Heavy particles, the Bragg curve and suppression of pituitary function in diabetic retinopathy. Diabetes, *12:*490–501, 1963.

47. Levy R.P., Fabrikant J.I., Frankel K.A., *et al.* Charged-particle radiosurgery of the brain. Neurosurg. Clin. North Am., *1:*955–990, 1990.

48. Levy R.P., Fabrikant J.I., Lyman J.T., *et al.* Clinical results of stereotactic helium-ion radiosurgery of the pituitary gland at Lawrence Berkeley Laboratory. In: *International Workshop on Proton and Narrow Photon Beam Therapy,* pp. 38–42, Oulu, Finland, 1989.

49. Linfoot J.A. Heavy ion therapy: Alpha particle therapy of pituitary tumors. In: *Recent Advances in the Diagnosis and Treatment of Pituitary Tumors,* edited by J.A. Linfoot, pp. 245–267, New York, Raven Press, 1979.

50. Linfoot J.A., Born J.L., Garcia J.F., *et al.* Metabolic and ophthalmological observations following heavy particle pituitary suppressive therapy in diabetic retinopathy. In: *Symposium on the Treatment of Diabetic Retinopathy,* edited by M.F. Goldberg, and S.L. Fine, pp. 277–289, Airlie House, Warrenton, VA (U.S. Public Health Service Publication No. 1890), Arlington, 1968.

51. Linfoot J.A., Lawrence J.H., Born J.L., *et al.* The alpha particle or proton beam in radiosurgery of the pituitary gland for Cushing's disease. N. Engl. J. Med., *269:*597–601, 1963.

52. Lopatkin N.A., Khazanov V.G., Minakova Ye.I., *et al.* Proton irradiation of the hypophysis in the combined antiandrogenical treatment of cancer of the prostate. Khirurgiia (Sofia) (in Bulgarian), *3:*1–3, 1988.

53. Luft R. The use of hypophysectomy in juvenile diabetes mellitus with vascular complications. Diabetes, *11:*461–462, 1962.

54. Lundbaek K., Malmros R., Anderson H.C., *et al.* Hypophysectomy for diabetic angiopathy: A controlled clinical trial. In: *Symposium on the Treatment of Diabetic Retinopathy,* edited by M.F. Goldberg, and S.L. Fine, pp. 291–311, Airlie House,

Warrenton, VA (U.S. Public Health Service Publication No. 1890), Arlington, 1968.

55. Lyass F.M., Minakova Ye.I., Rayevskaya S.A., Krymsky V.A., Luchin Ye.I., *et al.* The role of radiotherapy in the treatment of pituitary adenomas. Med. Radiol. (Mosk) (in Russian), *34(8):*12–24, 1989.

56. McDonald L.W., Lawrence J.H., Born J.L., *et al.* Delayed radionecrosis of the central nervous system. In: *Semiannual report. Biology and Medicine.* Donner Laboratory and Donner Pavilion. Fall 1967 (U.C.R.L. Report No. 18066), edited by J.H. Lawrence, pp. 173–192, Berkeley, Regents of the University of California, 1967.

57. Minakova Ye.I. Review of twenty years proton therapy clinical experience in Moscow. In: *Proceedings of the Second International Charged Particle Workshop,* pp. 1–23, Loma Linda, CA, 1987.

58. Minakova Ye.I., Kirpatovskaya L.Ye., Lyass F.M., *et al.* Proton therapy of pituitary adenomas. Med. Radiol. (Mosk) (in Russian), *28(10):*7–13, 1983.

59. Minakova Ye.I., Krymsky V.A., Luchin Ye.I., *et al.* Proton beam therapy in neurosurgical clinical practice. Med. Radiol. (Mosk) (in Russian), *32(8):*36–42, 1987.

60. Minakova Ye.I., Vasil'eva N.N., and Svyatukhina O.V. Irradiation of the hypophysis with single large dose of high energy protons for advanced breast carcinoma. Med. Radiol. (Mosk) (in Russian), *22(1):*33–39, 1977.

61. Moss W.T., Brand W.N., and Battifora H. The brain, spinal cord, and pituitary gland. In: *Radiation Oncology. Rationale, Technique, Results,* pp. 586–617, St. Louis, C.V. Mosby Company, 1979.

62. Orth D.N., and Liddle G.W. Results of treatment in 108 patients with Cushing's syndrome. N. Engl. J. Med., *285:*243–247, 1971.

63. Pistenma D.A., Goffinet D.R., Bagshaw M.A., *et al.* Treatment of acromegaly with megavoltage radiation therapy. Int. J. Radiat. Oncol. Biol. Phys., *1:*885–893, 1976.

64. Pistenma D.A., Goffinet D.R., Bagshaw M.A., *et al.* Treatment of chromophobe adenomas with megavoltage irradiation. Cancer, *35:*1574–1582, 1975.

65. Poulsen J.E. Diabetes and anterior pituitary insufficiency. Final course and postmortem study of a diabetic patient with Sheehan's syndrome. Diabetes, *15:*73–77, 1966.

66. Reichlin S. Neuroendocrinology. In: *Williams Textbook of Endocrinology,* edited by J.D. Wilson, and D.W. Foster, pp. 492–567, Philadelphia, W.B. Saunders Company, 1985.

67. Rodriguez A., Levy R.P., Fabrikant J.I. Experimental central nervous system injury after charged-particle irradiation. In: *Radiation Injury to the Nervous System,* edited by P.H. Gutin, S.A. Leibel, and G.E. Sheline, pp. 149–182, New York, Raven Press, 1991.

68. Ross D.A., *et al.* Results of transsphenoidal microsurgery for growth hormone-secreting pituitary adenoma in a series of 214 patients. J. Neurosurg., *68:*854–867, 1988.

69. Rush S.C., and Newall J. Pituitary adenoma: The efficacy of radiotherapy as the sole treatment. Int. J. Radiat. Oncol. Biol. Phys., *17:*165–169, 1989.

70. Samaan N.A., Maor M., Sampiere V.A., *et al.* Hypopituitarism after external irradiation of nasopharyngeal cancer. In: *Recent Advances in the Diagnosis and Treatment of Pituitary Tumors,* edited by J.A. Linfoot, pp. 315–330, New York, Raven Press, 1979.

71. Sheline G.E. The role of conventional radiation therapy in the treatment of functional pituitary tumors. In: *Recent Advances in the Diagnosis and Treatment of Pituitary Tumors,* edited by J.A. Linfoot, pp. 289–313, New York, Raven Press, 1979.

72. Sheline G.E., Goldberg M.B., and Feldman R. Pituitary irradiation for acromegaly. Radiology, *76:*70–75, 1961.

73. Sheline G.E., Grossman A., Jones A.E., *et al.* Radiation therapy for prolactinomas. In: *Secretory Tumors of the Pituitary Gland,* edited by P.M. Black, N.T. Zervas, E.D. Ridgway, and J.B. Martin, pp. 93–108, New York, Raven Press, 1984.

74. Sheline G.E., and Tyrrell J.B. Pituitary adenomas. In: *Radiation Oncology Annual,* edited by T.L., and D.A. Pistenmaa D.A., pp. 1–35, New York, Raven Press, 1983.

75. Styne D.M., Grumbach M.M., Kaplan S.L., *et al.* Treatment of Cushing's disease in childhood and adolescence by transsphenoidal microadenomectomy. N. Engl. J. Med., *310:*889–893, 1984.

76. Sutton M.L. Adult central nervous system. In: *The Radiotherapy of Malignant Disease,* pp. 215–236, New York, Springer-Verlag, 1985.

77. Tobias C.A. Pituitary radiation: Radiation physics and biology. In: *Recent Advances in the Diagnosis and Treatment of Pituitary Tumors,* edited by J.A. Linfoot, pp. 221–243, New York, Raven Press, 1979.

78. Tobias C.A., Lawrence J.H., Born J.L., *et al.* Pituitary irradiation with high-energy proton beams: A preliminary report. Cancer Res., *18:*121–134, 1958.

79. Tobias C.A., Roberts J.E., Lawrence J.H., *et al.* Irradiation hypophysectomy and related studies using 340-MeV protons and 190-MeV deuterons. In: *Proceedings of the International Conference on the Peaceful Uses of Atomic Energy,* pp. 95–106, Geneva, 1955.

80. Waltz T.A., Brownell B. Sarcoma: A possible late result of effective radiation therapy for pituitary adenoma: Report of two cases. J. Neurosurg., *24:*901–907, 1966.

81. Werner S., Trampe E., Palacios P., *et al.* Growth hormone producing pituitary adenomas with concomitant hypersecretion of prolactin are particularly sensitive to photon irradiation. Int. J. Radiat. Oncol. Biol. Phys., *11:*1713–1720, 1985.

82. Williams R.A., Jacobs H.S., Kurtz A.B., *et al.* The treatment of acromegaly with special reference to trans-sphenoidal hypophysectomy. Quart. J. Med., *44:*79–98, 1975.

83. Woodruff K.H., Lyman J.T., Lawrence J.H., *et al.* Delayed sequelae of pituitary irradiation. Hum. Pathol., *15:*48–54, 1984.

CHAPTER 19

Pituitary Tumors— Therapeutic Considerations: Surgical

EDWARD R. LAWS, JR., M.D., F.A.C.S.

Early in the 19th century, it was recognized that lesions in the region of the pituitary gland could affect vision. This information, along with the endocrine abnormalities that began to be discovered and described toward the end of the 19th century, tended to make the region of the pituitary an area of intense interest for surgeons. The most common problem for which surgery in the region of the sella is performed is the pituitary adenoma; the surgical management of this tumor and related abnormalities is the focus of this chapter. Pituitary tumors are among the most common benign neoplasms encountered in neurosurgical practice and, in many series, they represent up to 10% of all brain tumors surgically treated.

There are a number of epidemiological studies of brain tumors, but many of these have not included pituitary tumors. A comprehensive epidemiologic study was carried out at the Mayo Clinic investigating the occurrence of pituitary adenomas in the population of Olmsted County, MN. in the 1970's. The prevalence of all types of pituitary tumors was 14.7 per 100,000 per year, making this a regularly encountered clinical problem.

The incidence of clinically undetected pituitary adenomas has been addressed in a number of autopsy studies, wherein careful serial sectioning of the pituitary was performed on patients who died of nonpituitary problems and were subjected to postmortem examination (3). The detection rate for inci-

dental pituitary adenomas (usually microadenomas) ranges between 6% and 22%. Similarly, a number of radiographic studies have been performed. These imaging studies (tomograms of the sella turcica, CT scans of the head) in patients with no known pituitary disease have detected abnormalities suggestive of a pituitary tumor in 6% to 12% of patients studied. MRI studies may show an even higher incidence.

The relative incidence of different types of pituitary tumors has been addressed in a number of studies performed by pituitary surgeons or pituitary pathologists. The data from our series are given in Table 19.1.

The evaluation of patients with pituitary adenomas rests on a comprehensive interdisciplinary effort that continues to become more accurate (1). Endocrine diagnosis is based on the measurement of pituitary hormones and their effects on target organs. These measurements are made in basal and provoked states and are sensitive indicators of distributed pathophysiology (6).

Anatomic diagnosis, once based on plain radiograph and multidirectional polytomography, has become more accurate and more valuable as X-ray transmission computed tomography (CT) and MRI have been applied to pituitary lesions. Further development of imaging techniques such as MRI and positron emission computed tomography (PET) may permit metabolic–anatomic correlations in the future.

A neuro–ophthalmologic evaluation with

TABLE 19.1.
Transsphenoidal Surgery for Pituitary Tumors 1972–1990

Number of Patients	
Acromegaly	360
Prolactin adenomas	737
Cushing's disease	288
Nelson-Salassa syndrome	50
Nonfunctioning adenomas	608
Miscellaneous adenomas	9
Total	2052

careful recording of the visual fields is performed in all patients with visual complaints and all patients with tumors that extend outside the confines of a normal sella (8). A careful rhinologic assessment, including anatomic, cosmetic, and functional analysis is performed on patients who are candidates for transsphenoidal surgery.

At the time of surgery, an assessment of the actual size of the tumor and of the invasiveness of the lesion, evidenced by the involvement of the dura or bone, can be made. This assessment, in combination with imaging and pathologic findings, is the basis of the ultimate classification. (Fig. 19.1)

The evaluation of the results of any form of management of pituitary adenomas must address criteria that have become more and more rigorous as treatment has become in-

creasingly effective. It is wise for the treating physician to consider carefully and realistically the goals of an individual patient. When progressive visual loss occurs in an elderly patient, for example, a radical operation with attempt at "total" surgical removal may be less prudent than a satisfactory but less radical surgical decompression. A prolactin microadenoma in a woman who has no desire to become pregnant, has little or no galactorrhea, and does not wish to resume menstruating may need no treatment at all, but simply careful periodic follow–up evaluation.

Therapeutic options for pituitary adenoma currently include medical management, radiation therapy, and surgery. Drugs, such as bromocriptine (Parlodel) and related compounds that affect dopaminergic hypothalamic–pituitary relationships, are quite effective against prolactin adenomas and, to a lesser extent, against tumors associated with acromegaly. In addition to the potential for normalization of excess levels of Prl and GH, many of these tumors will decrease in size dramatically in response to bromocriptine therapy. Somatostatin analogues have become options for medical management of acromegaly. Deliberative preoperative medical treatment of GH and Prl macroadenomas is currently under evaluation.

The most common form of radiation ther-

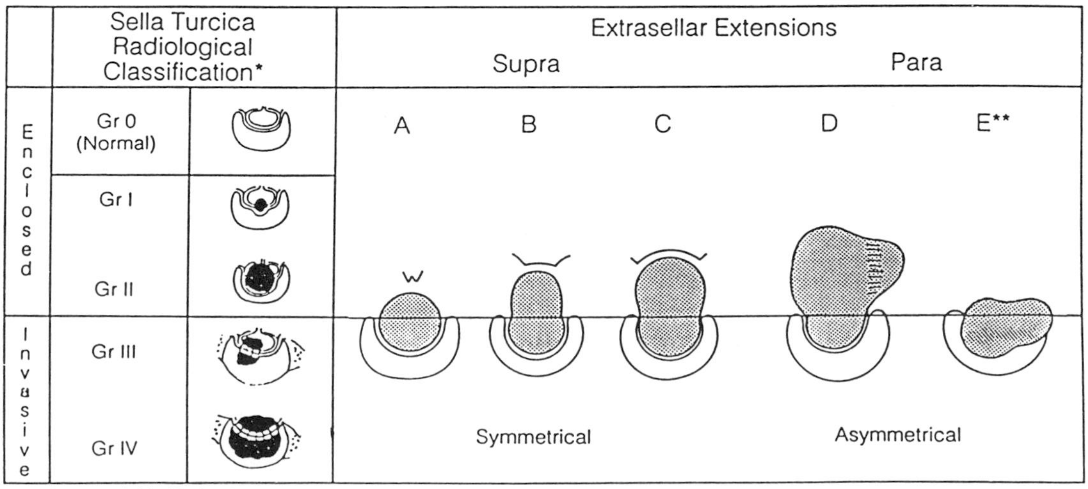

*J. Hardy and J.L. Vezina[9]
**As suggested by C.B. Wilson

Figure 19.1. Classification of Pituitary Adenomas (Reprinted with permission from Hardy, J. Transsphenoidal microsurgery of the normal and pathological pituitary. Clin. Neurosurg., *16:*185–217, 1969.)

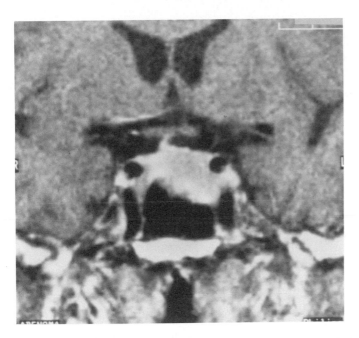

Figure 19.2. MRI study. AP views of an intrasellar pituitary adenoma in a patient with acromegaly. The lesion extends toward the left cavernous sinus.

apy used for the management of pituitary tumors is conventional teletherapy, using high-energy photons (gamma rays) generated by a linear accelerator to a total dose of 4500-5000 rads. Stereotactic teletherapy using multiple-focused radiation sources or a linear accelerator may also be utilized.

Surgical therapy of pituitary adenomas continues to include craniotomy for selected lesions; however, the vast majority of surgically treated cases are now managed by the transseptal transsphenoidal microsurgical approach (2, 5, 7).

This report will describe our experience with the surgical management of over 2000 patients with pituitary adenomas operated upon since 1972. Each type of tumor will be described separately.

ACROMEGALY

The clinical diagnosis of acromegaly is confirmed by elevation in the basal level of growth hormone (GH), a lack of suppression of GH levels after a glucose load, and lack of elevation of growth hormone after insulin-induced hypoglycemia. Prolactin (Prl) should be measured in all acromegalics, as hyperprolactinemia is present in about 30% to 50% of them. Somatomedin-C levels are another pre- and postoperative measure of the activity of clinical acromegaly. These tumors are more common in men (58%) than women. CT and MRI scans of the head are able to detect all large lesions and about 90% of smaller intrasellar tumors. (Fig. 19.2) Tumors have been categorized, as in Table 19.2, with GH levels generally correlating well with the stage of the tumor.

Criteria for successful management include resolution of symptoms and signs of acromegaly, and normalization of GH dynamics. Because the best results follow transsphenoidal surgical management, this mode of treatment is recommended for virtually all patients with active acromegaly. For practical purposes, successful results include a basal GH level of 5 ng/ml or less, or suppression to a level of less than 2 ng/ml during a glucose-tolerance test. Those patients with preoperative GH levels of less than 40 ng/ml have more successful results than those with levels that are higher (Table 19.3).

TABLE 19.2.
Categorization of Tumor in Acromegaly

Type of Tumor	Incidence	Mean GH (ng/ml)
Microadenoma (≤ 10 mm in diameter)	26%	29.1
Diffuse Adenoma	50%	56.2
Invasive Adenoma	24%	65.2

TABLE 19.3.
Results of Surgery in Acromegaly

Type of Tumor	Postoperative Normalization of GH
Microadenoma	85%
Diffuse adenoma	65%
Invasive adenoma	48%
All tumors, preoperative GH < 40 ng/ml	82%
All tumors, preoperative GH >40 ng/ml	35%

There have been no operative deaths; one case of CSF rhinorrhea and 3 cases of excessive bleeding comprise the significant complications in this series.

Radiation therapy is usually recommended in cases when the GH remains elevated after surgery, particularly in invasive tumors.

PROLACTIN ADENOMAS

The most common hypersecreting pituitary adenomas are those that secrete prolactin (Prl). These tumors are much more common in women (78%) than men, and they typically present with amenorrhea and galactorrhea (Forbes–Albright syndrome).

Men with Prl adenomas most commonly come to diagnosis with large tumors producing mass effect (headache and visual loss), though some may have relative hypopituitarism, impotence, azoospermia, infertility and, rarely, galactorrhea.

Endocrine diagnosis is made by confirmation of elevated basal Prl and dynamics are tested by response (stimulation) to TRH infusion. Pituitary tumors are not the only cause of hyperprolactinemia, but basal Prl levels over 200 ng/ml are virtually always associated with tumors. CT and MRI are positive in large tumors and are positive in 80% to 90% of microadenomas.

In our clinic, indications for surgical management include mass effect (progressive visual loss), apoplexy, and desire for fertility. Primary therapy with bromocriptine is usually recommended for management of small tumors in patients who do not desire fertility. Nine percent of our female patients had large tumors with suprasellar extension.

Criteria for successful management include resolution of mass effect, cessation of galactorrhea, normalization of Prl values as well as resumption of menses and successful pregnancy in women, and restoration of potency and spermatogenesis in men. Results are much better in patients with microadenomas than in those with large tumors, and they are better when the preoperative Prl level is less than 200 ng/ml (Table 19.4).

In patients with large tumors and in those who have persistent postoperative hyperprolactinemia, adjunctive treatment with bromocriptine is recommended. Radiation therapy is generally reserved for patients with invasive tumors, particularly those who do not respond to bromocriptine.

CUSHING'S DISEASE AND NELSON'S SYNDROME

In Cushing's disease, accurate endocrine diagnosis becomes most important, as it is essential to rule out ectopic sources of ACTH. The clinical diagnosis may be difficult in atypical cases. Alcoholism, depression, and obesity may all mimic some features of Cushing's disease. Hypokalemia is said to be frequently associated with ectopic sources of ACTH, such as bronchogenic carcinomas or pulmonary carcinoid tumors.

Laboratory diagnosis currently depends primarily on hypercortisolism as documented by measurement of 24-hr urinary free cortisol, loss of diurnal variation of blood corticosteroid levels, lack of suppression with high dose dexamethasone, and elevation of ACTH. The CT scan and the MRI study are frequently normal (40% to 60%), as the tumors are generally very small in size.

TABLE 19.4.
PRL Adenomas - Results of Surgery

Type of Tumor	Initial Normalization of PRL
Microadenoma	74%
Diffuse adenoma	53%
Invasive adenoma	28%
All tumors, preoperative PRL <200 ng/ml	83%
All tumors, preoperative PRL >200 ng/ml	43%

Normal scans of the adrenals and the lungs may be helpful in confirming the diagnosis of a pituitary–hypothalamic source of excess cortisol production. Petrosal vein sampling and analysis for ACTH after CRH administration can help to confirm the diagnosis of Cushing's disease and, in some cases, it can help to localize the tumor within the pituitary gland itself (9).

Surgery in these patients is more difficult because the sella is small and the sellar dura may contain many venous channels. Tumors are often centrally located, but may be found in any portion of the gland, including laterally and in the posterior lobe, so a thorough exploration is mandatory.

Results of surgery have been excellent and, as in the other endocrine active tumors, results are better with microadenomas than with large or invasive adenomas (Table 19.5). Criteria for success include the dramatic and prompt fall in blood corticosteroid levels and the eventual return to normal dynamics.

The pituitary tumors that become manifest after patients with Cushing's disease are treated by adrenalectomy generally produce hyperpigmentation (Nelson's syndrome). They tend to be active tumors and some may grow rapidly and recur even after thorough surgical removal.

In our surgically treated patients, hyperpigmentation improved in 50%, but normalization of ACTH was achieved in only 20% to 25%. The need for further therapy because of recurrence has been common.

NONFUNCTIONING AND NULL-CELL ADENOMAS

It should be noted that clinically nonfunctioning tumors comprise a diverse group of neoplasms. Although the majority are null–cell adenomas (some with oncocytic features on electron microscopic analysis), clinically silent ACTH and GH adenomas have been encountered. It is uncommon for the rare TSH adenoma to be clinically manifest and this is also true for the more common gonadotrophic (FSH/LH) adenoma. These latter three tumors (TSH, FSH, and LH adenomas), are composed of cells that produce glycoprotein hormones. All produce an identical α subunit of their characteristic hormone, and "α-subunit" tumors also exist.

The nonfunctioning or null–cell pituitary adenomas usually present with signs and symptoms of mass effect. The typical patient has a progressive bitemporal visual field defect and hypopituitarism. Many of these patients will have mild elevation of Prl, presumably secondary to a disturbance of the pituitary stalk, which alters the effect of hypothalamic prolactin-inhibiting factor (PIF) on the pituitary lactotrophs.

Imaging diagnosis is particularly important in these patients with large lesions and the relationship of the tumor to intracranial structures must be carefully studied.

Results of surgery have been quite satisfactory, with visual function improved or stabilized in 94% of the patients. Hypopituitarism improved postoperatively in about 16% of patients, and headache is usually relieved (4).

SUMMARY

As experience with endocrine diagnosis, radiologic evaluation, and transsphenoidal microsurgery has developed, more effective therapy has become available for patients suffering from pituitary adenomas. The amelioration of the various endocrinopathies and the potential for restoration of vision in patients with visual impairment make this aspect of modern neurosurgery most satisfying, both for the patient and the surgeon.

TABLE 19.5.
Results of Surgery - Cushing's Disease

Type of tumor	Initial Normalization
Microadenoma (confirmed)	91%
Macroadenoma	61%
All patients treated with transsphenoidal surgery	84%

REFERENCES

1. Abboud C.F., and Laws E.R. Jr. Clinical endocrinological approach to hypothalamic-pituitary disease. J. Neurosurg., *51*:271–291, 1979.
2. Cushing H. *The Pituitary Body and Its Disorders,* p. 297, Philadelphia, J.B. Lippincott Company, 1912.

3. Costello R.T. Subclinical adenoma of the pituitary gland. Am. J. Path., *12*:205–215, 1936.

4. Ebersold M.J., Quast L.M., Laws E.R. Jr., *et al.* Long-term results in transsphenoidal removal of nonfunctioning pituitary adenomas. J. Neurosurg., *64*:713–719, 1986.

5. Hardy J. Transsphenoidal microsurgery of the normal and pathological pituitary. Clin. Neurosurg., *16*:185–217, 1969.

6. Klibanski A., and Zervas N.T. Diagnosis and management of hormone-secreting pituitary adenomas. N. Engl. J. Med., *324*:822–831, 1991.

7. Laws E.R. Jr., Randall R.V., Kern E.B., Abboud C.F., eds. *Management of Pituitary Adenomas and Related Lesions,* p. 376. New York, Appleton-Century-Crofts, 1982.

8. Laws E.R. Jr., Trautmann J.C., Hollenhorst R.W. Jr. Transsphenoidal decompression of the optic nerve and chiasm: visual results in 62 patients. J. Neurosurg., *46*:717–722, 1977.

9. Oldfield E.H., Doppman J.L., Nieman L.K., *et al.* Petrosal sinus sampling with and without corticotropin-releasing hormone for the differential diagnosis of Cushing's syndrome. N. Engl. J. Med., *325*:897–905, 1991.

Index

Page numbers in *italics* denote figures; those followed by *t* denote tables.